IMAGING OF CHILDREN WITH CANCER

IMAGING OF CHILDREN WITH CANCER

MERVYN D. COHEN, M.B., Ch.B.

Professor of Radiology
Indiana University Medical Center

Director of Pediatric Radiology
James Whitcomb Riley Hospital for Children
Indiana University Medical Center

Chairman, Imaging Committee
Children's Cancer Study Group

Mosby Year Book

St. Louis Baltimore Boston Chicago London Philadelphia Sydney Toronto

Mosby Year Book
Dedicated to Publishing Excellence

Editor: George Stamathis
Developmental Editor: Ellen Thomas
Project Manager: Annette Hall
Production Editor: University Graphics

Printed in the United States of America

Mosby–Year Book, Inc.
11830 Westline Industrial Drive, St. Louis, MO 63146

Library of Congress Cataloging in Publication Data

ISBN 1-5566-4359-4
D-21774

92 93 94 95 96 UG/MY/MY 9 8 7 6 5 4 3 2 1

PREFACE

This book applies recent knowledge of the biology of pediatric tumors to tumor imaging. This book is *not* a comprehensive atlas of the radiographic appearance of all variations of every pediatric tumor, nor is it a comprehensive historical review of the imaging of pediatric tumors. It is a comprehensive review of the recent literature pertaining to pediatric tumors where relevant to the art of pediatric radiology. I hope it will be helpful to all those involved in the investigation and treatment of children with cancer.

ACKNOWLEDGMENTS

My grateful thanks to my secretary, Barbara Smith, who has devoted many hundreds of hours to the typing of many drafts of this book. Thank you, Barbara!

My warm thanks and appreciation are also due to the following:

The medical photographers of Indiana University who spent many hours faithfully reproducing the radiographic images into photographs for inclusion in the book. These individuals include Joe Demma, David Jaynes, John Murphy, Robert Coffer, Tex McCormick, and Phil Wilson.

Dr. John Kennedy and Professor Rob Gibson of the Department of Radiology, Christchurch Hospital, Christchurch, New Zealand. These individuals warmly welcomed me into their department for a 6-month sabbatical, during which time much of the work on this book was completed.

Dr. Mary Edwards and Dr. Todd Harris for assistance in selection of images for the central nervous system chapter.

Many pediatric radiology and other clinical colleagues throughout the world who have generously responded to my request for images of tumors to include in the book.

CONTENTS

INTRODUCTION

Each year in the United States approximately 6,000 children under the age of 15 years are diagnosed as having cancer[1] (Table 1). About 60 percent of these children will be cured of their cancer.

Imaging is exceedingly important in the management of these children with cancer. The role of imaging is to detect the disease, formulate a differential diagnosis, stage the tumor, monitor therapy, and detect complications.

The principles guiding the application of imaging are:

1. Imaging must contribute to patient management and, ideally, improve patient outcome. In other words, imaging must detect and provide meaningful information.
2. Although pathology, and not imaging, provides the final definitive diagnosis, the earlier the correct diagnosis is suspected the better, because additional imaging tests, and early therapeutic intervention, will often be guided by the "most likely" diagnosis provided by initial imaging.
3. In certain situations, imaging will be done for research purposes alone.
4. Imaging must be cost effective. It must be clearly understood and appreciated that the definition of "cost effective" is as much social and economic as medical. For this reason the question, "what is a cost effective study," is extremely difficult to answer.

The radiologist cannot fulfill his or her clinical obligations by having a knowledge only of the imaging appearance of the various tumors. The radiologist must have a thorough grasp of the biology of the tumor as well. He or she must understand the epidemiology, pathology, clinical manifestations, treatment, complications, and prognosis of each tumor. I make no apology, therefore, for including this information in the text. The information included has been chosen to provide all that is most relevant to the radiologist; additional information has been included because of its relevance to the radiologist's task. For example:

1. With testicular yolk sac tumor, recurrence of disease is extremely rare without a concomitant elevation in the serum concentration of alpha-fetoprotein. Therefore, it might be entirely appropriate to monitor patients with this tumor by estimating only the serum alpha-fetoprotein concentration and imaging the patients only when this tumor marker increases.
2. Relapse in patients with Hodgkin disease can frequently be cured, whereas in patients with rhabdomyosarcoma relapse is usually fatal. Therefore, the current application of imaging for detection of relapse with Hodgkin disease is reasonably appropriate. For rhabdomyosarcoma new techniques must be developed to permit earlier detection of recurrence, with the hope of improving survival.
3. The incidence of late recurrence of tumor varies between tumor types. For example, it is very low with germ cell tumor, osteogenic sarcoma, neuroblastoma, Wilms tumor, soft-tissue sarcoma, non-Hodgkin lymphoma, and astrocytoma. Late recurrence is more likely with Hodgkin disease, acute lymphocytic leukemia, medulloblastoma, and Ewing sarcoma. It is inappropriate to intensively investigate patients for late recurrence of tumor if the likelihood of such recurrence is very low.

It is clear that imaging cannot be properly planned unless the disease process is fully understood.

Imaging must be dynamic and respond to changes in imaging technology, cancer treatment, and survival. New therapies are altering the natural history of the cancers, and the complications of therapy are changing. For example:

1. Fifteen to 20 years ago abdominal masses were investigated using intravenous urography and barium studies, followed by laparotomy. None of these approaches is now applicable.
2. Initial presurgical chemotherapy is becoming the selected approach for many tumors, e.g., osteogenic sarcoma. This means that in many patients imaging is now required to monitor response of a tumor to this initial chemotherapy. Imaging must respond to this requirement. For example, it is no longer appropriate to assess tumors by measuring their diameters, because both computed tomography (CT) and magnetic resonance imaging (MR) can provide more accurate tumor volume estimations.
3. No longer is any particular tumor treated with a standard protocol. A variety of biological markers are used to identify selected subgroups of high-risk, poor-prognosis patients with each tumor. These patients are

TABLE 1
Annual Number of New Cancers per Year in Children under 15 Years

Type of Cancer		Number
Leukemia		1,800
Central nervous system		1,100
Glioma	725	
Medulloblastoma	240	
Ependymoma	100	
Other	35	
Lymphoma		700
Hodgkin	320	
Non-Hodgkin	385	
Neuroblastoma		390
Wilms		360
Retinoblastoma		150
Bone		270
Osteosarcoma	140	
Ewing	110	
Chondrosarcoma	10	
Other	10	
Soft-tissue sarcoma		360
Rhabdomyosarcoma	190	
Other	170	
Ovary		60
Testis		50
Nongonadal cell		70
Teratoma	25	
Embryonal carcinoma	25	
Germinoma	20	
Liver		60
Melanoma		50
Other		350
		5,770

treated with much more aggressive therapeutic protocols. Therapy complications (and their detection by imaging) are, therefore, much more likely in this subgroup of patients than in the excellent-prognosis groups for whom less toxic therapy is used.

4. Prior to the 1960s all children with leukemia died. Now well over half of these patients survive. Although these survivors are cured of their tumor, they have a large number of long-term problems, including disturbances of growth, endocrine function, central nervous system function, and second malignancy. This provides new challenges for imaging technology.

Oncologic imaging can be divided into two divisions: imaging of a known tumor mass and screening. Screening is the surveillance of a patient for the early detection of tumor. This may involve screening of a high-risk population for initial detection of a primary tumor, seeking metastases on initial presentation of a tumor, and seeking local recurrence or metastatic spread after initiation of therapy. Appropriate patient screening requires answering four questions all beginning with the letter "W". These are *whom* to screen, with *what* imaging modality, *when* to screen, and *which* anatomical area to survey? There are many problems in determining the most appropriate screening methods. Some of these are:

1. Most existing recommendations for follow-up screening imaging are relatively dogmatic, utilizing predefined imaging techniques at fixed, predetermined time intervals. Many of these recommendations are ad hoc and not based on scientific data. In defense of this method, it has worked reasonably well and has been the best method available, but we can now do much better. Screening protocols need to be much more flexible.
2. It is often difficult to define the benefits of screening. In other words, how much earlier is relapse detected with testing than without it and what impact does this have on patient outcome?
3. It is impossible to define the optimal frequency of repetition of imaging. Clearly, to perform no imaging is absurd. Equally absurd would be comprehensive imaging repeated every week. Somewhere between these extremes lies an acceptable compromise.
4. As the yield from a screening procedure decreases, what should we do? Should the screening be abruptly stopped, should the intensity (e.g., chest radiograph rather than chest CT) be decreased, should the frequency be decreased, or should a combination of the latter two alternatives be utilized?
5. How should children be screened for long-term complications? Patients are lost to follow-up, the yield from screening is very low, and the cost is high.
6. A cost-effective analysis of any screening protocol often results in a conflict as to what is best for the patient, when compared to what is best for society as a whole.

Screening protocols must be customized, taking into account the institutional expertise, therapeutic protocols utilized in an institution, knowledge of the biology of the tumor under consideration, and consideration of the needs of the individual patient and his or her family. The following guidelines should permit a reasonable protocol to be developed for each patient. The word "reasonable" is deliberately used, as there are too many gaps in our scientific knowledge to make optimal use of expensive imaging technology. The guidelines for screening are:

1. All studies must have a minimal acceptable positive yield. I would suggest adoption of an arbitrary standard stating that, to be used for screening, an imaging modality must have a minimum yield of 5 percent over a 2-year period, and that the yield must be meaningful in terms of patient management. I think this is a very conservative definition of minimum standards. At first it may be strange to accept such an arbitrary standard in imaging, but we are all very comfortable with acceptance of other arbitrary criteria such as 2-year disease-free survival being equated, for many tumors, with long-term survival.
2. On initial diagnosis of a tumor, maximal intensity of investigation must be utilized. At this time it is appropriate to utilize all modalities that provide additional in-

formation even if this additional information is small. The importance of accurate definition of the total extent of disease on initial diagnosis should be obvious. Staging, therapy, and prognostic predictions are all based on this initial evaluation. In addition, research protocols depend heavily on assigning patients to particular stages and, if this is incorrect, the results of the study are diminished in accuracy. Current knowledge of the biology of many tumors permits definition of specific high-risk subgroups. This means that in many patients screening for a particular location of disease can be confined to these subgroups. An excellent example of this is Wilms tumor; it is now known that bone metastases only occur with the rare clear-cell histology, occasionally with rhabdoid histology, but virtually never with the common classic histology.

3. There is a need to relate the prognosis of the tumor with imaging. For example, if salvage is excellent, early detection is less critical. Of equal significance, if a particular tumor has an excellent prognosis even if diagnosed when large, early detection is less critical. For example, most Wilms tumors have an extremely good prognosis even though the vast majority are large at the time of detection. Does this mean that many of the screening protocols used to detect Wilms tumor in high-risk population groups are applied too aggressively with the object of detecting small tumors?
4. Knowledge of tumor biology is essential. For example, it is known that there is a very high incidence of Wilms tumor in patients with aniridia, and these patients should be screened. It must be appreciated that this only applies to patients with sporadic aniridia and that it is entirely inappropriate to screen patients with familial aniridia.
5. Which modality to utilize in a particular anatomic area is determined from knowledge of scientific publications and current trends. In some situations, there is fairly universal agreement (e.g., bone scanning for seeking bone metastases), but in others the choice is much less well defined (e.g., CT versus MR for pelvic tumors).
6. Studies should be performed on initial diagnosis, when therapy is stopped, when therapy is changed, a couple of months after an alteration in therapy to establish the response to the change, if tumor is detected in another site, or if there are positive clinical indicators (e.g., localized pain, new mass, or positive lab findings for tumor markers). Studies should be stopped if meaningful yield drops below 5 percent over a 2-year period.
7. The concept of baseline studies is important. After a therapeutic intervention, even if it is suspected that no tumor will be found, it is extremely helpful to establish a baseline study for comparative purposes in the future.

Screening imaging is based on yield, rate of tumor growth, natural history of the tumor, treatment response, and the ability to act on the information provided.

Imaging faces many challenges for the future and has many problems. Some of these are:

1. Can imaging define any new criteria for predicting prognosis?
2. Imaging is frequently nonspecific in findings and the importance of pathologic and histologic confirmation of imaging findings cannot be stressed too much.
3. Can early promise of new technology such as MR spectroscopy be matured into routine use?
4. Can we define tumor response by criteria other than alteration in tumor size?
5. There are great problems in performing studies comparing various modalities with regard to their relative accuracy.
6. It is difficult to evaluate the precise impact of a positive imaging finding on patient outcome.
7. With the increasing effectiveness of chemotherapy we are being faced more frequently with the problem of the sterilized residual tumor or metastasis. Can we differentiate without the need for surgery between a small volume of residual active tumor and fibrosis? As imaging can never evaluate at the cellular level, we may never be able to differentiate accurately between a totally nonviable residual mass and a similar mass with a small number of viable tumor cells.
8. Following surgery, even with gadolinium-enhanced MR, we have difficulty in differentiating edema, hemorrhage, infection, and residual tumor.
9. Costs to a family of a child with cancer can be astronomical and imaging contributes significantly to these costs.
10. In a very broad sense, it is very difficult to define accurately our end point of cure. This is taken by many to mean the long-term elimination of tumor, but this is frequently not synonymous with a return to prior baseline health status.
11. Because childhood tumors are rare, scientific studies require multi-institution cooperation. From an imaging viewpoint, this creates difficulties in that the imaging requirements and recommendations of any particular protocol must be lowered to the ability and resources of the smallest participating institution.

Reference

1. Miller RW. Frequency and environmental epidemiology of childhood cancer. In: Pizzo PA, Poplack DG, eds. Principles and practice of pediatric oncology. Philadelphia: JB Lippincott, 1989:3–18.

CHAPTER 1
CARDIOVASCULAR TUMORS

All tumors of the heart are extremely rare. In children, about three-fourths of these tumors will be benign.[1,2] The benign tumors include rhabdomyoma, fibroma, myxoma, teratoma, and hemangioma[1,3]; rhabdomyoma is the most common.[2,3] Almost all malignant tumors are either sarcomas or metastases.[3] The symptoms from all cardiac tumors are very nonspecific. The tumors may sometimes be identified incidentally on a chest radiograph. Presenting symptoms in other children include arrhythmia, pericardial effusion, valve function abnormality, and congestive cardiac failure.[1]

Comment: Heart tumors are exceedingly rare.

BENIGN TUMORS

Rhabdomyomas are usually multiple.[2] They are frequently associated with the presence of tuberosclerosis.[4] About two-thirds will occur in children under the age of 3 years.[2] The tumors are most often in the ventricular walls, but can occur in other sites.[2] Symptoms are arrhythmia or cardiac failure from obstruction as the tumor projects into the lumen of the cardiac chambers.[2]

Fibromas occur most commonly in children under the age of 1 year. They are most often located in the wall of the left ventricle, are usually single, and can occasionally calcify.[2]

Lipomas usually occur in adults and are very rare in children. They are most commonly subendocardial and project into the lumen, but can occasionally occur in the wall or in the epicardial surface of the heart.[2]

Myxomas are rare in children and more common in adults. Two-thirds occur in the left atrium. They are gelatinous tumor masses attached to the atrial wall by a stalk. Symptoms are caused by obstruction or embolization.[2]

METASTASES

Cardiac metastases are over 20 times more common than primary malignant cardiac tumors.[1] Almost any malignant tumor can metastasize to the heart or pericardium. Table 1–1 shows the relative site of origin of metastases in 59 children.[3] Lymphoma is the most common malignancy to secondarily involve the heart (Fig. 1–1). Of the tumors spreading into the heart via the venous system, Wilms is the most common. Hepatocellular carcinoma, adrenal cell carcinoma, and yolk sac tumor also may spread via this route. Cardiac metastases may calcify and may cause pericardial effusions.[5] Most of the metastases are asymptomatic. They can be identified as nonspecific, focal, or more diffuse masses with computed tomography (CT), ultrasound, magnetic resonance imaging (MR). Most will not be identified on chest radiograph. The heart is rarely the first site of metastatic spread of a tumor. Most patients have evidence of metastatic disease in other locations when they develop cardiac metastases.[6] The metastases may involve any segment of the heart. In one study of 8 patients, the pericardium was involved in all 8, the myocardium in 7, and endocardium in 6.[6]

TABLE 1–1
Origin of Cardiac Metastases in 59 Children[1]

Metastasis	Percentage
Non-Hodgkins lymphoma	36
Neuroblastoma	22
Wilms tumor	20
Sarcoma	12
Spread via venous invasion	14

Reference
1. Chan HSL, Sonley MJ, Moes CAF, et al. Primary and secondary tumors of childhood involving the heart, pericardium and great vessels. Cancer 1985;56:825–836.

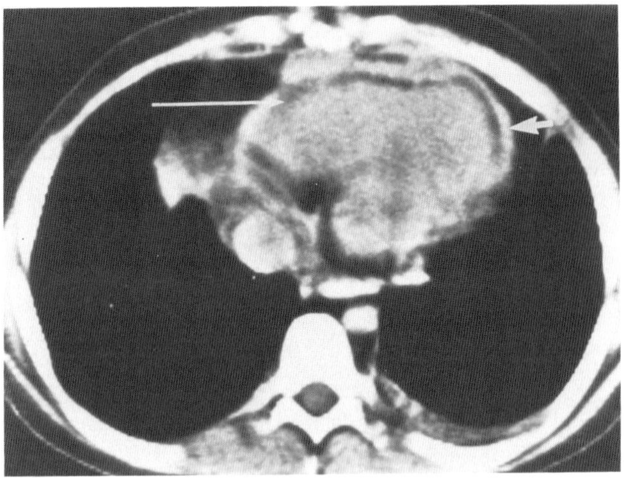

Figure 1-1. Diagnosis: Non-Hodgkin lymphoma of the pericardium.
The pericardium is extensively thickened due to tumor infiltration *(short arrow).* There is a small pericardial effusion *(long arrow).*

Figure 1-2. Diagnosis: Rhabdomyosarcoma of the heart.
A, Chest radiograph. A large mediastinal mass *(arrow)* is contiguous with the right heart border. ***B,*** Ultrasound. The large tumor (*T*) involves the mediastinum and wall of the right atrium *(RA)* and also projects into the lumen of the right atrium. *S* = Superior vena cava. ***C,*** Axial CT. The mediastinal extension of the tumor (*T*) is very large. It separates the superior vena cava (*S*) from the pulmonary artery (*P*) and displaces the ascending aorta (*A*). ***D,*** Axial MR. The appearance is almost identical to that seen on the CT in image ***C***.

A B C D

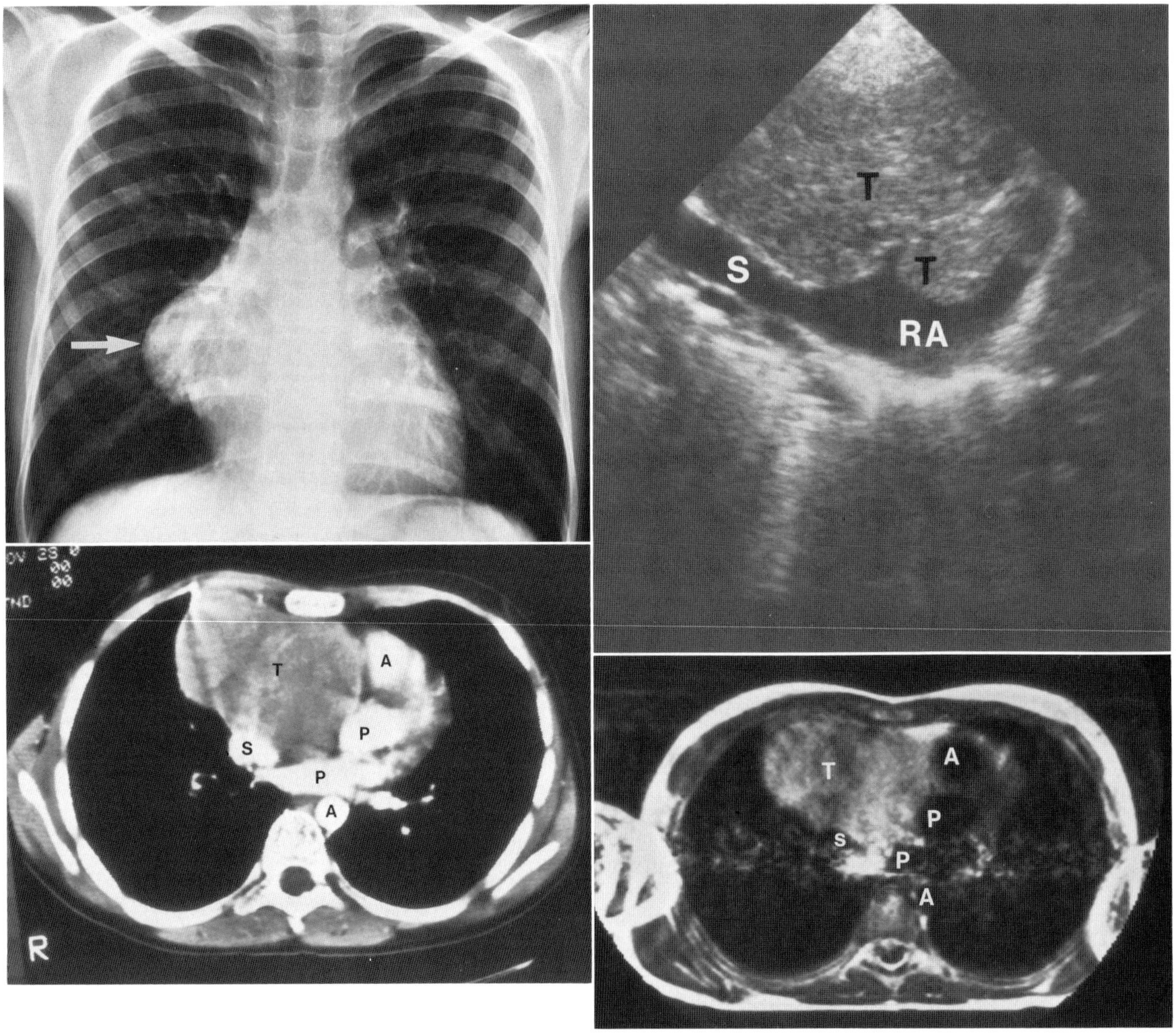

SARCOMA

Sarcomas of the heart are mainly rhabdomyosarcomas. In a literature review of 61 patients, the tumors were found to arise in the wall of the heart, with most growing large enough to enter the lumen. Symptoms included congestive failure in 70 percent and arrhythmias in 40 percent of patients.[7] Ultrasound, CT, or MR will identify the lesion (Fig. 1–2).

Other sarcomas are exceedingly rare[2] (Fig. 1–3). These include hemangiopericytoma, which has been identified in the pulmonary artery in 2 children.[8] These tumors were seen on ultrasound as mass lesions projecting into the lumen of the vessel.[8]

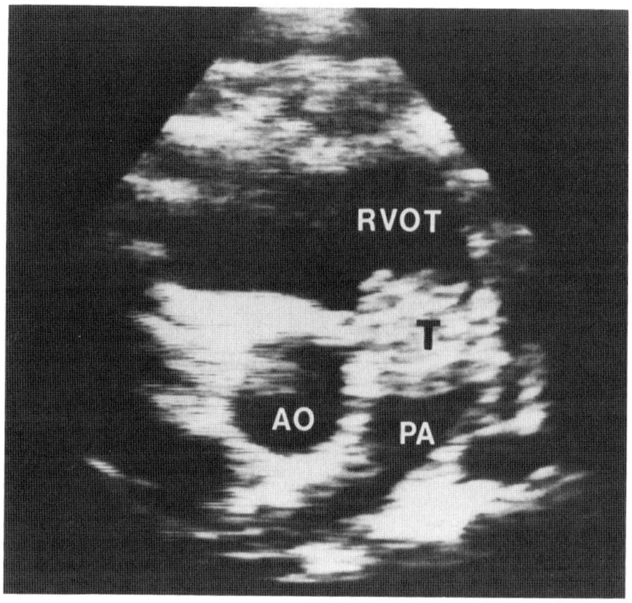

Figure 1-3. **Diagnosis: Pulmonary artery sarcoma. Ultrasound. A large tumor mass (*T*) lies in the proximal pulmonary artery *(PA)*. *RVOT* = right ventricular outflow tract; *AO* = ascending aorta. (From Farooki Z. Primary pulmonary artery sarcoma in two children. Pediatr Cardiol 1988;9:243.)**

> *Comment:* Rhabdomyosarcoma is the most common primary malignant heart tumor.

TERATOMA

Cardiac teratomas usually occur in the pericardium in newborn babies.[9] Most of these tumors are benign, but they can be malignant. There is a high mortality because of the location of the tumor.[10] Symptoms include cardiomegaly, a murmur, congestive failure, and hydrops.[1,9–12] Serum alpha-fetoprotein concentration is elevated.[11] Pericardial effusions are common.[9,11] Ultrasound will show the effusion and will usually show a mass lesion projecting into the pericardium.[11]

References

1. Arshadi S, Watson DG. Teratocarcinoma of the heart. Am J Dis Child 1966;112:87–91.
2. Arciniegas E, Hakimi M, Farooki ZQ, et al. Primary cardiac tumors in children. J Thorac Cardiovasc Surg 1980;79:582–591.
3. Chan HSL, Sonley MJ, Moses CAF, et al. Primary and secondary tumors of childhood involving the heart, pericardium and great vessels. Cancer 1985;56:825–836.
4. Riemuller R, Lloret JL, Tiling R, et al. MR imaging of pediatric cardiac tumors previously diagnosed by echocardiography. J Comput Assist Tomog 1989;13:621–626.
5. Widdowson DJ, Bradley MJ. Peribronchial calcification and ossification—an unusual pattern of metastatic osteosarcoma. Pediatr Radiol 1988;18:490.
6. Pratt CB, Dugger DL, Johnson WW, et al. Metastatic involvement of the heart in childhood rhabdomyosarcoma. Cancer 1973;31:1492–1497.
7. Schmaltz AA, Apitz J. Primary rhabdomyosarcoma of the heart. Pediatr Cardiol 1982;2:73–75.
8. Farooki ZQ, Chang CH, Jackson WL, et al. Primary pulmonary artery sarcoma in two children. Pediatr Cardiol 1988;9:243–251.
9. Dehner LP. Gonadal and extragonadal germ cell neoplasia of childhood. Hum Pathol 1983;14:493–511.
10. Sumner TE, Crowe JE, Klein A, et al. Intrapericardial teratoma in infancy. Pediatr Radiol 1980;10:51–53.
11. Nelson E, Stenzel P. Intrapericardial yolk sac tumor in an infant girl. Cancer 1987;60:1567–1569.
12. Banfield F, Dick M, Behrendt D, et al. Intrapericardial teratoma: a new and treatable cause of hydrops fetalis. Am J Dis Child 1980;134:1174–1175.

CHAPTER 2 RESPIRATORY TUMORS

Primary tumors of the lung in children are extremely rare. Benign tumors include adenoma, hamartoma, neuroma, leiomyoma, and teratoma.[1] Malignant tumors include blastoma, mucoepidermoid carcinoma, bronchogenic carcinoma, leiomyosarcoma, rhabdomyosarcoma, hemangiopericytoma, lymphoma, and malignant teratoma.[1] In addition to the lung, malignant tumors of the respiratory system may occur in the larynx or the nasal cavity.

Symptoms from tumors of the lung are very nonspecific, but include cough or obstruction. The tumors may be identified incidentally on chest radiograph without causing any symptoms. The lesions may cause collapse and secondary infection of lung segments, and the patient may, therefore, present with pneumonia. The tumors cannot be differentiated on the basis of symptoms. Similarly, the imaging appearance of tumors in the lung is very nonspecific. They may be small or large, focal or more diffuse, and will frequently have signs of secondary pulmonary collapse with or without infection.

Reference

1. Hartman GE, Shohat SJ. Primary pulmonary neoplasms of childhood: a review. Ann Thorac Surg 1983;36:108–119.

NASOPHARYNGEAL CARCINOMA

Epidemiology

There are two large and several smaller reports of nasopharyngeal carcinoma in children. The largest report is from the Children's Cancer Study Group (CCSG), reviewing 199 patients.[1] Another study reviewed 27 children with this tumor.[2] There is a strong association with Epstein-Barr virus infection.[3,4]

Pathology

Nasopharyngeal carcinoma is also called lymphoepithelioma or epidermoid carcinoma.[3] The tumors arise in the fossa of Rosenmuller.[3] They can invade locally, including penetration through the base of the skull. Local spread to neck lymph nodes is extremely common at the time of presentation.[3] In the study of 119 patients, the primary tumor mass at the time of diagnosis was confined to the nasopharynx in 41, extended into the rest of the nose or oropharynx in 19, and invaded the base of the skull in 43.[1] In the same study, node metastases were present in 74 patients at the time of diagnosis. Distant metastases can occur, especially to the lung, mediastinum, bones, and liver.[3,4] They are, however, unusual at the time of diagnosis, being present in only 3 of 119 patients.[1]

Histologically, the tumors are undifferentiated carcinoma.

Figure 2-1. **Diagnosis: Nasopharyngeal carcinoma. CT. The nasopharyngeal carcinoma (*N*) fills most of the nasopharynx and extends to involve the muscles medial to the mandibular ramus (*M*). There is erosion of the medial and lateral and pterygoid *(closed arrow)* and of the posterior wall of the left maxillary sinus *(open arrow)*.**

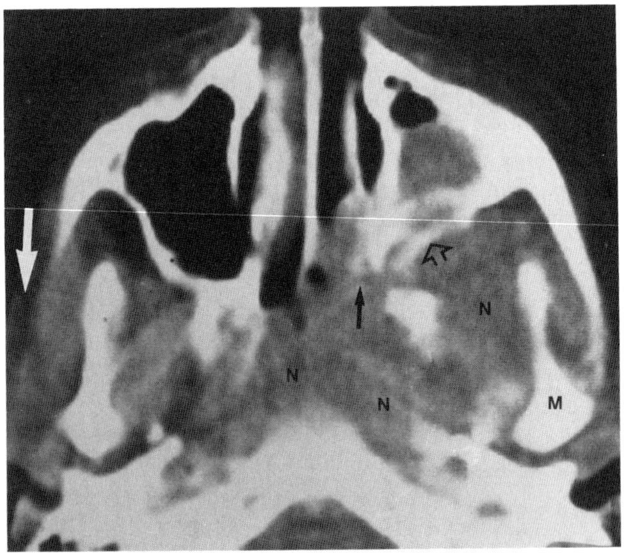

A B C D

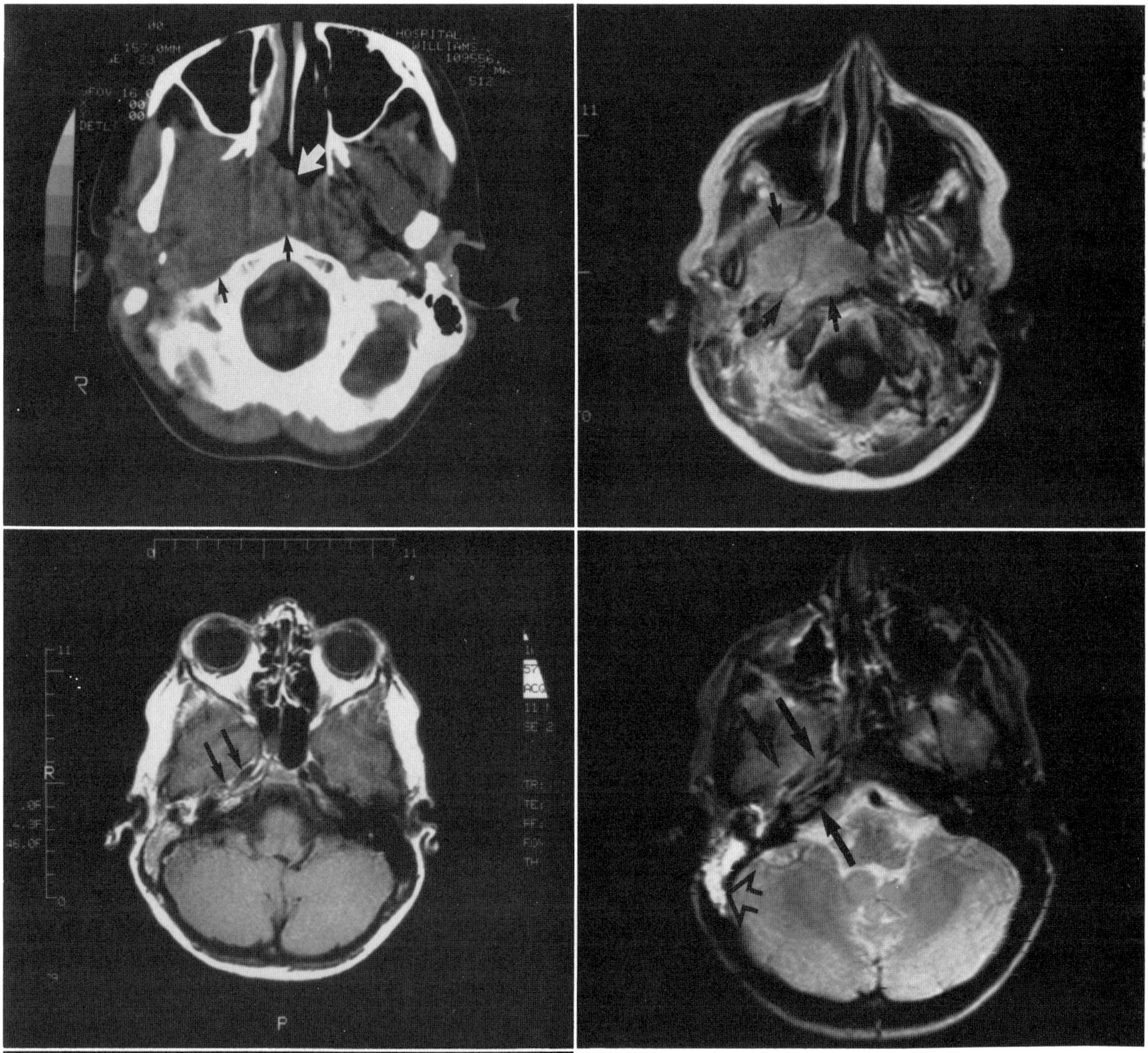

E

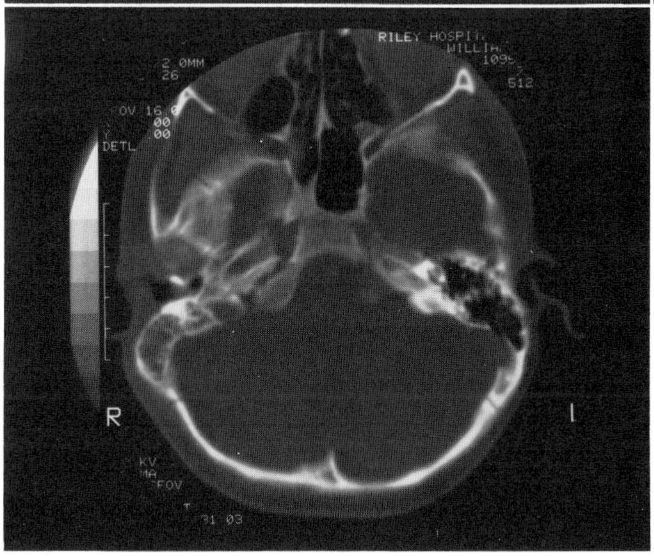

Figure 2-2. Diagnosis: Nasopharyngeal carcinoma. ***A,*** CT. There is a large right nasopharyngeal mass *(arrows).* ***B,*** MR. T1 weighted after gadolinium-DTPA injection. The mass is well seen *(arrows).* ***C*** and ***D,*** MR. T1 weighted image with gadolinium-DTPA and T2 weighted image. Subtle tumor encasement of the internal carotid artery *(arrows)* is seen. Strong signal *(open arrow)* in the mastoid sinus is fluid from obstruction of the Eustachian tube. ***E,*** CT. The tumor encasing the carotid artery is not appreciated.

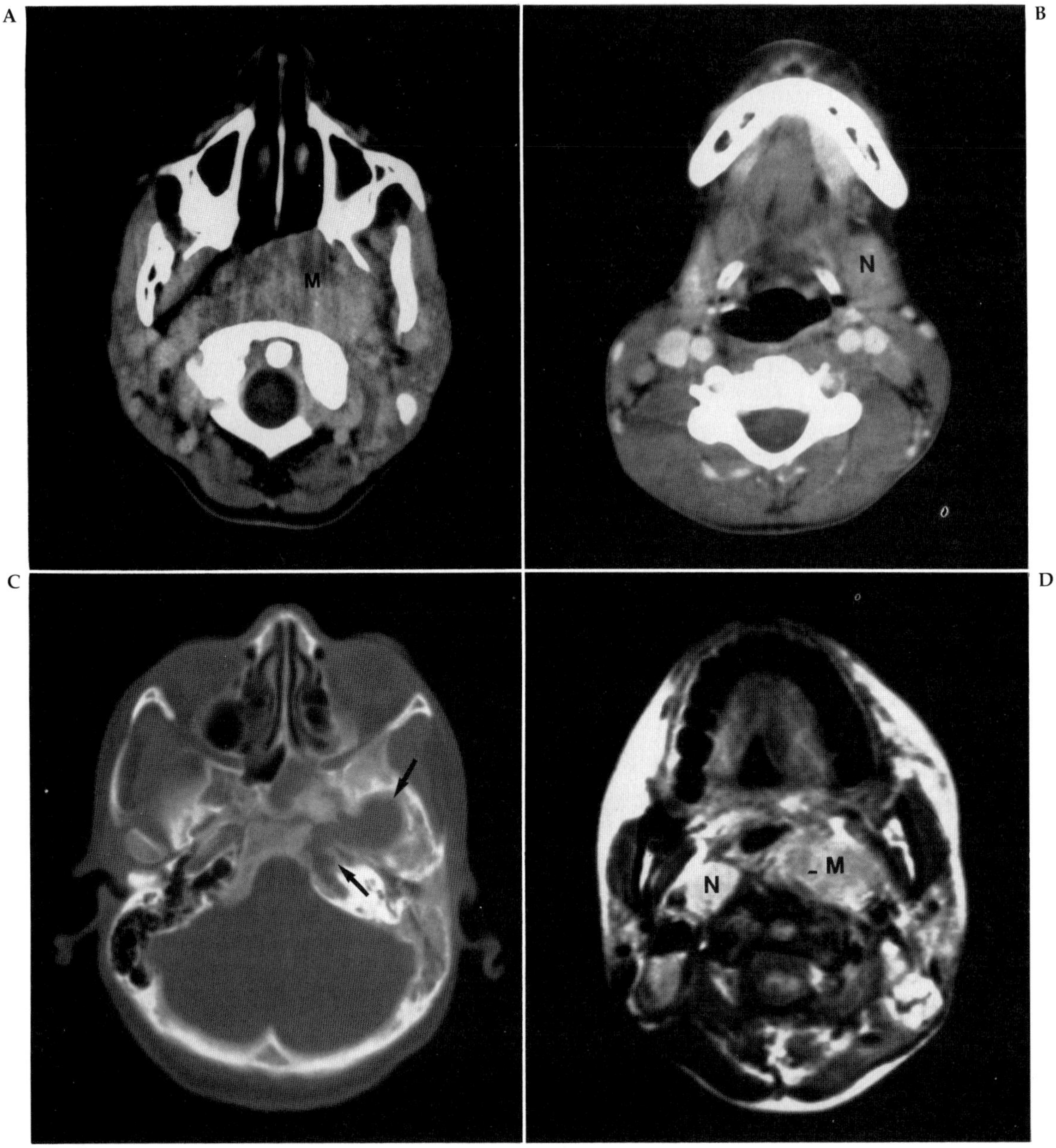

Figure 2-3. **Diagnosis: Nasopharyngeal carcinoma.**
***A, B,* and *C*: CT after contrast injection. There is a large tumor mass (*M*) in the nose, bone destruction *(arrows),* and node (*N*) metastasis. *D,* MR. T2 weighted image shows tumor mass (*M*) and node (*N*) metastasis.**

Clinical Presentation

The signs and symptoms at the time of diagnosis may be related to the tumor, local spread, or nodal metastases. Enlarged lymph nodes in the neck are extremely common.[1,3] Epistaxis is also extremely common, being identified in 14 of 27 patients in one study.[2] Local spread may cause cranial nerve palsy.[3] Obstruction of the Eustachian tube or spread along the tube will cause decrease in hearing in up to 40 percent of patients.[2,3,5] Patients may mistakenly be thought to have otitis media. Patients may very rarely present with osteoarthropathy and joint pain,[3,4] or local facial pain due to secondary sinusitis.[4]

Imaging Studies

Plain film radiographs show a soft-tissue mass in the nasopharynx. Bone erosion may be identified[5] (Fig.

2–1). Computed tomography (CT) and magnetic resonance imaging (MR) are excellent for evaluation of the tumor. They will show a nonspecific soft-tissue mass in the nasopharynx with its epicenter in the region of the fossa of Rosenmuller (Figs. 2–2 and 2–3). Both modalities will show the extent of soft-tissue spread within the nose (Fig. 2–4) and into base of the skull (Fig. 2–2). Both modalities will also show the extent of lymph node enlargement in the neck (Figs. 2–2 and 2–3). CT will be better than MR for definition of bone erosion. MR will be better for defining tumor margins and showing vessel encasement (Fig. 2–3). Sinus, middle ear, and mastoid fluid may be seen as well (Figs. 2–2 and 2–3). Because distant metastatic spread is rare, limited imaging should be performed seeking distant metastases. Chest radiograph and probably chest CT scan should be obtained. The bones and abdomen should probably not be imaged unless the patients have symptoms.

Differential Diagnosis

Differential diagnosis includes rhabdomyosarcoma, lymphoma, angiofibroma,[5] and rarely primary bone tumors.

Therapy and Prognosis

Treatment has been predominantly with radiation therapy and in most series, all patients have received such treatment. Chemotherapy has only been utilized in a small number of patients; for example, it was used in only 12 of 119 patients.[1] The exact role of chemotherapy is, therefore, not known. Because of the location of the tumor, surgery has little role to play apart from initial biopsy.

Survival of patients with nasopharyngeal carcinoma is in the region of 40 to 50 percent. After initial remission, subsequent relapse is associated with a dismal survival of only 17 percent.[1]

Figure 2-4. **Diagnosis: Nasopharyngeal carcinoma. CT. There is extension of the carcinoma into the nasal cavity on the left side *(white arrow).***

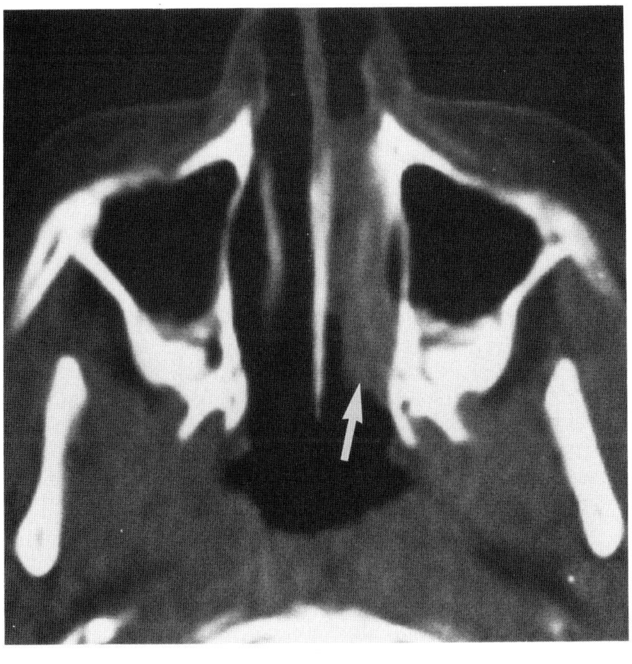

References

1. Jenkin RDT, Anderson JR, Jereb B, et al. Nasopharyngeal carcinoma—a retrospective review of patients less than thirty years of age: a report from Childrens Cancer Study Group. Cancer 1981;47:360–366.
2. Vita HC, Mendiondo OA, Shaw DL, et al. Nasopharyngeal carcinoma in the second decade of life. Radiology 1983;148:253–256.
3. Pratt CB, Douglas EC. Management of the less common cancers of childhood. In: Pizzo PA, Poplack DG, eds. Principles and practice of pediatric oncology. Philadelphia: JB Lippincott, 1989:759–782.
4. Bass IS, Haller JO, Berdon WE, et al. Nasopharyngeal carcinoma: clinical and radiographic findings in children. Radiology 1985;156:651–654.
5. Baker SR, McClatchey KD. Carcinoma of the nasopharynx in childhood. Otolaryngol Head Neck Surg 1981;89:555–559.

CARCINOMA OF THE LARYNX

Very few pediatric patients have been reported with squamous carcinoma of the larynx. Fewer than 100 patients have been reported in the literature. Two literature reviews,[1,2] together with case presentations, indicate that the pathology of these tumors is similar to that seen in adults. The lesions occur mainly on the vocal cord. There is frequently a prior history of radiation therapy for papillomatosis, and residual papillomas may still be present. The tumors can occur at any age in children, but the children are most commonly over the age of 10. Eighty-five percent of the tumors are limited to the larynx. Fifty percent of tumors cause fixation of the vocal cords.

Symptoms are nonspecific and include obstruction, hoarseness, and cough. CT is the imaging modality of choice, with the role of MR yet to be defined. CT will identify the tumor and define its extent. The treatment is surgery and radiation therapy.[1] Differential diagnosis includes hemangioma and papilloma, both of which are more common than malignant lesions of the larynx. Other laryngeal malignancies include rhabdomyosarcoma.[3,4] The history of papillomatosis with possible prior radiation therapy and the location of the tumor in the vocal cord should suggest the correct diagnosis.

References

1. Gindhart TD, Johnston WH, Chism SE, et al. Carcinoma of the larynx in childhood. Cancer 1980;46:1683–1687.
2. Laurian N, Sadov R, Strauss M, et al. Laryngeal carcinoma in childhood. Report of a case and review of the literature. Laryngoscope 1984;94:684–687.

3. Abramowsky CR, Witt WJ. Sarcoma of the larynx in a newborn. Cancer 1983;51:1726–1730.
4. Pratt CB, Douglas EC. Management of the less common cancers of childhood. In: Pizzo PA, Poplack DG, eds. Principles and practice of pediatric oncology. Philadelphia: JB Lippincott, 1989:759–782.

BLASTOMA

Epidemiology

Blastomas usually occur in young children. In one study, 60 percent were under the age of 4 years.[1]

Pathology

This tumor is also called pulmonary blastoma or thoracopulmonary blastoma. These are tumors that arise in the lung or on the lung surface. They are completely different from blastomas in adults. Macroscopically, they are single tumors located peripherally in the lung. Because of this they do not cause early symptoms of bronchial obstruction and are frequently very large at the time of diagnosis. Large areas of hemorrhage and necrosis are common. These may rarely develop cavitation.[2–4] Microscopically, they are embryonal tumors, resembling fetal lung.[3,5] They contain both mesenchymal and epithelial elements[5] and, therefore, one may identify within these tumors areas of rhabdomyosarcoma, chondrosarcoma, liposarcoma, cartilage, smooth muscle, or glands.[4,5]

Metastases occur to the opposite lung, liver, bone, or brain.[4,6] Bilateral tumors are extremely rare; lymph node metastases are rare.[4]

Clinical Presentation

Symptoms are nonspecific and will include pain, distress, hemoptysis, fever, nonspecific illness, and cough.[4,5] The tumors may occasionally be identified, without symptoms, on a chest radiograph.[4]

Imaging Studies

A very large tumor is revealed by imaging (Figs. 2–5 and 2–6). Chest radiograph shows a homogenous soft-tissue mass that may fill the entire hemithorax (Figs. 2–5 and 2–6). There is displacement of mediastinum to the opposite side. Pneumothorax was identified in 2 of 16 patients in one study.[7] Ultrasound will show a nonspecific echogenic mass. CT shows a massive chest tumor with displacement of the mediastinum. Areas of hemorrhage and necrosis will be seen as low attenuation (Fig. 2–6). CT clearly differentiates the tumor from pleural effusion with mediastinal displacement.[5] Invasion of the mediastinum can be identified occasionally with CT[8] (Fig. 2–6). Cystic components, the result of hemorrhage, may be identified in up to a third of patients.[5] Occasionally, calcification, which is curvilinear, may be seen.[2]

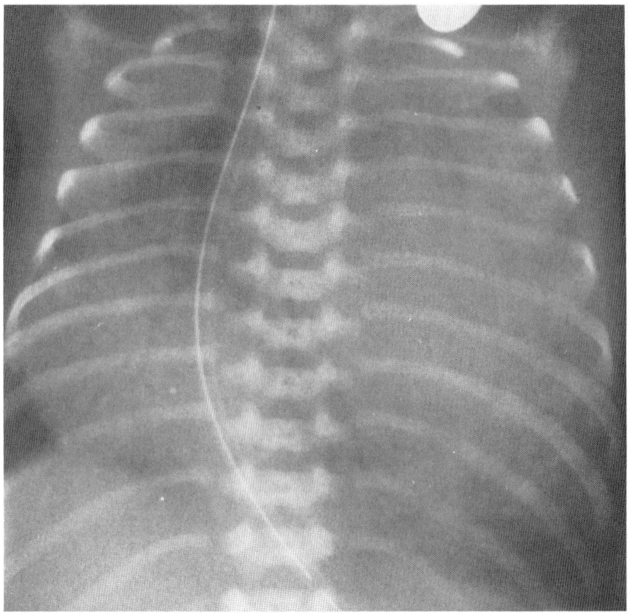

Figure 2–5. **Diagnosis: Pulmonary blastoma. Chest radiograph. There is a very large mass lesion occupying most of the left hemithorax. A little air is seen in the base of the left lung. The heart and mediastinum are displaced to the right by this very large tumor.**

Therapy and Prognosis

Treatment is surgery, but because of the tumor's very large size, resection may be difficult and prognosis is often poor.[3] In one study, recurrence occurred in 9 of 11 patients within a year of initial surgery.[5] Prognosis has been reported as ranging from less than 20 percent survival[2] to over 40 percent survival.[1]

References
1. Hartman GE, Shochat SJ. Primary pulmonary neoplasms of childhood: a review. Ann Thorac Surg 1983;36:108–119.
2. Solomon A, Rubinstein ZJ, Rogoff M, et al. Pulmonary blastoma. Pediatr Radiol 1982;12:148–149.
3. Capp MP, Strautman PR. Image interpretation session. RadioGraphics 1990;10:131–156.
4. Sumner TE, Phelps CR, Crowe JE, et al. AJR 1979;133:147–148.
5. Manivel JC, Priest JR, Watterson J, et al. Pleuropulmonary blastoma. The so-called pulmonary blastoma of childhood. Cancer 1988;62:1516–1526.
6. Dehner LP. Pediatric surgical pathology, 2nd ed. Baltimore: Williams & Wilkins, 1987:292.
7. Ohtomo K, Araki T, Yashiro N, et al. Pulmonary blastoma in children. Radiology 1983;147:101–104.
8. Ivancev K, Halldorsdottir A, Laurin S, et al. Computed tomography in the diagnosis and treatment of mediastinal abnormalities in children. Acta Radiol 1988;29:115–120.

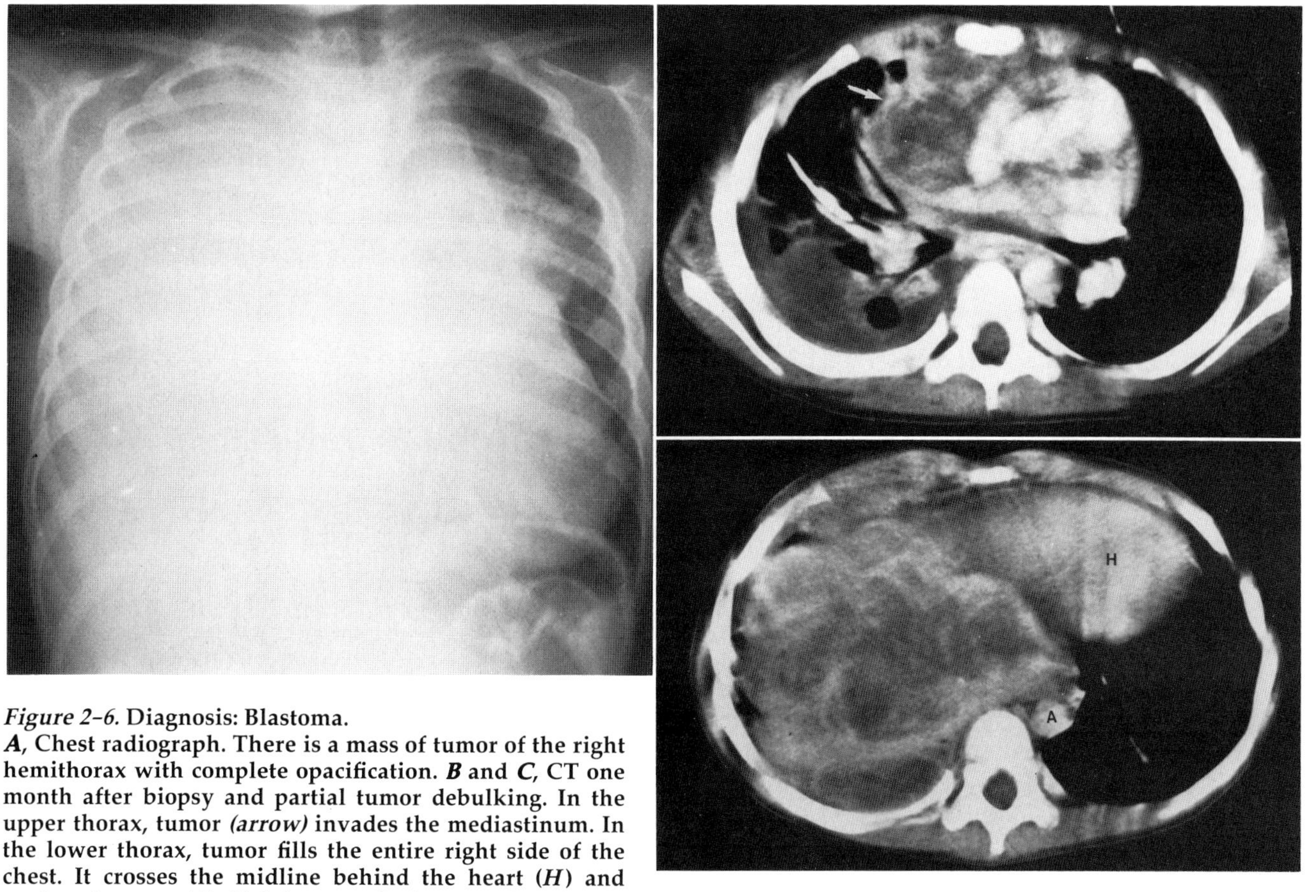

Figure 2-6. Diagnosis: Blastoma.
A, **Chest radiograph. There is a mass of tumor of the right hemithorax with complete opacification. *B* and *C*, CT one month after biopsy and partial tumor debulking. In the upper thorax, tumor *(arrow)* invades the mediastinum. In the lower thorax, tumor fills the entire right side of the chest. It crosses the midline behind the heart (*H*) and pushes the aorta (*A*) slightly posteriorly. Many low-intensity regions of the tumor are due to hemorrhage and necrosis.**

MUCOEPIDERMOID CARCINOMA

Epidemiology

Mucoepidermoid carcinoma is a rare tumor, with probably fewer than 50 cases being reported.[1–5]

Pathology

There is some debate regarding the histology of this tumor. The histology is described as being low grade in all patients, or low grade in most patients with occasional patients having a high-grade (more malignant) histology.[2] The tumors are polypoid masses projecting into the lumen of the bronchus[1,4]; they can penetrate through the wall of the bronchus.[4]

Clinical Presentation

Symptoms include hemoptysis caused by hemorrhage from the tumor, wheezing due to airway narrowing, pulmonary collapse, and recurrent pneumonia.[1,3,4]

Imaging Studies

On plain film radiograph, the mass may occasionally be identified (Fig. 2–7), but frequently it is not. The secondary signs of more peripheral collapse and infection are commonly identified. Very often the patients will have recurrent areas of pulmonary consolidation and collapse, which may clear for many months between acute episodes. CT scan will show the secondary collapse and infection, and will in most cases identify the tumor within the bronchus and also the extension beyond the wall of the bronchus (Fig. 2–7). These tumors grow very slowly. Recurrent episodes of abnormality may, therefore, be seen for many years, if the diagnosis is not suspected.

Differential Diagnosis

This includes chronic inflammatory disorders such as cystic fibrosis. The persistence of the abnormality in one segment of the lung on serial chest radiographs should suggest bronchial obstruction. Clinically and radiographically, it may be extremely difficult to differentiate the tumor from an inhaled foreign body. Other bronchial and tracheal tumors such as adenoma will appear

A B

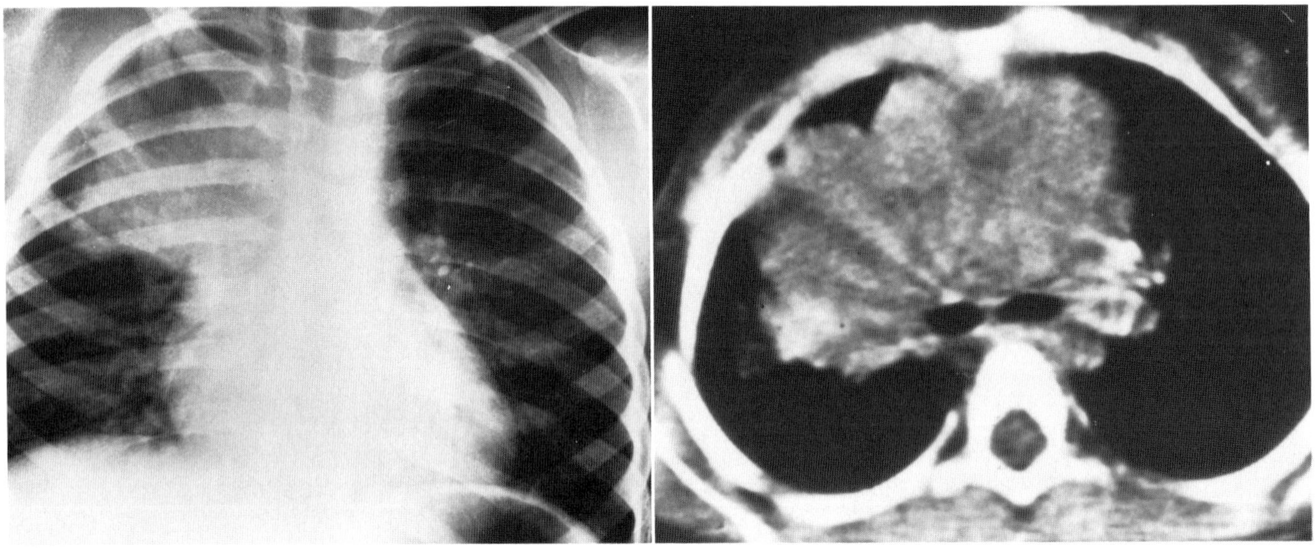

Figure 2-7. Diagnosis: Mucoepidermoid carcinoma of the lung.
***A**,* Chest radiograph. A large density spreads from the hilum into the upper half of the right chest. Tumor cannot be differentiated from collapse and consolidation in the right upper lobe. ***B**,* The abnormality on the chest radiograph has a lobulated contour and it is comprised predominantly of tumor that has grown through the bronchus, invading the mediastinum and lung. This child had been treated for recurrent episodes of pneumonia of the right upper lung for many years.

Figure 2-8. Diagnosis: Tracheal adenoma.
***A**,* Chest radiograph. A subtle but definite mass *(arrows)* is seen within the trachea. ***B**,* CT. This clearly shows a large mass (*M*) lesion projecting into the lumen of the trachea. This child was treated for several years with a diagnosis of asthma.

A B

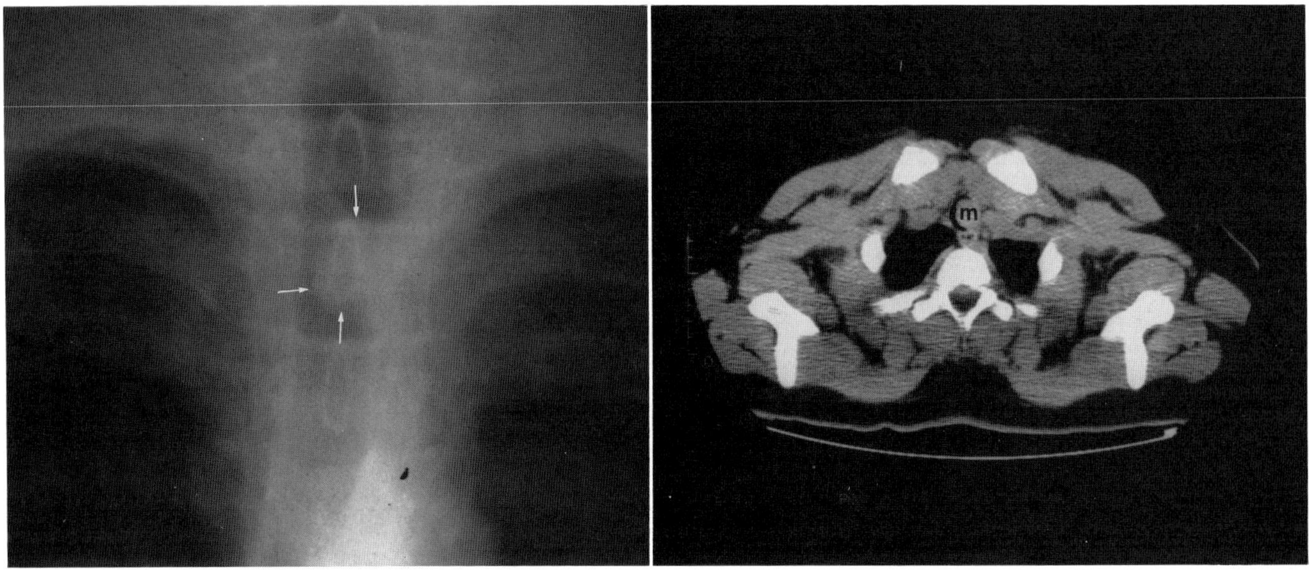

similar (Fig. 2–8). The most important factor in making the correct diagnosis is to think of the possibility of a bronchial tumor in all patients with recurrent focal pulmonary abnormality and to perform relatively early bronchoscopy.

Therapy and Prognosis

Diagnosis is confirmed by bronchoscopy and biopsy; with wide surgical resection, the prognosis is excellent.

> *Comment:* Consider a bronchial tumor or foreign body as the cause of recurrent localized "pneumonia."

References

1. Breyer RH, Dainauskas JR, Jensik RJ, et al. Mucoepidermoid carcinoma of the trachea and bronchus: the case for conservative resection. Ann Thorac Surg 1979;29:197–204.
2. Heitmiller RF, Mathisen DJ, Ferry JA, et al. Mucoepidermoid lung tumors. Ann Thorac Surg 1989;47:394–399.
3. Mullins JD, Barnes RP. Childhood bronchial mucoepidermoid tumors. Cancer 1979;44:315–322.
4. Nakagawara A, Ikeda K, Ohgami H. Mucoepidermoid tumor of the bronchus in an infant. J Pediatr Surg 1979;14:608–609.
5. Hartman GE, Shochat SJ. Primary pulmonary neoplasms of childhood: a review. Ann Thorac Surg 1983;36:108–119.

ADENOID CYSTIC CARCINOMA

Adenoid cystic carcinoma has been reported in only 4 children.[1] These children presented with cough, hemoptysis, and recurrent infection. The tumors were seen as polypoid masses penetrating through the bronchial wall into the lung. Treatment is surgical resection, and there is a tendency to local recurrence. Radiographic findings are the same as those for mucoepidermoid carcinoma.

Reference

1. Hartman GE, Shochat SJ. Primary pulmonary neoplasms of childhood: a review. Ann Thorac Surg 1983;36:108–119.

CARCINOID

Carcinoid is an unusual tumor in children.[1–4] The tumors are located in the bronchial airway and symptoms include cough, infection, and hemoptysis.[3] The carcinoid syndrome is said never to occur in children.[2,3] Metastases have been described in between 8 and 27 percent of patients.[2–4] As with mucoepidermoid carcinoma and adenoid cystic carcinoma, imaging findings are nonspecific, with signs of distal pulmonary collapse and infection occurring intermittently, and possible demonstration of the polypoid mass in the airway with CT. Diagnosis is by bronchoscopy and biopsy. Hemorrhage following biopsy is common.[3] With surgical resection there is over 90 percent survival.[2,3]

References

1. Dehner LP. Pediatric surgical pathology, 2nd ed. Baltimore: Williams & Wilkins, 1987:289.
2. Scully RE, Mark EJ, McNeely WF, et al. Weekly clinicopathological exercise. New Engl J Med 1989;321:1665–1672.
3. Hartman GE, Shochat SJ. Primary pulmonary neoplasms of childhood: a review. Ann Thorac Surg 1983;36:108–119.
4. Lack EE, Harris GBC, Eraklis AJ, et al. Primary bronchial tumors in childhood. Cancer 1983;51:492–497.

BRONCHOGENIC CARCINOMA

Bronchogenic carcinoma, common in adults, is rare in children.[1,2] In a literature review of 46 cases in children, 20 percent were less than 3 years of age.[2] About 80 percent of cases were adenocarcinomas, with most of the rest being squamous carcinomas. Two of the tumors arose in a congenital cystic pulmonary abnormality. Most of the children had metastases at the time of diagnosis. Clinical symptoms include cough and recurrent pneumonia. Chest radiograph findings are nonspecific and reveal the presence of a mass lesion. The adenocarcinomas tend to be smaller and have a better resectability than the squamous carcinomas.[1]

References

1. Dehner LP. Pediatric surgical pathology, 2nd ed. Baltimore: Williams & Wilkins, 1987:289.
2. Hartman GE, Shochat SJ. Primary pulmonary neoplasms of childhood: a review. Ann Thorac Surg 1983;36:108–119.

RHABDOMYOSARCOMA

Rhabdomyosarcoma is also a rare tumor of the lung in children. It can occur at any age.[1,2] The tumor may be endobronchial in location or can occur within existing congenital cystic pulmonary abnormalities.[1–3] It can cause airway occlusion with peripheral collapse and infection. Findings on imaging are the appearance of either a mass lesion or secondary collapse and consolidation. There are no specific features. The association of a growing mass lesion with a cystic malformation of the lung might suggest the correct diagnosis.

References
1. Krous HF, Sexauer CL. Embryonal rhabdomyosarcoma arising within a congenital bronchogenic cyst in a child. J Pediatr Surg 1981;16:506–508.
2. Hartman GE, Shochat SJ. Primary pulmonary neoplasms of childhood: a review. Ann Thorac Surg 1983;36:108–119.
3. Dehner LP. Pediatric surgical pathology, 2nd ed. Baltimore: Williams & Wilkins, 1987:291.

MALIGNANCY IN PULMONARY CYSTS

There is an increasing number of reports of malignant disease occurring in association with lung cysts.[1-3] These may be simple cysts or cystic adenomatoid malformation, and the malignancy may occur before cyst resection or in the location of a previously resected cyst. One literature review identified 14 cases of malignancy occurring in relation to pulmonary cysts.[2] Most of the children were in the age range of 2 to 4 years. In most patients, imaging was not able to identify the malignancy accurately, but in some cases showed a nodule. Tumors that have been reported in association with pulmonary cysts include mesenchymal sarcoma,[2] bronchogenic carcinoma,[1] pulmonary blastoma,[2] and rhabdomyosarcoma.[1-4]

Comment: All congenital pulmonary cysts should be resected, even if asymptomatic, because of the risk of malignancy developing in the cyst.

References
1. Hartman GE, Shochat SJ. Primary pulmonary neoplasms of childhood: a review. Ann Thorac Surg 1983;36:108–119.
2. Hedlund GL, Bisset GS, Bove KE. Malignant neoplasms arising in cystic hamartomas of the lung in childhood. Radiology 1989;173:77–79.
3. Krous HF, Sexauer CL. Embryonal rhabdomyosarcoma arising within a congenital bronchogenic cyst in a child. J Pediatr Surg 1981;16:506–508.
4. Dehner LP. Pediatric surgical pathology, 2nd ed. Baltimore: Williams & Wilkins, 1987:248.

MALIGNANT FIBROUS HISTIOCYTOMA

There have been a few cases of malignant fibrous histiocytoma reported in adults and one case in a 12-year-old child (R-16). This child had a 9 cm right upper lung mass. On CT scan, the mass was moderately well defined, heterogenous with large areas of necrosis, and contained stippled calcification. At the time of diagnosis metastases were present in the opposite lung and brain.

Reference
1. Ismailer I, Khan A, Leonidas JC, et al. Computed tomography of primary malignant fibrohistiocytoma of the lung. Computerized Radiol 1987;11:37–40.

LEIOMYOSARCOMA

A literature review identified 9 children with leiomyosarcoma[1]; 78 percent were under the age of 4 years. The tumor can occur within the tracheobronchial tree or in the lung parenchyma.[1,2] Chest radiograph may show a single nodule or signs of pulmonary collapse and infection.[2] There are no specific diagnostic features. Diagnosis is usually made at surgery.

References
1. Hartman GE, Shochat SJ. Primary pulmonary neoplasms of childhood: a review. Ann Thorac Surg 1983;36:108–119.
2. Sweet RS. Pulmonary leiomyoma. AJR 1969;107:823–826.

METASTASES

The consideration of metastatic disease to the lung is of considerable importance, because the lung is the most common site of metastatic spread for the vast majority of pediatric malignant tumors. In many patients, it is the only site of metastatic disease. In other patients, it is frequently the first site of metastatic disease. The detection of lung metastases greatly influences therapy and prognosis. The following principles and comments should be considered in evaluation of any child with potential pulmonary metastases.

1. Very few pediatric tumors present with the incidental finding of a pulmonary metastasis. This is probably because routine radiographs are much less frequently performed in children than in adults. In contrast to adults, in whom incidental pulmonary nodules frequently require biopsy to make an initial diagnosis, most children do not require this procedure. An incidental nodule on a chest radiograph in a child is most likely to be benign, and every effort, such as history, measurement of histoplasma serum titers, and follow-up, should be made to confirm that the lesion is benign and to avoid unnecessary biopsy.
2. In a child with known malignant disease, the development of a single lung nodule cannot and must not be assumed to represent malignant disease. In one study of 39 children with cancer, 13 of 39 new nodules developing after the commencement of therapy were benign.[1] The radiologist must be willing to adopt an aggressive approach to biopsy these lesions. Obviously, if there is widespread metastatic disease in other anatomic regions of the body, the need to biopsy the lung lesion becomes much less critical. If, however, the lung lesion is the only site of potential metastatic dis-

ease, and especially if therapeutic changes will be made if the lesion is a metastasis, biopsy should be encouraged.

3. Multiple lung nodules, in a child with known cancer, are much much more likely to be malignant than a single nodule.
4. Most but not all pulmonary metastases are round and well defined. Metastases may be diffuse and infiltrating; this pattern is seen, for example, with neuroblastoma. The metastasis may also be distorted by other underlying lung disease and in these patients the correct diagnosis may easily be missed.
5. There are no imaging criteria by which diagnosis of metastasis can be made with 100 percent confidence.
6. Diffuse metastases may appear as small or large nodules. The nodules may be of similar size or may vary in size. On the chest radiograph, take care not to confuse chest wall masses with lung metastases (Fig. 2–9).
7. Benign and malignant nodules can occur in the same patient. This is particularly true in regions of the United States where histoplasmosis is common. Benign and malignant nodules may be separate in location, or metastasis may occur immediately adjacent to a benign nodule.
8. Calcification is not an indication that a lesion is benign. For example, osteogenic sarcoma metastases will frequently calcify. In addition, calcified histoplasma nodules may occur in continuity with metastatic nodules.
9. For the identification of pulmonary nodules, increasing accuracy is found with the chest radiograph, whole lung tomography, chest CT, and finally surgery. There is no longer any place for whole lung tomography in evaluation of children for pulmonary metastases. Early studies with CT consistently showed superiority of surgery over CT for identification of pulmonary nodules. There are no reports in the last few years comparing the new high-resolution CT scanners with surgery.
10. When performing CT scanning for detection of pulmonary metastases, intravenous contrast is not required. Contiguous 1 cm or thinner slices should be obtained through the lung. In most children, it is best to let the child breathe spontaneously. Attempts to get the child, particularly under the age of about 8 years, to hold his or her breath will frequently result in deeper respiratory excursions and more motion artifact than if the child is allowed to breathe spontaneously. In the intrepretation of pulmonary CT, it must be borne in mind that some respiratory motion will occur between slices. This, together with partial volume effect, means that occasionally very small nodules will be missed. In addition, some nodules may appear smaller than they actually are. This must be remembered in evaluating the response of nodules to therapy. If a new tiny nodule is identified on a CT scan, it may not be present on the previous study, but review of earlier studies may sometimes show the presence of this lesion. Before diagnosing a new nodule on follow-up studies, it is always prudent to review not only the previous scan but also, if available, earlier studies.
11. There is no doubt that chest CT is more sensitive than chest radiograph for detection of pulmonary nodules. However, in some situations, it may be entirely appropriate to follow children with a chest radiograph rather than CT, because of the lower cost and radiation dose of the chest radiograph. In general, CT should be performed if the earlier diagnosis of a nodule will alter therapy in any way. Thus, CT should always be performed on initial presentation, because therapy depends on accurate staging. Even if widespread nodules are identified on the chest radiograph, on initial presentation, I would still recommend a CT to obtain an accurate baseline for the presence of smaller nodules not seen on the chest radiograph, and also to identify additional disease not shown on the chest radiograph, such as lymph node involvement or calcification in some of the nodules. CT should also be performed any time chemotherapy is stopped. CT should also be performed in a child who has had pulmonary metastases responding to treatment, and in whom the chest radiograph shows apparent complete resolution. CT should be performed any other time earlier detection of nodules will affect therapy. This is particularly true for those diseases such as osteogenic sarcoma where therapeutic protocols include aggressive surgical resection of pulmonary nodules, if identified. When can the chest radiograph alone be utilized? In tumors in which very early detection of nodules does not affect therapy (i.e., they are not resected), and in which a child is on a therapeutic protocol that will not alter immediately even if nodules are detected, a chest radiograph rather than CT is appropriate. In addition, for the long-term follow-up of children, after successful conclusion with chemotherapy, and with the child in complete remission, chest radiograph is probably most appropriate, particularly in those situations where the expected detection of nodules is extremely low.
12. The response of pulmonary metastases to therapy is usually that of complete resolution of the nodule, when therapy is successful. Occasionally, however, a small residual fibrotic scar may remain, or the nodule may cavitate before it resolves (Fig. 2–10). Not every small residual abnormality represents residual disease.

***Figure 2-9.* Diagnosis: Pseudopulmonary metastasis. Chest radiograph. Apparent metastatic nodules *(arrows)* in both lung fields are in fact rib metastases from a neuroblastoma.**

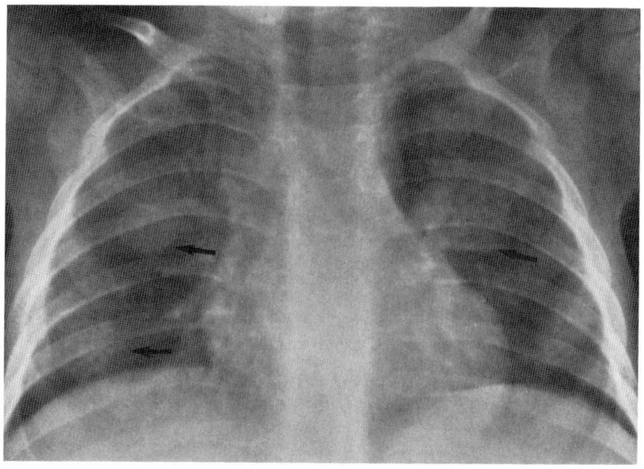

A

B

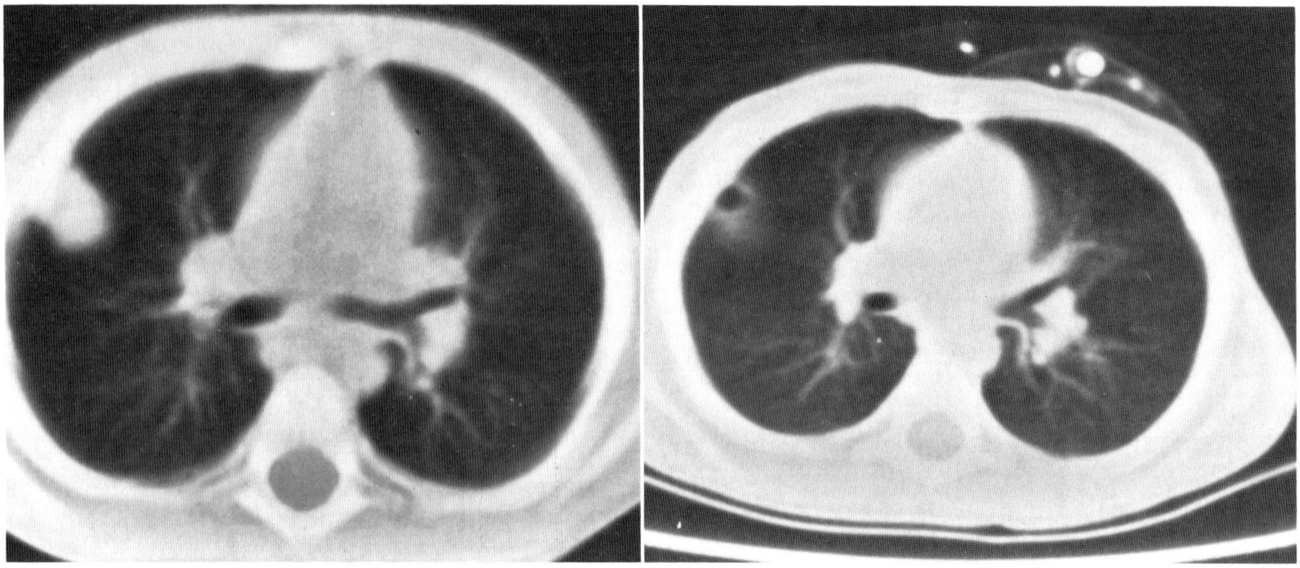

Figure 2–10. **Diagnosis: Cavitation of metastases from Wilms tumor following chemotherapy. *A*, CT. There is a well-defined metastatic nodule in the right chest. *B*, CT. After chemotherapy, the nodule is not resolved but remains as a thin-walled cavity. A tumor cannot be differentiated from fibrosis in the wall of this cavity.**

In 3 children with malignant bone tumors, residual nodules were resected after chemotherapy. In 2 patients, the nodules revealed only fibrous tissue, and in the third patient tumor was present.[2] I do not believe that any imaging modality, including MR, can always accurately differentiate fibrosis from residual tumor.

13. Some of the disorders to be considered in the differential diagnosis of pulmonary metastases are listed in Table 2–1. In some patients, it may not be possible to differentiate the benign disorder from a metastasis without a biopsy. In other disorders, careful imaging can be helpful. For example, with round atelectasis the nodule is always pleural based, there is a pleural scar, and the vessels crowd together as they converge on the area of collapse.[3] Arteriovenous malformations may show the presence of enlarged feeding and draining

TABLE 2–1
Differential Diagnosis of Lung Metastases

Infection	Tumor
Histoplasma	Primary lung malignancy (rare)
Other fungal infection	Hamartoma[2,3]
Abscess	Inflammatory pseudotumor[2,4]
Round pneumonia	Neurofibroma[2]
Congenital	Therapy
Arteriovenous malformation	Bleomycin induced nodules[5]
Mechanical, trauma	Nodules after radiation therapy[6]
Hematoma	
Round atelectasis[1]	

References

1. Schneider HJ, Felson B, Gonzalez LL. Rounded atelectasis. AJR 1980;134:225–232.
2. Hartman GE, Shochat SJ. Primary pulmonary neoplasms of childhood: a review. Ann Thorac Surg 1983;36:108–119.
3. Haller JO, Kauffman SL, Kassner EG. Congenital mesenchymal tumour of the lung. Br J Radiol 1977;50:217–219.
4. Schwartz EE, Katz SM, Mandell GA. Postinflammatory pseudotumors of the lung: fibrous histiocytoma and related lesions. Radiology 1980;136:609–613.
5. Scharstein R, Johnson JF, Cook BA, et al. Bleomycin nodules mimicking metastatic osteogenic sarcoma. Am J Pediatr Hematol/Oncol 1987;9:219–221.
6. Cohen MD, Mirkin DL, Provisor A, et al. Lung nodules after whole lung radiation. Am J Pediatr Hematol/Oncol 1983;5:283–286.

vessels. The age of the patient may be helpful. For example, inflammatory pseudotumors are uncommon under the age of 5 years.[4]

14. Surgical resection of pulmonary metastases is a new form of therapy.[5–8] In one study of 22 children with surgical resection of metastases, there was significant survival. Of 10 children with osteogenic sarcoma lung metastases, 5 survived at 5 years. Of 5 children with Wilms tumor, 4 survived 8 years after surgical resection of lung metastases. From a technical point of view wedge resection is usually performed, and bilateral metastases are approached in two staged sessions.[9] Imaging is extremely important in selection of patients for surgical resection. The criteria to be met are:

    - The tumor type should be such that the lung is known to be the only site of metastasis in a significant number of patients.
    - Metastases appearing late after initial diagnosis are more likely to be slow growing and, therefore, have a much better likelihood of cure following surgical resection.[8,10]
    - Mediastinal disease must be excluded.[9] Careful evaluation with CT scan is, therefore, important.
    - Imaging must show good control of the primary tumor.
    - Metastases must be confined to the lung.[9] Ideally, there should be only a few nodules present.[10] Prognosis, after metastatic resection, is much better in patients with less than 4 nodules than in patients with more than 4 nodules.[6]

> *Comment:* The lungs are the most common site of metastases from pediatric cancers. Not all lung nodules are, however, malignant.

References

1. Cohen MD, Smith WL, Weetman R, et al. Pulmonary pseudometastases in children with malignant tumors. Radiology 1981;141:371–374.
2. Hidalgo H, Korobkin M, Kinney TR, et al. The problem of benign pulmonary nodules in children receiving cytotoxic chemotherapy. AJR 1983;140:21–24.
3. Schneider HJ, Felson B, Gonzalez LL. Rounded atelectasis. AJR 1980;134:225–232.
4. Schwartz EE, Katz SM, Mandell GA. Postinflammatory pseudotumors of the lung: fibrous histiocytoma and related lesions. Radiology 1980;136:609–613.
5. Solomon A, Rubinstein ZJ, Rogoff M, et al. Pulmonary blastoma. Pediatr Radiol 1982;12:148–149.
6. Roth JA, Putnam JB, Wesley MN, et al. Differing determinants of prognosis following resection of pulmonary metastases from osteogenic and soft tissue sarcoma patients. Cancer 1985;55:1361–1366.
7. Holmes EC, Ramming KP, Eiber FR, et al. The surgical management of pulmonary metastases. Semin Oncol 1977;4:65–69.
8. Huth JF, Holmes EC, Vernon SE, et al. Pulmonary resection for metastatic sarcoma. Am J Surg 1980;140:9–16.
9. Di Lorenzo M, Collin PP. Pulmonary metastases in children: results of surgical treatment. J Pediatr Surg 1988;23:762–765.
10. Hudson M, Jaffe MR, Jaffe N, et al. Pediatric osteosarcoma. Therapeutic strategies, results and prognostic factors derived from 10 year experience. J Clin Oncol 1990;8:1988–1993.

CHAPTER 3 GASTROINTESTINAL TUMORS

LIVER TUMORS

HEPATOMA (Hepatoblastoma, Hepatocellular Carcinoma)

In a discussion of hepatoblastoma and hepatocellular carcinoma, it is difficult to know whether to separate these two tumors or discuss them under a single heading. There are clear differences between hepatoblastoma and hepatocellular carcinoma, as outlined in Table 3–1. From an imaging standpoint, however, there are no criteria for differentiating these two tumors unless the patient's age is known. If the patient is under the age of 5, the abnormality is likely to be hepatoblastoma; if the patient is over the age of 5, it is most likely to be hepatocellular carcinoma.

The approach to planning an imaging protocol, the appearance of the primary tumor, and the pattern of metastatic spread are the same for each of these two tumors. For this reason I have chosen to discuss them together under the general term hepatoma, and I will emphasize any differences as they occur.

> *Comment:* Hepatoblastoma and hepatocellular carcinoma have many similarities.

Epidemiology

Hepatomas are the most common malignant liver tumors in children.[1,2] Hepatoblastoma is more common than hepatocellular carinoma.[1,2] In the liver, benign tumors are much less common than malignant tumors, with about two-thirds of liver masses in children being malignant.[3,4] Hepatomas account for about 2 percent of

TABLE 3–1
Differences between Hepatoblastoma and Hepatocellular Carcinoma

Criterion	Hepatoblastoma	Hepatocellular Carcinoma
Age	Usually <5 yrs old	Usually > 5 yrs old
Sex distribution	Definite male dominance	Slight male dominance
Relative incidence in children under 15 yrs	75%	25%
Associated liver disease	No	Increased incidence with any chronic liver disease
Elevated serum alpha-fetoprotein concentration	Almost all	Most
Relative prognosis	Better	Worse
Multifocal	Less likely	More likely
Local invasion including veins	Less likely	More likely
Involvement of right & left lobes of liver	Less likely	More likely
Resectable at time of presentation	More likely	Less likely
Location	Right lobe much more common	Right lobe slightly more common

all pediatric malignancy and occur in about 0.6 children per million children per year.[5]

All hepatoblastomas occur under the age of 5 years, with 45 percent occurring under the age of 1 year[6] and 66 percent under the age of 2 years.[4] They are rare over the age of 3 years,[7] and the mean age at presentation is about 16 months.[8] They can, rarely, be congenital, being diagnosed in the newborn.[9,10] In contrast, hepatocellular carcinoma in children is found in the age range between 5 to 15 years, with a peak over the age of 10 years.[6,7,11]

There is a sex difference with hepatoma. Hepatoblastoma is much more common in boys than girls, with the ratio of boys to girls being reported as high as 2:1.[6,7,9,12] Hepatocellular carcinoma has been reported as having an equal sex incidence[6] or a moderate male predominance.[2] Hepatoblastoma occurs in a previously normal liver. There are few consistently recognized strong predisposing factors to hepatoblastoma. Hepatoblastoma has been reported in siblings,[13] with trisomy 18,[18] and has an increased incidence with occupational exposure of mothers to metals, petroleum products, or paints.[15] There is a definite association of hepatoblastoma with polyposis coli (familial adenomatous polyposis). In one study, there was a family history of polyposis in 26 children with hepatoblastoma.[16] The hepatoblastoma occurs at the usual young age.[17] In 6 of 7 survivors of hepatoblastoma, with a positive history of polyposis coli, 6 children developed colon polyps on long-term follow-up.[16]

Hepatocellular carcinoma has a definite association with chronic liver disease.[9,18] It can occur with any chronic liver disease, but is particularly common with cirrhosis, glycogen storage disease type I, tyrosinemia, biliary atresia, or chronic hepatitis.[2,18] The treatment of Fanconi anemia with anabolic steroids can result in the production of adenomas in the liver, and also, rarely, hepatocellular carcinoma.

A 1991 review of 2,438 patients with Wilms tumor identified 4 cases of hepatocellular carcinoma 9 to 16 years after initial diagnosis of the Wilms tumor.[19] In all 4 children, the tumor occurred in the right lobe of the liver. All had had prior radiation therapy involving that segment of the liver.

Comment: Young children in families with familial adenomatous polyposis should be carefully observed for hepatoma. Children with chronic liver disease causing cirrhosis should be carefully observed for development of hepatocellular carcinoma.

References

1. Filler RM, Hagen J. Liver tumors. Surg Clin N Am 1981;61:1209–1217.
2. Lack EE, Neave C, Vawter CF. Hepatocellular carcinoma. Review of 32 cases in childhood and adolescence. Cancer 1983;52:1510–1515.
3. Smith WL, Franken EA, Mitros FA. Liver tumors in children. Semin Roentgenol 1983;18:136–148.
4. Guzetta PC, Randolph JG. Pediatric hepatic surgery. Surg Clin N Am 1989;69:251–257.
5. Greenberg M, Filler RM. Hepatic tumors. In: Pizzo PA, Poplack DG, eds. Principles and practice of pediatric oncology. Philadelphia: JB Lippincott, 1989:569–582.
6. Haas JE, Muczynski KA, Krailo M, et al. Histopathology and prognosis in childhood hepatoblastoma and hepatocarcinoma. Cancer 1989;64:1082–1095.
7. Exelby PR, Filler RM, Gorsfeld JL. Liver tumors in children in the particular reference to hepatoblastoma and hepatocellular carcinoma: American Academy of Pediatrics Surgical Section Survey–1974. J Pediatr Surg 1975;10:329–337.
8. Dachman AH, Pakter RL, Ros PR, et al. Hepatoblastoma: radiologic-pathologic correlation in 50 cases. Radiology 1987;164:15–19.
9. Weinberg AG, Finegold MJ. Primary hepatic tumors of childhood. Human Pathol 1983;14:512–537.
10. Kazzi NJ, Chang CH, Roberts EC, et al. Fetal hepatoblastoma presenting as nonimmune hydrops. Am J Perinatol 1989;6:278–280.
11. Farhi DC, Shikes RH, Murari PJ, et al. Hepatocellular carcinoma in young people. Cancer 1983;52:1516–1525.
12. Hartley AL, Birch JM, Kelsey AM, et al. Epidemiological and familial aspects of hepatoblastoma. Med Pediatr Oncol 1990;18:103–109.
13. Surendran N, Radhakrishna K, Chellam VG. Hepatoblastoma in siblings. J Pediatr Surg 1989;24:1169–1171.
14. Mamlok V, Nichols M, Lockhart L, et al. Trisomy 18 and hepatoblastoma. Am J Med Genet 1989;33:125–126.
15. Buckley JD, Sather H, Ruccione K, et al. A case—control study of risk factors for hepatoblastoma. Cancer 1989;74:1169–1176.
16. Phillips M, Dicks-Mireaux C, Kingston J, et al. Hepatoblastoma and polyposis coli (familial adenomatous polyposis). Med Pediatr Oncol 1989;17:441–447.
17. LeSher AR, Castronuovo JJ, Filippone AL. Hepatoblastoma in a patient with familial polyposis coli. Surgery 1989;105:668–670.
18. Chen WJ, Lee JC, Hung WT. Primary malignant tumor of liver in infants and children in Taiwan. J Pediatr Surg 1988;23:457–461.
19. Kovalic JJ, Thomas PRM, Beckwith JB, et al. Hepatocellular carcinoma as second malignant neoplasms in successfully treated Wilms' tumor patients. A National Wilms' Tumor Study Report. Cancer 1991;67:342–344.

Pathology

Both hepatoblastoma and hepatocellular carcinoma are more common in the right lobe of the liver. This right-sided dominance is more marked with hepatoblastoma. Hepatocellular carcinoma is commonly found involving both lobes of the liver either because of direct invasion or because the carcinoma is multifocal. In one study of 32 patients, both lobes were involved in 72 percent,[1] and in another study, 23 of 30 patients had both lobes involved.[2] In a third study, both lobes were involved in 33 percent of 98 patients.[3] With hepatoblastoma both lobes have been reported as being involved in 4 of 10 patients,[2] 4 of 34 patients,[4] and the tumor was multifocal in 15 percent of 129 patients.[3]

Hepatomas are almost always large at the time of diagnosis, being over 5 cm in diameter in almost all patients in one study of 227 children.[3] In this study, over half of the tumors were greater than 10 cm in diameter. The tumors often contain areas of hemorrhage and necrosis.

Microscopically, hepatocellular carcinomas are seen as malignant liver cells. There is no difference between the appearance in children and adults.[5] Hepatoblastomas are classified according to the epithelial cell type seen.[5,6] This classification is summarized in Table 3–2. Note that the term fetal tumor is used only if all the cells are of the fetal type. If mixed fetal and embryonal cells are present, the tumor is termed an embryonal cell tumor. The tumors may contain mesenchymal elements such as osteoid, cartilage, or muscle, and areas of hemopoiesis may be identified.[4] Calcification may be identified in up to 50 percent of patients.[4]

There is no universally agreed staging system for hepatomas. Two classification systems that have been used are summarized in Table 3–3. In one study in the United Kingdom, using the second classification system of Table 3–3, 11 of 25 patients were stage I and II, while 14 patients were stage III or IV. Because hepatocellular carcinomas are more likely to be multifocal and involve both lobes of the liver, they are less likely to be resectable than hepatoma and will in general have a worse stage.

> *Comment:* Hepatomas can be multifocal and involve both lobes of the liver. This is important in planning surgical resection of these tumors.

Normal liver anatomy must be understood by the radiologist. Surgical resection of liver tumors occurs along planes separating lobes, segments, or subsegments. Accurate localization of tumor within the liver lobes, segments, and subsegments is, therefore, critical. Division of the liver into lobes and segments occurs predominantly along planes of the hepatic veins. These relationships are summarized in Table 3–4.

TABLE 3–2
Classification of Hepatoblastoma

Fetal
Embryonal
Small cell undifferentiated (anaplastic)

Notes:
1. Fetal and embryonal cells may both be present—if so, the tumor is classified as embryonal.
2. Macrotubular is used to describe any of the above types if the cells are arranged in trabeculae.
3. Mixed is used to describe any of the above types if mesenchymal elements (osteoid, cartilage, muscle) are present in the tumor.

References
1. Dehner LP. Pediatric surgical pathology, 2nd ed. Baltimore: Williams & Wilkins, 1987:433–499.
2. Haas JE, Muczynski KA, Krailo M, et al. Histopathology and prognosis in childhood hepatoblastoma and hepatocarcinoma. Cancer 1989;64:1082–1095.

References
1. Lack EE, Neave C, Vawter GF. Hepatocellular carcinoma. Review of 32 cases in childhood and adolescence. Cancer 1983;52:1510–1515.
2. Chen WJ, Lee JC, Hung WT. Primary malignant tumor of liver in infants and children in Taiwan. J Pediatr Surg 1988;23:457–561.
3. Exelby PR, Filler RM, Grosfeld JL. Liver tumors in children in the particular reference to hepatoblastoma and hepatocellular carcinoma: American Academy of Pediatrics Surgical Section Survey–1974. J Pediatr Surg 1975;10:329–337.
4. Dachman AH, Pakter RL, Ros PR, et al. Hepatoblastoma: radiologic-pathologic correlation in 50 cases. Radiology 1987;164:15–19.
5. Haas JE, Muczynski KA, Krailo M, et al. Histopathology and prognosis in childhood hepatoblastoma and hepatocarcinoma. Cancer 1989;64:1082–1095.
6. Dehner LP. Pediatric surgical pathology, 2nd ed. Baltimore: Williams & Wilkins, 1987:433–499.

Clinical Presentation

Early signs and symptoms of hepatoma are very uncommon, and it is for this reason that these tumors are often large at the time of presentation. The most common presenting sign is, in fact, a right upper quadrant abdominal mass. This has been reported in from two-thirds to over 90 percent of patients.[1–5] The next most common sign is local pain or discomfort, and this occurs in up to two-thirds of patients.[1] Other local signs are very uncommon. Jaundice is unusual, and is slightly more common with hepatocellular carcinoma than hepatoblastoma.[3] Systemic signs are quite common. These include vomiting, weight loss, irritability, anorexia, lethargy, and fatigue.[4,7] Bleeding will rarely be found. Fetal hydrops has been described in one newborn with hepatoblastoma.[8]

The tumors may occasionally present with syndromes caused by the production of hormones.[4] These include male sexual precocity, polycythemia, thrombocytosis, hypoglycemia, osteomalacia, hyperlipidemia, or hypercalcemia. Hepatocellular carcinomas may have signs of associated chronic liver disease.

Large, rapidly growing tumors may present with a tumor lysis syndrome with elevation of serum uric acid and potassium concentrations; in one patient, fatal hyperkalemia occurred because of tumor handling at surgery.[9]

> *Comment:* Hepatocellular carcinoma and hepatoblastoma cannot be differentiated on the basis of symptoms. Symptoms are nonspecific in most patients. Unusual symptoms result from hormone production.

Alpha-fetoprotein is a very useful marker for hepatoma. Its concentration is elevated in the serum in over 90 percent of patients with hepatoblastoma.[2,10] With hepatocellular carcinoma, alpha-fetoprotein is also elevated. The number of patients in whom it is elevated is

TABLE 3–3
Two Classifications for Staging of Hepatoma

Stage	Ref 1	Ref 2 and 3
I	Completely resected	Completely resected
II A	Resected with marginal residual	Resectable after chemotherapy or radiation therapy
II B	Resected with regional residual	Residual in one lobe
III A	Unresectable ± rupture	Residual in both lobes
III B	Same as IIIA	Local nodes involved
IV	Distant metastases	Distant metastases

References
1. Guzetta PC, Randolph JG. Pediatric hepatic surgery. Surg Clin N Am 1989;69:251–257.
2. Link MP, Eilber F. Osteosarcoma. In: Pizzo PA, Poplack DG, eds. Principles and practice of pediatric oncology. Philadelphia: JB Lippincott, 1989:689–711.
3. Evans AE, Land VJ, Newton WA, et al. Combination chemotherapy (vincristine, adriamycin, cyclophosphamide, and 5-fluorouracil) in the treatment of children with malignant hepatoma. Cancer 1982;50:821–826.

TABLE 3–4
Normal Surgical Anatomy of the Liver[1,2]

Structure	Lies Between
Middle hepatic vein	Right and left lobes
Right hepatic vein	Anterior and posterior segments of right lobe
Left hepatic vein	Medial and lateral segments of left lobe
A line from gallbladder to inferior vena cava	Right and left lobes
A line from ligamentum teres to falciform ligament	Medial and lateral segments of left lobe
Proximal left portal vein	Medial and lateral segments of left lobe

Notes:
1. Each of the above segments can be divided into two subsegments.
2. Hepatic veins run between lobe and segments.
3. Hepatic artery, portal vein branches, and bile ducts run within segments.

References
1. Lorigan JG, Charnsangavej C, Carrasco CH, et al. Atrophy with compensatory hypertrophy of the liver in hepatic neoplasms: radiographic findings. AJR 1988;150:1291–1295.
2. Mukai JK, Stack CM, Turner DA, et al. Imaging of surgically relevant hepatic vascular and segmental anatomy. Part 1. Normal anatomy. AJR 1987;149:287–292.

variable, with some studies reporting elevation in up to 90 percent of patients.[1,11] In most patients, estimation of serum alpha-fetoprotein can be utilized to monitor for disease recurrence after inital successful therapy. In a very few patients, it is important to note that alpha-fetoprotein levels may be normal with development of metastases, even when they were elevated before resection of the primary tumor.[11] Also remember that alpha-fetoprotein may be increased with benign liver tumors or other nonhepatic tumors such as yolk sac tumor. A recent report suggests that the alpha-fetoprotein produced by these tumors is different and that these differences can be detected.[12]

Comment: Alpha-fetoprotein is a very useful tumor marker for hepatoma and can be used to monitor therapy in most patients.

References

1. Chen WJ, Lee JC, Hung WT. Primary malignant tumor of liver in infants and children in Taiwan. J Pediatr Surg 1988;23:457–461.
2. Dachman AH, Pakter RL, Ros PR, et al. Hepatoblastoma: radiologic-pathologic correlation in 50 cases. Radiology 1987;164:15–19.
3. Exelby PR, Filler RM, Grosfeld JL. Liver tumors in chil-

dren in the particular reference to hepatoblastoma and hepatocellular carcinoma: American Academy of Pediatrics Surgical Section Survey–1974. J Pediatr Surg 1975;10:329–337.
4. Filler RM, Hagen J. Liver tumors. Surg Clin N Am 1981;61:1209–1217.
5. Lack EE, Neave C, Vawter GF. Hepatocellular carcinoma. Review of 32 cases in childhood and adolescence. Cancer 1983;52:1510–1515.
6. Barton JW, Keller MS. Liver transplantation for hepatoblastoma in a child with congenital absence of the portal vein. Pediatr Radiol 1989;20:113–114.
7. Amendola MA, Blane CE, Amendola BE, et al. CT findings in hepatoblastoma. J Comput Assist Tomogr 1984;18:1105–1109.
8. Kazzi NJ, Chang CH, Roberts EC, et al. Fetal hepatoblastoma presenting as nonimmune hydrops. Am J Perinatol 1989;6:278–280.
9. Lobe TE, Karkera MS, Custer MD, et al. Fatal refractory hyperkalemia due to tumor lysis during primary resection for hepatoblastoma. J Pediatr Surg 1990;25:249–250.
10. Haas JE, Muczynski KA, Krailo M, et al. Histopathology and prognosis in childhood hepatoblastoma and hepatocarcinoma. Cancer 1989;64:1082–1095.
11. Weinberg AG, Finegold MJ. Primary hepatic tumors of childhood. Human Pathol 1983;14:512–537.
12. Tsuchida Y, Kaneko M, Fukui M, et al. Three different types of alpha-fetoprotein in the diagnosis of malignant solid tumors: use of a sensitive lectin-affinity immunoelectrophoresis. J Pediatr Surg 1989;24:350–355.

Imaging Studies

The aims of imaging in hepatoma are summarized in Table 3–5. The first objective is to characterize the abnormality in the liver. This is discussed later in some detail in the section on differential diagnosis. However, it is important to note at this stage that, contrary to some reports, I believe that there are no specific imaging features of hepatoma by which a specific prebiopsy diagnosis can be made. The only situations in which malignancy can definitely be diagnosed are if metastases have been identified, the alpha-fetoprotein level is elevated, or both. The appearance of hepatoma is nonspecific, and many benign lesions may appear similar on many of the imaging modalities. Even if a classic imaging appearance for hepatoma could be defined, there would still be a large number of patients in whom atypical variations would occur. For this reason it is almost always advisable to perform a fairly wide range of imaging tests on initial presentation. As soon as the tests have been performed it is important to correlate the findings with laboratory data such as alpha-fetoprotein estimations, clinical findings, and the patient's age. The most important objective of imaging is to define resectability of the tumor. This is particularly important with hepatoma, as the prognosis is directly related to tumor resection. Finally, imaging is required to monitor therapy.

TABLE 3–5
Imaging Objectives in Hepatoma

Differential diagnosis
Solid or cystic
Vascularity
Enhancement patterns
Resectability
Size
Single or multifocal
Segmental localization
Sharp margins or infiltrating
Large areas of hemorrhage or necrosis
Invasion of portal or hepatic veins
Invasion of inferior vena cava
Relationship to porta hepatis
Local lymph node
Other liver disease
Metastases
Monitor therapy
Is resection complete
Response to chemotherapy (if not initially resectable)
Recurrence

Before each of the different imaging modalities is described a few general comments with regard to hepatoma can be made.

1. Calcification is a nonspecific and not uncommon finding and is not particularly helpful in differential diagnosis.
2. If a vessel defect is identified on any imaging modality, this is much more likely to be tumor invasion than simple clot.[1]
3. Especially in patients with hepatocellular carcinoma, diffuse, preexisting liver disease may be present and this should not be confused with tumor.
4. Atrophy or hypertrophy of normal liver can occur before or after starting therapy. Hypertrophy is usually identified in the opposite normal lobe. Atrophy of part of the normal liver occurs distal to the tumor as a result of vessel occlusion (either portal or hepatic vein) by the tumor.

Abdominal Radiograph. This should be performed in all patients. In one study of 277 patients, it was abnormal in 85 percent.[2] The abdominal radiograph will usually show evidence of hepatomegaly. Occasionally, metastases may be seen in the bones. Calcification may be identified. As previously stated, this is not helpful in differentiating benign from malignant liver tumors. Very occasionally, gas may be identified; this would be strong evidence for the presence of a hepatic abscess rather than a tumor.

Nuclear Medicine Studies. Sulfur colloid technetium 99m will be very sensitive for detecting large hepatomas, which are seen as cold areas in the liver. Very small lesions, less than 2 cm in diameter, or lesions deeply located in the liver may be missed.[3] Most hepatomas are very large and, therefore, easily identifiable with sulfur colloid scanning, but second smaller foci of tumor may be missed. This study is now, therefore, little used,[4] as other modalities are better. Advantages of computed tomography (CT), ultrasound, and magnetic resonance imaging (MR) are that they all evaluate other areas of the abdomen in addition to the liver.[3] Very occasionally, a primary hepatoblastoma may show uptake of sulfur colloid.[5] Primary hepatomas may also occasionally take up MDP or labeled red blood cells.[6,7] The most useful nuclear medicine study is an isotope labeled red blood cell study. This is particularly helpful in differentiation of hepatoma from hemangioendothelioma.

Ultrasound. Most hepatomas will have mixed pattern of predominantly increased echoes compared to normal liver. In one study of 23 patients, the tumors were usually echogenic, with low echo areas owing to hemorrhage and necrosis.[8] In other studies, the tumors have been reported as being echogenic or mixed.[9,10] They are usually nonhomogenous in internal structure.[1,9,11] Some tumors will, however, be of low echotexture compared to normal liver (Fig. 3–1). In one study of 29 patients, 5 tumors were of low echogenicity.[1] The margins of the tumor are variable (Fig. 3–1). They have been unidentifiable in up to 50 percent of patients.[9,11] Some studies report a relatively high incidence of a well-defined low echogenic rim. This was seen in 8 of 15 patients.[12] From all of these reports it can be seen that the appearance of the tumor is very variable. A heterogenous echogenic mass with good or poorly defined margins is the most typical finding. Ultrasound, particularly with the use of color Doppler, is extremely good for evaluation of hepatic veins, portal veins, and inferior vena cava for tumor invasion of the veins. Doppler studies in 3 children with hepatoblastoma showed a marked increase in flow in systole together with antegrade diastolic flow.[13]

Problems with ultrasound are the nonspecific appearance of the lesions, the fact that certain areas of the liver may be obscured by bone or bowel gas and not visualized,[3] and the fact that very large tumors may cause distortion so that the vessel anatomy cannot accurately be appreciated.[14] Ultrasound has not proved accurate for defining resectability of tumors, being accurate in only 72 percent of patients in one study.[8] This is mainly because of the difficulty in defining the margins of the tumor.

Occasionally, ultrasound is fairly specific in differential diagnosis. This is true with simple liver cysts and some hemangioendotheliomas. One report suggests that ultrasound is particularly helpful in accurately identifying malignancy. In 15 of 16 patients, the absence of one branch of the portal vein in the area of the tumor has been taken as evidence of malignancy.[12] This is because the tumor occludes the vessel. With benign lesions these vessels should be displaced but still visible. Such accuracy in identification of the presence of subbranches of the portal vein is, however, tedious and difficult, and not everyone is able to reproduce these results. From a practical point of view a definite diagnosis of benign or malignant should rarely be made on the ultrasound findings of a liver mass.

CT. CT is the most appropriate modality for evaluation of hepatoma and is very helpful in predicting resectability. It is not as good as ultrasound for identification of tumor invasion of vessels and, therefore, these two modalities should be used in a complementary fashion. Prior to the advent of CT, angiography was widely utilized to define resectability of hepatoma.

Figure 3–1. **Diagnosis: Hepatocellular carcinoma.**
A, **Ultrasound. There is very large mass occupying most of the posterior part of the right lobe of the liver. The mass is of lower echo intensity than normal liver, which lies anterior to the mass. The interface between tumor and normal liver is fairly well defined *(arrows).* *B,* CT after IV contrast. The large mass in the posterior part of the right lobe of the liver is enhanced less than normal liver. The tumor is multifocal with a smaller low-intensity segment identified anteriorly in the right lobe.**

A

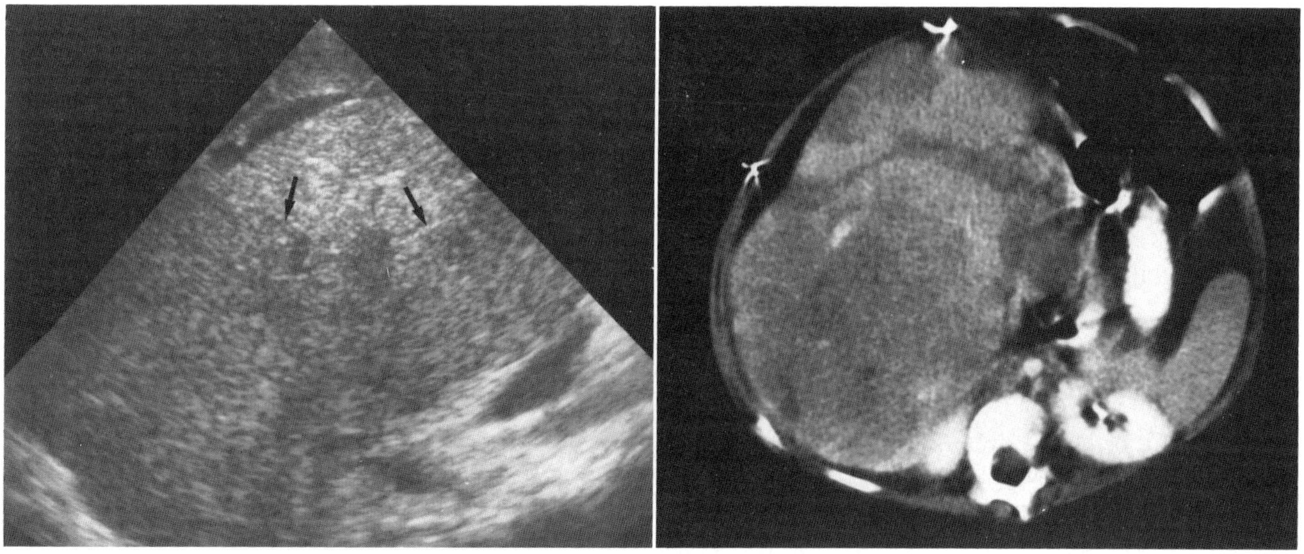

B

Early reports of CT studies of hepatoma attested to its usefulness in defining tumor resectability,[15] and modern CT is extremely accurate in predicting resectability. This is true in most cases. For example, a small tumor localized to one segment is clearly resectable (Fig. 3–2), whereas diffuse tumor involving the entire liver is clearly nonresectable. There do remain, however, a number of cases in which the tumor extends close to the boundaries of a segment and in which final decision regarding actual resectability is deferred to the time of laparotomy. Even in these patients, however, CT is extremely helpful to the surgeon in identifying the zone of questionable tumor extent.

More and more patients in whom initial CT evaluation identified either questionable or potentially very difficult resectability are being treated with initial chemotherapy to shrink the tumor (Figs. 3–3 and 3–4). In these patients, CT is extremely valuable in evaluating the response of the tumor to chemotherapy and in identifying the optimum time for surgical intervention. The appearance of hepatoma on CT is variable. Most of the tumors are of lower intensity than adjacent normal liver prior to contrast injection.[1,6–9,15] Most of the tumors are nonhomogeneous owing to areas of hemorrhage or necrosis within them. Following administration of intravenous contrast, there will be some enhancement of the

A

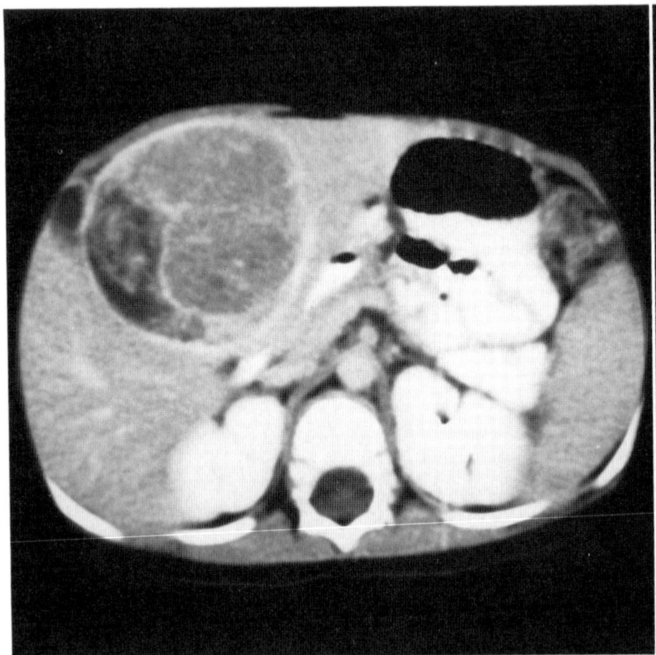

B

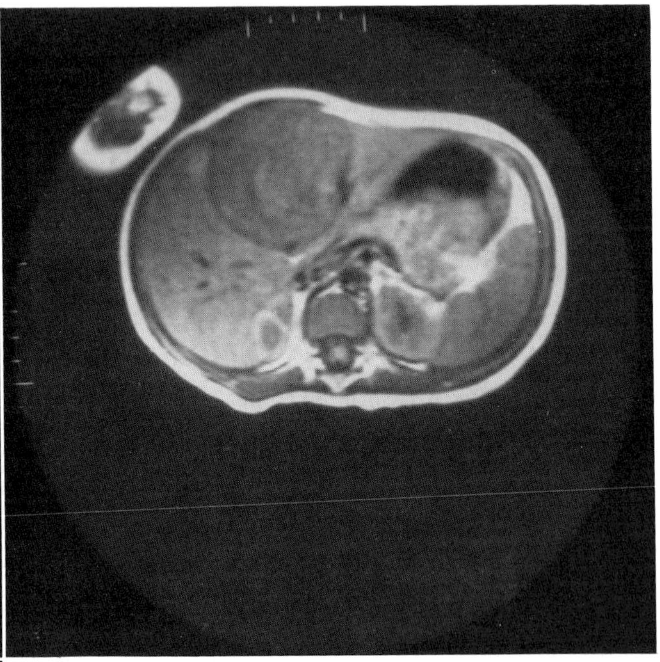

C

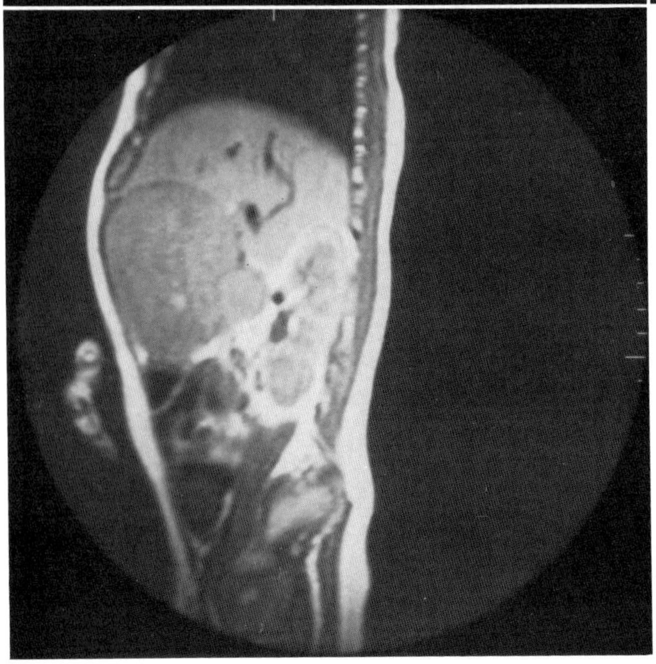

Figure 3–2. **Diagnosis: Hepatoblastoma. The tumor is confined to the medial segment of the left lobe of the liver. *A*, CT after bolus of intravenous contrast. A well-defined mass is seen in the medial segment of the left lobe. It enhances less than normal liver. There is a rim of brightly enhancing compressed normal liver tissue. Very low-intensity areas in the tumor are caused by hemorrhage, necrosis, or both. *B* and *C*, Axial and sagital MR, T1 weighted. A focal mass lesion is again well shown.**

A B C

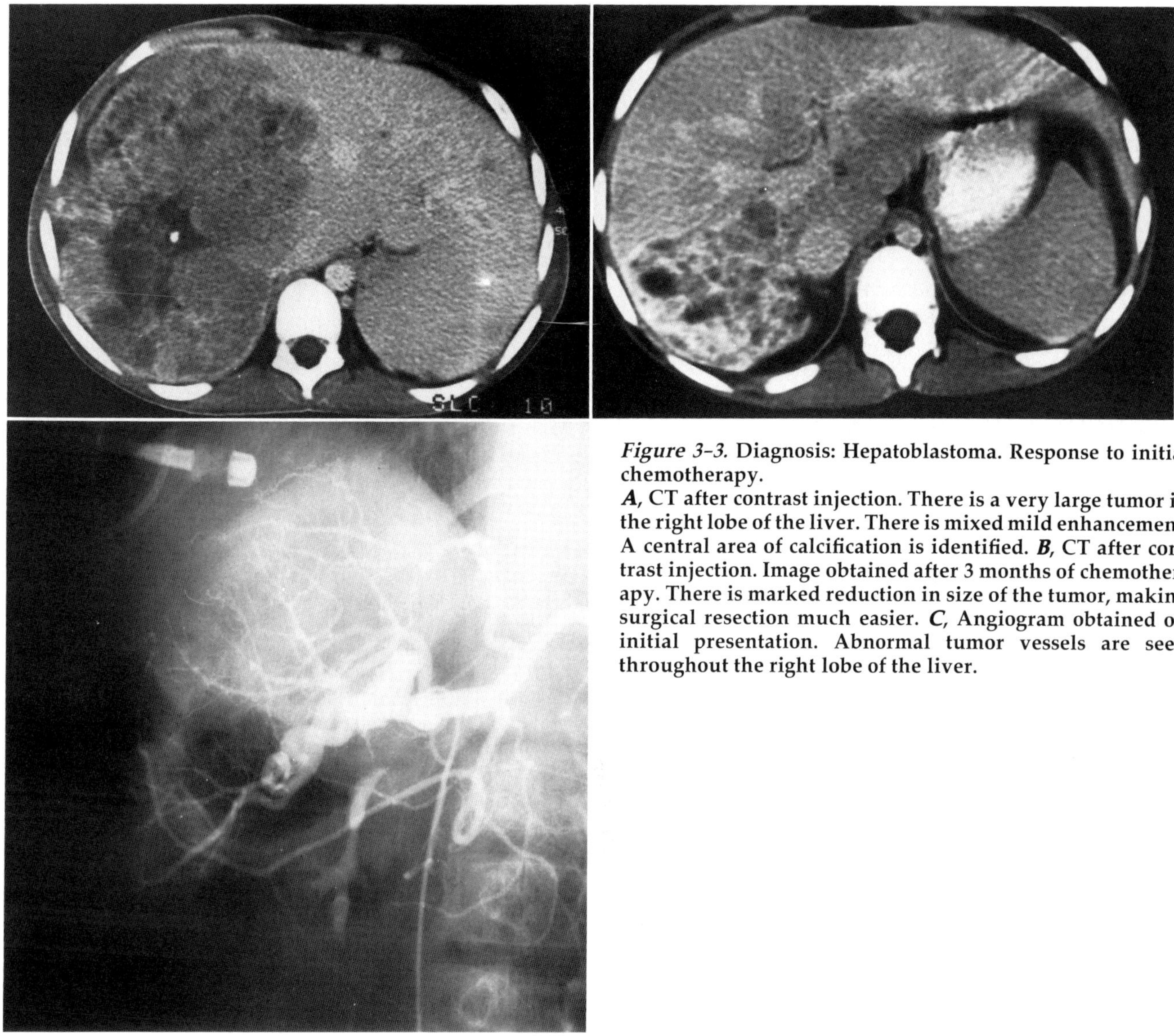

Figure 3-3. **Diagnosis: Hepatoblastoma. Response to initial chemotherapy.**
A, **CT after contrast injection. There is a very large tumor in the right lobe of the liver. There is mixed mild enhancement. A central area of calcification is identified.** ***B,*** **CT after contrast injection. Image obtained after 3 months of chemotherapy. There is marked reduction in size of the tumor, making surgical resection much easier.** ***C,*** **Angiogram obtained on initial presentation. Abnormal tumor vessels are seen throughout the right lobe of the liver.**

tumor (Fig. 3–3). In 21 patients, this was described as minimal in each patient.[8] In almost all patients, the enhancement will be less than that of adjacent normal liver (see Figs. 3–1 and 3–2). The enhancement pattern will also be variable, particularly if there are areas of hemorrhage and necrosis. The appearance of the enhancement will vary depending on the type of contrast bolus injected, the volume of contrast injected, and the delay before imaging. Some tumors may show a peripheral rim of enhancement in the early arterial phase if rapid bolus and early dynamic scan are used[8] (see Fig. 3–2). The pattern of enhancement is nonspecific and a definite diagnosis of malignancy cannot be made from it. The only exception to this is in the differentiation of hemangioendothelioma from hepatoblastoma in young infants. This is discussed further in the differential diagnosis section.

The technique utilized for CT scanning of the liver with hepatoma requires some compromises. In general, contiguous slices should be obtained through the liver prior to the administration of intravenous contrast. Occasionally, some areas of tumor may be better visualized on these images. Intravenous contrast should always be utilized. If the main consideration is differentiation of hepatoblastoma from hemangioendothelioma, dynamic bolus scanning at one level should be performed, with serial images obtained at the same level over a period of about one-half hour to follow the pattern of enhancement. This technique means that the entire liver is not visualized following the bolus contrast injection. If the diagnosis of malignancy is already known, it would be more useful to give a bolus injection and scan rapidly through the entire liver. This will maximize contrast differences between tumor and normal liver and aid in more accurately identifying the total extent of tumor. In addition, the best opportunity for visualizing tumor invasion of the liver vessels is during bolus injection of contrast (Fig. 3–5). Following the

A

B

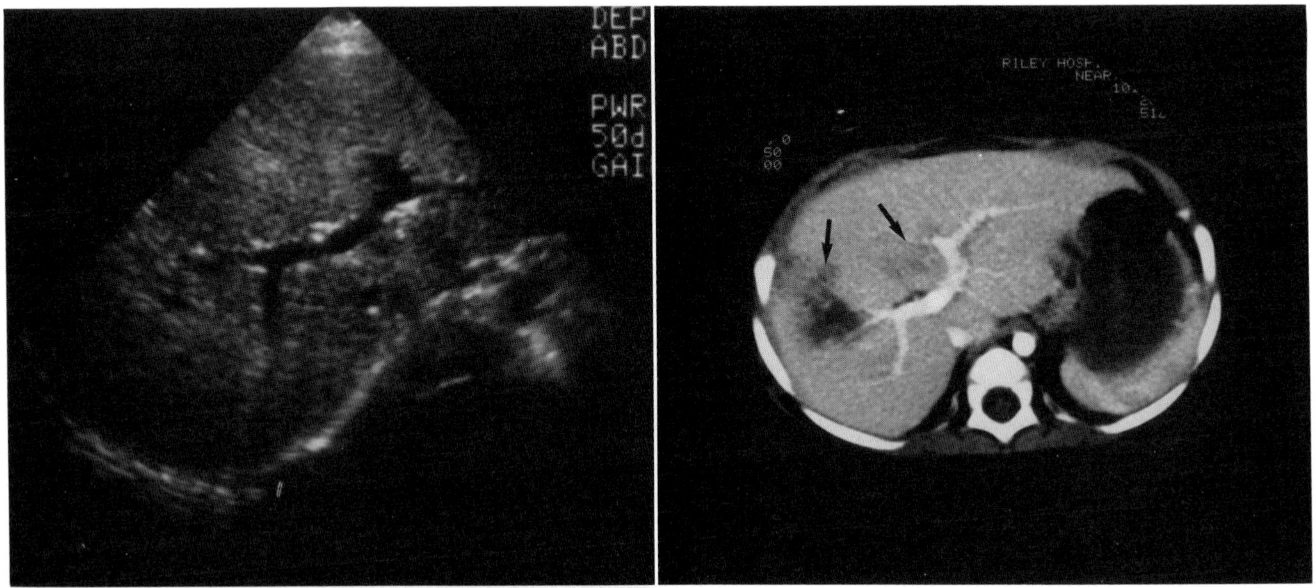

C

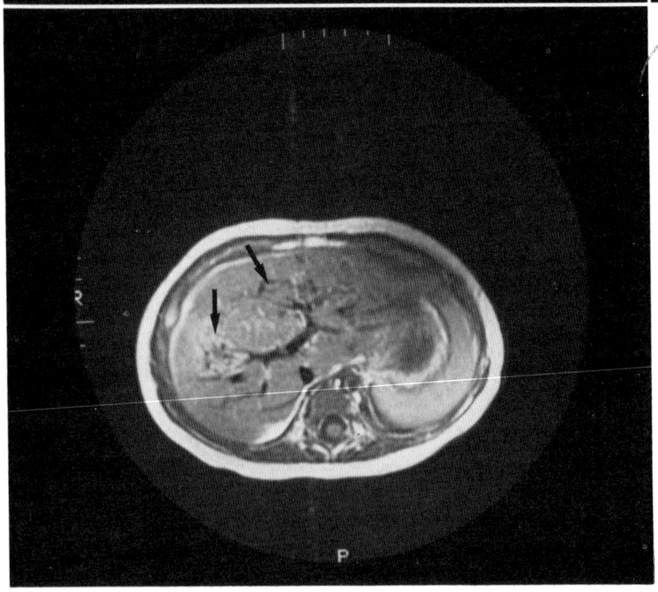

Figure 3–4. **Diagnosis: Residual hepatoblastoma following chemotherapy. Comparison of ultrasound, CT, and MR. All images are axial obtained at the level of the portal vein.**
***A*, Ultrasound echoes are nonhomogeneous, but margins of residual tumor are extremely difficult to define. *B*, CT. Residual tumor *(arrows)* is well identified. *C*, MR, T1 weighted after gadolinium-DTPA. The tumor *(arrows)* is not quite as sharply defined as with CT. Enhancement with gadolinium-DTPA suggests tumor activity rather than fibrosis.**

liver scanning, the rest of the abdomen should be scanned for evidence of tumor spread. CT scan of the chest should also be performed.

Several experimental CT techniques have been utilized in adults and their utility in children is completely unknown. The first technique involves a slow injection of contrast via a catheter into the superior mesenteric artery during CT scanning. About 2 ml per kg of 30 percent iodine contrast is injected at a rate of about 3 ml per sec.[16,17] Using this technique, and comparing results with surgical specimens, CT was able to identify 94 percent of the main tumor masses and 38 percent of secondary tumor nodules. Most of the missed nodules were less than 5 mm in size. Another new technique involves catheter arterial injection of an iodine-containing oil emulsion followed by CT scanning after a delay of between 1 and 4 weeks. The tumor cells take up this emulsion and appear bright on the CT images.[17]

Figure 3–5. **Diagnosis: Hepatoblastoma. Portal vein obstruction.**
Axial CT image with bolus contrast injection. There is a massive tumor involving most of the visualized segments of the liver. Enhancement of the tumor is variable, with intermediate- and low-intensity areas identified. In the region of the porta hepatis, multiple collateral vessels are opacified with contrast *(arrow)*. The portal vein was occluded by tumor.

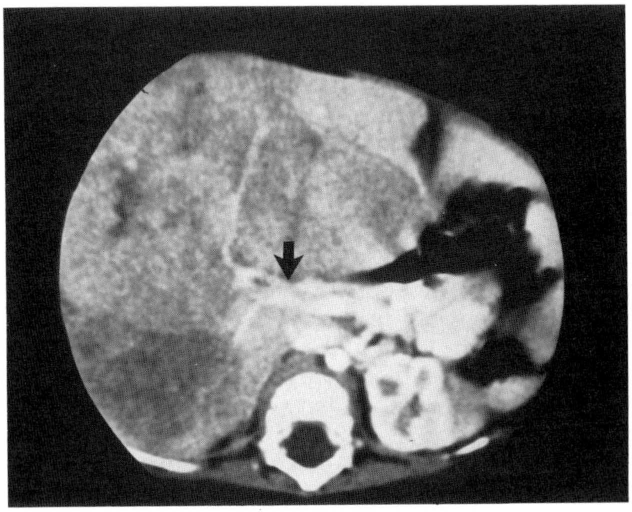

MR. There are a number of reports of MR evaluation of hepatoma, mostly in adults. The results indicate that MR is sensitive for detection of hepatic tumors. The appearance of most of the tumors is nonspecific. The multiplanar imaging potential of MR, and the excellent visualization of blood vessels, could potentially make it extremely valuable for predicting tumor resectability. In most patients, the tumors show signal characteristics consistent with prolongation of T1 and T2 relaxation times, appearing darker than normal liver on T1 weighted images and brighter than normal liver on T2 weighted images[4,18,19] (Fig. 3–6), whereas hemorrhage and necrosis will show a more varied appearance.

From the point of view of technique some reports suggest that short TE short TR, T1 weighted images, or STIR images will best detect tumor[20] while others recommend T2 weighted sequences for optimal visualization of tumor.[21] These differences are not surprising in view of the wide range of different imaging machines available, different field strengths, and different techniques for motion suppression. Therefore, no definite statements regarding technique can be made. Each radiologist must experiment to determine what is best for his or her equipment and patient population. Another study suggests that the T2 weighted images will be preferable at high field strengths (1.5 Tesla) while T1 weighted images will be better at lower field strengths (0.6 Tesla).[22] Most of the tumors will be well identified. The margins may be sharply defined (see Fig. 3–2) or infiltrating. A pseudocapsule of compressed tissue may be identified. Septa may be seen throughout the tumor. Vessel invasion may be identified (Fig. 3–7). Portal vein occlusion will be suggested by the identification of enlarged collateral vessels in the region of the porta hepatis together with the presence or absence of varices.[4]

Gadolinium-DTPA has been utilized to study a number of patients. In one study of 28 patients given a bolus injection of gadolinium-DTPA, the enhancement pattern was very varied, involving the periphery, central areas, a mixed pattern, or the entire tumor. Comparison with pathological specimens showed some correlation between tumor vascularity and the degree of enhancement following bolus injection of contrast (Fig. 3–7). On delayed images, most tumors (21 of 28) showed no alteration in signal pattern, 5 showed mixed enhancement, and 2 peripheral enhancement. Two other studies[23,24] suggest that the enhancement pattern following a bolus of gadolinium-DTPA can differentiate hepatoma from cavernous hemangioma in up to 80 percent of patients. An early peak of enhancement with rapid fading is seen with hepatoma, whereas a later peak with persistence of enhancement is seen with hemangioma.[23,24] Although this early work is encouraging, these patterns of enhancement should not, I believe, be relied on to make a definitive diagnosis.

The main role of MR should, I believe, be in defining tumor extent rather than differentiating between malignant and benign conditions. Like CT, MR can also be utilized to follow the response of tumor to initial chemotherapy. At the present time there is no evidence to suggest that MR can accurately differentiate residual active tumor from residual inflammatory tissue. Following surgery, again there is no definite evidence to suggest that MR can identify residual tumor in the surgical margins and differentiate this from surgical edema and inflammation. With regard to tumor recurrence the presence of a new mass lesion is strong evidence of recurrent disease. In patients with a rising concentration of alpha-

Figure 3-6. **Diagnosis: Hepatoblastoma.**
***A*, Axial MR, T1 weighted. There is a large hepatoblastoma (*H*) that involves both the right and left lobes of the liver. It is of slightly lower intensity than normal liver. *B*, Coronal MR, T2 weighted. There is an increase in signal intensity from the hepatoma (*H*). The lesion is very nonhomogeneous, probably as a result of areas of hemorrhage and necrosis within it.**

A

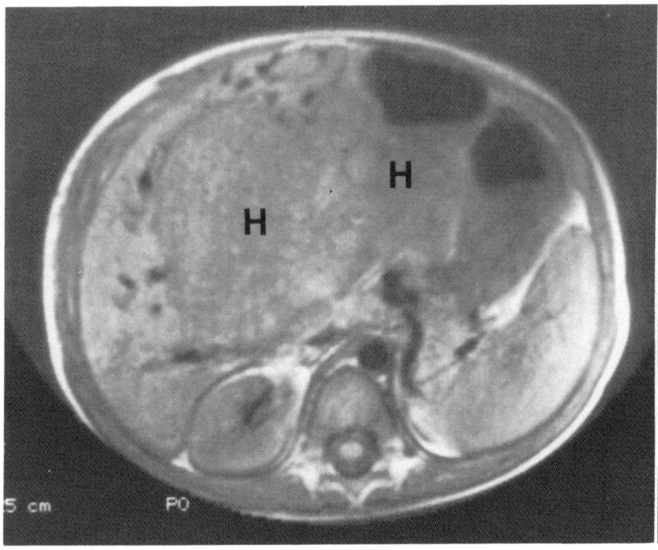

B

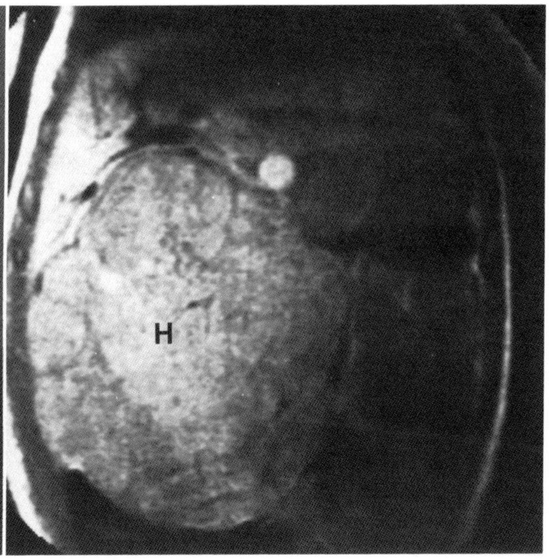

A B

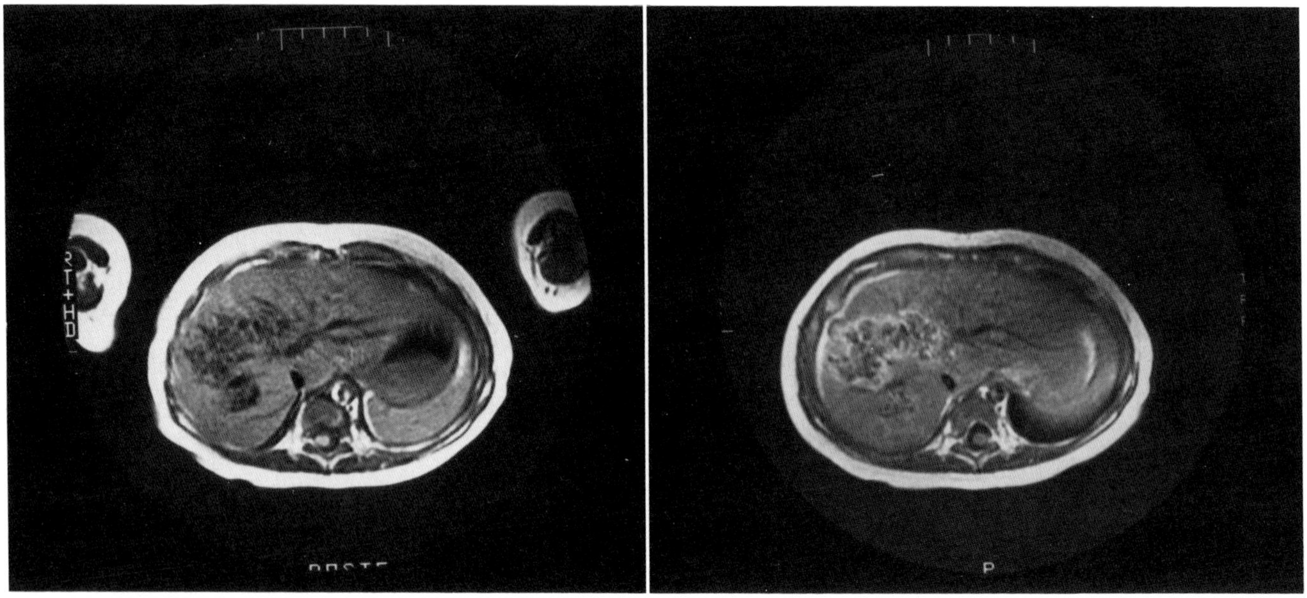

Figure 3-7. **Diagnosis: Hepatoblastoma. Gadolinium enhancement of residual tumor after initial chemotherapy.**
***A*, Axial MR, T1 weighted. There is a mixed low-intensity lesion occupying the middle part of the right lobe of the liver. On this image it is impossible to differentiate residual fibrosis from residual active tumor. *B*, Same image obtained after gadolinium-DTPA administration. There is marked enhancement of the rim of the lesion, with little enhancement of the central area. This correlated well with the surgical specimen. The rim of the lesion contained some residual active tumor. The central area was necrotic and fibrotic.**

fetoprotein after tumor resection, I do not believe that MR can differentiate residual inflammation from early recurrence in the absence of actual formation of a focal mass. In this regard, there is no evidence that MR is any better than CT for early detection of recurrent disease.

Angiography. Angiography, 15 to 20 years ago, was used almost routinely in most patients with hepatoma. With the advent of ultrasound, CT, and more recently MR, angiography is now rarely performed, particularly in children. One role for angiography might be in differentiating malignant tumors from benign conditions[25] (Fig. 3–8). There are some reports that suggest that the features of malignancy are fairly characteristic on angiography. Other workers, however, do not agree and my own view is that the findings on angiography are so variable that it should not be utilized to attempt differential diagnosis. Angiography has also been utilized to define tumor extent. Because imaging with angiography is limited to frontal, oblique, or lateral planes, accurate segmental localization of tumors is not possible. In addition, inaccuracies also occur, because many of the tumors are not particularly vascular. CT and MR should now replace angiography for defining tumor extent.

Angiography may show venous obstruction (see Fig. 3–8). Another reason for performing angiography was to identify unusual location of origin of major hepatic vessels. Most surgeons today do not require this to be done and will identify the origin of the hepatic artery and its major branches from the aorta, celiac artery, or superior mesenteric artery at the time of surgery. Alternatively, ultrasound or MR can provide this information. Angiography may also be utilized for tumor embolization prior to surgical resection. In recent years, chemotherapy has become the method of choice for reducing the size of very large tumors prior to attempted surgical reduction. The only remaining role for angiography would be for the intra-arterial administration of chemotherapeutic agents. This has been used in adults but not in children.

If angiography is performed, the findings of hepatoma will include increased vascularity or decreased vascularity[8]; there may be arteriovenous shunts, contrast pooling, neovascularity, and distortion and displacement of vessels[25–27] (see Fig. 3–3).

Image Comparison. A few studies have compared the various imaging modalities. In one study of 23 children, CT and MR were compared.[4] Neither was accurate in differentiating benign from malignant lesions; both were excellent for identification of the extent of tumor. MR was positive in 3 patients for suspected tumor recurrence. CT was negative in these 3 patients. MR was correct in 2 patients but falsely positive in one patient in whom there was inflammatory fibrosis. In another study of 39 adults,[28] it was concluded that MR was slightly better than CT or ultrasound, but that the best information was obtained by utilizing multiple modalities. A 1990 study compared CT and MR for predicting resectability of liver tumors.[29] MR was better than CT for evaluation of the hepatic vein, portal vein, and inferior vena cava. When compared to surgery, MR identified the parenchymal extent of the tumor accurately in all 8 patients. CT underestimated parenchymal tumor in

A B

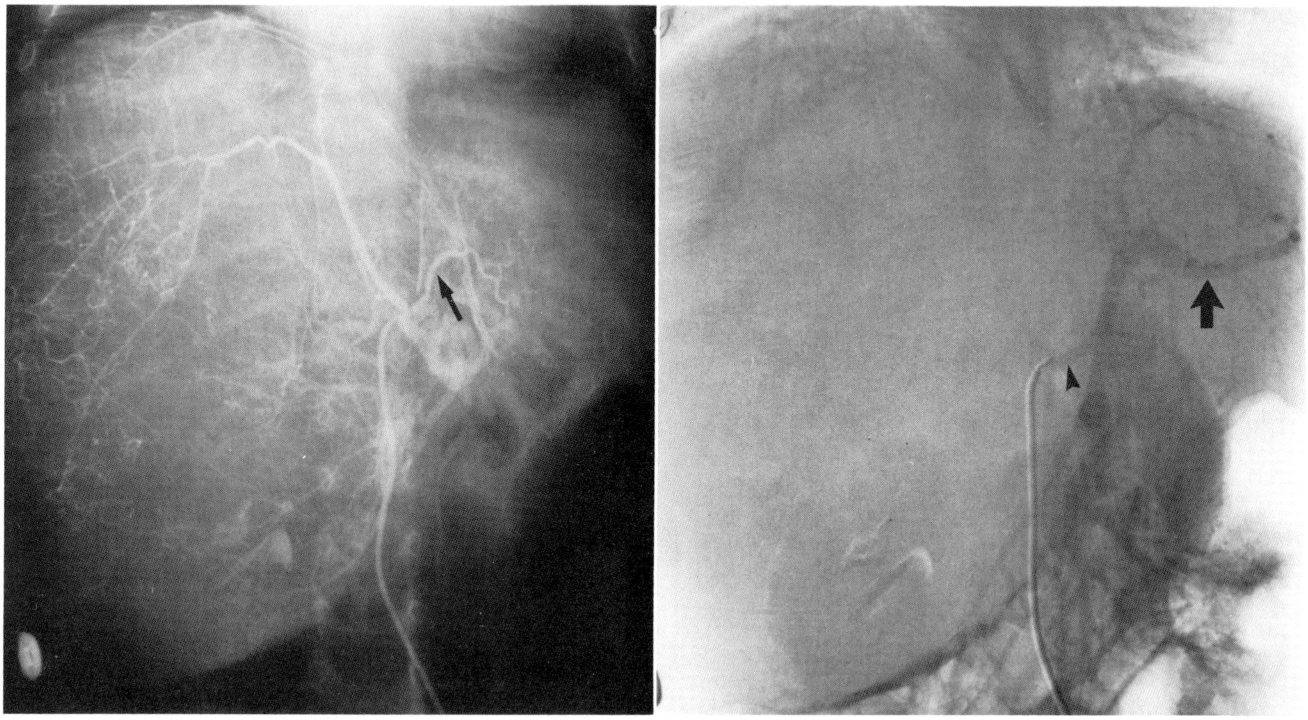

Figure 3–8. **Diagnosis: Hepatoblastoma. Angiographic findings.**
***A*, Selective celiac injection. There is diffuse neovascularity and encasement of the right hepatic artery with a small normal left hepatic artery *(arrow)*. *B*, Subtracted venous phase. The splenic vein is normal *(arrow)*. The left portal vein is displaced but patent *(arrowhead)*. The right portal vein is occluded. (From Tonkin ILD, Wrenn EL, Hollabaugh RS. The continued value of angiography in planning surgical resection of hepatic tumors in children. Pediatr Radiol 1988; 18:35–44.)**

2 of 8 patients. MR was also better than CT in identification of the margins of the tumor. Ultrasound was found to be poor for demonstrating parenchymal extent of the tumor (Fig. 3–9). This study[29] also cautioned that increased signal seen in the region of the porta hepatis on MR imaging can be caused, on T2 weighted images, by tumor or reactive nodes.

Another recent study cautions against the too-ready acceptance of data from any one study; I very strongly agree with this conclusion. There are many variables in the way in which the various imaging modalities are performed or interpreted. In 43 adults, CT with arterial injection of contrast was found to be better than CT obtained after a delay following contrast injection. In general, because of the variability and nonspecificity of the various imaging modalities, it would seem that use of both CT and ultrasound is always appropriate. Ultrasound will be better than CT in most patients for identification of vessel invasion, while CT will be better than ultrasound for identification of total tumor extent (see Fig. 3–4). MR, particularly when obtained in different imaging planes, will at a minimum be complementary to CT and ultrasound, and should, I suspect, add additional useful information in some patients (see Figs. 3–4 and 3–9). There is insufficient experience with MR to recommend replacement of CT or ultrasound by MR. Nuclear medicine studies, such as red blood cell study in hemangioendothelioma, should be reserved for selected patients.

At the time of initial presentation, patients should, therefore, have ultrasound and CT of the liver and abdomen, MR of the liver and abdomen, and CT scan of the chest. An abdominal radiograph should be obtained. The reason for the chest CT is that the lung is the most common site of metastases from hepatoma, and such lesions may be expected in about 10 percent of patients at initial diagnosis[2,9] (Figs. 3–9 and 3–10). The next most common site of metastatic spread is portal or periaortic abdominal lymph nodes. These will be imaged by ultrasound and CT, with or without MR. Other sites of metastic spread of hepatoblastoma are the bone[9,30] (Figs. 3–10 and 3–11), bone marrow,[30] and brain.[2] The incidence of metastatic spread to these sites is low and it is difficult to know whether or not to perform imaging. In the absence of any symptoms, I do not suggest screening the central nervous system for metastases. On initial presentation, it is probably worthwhile to perform an MDP technetium 99m bone scan to identify those few patients with bone metastases. If MR is performed, it is probably worthwhile to include the pelvis and upper femurs together with the upper abdominal images. This will show a significant percentage of the bone marrow of the body.

Insufficient information regarding patterns of metastatic spread with relapse is available to make clear-cut recommendations for follow-up of hepatoma. Known areas of metastasis should obviously be followed at intervals of between 2 and 3 months until they have re-

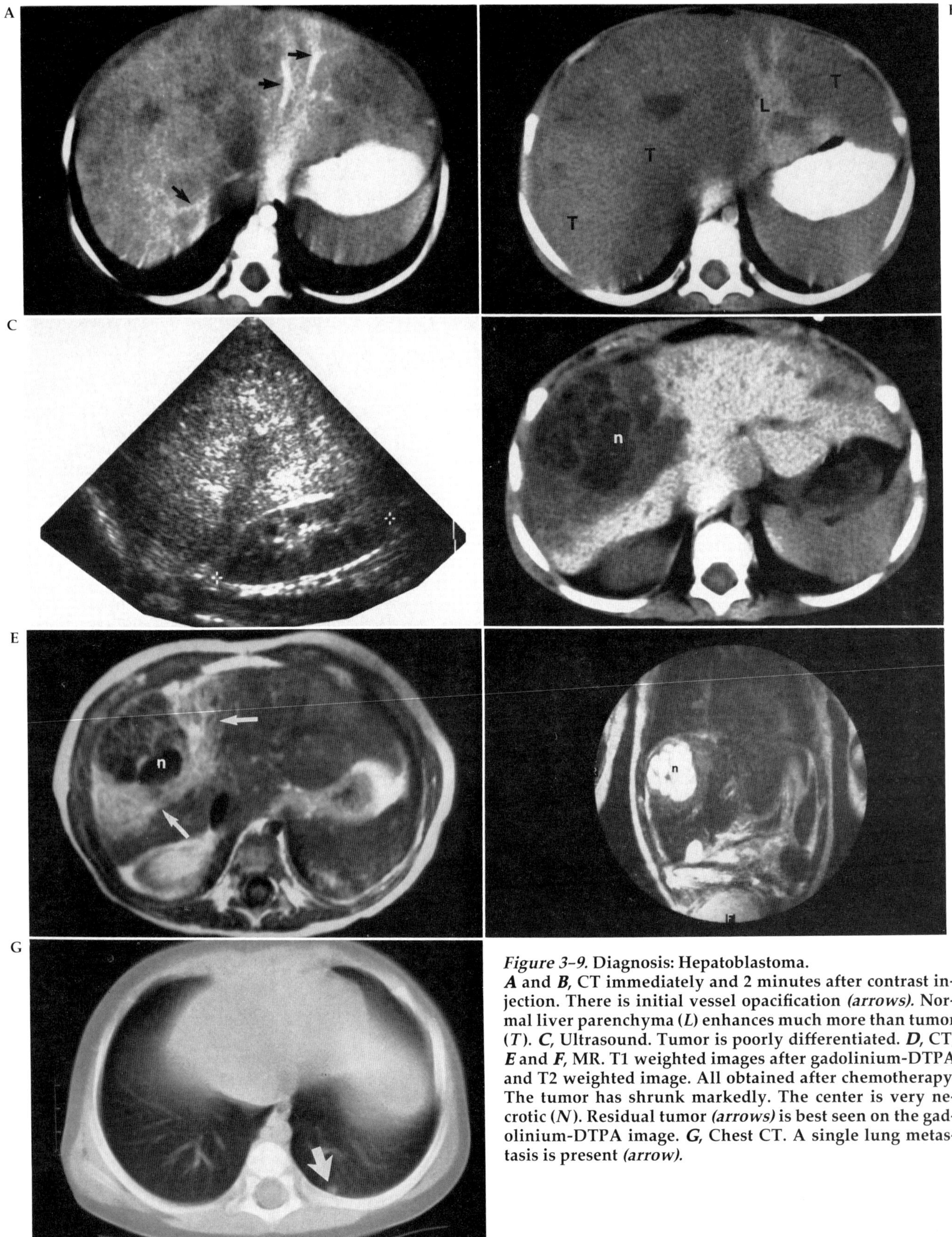

Figure 3–9. Diagnosis: Hepatoblastoma.
A and ***B***, CT immediately and 2 minutes after contrast injection. There is initial vessel opacification *(arrows)*. Normal liver parenchyma (*L*) enhances much more than tumor (*T*). ***C***, Ultrasound. Tumor is poorly differentiated. ***D***, CT; ***E*** and ***F***, MR. T1 weighted images after gadolinium-DTPA and T2 weighted image. All obtained after chemotherapy. The tumor has shrunk markedly. The center is very necrotic (*N*). Residual tumor *(arrows)* is best seen on the gadolinium-DTPA image. ***G***, Chest CT. A single lung metastasis is present *(arrow)*.

A B C

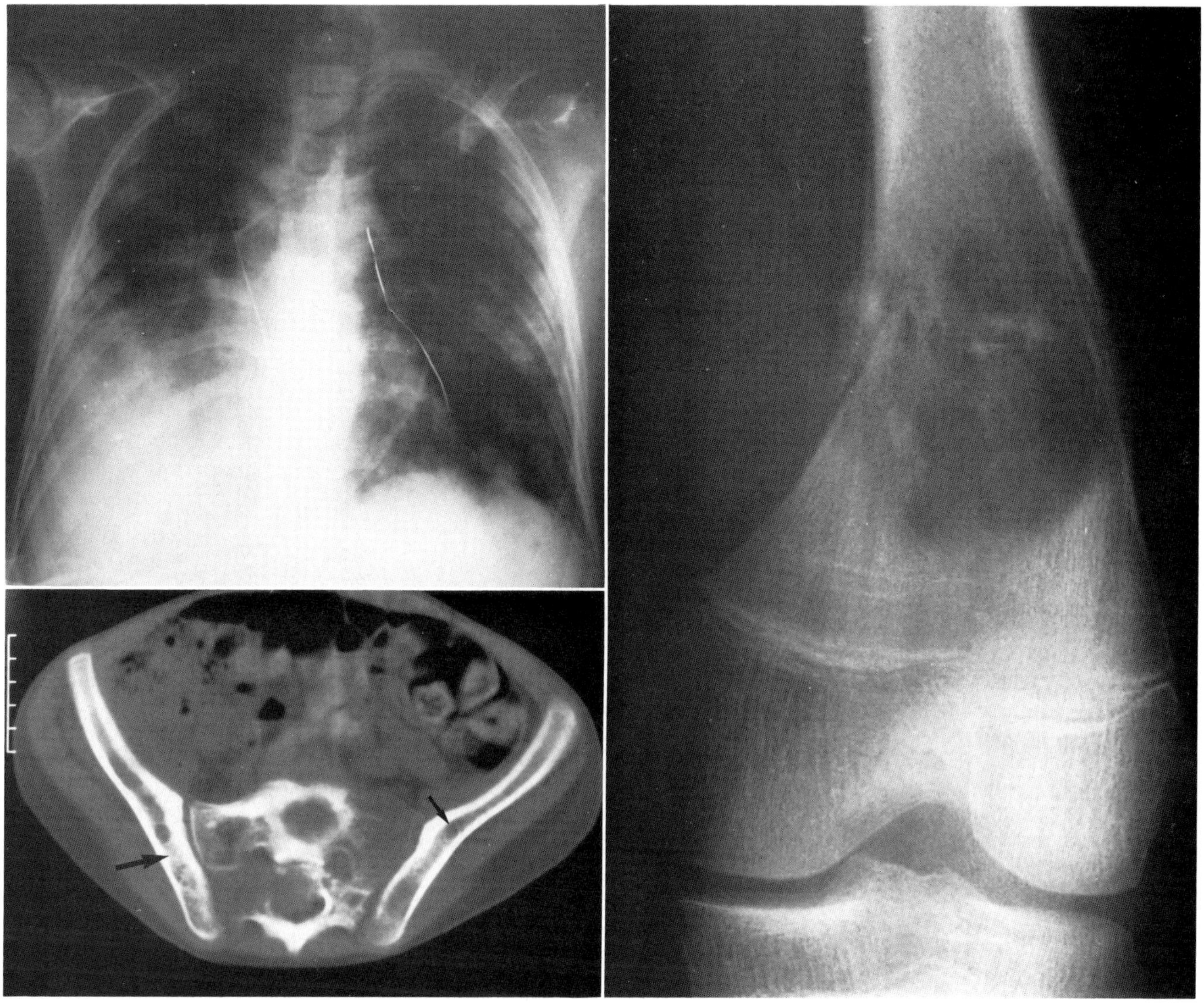

Figure 3–10. **Diagnosis: Metastases from a hepatoblastoma.**
***A*, Multiple lung nodules of varying size are identified. *B*, Distal femur. There is a large destructive lytic lesion in the metaphysis. There is a pathological fracture through the metastasis. *C*, There is extensive destruction of the sacrum owing to metastases. Several lytic (*small arrows*) and blastic (*large arrows*) metastatic lesions are seen in both iliac wings.**

solved. With regard to routine screening, in the absence of symptoms, I would perform chest screening only. Whether CT, chest radiographs, or both should be performed is difficult to say. In most situations, chest radiograph is probably adequate. I would suggest CT of the chest at critical time periods, such as prior to any abdominal surgery or as a baseline at the completion of chemotherapy.

Follow-up of the liver will be determined by the therapeutic protocol utilized. If the tumor is initially resected, a baseline follow-up CT scan should be obtained about 1 to 2 months after the surgery. If the tumor is not initially resected, initial response to chemotherapy should be evaluated at approximately 1 month. Further studies could be performed at intervals of 1 to 2 months, depending on the rate of further response. Following ultimate surgical resection, or maximal response to chemotherapy, it may be reasonable to follow the patients only with estimations of serum alpha-fetoprotein concentrations (if these were elevated at the time of initial diagnosis). Further imaging of the liver, lungs, and bones could be performed only at times that the alpha-fetoprotein concentration increased above normal.

Recurrence with hepatoma usually occurs within 3 years from initial diagnosis, but can be later than this.[31]

Comment: The appearance of hepatoma is usually nonspecific on all imaging studies and malignancy must be confirmed by biopsy. One major role for imaging is to plan resectability of the hepatoma. MR may prove to be the best modality for this. Ultrasound underestimates parenchymal extent of tumor quite significantly. Hepatomas can be multifocal.

A B

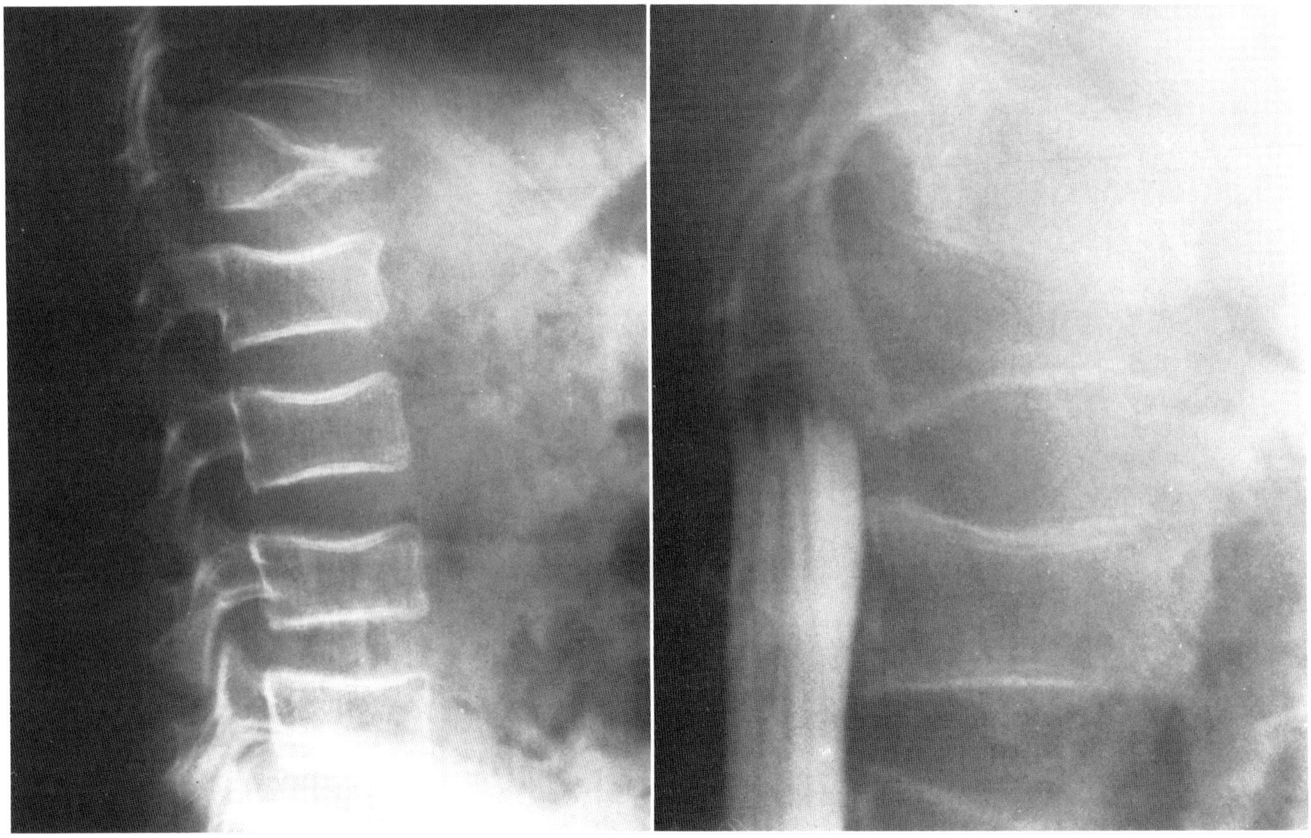

Figure 3-11. **Diagnosis: Bone metastasis from hepatocellular carcinoma. Diffuse osteoporosis as well. *A,* Lateral spine radiograph. There is diffuse osteoporosis with loss of height of many vertebra. There is a collapse of one of the lower thoracic vertebrae caused by metastatic spread. *B,* Myelogram. This shows complete block at the level of the collapsed vertebra because of tumor spread into the spinal canal.**

References

1. LaBerge JM, Laing FC, Federle MP, et al. Hepatocellular carcinoma: assessment of resectability by computed tomography and ultrasound. Radiology 1984;152:485–490.
2. Exelby PR, Filler RM, Grosfeld JL. Liver tumors in children in the particular reference to hepatoblastoma and hepatocellular carcinoma: American Academy of Pediatrics Surgical Section Survey–1974. J Pediatr Surg 1975; 10:329–337.
3. Bernardino ME, Lewis E. Imaging hepatic neoplasms. Cancer 1982;50:2666–2671.
4. Boechat MI, Kangarloo H, Ortega J, et al. Primary liver tumors in children: comparison of CT and MR imaging. Radiology 1988;169:727–732.
5. Diament MJ, Parvey LS, Tonkin ILD, et al. Hepatoblastoma: technetium sulfur colloid uptake simulating focal nodular hyperplasia. AJR 1982;139:168–171.
6. Miller JH, Greenspan BS. Integrated imaging of hepatic tumors in childhood. Part I: malignant lesions (primary and metastatic). Radiology 1985;154:83–90.
7. Evans AE, Land VJ, Newton WA, et al. Combination chemotherapy (vincristine, adriamycin, cyclophosphamide, and 5-fluorouracil) in treatment of children with malignant hepatoma. Cancer 1982;50:821–826.
8. Dachman AH, Pakter RL, Ros PR, et al. Hepatoblastoma: radiologic-pathologic correlation in 50 cases. Radiology 1987;164:15–19.
9. Amendola MA, Blane CE, Amendola BE, et al. CT findings in hepatoblastoma. J Comput Assist Tomogr 1984;18:1105–1109.
10. Smith WL, Franken EA, Mitros FA. Liver tumors in children. Semin Roentgenol 1983;18:136–148.
11. Barton JW, Keller MS. Liver transplantation for hepatoblastoma in a child with congenital absence of the portal vein. Pediatr Radiol 1989;20:113–114.
12. Brunelle F, Chaumont P. Hepatic tumors in children: ultrasonic differentiation of malignant from benign lesions. Radiology 1984;150:695–699.
13. Bates SM, Keller MS, Ramos IM, et al. Hepatoblastoma: detection of tumor vascularity with duplex Doppler US. Radiology 1990;176:505–107.
14. deCampo M, deCampo JF. Ultrasound of primary hepatic tumours in childhood. Pediatr Radiol 1988;19:19–24.
15. Korobkin M, Kirks DR, Sullivan DE, et al. Computed tomography of primary liver tumors in children. Radiology 1981;139:431–435.
16. Nelson RC, Chezmar JL, Sugarbaker PH, et al. Hepatic tumors: comparison of CT during arterial portography, delayed CT, and MR imaging for preoperative evaluation. Radiology 1989;172:27–34.
17. Merine D, Takayasu K, Wakao F. Detection of hepatocellular carcinoma: comparison of CT during arterial portography with CT after intraarterial injection of iodized oil. Radiology 1990;175:707–710.

18. Boechat MI, Kangarloo H, Gilsanz V. Hepatic masses in children. Semin Roentgenol 1988;23:185–193.
19. Ohtomo K, Itai Y, Yoshikawa K, et al. Hepatic tumors: dynamic MR imaging. Radiology 1987;163:27–31.
20. Kressel HY. Strategies for magnetic resonance imaging of focal liver disease. Radiol Clin N Am 1988;26:607–615.
21. Rummeny E, Weissleder R, Stark DD, et al. Primary liver tumors: diagnosis by MR imaging. AJR 1989;152:63–72.
22. Foley WD, Kneeland JB, Cates JD, et al. Contrast optimization for the detection of focal hepatic lesions by MR imaging at 1.5 T. AJR 1987;149:1155–1160.
23. Van Beers B, Demeure R, Pringot J, et al. Dynamic spin-echo imaging with Gd-DTPA: value in the differentiation of hepatic tumors. AJR 1990;154:515–519.
24. Yoshida H, Itai Y, Ohtomo K, et al. Small hepatocellular carcinoma and cavernous hemangioma: differentiation with dynamic flash MR imaging with Gd-DTPA. Radiology 1989;171:339–342.
25. Tonkin ILD, Wrenn EL, Hollabaugh RS. The continued value of angiography in planning surgical resection of benign and malignant hepatic tumors in children. Pediatr Radiol 1988;18:35–44.
26. Macpherson RI, Saldana JA, Cone RM, et al. Primary liver masses in infants. J Canad Assoc Radiol 1981;32:81–87.
27. Moss AA, Clark RE, Palubinskas AJ, et al. Angiographic appearance of benign and malignant hepatic tumors in infants and children. AJR 1971;113:61–69.
28. Curati WL, Halevy A, Gibson RN, et al. Ultrasound, CT, and MRI comparison in primary and secondary tumors of the liver. Gastrointest Radiol 1988;13:123–128.
29. Finn JP, Hall-Craggs MA, Dicks-Mireaux C, et al. Primary malignant liver tumors in childhood: assessment of resectability with high-field MR and comparison with CT. Pediatr Radiol 1990;21:34–38.
30. Lack EE, Neave C, Vawter GF. Hepatocellular carcinoma. Review of 32 cases in childhood and adolescence. Cancer 1983;52:1510–1515.
31. Weinberg AG, Finegold MJ. Primary hepatic tumors of childhood. Human Pathol 1983;14:512–537.

Differential Diagnosis

Most liver masses in children will be malignant.[1] In a review of 1237 patients, 66 percent were malignant (Table 3–6). A number of conditions should, however, be considered in the differential diagnosis of hepatoma.

Hemangioendothelioma. Hemangioendotheliomas will often present in the newborn period with hepatomegaly. Clinically, they will often cause congestive failure. With imaging studies they can usually be differentiated from hepatoma. Calcification, if present, tends to be finer.[2] Like hepatoma, these lesions may be single or multifocal and may be well defined or diffuse. They are much more likely to have many areas of low echogenicity on ultrasound.[2,3] If a bolus of contrast material is injected and serial CT images obtained at one level in the liver, hemangioendothelioma will typically show early rim enhancement with delayed opacification of the center of the tumor over a period of between a few minutes to half an hour. This pattern will not be clearly seen if early images after bolus injection or adequate delayed images are not obtained.[4,5] In addition, if there is thrombosis or fibrosis in the center of the tumor, this typical enhancement pattern will not be seen and the hemangioendotheliomas will be much more difficult to differentiate from hepatoma.[6] Hepatoma will typically show more uniform early enhancement. On ultrasound, it is sometimes difficult to differentiate the hemangioendothelioma from hepatoma.[7] Because of the vascular shunt in the hemangioendothelioma, ultrasound may identify enlargement of the celiac and hepatic arteries with reduction in caliber of the aorta below the level of the celiac artery. This finding is strongly suggestive of hemangioendothelioma. It will not be present in all cases, occurring only if there is a large shunt through the tumor. As mentioned above, congestive cardiac failure, if present, is helpful in differentiating hepatoma from hemangioendothelioma. It is, however, only present in 25 percent of affected babies.[5] Another helpful finding suggesting the diagnosis of hemangioendothelioma are skin hemangiomas. These were, unfortunately, present in only 37 percent of patients in one study.[5]

TABLE 3–6
Incidence of Liver Tumors in Children: Review of 1237 Cases[1]

Tumor	Percentage
Hepatoblastoma	43
Hepatocellular carcinoma	23
Benign vascular	13
Mesenchymal hamartoma	6
Malignant mesenchymoma	6
Adenoma	2
Focal nodular hyperplasia	2
Other	5

Reference
1. Weinberg AG, Finegold MJ. Primary hepatic tumors of childhood. Human Pathol 1983;14:512–537.

Technetium 99m labeled red blood cells, injected intravenously, show delayed accumulation in hemangioendotheliomas and this appearance is fairly characteristic.

Mesenchymal Hamartoma. Mesenchymal hamartomas are single benign liver tumors usually occurring in the right lobe[8] (Fig. 3–12). They can be very large and often require resection because of their size[9] (Fig. 3–13). They usually have cysts of varying size[10–14] separated by septa. The cysts may contain a mucoid material. Occasionally, no cysts will be identified[9,15,16] This is particularly true in the very young. The median age at presentation is about 11 months, similar to that for hepatoblastoma. Like hepatoblastoma the most common presenting sign is an abdominal mass. CT and ultrasound will show a well-defined mass lesion. The cysts can be easily identified. They will vary in size.[14] There have been occasional reports of shunt through these tumors with congestive cardiac failure,[3] but not all workers believe that these patients did in fact have mesenchymal hamartomas. On MR, the cysts appear of

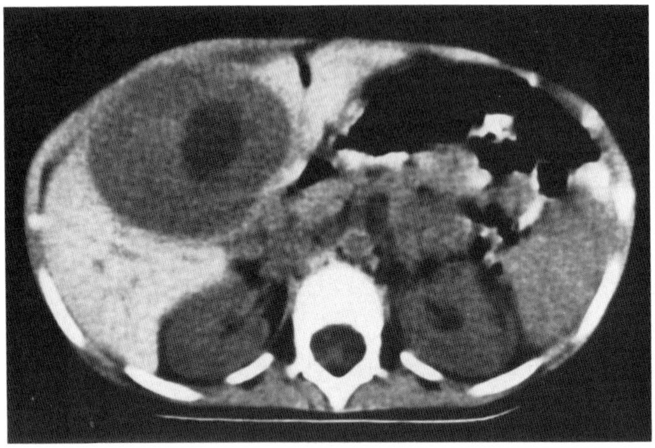

Figure 3–12. **Diagnosis: Mesenchymal hamartoma. CT. There is a well-defined liver mass lesion with a central low-intensity necrotic region. There are no features to distinguish this benign tumor from hepatoblastoma. (From Leary DL, Weiskittel DA, Blane CE, et al. Follow-up imaging of benign pediatric liver tumors. Pediatr Radiol 1989; 19:234–236.)**

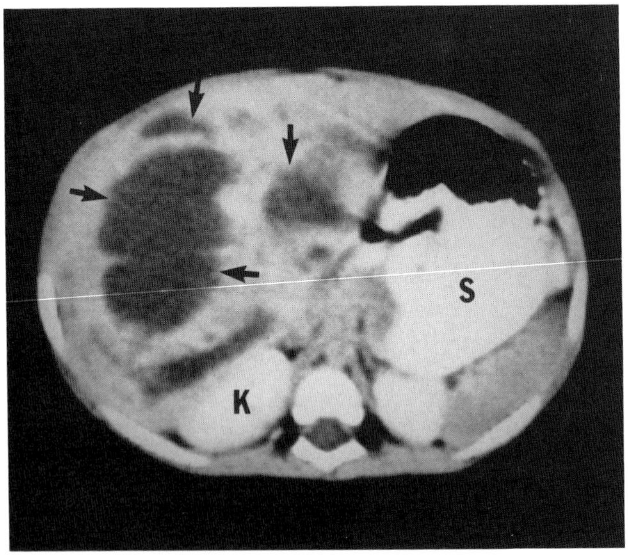

Figure 3–13. **Diagnosis: Mesenchymal hamartoma. CT. There is a large cystic lesion in the right lobe. Multiple septated low-density areas are identified *(arrows). K* = Kidney, *S* = stomach. (From Tonkin ILD, Wrenn EL, Hollabaugh RS. The continued value of angiography in planning surgical resection of hepatic tumors in children. Pediatr Radiol 1988; 18:35–44).**

very low signal on T1 and very bright signal on T2 weighted images,[17] and the margins of the lesion are well defined. The correct diagnosis can frequently be suggested by the presence of a well-defined large lesion in a young child with clear cysts and septa. Hemorrhage into the cysts may cause confusion. Areas of necrosis and hemorrhage in tumors may also cause confusion. Knowledge of alpha-fetoprotein concentrations is often particularly helpful in differentiating hamartoma from hepatoma.

Stage IV-S Neuroblastoma. Stage IV-S neuroblastoma is usually diffuse and infiltrating, involving the entire liver. It is very rare for a hepatoma to have such diffuse involvement of the liver, although occasionally this may occur. The diagnosis of neuroblastoma is usually, however, readily made from detection of the primary tumor, bone marrow metastases, and elevation of catecholamines such as VMA and HVA in the blood or urine.

Cavernous Hemangioma. In the neonate, the distinction between cavernous hemangioma and hemangioendothelioma is not made. In older children and adults, cavernous hemangiomas are well-defined lesions of varying size. They are often lobulated. Ultrasound or CT will show areas of fluid within them and also good margins.[18] MR shows a characteristic appearance of a smooth homogenous lobulated mass that is often isointense to normal liver on T1 weighted images but extremely bright on T2 weighted images.[19,20] Larger lesions, however, may not be typical, owing to areas of clot or fibrosis, and in these patients differentiation from hepatoma may be difficult. Technetium 99m labeled red blood cell studies will characteristically show increased isotope uptake in cavernous hemangiomas on delayed images.[18]

Adenomas. Adenomas are benign tumors and are made up of liver cells but contain no reticuloendothelial cells. They are usually single masses.[21] They may occur spontaneously or in disorders such as glycogen storage disease.[1,11] or in patients with Fanconi anemia treated with anabolic steroids.[11] It may be difficult to differentiate them from hepatoma with imaging. When induced by anabolic steroids, they may show spontaneous resolution when the steroids are stopped.

Focal Nodular Hyperplasia. Focal nodular hyperplasia are single well-defined liver masses. They are often subcapsular with radial scars.[11] Up to 20 percent will be multifocal.[21] On MR, they are often isointense with normal liver on both T1 and T2 weighted pulse sequences, or show mild increase in signal on T2 pulse sequences, or show mild increase in signal on T2 weighted pulse sequences, less than is seen with malignancy. A central area of low signal on all pulse sequences may be seen.[1,22] They may enhance with gadolinium-DTPA.[22] Forty percent of these lesions will show uptake of sulfur colloid technetium 99m,[23] which, when present, is helpful in characterizing them. It may not always be possible to make the diagnosis prior to biopsy.

Simple Cyst. Simple cysts can grow quickly. They are easily diagnosed with ultrasound or CT.[24]

Inflammatory Pseudotumor. Inflammatory pseudotumor of the liver has recently been reported in 9 adults,[25] with 9 children being reviewed from the literature. These patients present with fever, abdominal pain, and weight loss, findings that may mimic tumor. They have single or multiple well-defined lesions in the liver that appear as focal areas of low density on CT scanning and decreased vascularity if angiography is performed. It may not be possible to differentiate inflammatory pseudotumor from tumor by imaging alone.[25]

Choledochal Cyst. There should be no difficulty in di-

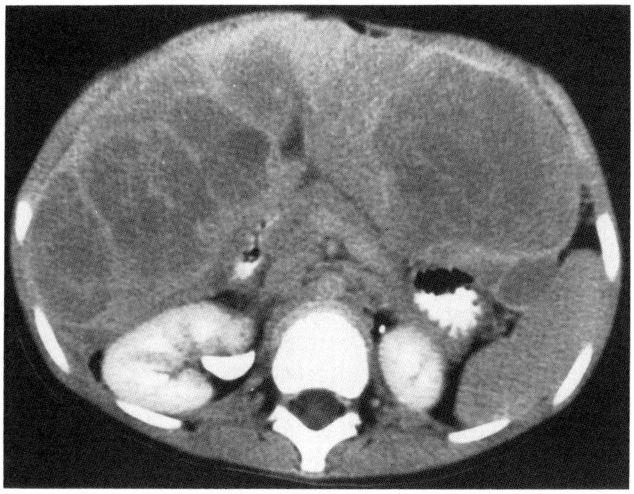

Figure 3-14. **Diagnosis: Liver lymphomas.**
CT after IV contrast. Multiple low-intensity nodules are identified throughout both lobes of the liver. These cannot be distinguished from other liver lesions such as hepatocellular carcinoma.

agnosis of choledochal cysts. They do not usually present as masses. They are easily diagnosed with ultrasound and CT together with isotope-labeled IDA studies.[13] It is, however, important to note that malignancy can develop in the wall of a choledochal cyst, which is one reason these cysts should always be surgically resected. These malignancies are usually adenocarcinomas. While it usually does not present until adult life, an adenocarcinoma in the wall of a choledochal cyst has recently been reported in a 12-year-old.[26]

Abscess. It may be difficult to differentiate abscess from liver tumors solely by the imaging appearance. The differentiation should, however, be easy when the clinical findings and laboratory investigation such as white blood cell study are taken into account. Gas seen in a lesion on CT scan is fairly good evidence for the presence of an abscess.[13]

Hematoma. The diagnosis should be evident because of the history of trauma.

Rhabdomyosarcoma. Rhabdomyosarcoma very rarely occurs in the liver. It is associated with biliary tree and is usually extrahepatic in location. When within the liver parenchyma, it cannot be differentiated from hepatoma.

Lymphoma. Areas of lymphoma within the liver characteristically have low echoes on ultrasound. There are few other distinguishing features to differentiate them from hepatoma. On CT, they are seen as masses on lower intensity than normal liver (Fig. 3–14). Again the consideration of clinical findings and the presence of disease in other locations in the body should help in the differential diagnosis.

Comment: There is a very large differential diagnosis for hepatoblastoma and hepatocellular carcinoma. Lesions containing pure cysts are usually easily differentiated with imaging. With other lesions careful attention to clinical findings and laboratory data greatly aids with differential diagnosis. In many patients, hepatoma can be differentiated from other liver masses only by biopsy.

References

1. Weinberg AG, Finegold MJ. Primary hepatic tumors of childhood. Human Pathol 1983;14:512–537.
2. Dachman AH, Pakter RL, Ros PR, et al. Hepatoblastoma: radiologic-pathologic correlation in 50 cases. Radiology 1987;164:15–19.
3. Abramson SJ, Lack EE, Teele RL. Benign vascular tumors of the liver in infants: sonographic appearance. AJR 1982;138:629–632.
4. Freeny PC, Marks WM. Patterns of contrast enhancement of benign and malignant hepatic neoplasms during bolus dynamic and delayed CT. Radiology 1986;160:613–618.
5. Mahboubi S, Sunaryo FP, Glassman MS, et al. Computed tomography, management, and follow-up in infantile hemangioendothelioma of the liver in infants and children. J Comput Tomogr 1987;11:370–375.
6. Exelby PR, Filler RM, Grosfeld JL. Liver tumors in children in the particular reference to hepatoblastoma and hepatocellular carcinoma: American Academy of Pediatrics Surgical Section Survey–1974. J Pediatr Surg 1975;10:329–337.
7. Kaude JV, Felman AH, Hawkins IF Jr. Ultrasonography in primary hepatic tumors in early childhood. Pediatr Radiol 1980;9:77–83.
8. Ros PR, Goodman AD, Ishak KG, et al. Mesenchymal hamartoma of the liver: radiologic-pathologic correlation. Radiology 1986;158:619–624.
9. Leary DL, Weiskittel DA, Blane CE, et al. Follow-up imaging of benign pediatric liver tumors. Pediatr Radiol 1989;19:234–236.
10. Stanley P, Hall TR, Woolley MM, et al. Mesenchymal hamartomas of the liver in childhood: sonographic and CT findings. AJR 1986;147:1035–1039.
11. Smith WL, Franken EA, Mitros FA. Liver tumors in children. Semin Roentgenol 1983;18:136–148.
12. Amendola MA, Blane CE, Amendola BE, et al. CT findings in hepatoblastoma. J Comput Assist Tomogr 1984;18:1105–1109.
13. Boechat MI, Kangarloo H, Gilsanz V. Hepatic masses in children. Semin Roentgenol 1988;23:185–193.
14. Ros PR, Goodman AD, Ishak KG, et al. Mesenchymal hamartoma of the liver: radiologic-pathologic correlation. Radiology 1986;158:619–624.
15. Guzetta PC, Randolph JG. Pediatric hepatic surgery. Surg Clin N Am 1989;69:251–257.
16. Lack EE. Mesenchymal hamartoma of the liver. A clinical and pathologic study of nine cases. Am J Pediatr Hematol/Oncol 1986;8:91–98.
17. Kressel HY. Strategies for magnetic resonance imaging of focal liver disease. Radiol Clin N Am 1988;26:607–615.
18. Brown RKJ, Gomes A, King W, et al. Hepatic hemangiomas: evaluation by magnetic resonance imaging and technetium-99m red blood cell scintigraphy. J Nucl Med 1987;28:1683–1687.
19. Li KC, Glazer GM, Quint LE, et al. Distinction of hepatic cavernous hemangioma from metastases with MR imaging. Radiology 1988;169:409–415.
20. Ros PR, Lubbers PR, Olmsted WW, et al. Hemangioma of

the liver: heterogeneous appearance on T2-weighted images. AJR 1987;149:1167–1170.

21. Dehner LP. Pediatric surgical pathology, 2nd ed. Baltimore: William & Wilkins, 1987:433–499.
22. Van Beers B, Demeure R, Pringot J, et al. Dynamic spin-echo imaging with Gd-DTPA: value in the differentiation of hepatic tumors. AJR 1990;154:515–519.
23. Diament MJ, Parvey LS, Tonkin ILD, et al. Hepatoblastoma: Technetium sulfur colloid uptake simulating focal nodular hyperplasia. AJR 1982;139:168–171.
24. Byrne WJ, Fonkalsrud EW. Congenital solitary nonparasitic cyst of the liver: a rare cause of rapidly enlarging abdominal mass in infancy. J Pediatr Surg 1982;17:316–317.
25. Horiuchi R, Uchida T, Kojima T, et al. Inflammatory pseudotumor of the liver. Cancer 1990;65:1583.
26. Iwai N, Deguchi E, Yanagihara J, et al. Cancer arising in a choledochal cyst in a 12-year-old girl. J Pediatr Surg 1990;25:1261–1263.

Therapy and Prognosis

In a study of 227 children with hepatoma reported in 1975, there were no survivors unless complete surgical resection of the tumor had been achieved.[1] Even with improvement in chemotherapy since that time, it still remains true that survival with hepatoma is extremely unlikely unless the tumor has been resected completely. This resection may take place on initial presentation or following chemotherapeutic tumor reduction. Hepatocellular carcinoma is not resectable in between 70 to 85 percent of patients on initial presentation.[2–6] Hepatoblastoma is more favorable, with between 50 to 65 percent of tumors being resectable on initial presentation.[7,8] The current approach is to resect the tumor on initial presentation if this is possible without excessive risks. Because most tumors will respond to chemotherapy and shrink significantly in size, more and more patients with large tumors are being treated initially with chemotherapy followed by delayed surgical resection.[9,10] Prior to effective chemotherapy, the surgeon had to be extremely aggressive to attempt removal of tumor, and operative complications were high. Complications are much reduced, with large tumors, if the tumor is initially shrunk with chemotherapy. Imaging has an important role to play in the initial assessment of potential resectability of the tumor and in monitoring the response to chemotherapy if the tumor is not initially resected. The following definitions of tumor resectability are helpful[11]:

1. Readily resectable. The tumor is confined to the liver and involves three or less segments.
2. Potentially resectable. There is contiguous spread of the tumor to the wall of the inferior vena cava, portal vein, or hepatic veins, or local spread of the tumor outside the liver.
3. Unresectable. The tumor involves all four segments of the liver. The tumor encases or invades the main portal vein, hepatic artery, or hepatic duct. There is tumor in the lymph nodes of the porta hepatis. There are distant metastases.
4. Inoperable. The patient has cirrhoses, portal hypertension, or ascites.[4,11] There are some contraindications to surgery that may not be identified by imaging. Imaging cannot show tumor in small lymph nodes in the porta hepatis, and also is extremely poor at identification of peritoneal seeding with tumor.[12]

Because imaging is important in planning surgical resection, and in following the liver after resection, it is important for the radiologist to understand the surgical procedures that are performed. Up to 3 of the 4 segments of the liver can be resected. The surgeon must leave adequate liver volume for the child to live, and the residual liver must have a vascular supply, and venous and biliary drainage. Actual resections are not through the hepatic veins dividing the liver segments, but are intrasegmental close to the boundary outlined by the veins. In general, the resection is done just to the side of the vessel forming the boundaries. The vessel is left behind. Thus, with a right lobectomy the resection extends along a plane from the gallbladder to the inferior vena cava, up to the middle hepatic vein, which is left in position. It is also important for the radiologist to note that the resection is not a straight line but will contour as the patient's anatomy and tumor permit. This is particularly true as the line of resection approaches the porta hepatis.[11]

All patients with stage I, II, III, or IV tumor will receive chemotherapy. Radiation therapy is predominantly used for patients with stage II or III disease. Surgical resection is attempted whenever possible in patients with stage I, II, or III disease and for stage IV disease if initial chemotherapy achieves control of metastases.[7]

Chemotherapy is usually given systemically. Intraarterial chemotherapy has not been widely attempted in children. Recent experimental therapy involves intraarterial injection of a suspension of chemotherapy and Lipiodol. Injected into the hepatic artery, this mixture is selectively taken up by the tumor cells. It has been attempted in two children with hepatoblastoma.[13] Transplantation has also been attempted, but a literature review[7] indicates that over 85 percent of patients will die.

The prognosis with hepatoma is directly proportional to the resectability of the tumor. In a 1982 combined CCSG and POG study, there was 83 percent survival in those children in whom complete resection of the primary tumor was achieved. Unfortunately, many children do not have resectable tumors. In one study reported in 1983, 11 of 16 children were stage III and IV on initial presentation. In another study from the United Kingdom, 8 of 11 children with stage I and II tumors lived, but all 14 children with stage III or IV tumors died. The potential of recent chemotherapy to reduce tumor size and increase the number of children in whom delayed resection is possible should, in the future, improve prognosis.

Hepatocellular carcinoma has a worse prognosis than hepatoblastoma. For any given stage the prognosis for these two tumors is the same.[6] The difference in prognosis is because hepatoblastomas are much more likely to be resectable than the hepatocellular carcinoma. A study in 1989 indicates that prognosis can be improved from less than 20 percent to about 50 percent in those patients in whom delayed resection is performed after chemotherapy.[7] Prognosis may also be affected by histology. The unusual small cell/anaplastic tumors have a worse prognosis than the other cell types.[14] There is some conflicting data concerning the prognosis of patients with pure fetal histology.[14] A study published in 1989 and involving 196 children clearly showed a better prognosis for children with pure fetal histology. When resection of the tumor was complete, the survival with pure fetal histology was 92 percent at 2 years compared to 57 percent for children, also with complete resection, but without pure fetal histology.[15]

Prognosis with hepatocellular carcinoma or hepatoma is excellent when complete resection of the tumor is possible. Even with modern chemotherapy prognosis is poor unless the tumor is resected. The main impact of chemotherapy is to reduce tumor size and increase the number of children in whom complete resection can be achieved.

> *Comment:* Surgical resection, either before or after initial chemotherapy, still remains the most important factor determining long-term prognosis in children with hepatoma.

References

1. Exelby PR, Filler RM, Grosfeld JL. Liver tumors in children in the particular reference to hepatoblastoma and hepatocellular carcinoma: American Academy of Pediatrics Surgical Section Survey–1974. J Pediatr Surg 1975; 10:329–337.
2. Boechat MI, Kangarloo H, Gilsanz V. Hepatic masses in children. Semin Roentgenol 1988;23:185–193.
3. Chen WJ, Lee JC, Hung WT. Primary malignant tumor of liver in infants and children in Taiwan. J Pediatr Surg 1988;23:457–461.
4. LaBerge JM, Laing FC, Federle MP, et al. Hepatocellular carcinoma: assessment of resectability by computed tomography and ultrasound. Radiology 1984;152:485–490.
5. Lack EE, Neave C, Vawter GF. Hepatocellular carcinoma. Review of 32 cases in childhood and adolescence. Cancer 1983;52:1510–1515.
6. Weinberg AG, Finegold MJ. Primary hepatic tumors of childhood. Human Pathol 1983;14:512–537.
7. Guzetta PC, Randolph JG. Pediatric hepatic surgery. Surg Clin N Am 1989;69:251–257.
8. Pierro A, Langevin AM, Filler RM, et al. Preoperative chemotherapy in "unresectable" hepatoblastoma. J Pediatr Surg 1989;24:24–29.
9. Herlin T, Norup K, Storm K. Treatment of unresectable hepatoblastoma with cisplatin, vincristin and 5-fluorouracil. Eur J Pediatr 1988;147:514–515.
10. Tsuchida Y, Bastos JC, Honna T, et al. Treatment of disseminated hepatoblastoma involving bilateral lobes. J Pediatr Surg 1990;25:1253–1255.
11. Mukai JK, Stack CM, Turner DA, et al. Imaging of surgically relevant hepatic vascular and segmental anatomy. Part 2. Extent and resectability of hepatic neoplasms. AJR 1987;149:293–297.
12. Sugarbaker PH. Surgical decision making for large bowel cancer metastatic to the liver. Radiology 1990;174:621–626.
13. Sue K, Ikeda K, Nakagawara A, et al. Intrahepatic arterial injections of cisplatin-phosphyatidylocholine-lipiodol suspension in two unresectable hepatoblastoma cases. Med Pediatr Oncol 1989;17:496–500.
14. Dehner LP, Manivel JC. Hepatoblastoma: an analysis of the relationship between morphologic subtypes and prognosis. Am J Pediatr Hematol/Oncol 1988;10:301–307.
15. Haas JE, Muczynski KA, Krailo M, et al. Histopathology and prognosis in childhood hepatoblastoma and hepatocarcinoma. Cancer 1989;64:1082–1095.

FIBROLAMELLAR HEPATOCELLULAR CARCINOMA

This tumor is a hepatocellular carcinoma, but is discussed separately because it has several characteristic differentiating features. Fibrolamellar hepatocellular carcinoma is differentiated from other hepatocellular carcinomas by the age of the patients, the pathology, the absence of associated liver disease, and a better prognosis.

Epidemiology

Fibrolamellar hepatocellular carcinoma occurs in the age range of 5 to 30 years[1,2] with a mean of approximately 20 years.[3] It is not uncommon, being identified in 5 of 32 children with hepatocellular carcinoma.[4]

Incidence among males and females is equal.[2] Unlike conventional hepatocellular carcinoma, fibrolamellar hepatocellular carcinoma has no association with chronic liver disease such as cirrhosis.[5–8] Metastases can occur.[2]

Pathology

Grossly, the tumors are invariably large. In two series, the smallest tumor was 7 cm in diameter.[7,9] The lesions are frequently single,[2,5] but satellite nodules can occur.[5,6] They are almost always sharply defined and do not show the local permeative invasion seen with other hepatocellular carcinomas. In addition, a central fibrotic scar is present in a large number of patients. In one series, it was seen in over 60 percent of CT scans.[5] Central calcification may occur in the scar.[5,9] In one study, it was present in up to 40 percent of patients.[3]

Clinical Presentation

The symptoms are nonspecific. In 23 patients, pain was identified in 74 percent, malaise in 32 percent.[2] Pain, fever, and weight loss are the most common symptoms.[5] The symptoms are the same as with conventional hepatocellular carcinoma.[8] Serum alpha-fetoprotein concentration, however, is usually normal,[2,3,8] although there have been some reports of a mild elevation.[3,6]

Imaging Studies

On imaging, these tumors may have a characteristic appearance. On ultrasound, increase in echogenicity is the most common finding, being found in all 9 patients in one study.[3] The tumors usually have sharp margins. They may be homogenous or of mixed intensity. Although an increase in echoes is the most common finding,[6] areas of isointensity or decreased intensity compared to liver may be found. The central scar may be visualized as a region of strong echoes with a shadow.

On CT scan, these tumors are usually of lower intensity than normal liver on precontrast scan. They may occasionally be of iosintensity.[6] Well-defined calcification is more commonly seen than with conventional hepatocellular carcinoma. A central scar is frequently identified. This usually shows no enhancement with contrast, but may show very minimal enhancement.[5] The rest of the tumor shows only mild to moderate enhancement after intravenous contrast and always enhances less than normal liver tissue.

On MR imaging, the tumor is of lower signal intensity than normal liver on T1 weighted images with some increase on T2 weighted images. The scarred areas increase minimally with increased T2 weighting. Sulfur colloid nuclear medicines scan shows a cold region corresponding to the tumor.[6] On angiography, these tumors are either vascular or very vascular.[5,7,8] Arterovenous shunting may be present[10] or absent.[8] The veins usually appear normal.[8] The vessels are sometimes characteristically arranged in a radiating pattern.[5]

Therapy and Prognosis

The prognosis of fibrolamellar hepatocellular carcinoma is much better than with other hepatocellular carcinomas. This probably is a reflection of the fact that these tumors are much more commonly well defined and, therefore, much more commonly amenable to complete surgical resection. Resection rate varies from between 48 percent of 23 patients[2] to over 60 percent of patients.[6,11] The prognosis is much better than with conventional hepatocellular carcinoma.[1,5]

> *Comment:* Fibrolamellar hepatocellular carcinoma occurs in older children, is better defined, is more readily surgically resectable, and has a characteristic central scar, and a better prognosis than hepatocellular carcinoma.

References

1. Farhi DC, Shikes RH, Murari PJ, et al. Hepatocellular carcinoma in young people. Cancer 1983;52:1516–1525.
2. Craig JR, Peters RL, Edmondson HA, et al. Fibrolamellar carcinoma of the liver: a tumor of adolescents and young adults with distinctive clinico-pathologic features. Cancer 1980;46:372–379.
3. Friedman AC, Lichtenstein JE, Goodman Z, et al. Fibrolamellar hepatocellular carcinoma. Radiology 1985; 157:583–587.
4. Haas JR, Muczynski KA, Krailo M, et al. Histopathology and prognosis in childhood hepatoblastoma and hepatocarcinoma. Cancer 1989;64:1082–1095.
5. Brandt DJ, Johnson CD, Stephens DH, et al. Imaging of fibrolamellar hepatocellular carcinoma. AJR 1988;151: 295–299.
6. Titelbaum DS, Burke DR, Meranze SG, et al. Fibrolamellar hepatocellular carcinoma: pitfalls in nonoperative diagnosis. Radiology 1988;167:25–30.
7. Adam A, Gibson RN, Soreide O, et al. The radiology of fibrolamellar hepatoma. Clin Radiol 1986;37:355–358.
8. Francis IR, Agha FP, Thompson, NW, et al. Fibrolamellar hepatocarcinoma: clinical, radiologic, and pathologic features. Gastrointest Radiol 1986;11:67–72.
9. LeSher AR, Castronuovo JJ, Filippione AL. Hepatoblastoma in a patient with familial polyposis coli. Surgery 1989;105:668–670.
10. Wong LK, Link DP, Frey CF, et al. Fibrolamellar hepatocarcinoma: radiology, management, and pathology. AJR 1982;139:172–175.
11. Lack EE, Neave C, Vawter GF. Hepatocellular carcinoma. Review of 32 cases in childhood and adolescence. Cancer 1983;52:1510–1515.

ANGIOSARCOMA

Angiosarcoma is a very rare liver tumor in children. It is also called a malignant hemangioendothelioma. In one report, all 4 children with this disorder died.[1] All 4 children were females under the age of 3 years; 3 presented with a mass and 1 with congestive cardiac failure. In all 4 children, a significant component of the tumor mass was benign hemangioendothelioma, and it is believed that angiosarcoma arises in a preexisting hemangioendothelioma. Two of the 4 children reported had lung metastases. There are no reports of imaging of these tumors, but apart from the identification of pulmonary metastases I suspect that there were no specific features that would enable them to be differentiated from benign hemangioendothelioma.

Reference

1. Falk H, Herbert JT, Edmonds L, et al. Review of four cases of childhood hepatic angiosarcoma—elevated environmental arsenic exposure in one case. Cancer 1981;47:382–391.

MALIGNANT MESENCHYMOMA

Malignant mesenchymoma is also called an undifferentiated sarcoma. It occurs only in children, usually between the age of 5 and 10 years.[1–3] The incidence in males and females is approximately equal. It is a very aggressive tumor with a poor prognosis.

The tumor almost always involves the right lobe of the liver. It is a large single mass with sharp margins and microscopic infiltration of the adjacent liver tissue.[1,4] It frequently has cystic areas containing a gelatinous material.[1,4] Hemorrhage and necrosis are common[3,4] (Fig. 3–15).

Symptoms are nonspecific, with mass and pain being the most common.[1,2]

Ultrasound shows a complex mass lesion with areas of increased echogenicity and some cystic areas.[2] On CT, the masses may appear solid or cystic[2] and are well defined. In one patient, angiography showed reduced vascularity.[2]

Treatment of the condition is surgical. The tumor is extremely aggressive and prognosis is very poor.[1,3] In a review of 43 patients in the literature,[2] 39 died.

References

1. Guzetta PC, Randolph JG. Pediatric hepatic surgery. Surg Clin N Am 1989;69:251–257.
2. Newman KD, Schisgall R, Reaman G, et al. Malignant mesenchymoma of the liver in children. J Pediatr Surg 1989;24:781–783.

Figure 3–15. **Diagnosis: Malignant mesenchymoma of the liver.**
CT image after contrast injection. There is a large solitary mass in the right lobe. Very-low-intensity areas represent cysts and hemorrhage. (From Guzetta P, Randolph JG. Pediatric hepatic surgery. Surg Clin N Amer 1989; 89:251–257.)

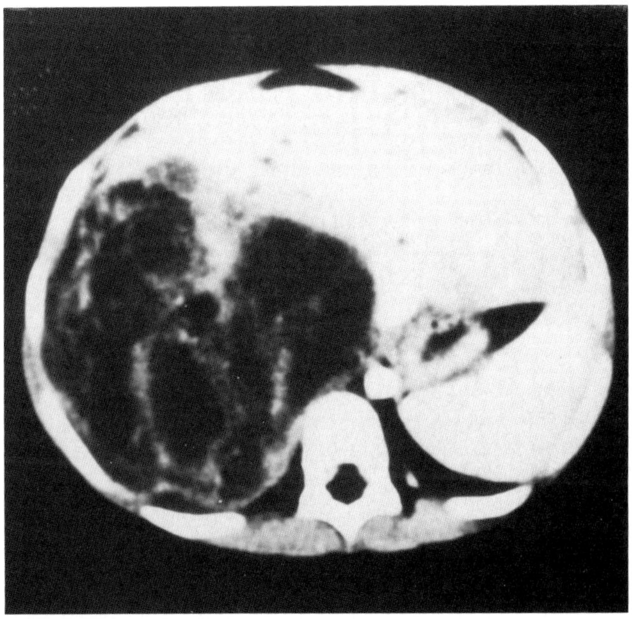

3. Dehner LP. Pediatric surgical pathology, 2nd ed. Baltimore: Williams & Wilkins, 1987:433–499.
4. Weinberg AG, Finegold MJ. Primary hepatic tumors of childhood. Human Pathol 1983;14:512–537.

HEPATOBILIARY CYST ADENOMA

Hepatobiliary cyst adenoma is a very rare multilocular cystic tumor that usually occurs in adults.[1] It was, however, recently reported in one 3-year-old and a review of literature identified 3 other cases in children.[1] The lesions are multilocular cysts with soft-tissue components. They are lined by columnar, mucin-secreting epithelium. They can recur if not completely resected and can develop carcinoma in the wall of the cyst.

Reference

1. Williams JG, Newman BM, Sutphen JL, et al. Hepatobiliary cystadenoma: a rare hepatic tumor in a child. J Pediatr Surg 1990;25:1250–1252.

LIVER METASTASES

In children, many tumors can metastasize to the liver, and metastatic spread from virtually any primary pediatric malignant tumor should be considered in the differential diagnosis of a suspected liver metastasis. The metastases are single or multiple and most commonly well defined (Fig. 3–16). With stage IV-S neuroblastoma, however, it is much more common to identify diffuse infiltrating metastatic spread involving the entire liver.

The appearance of metastases on imaging is nonspecific and the differential diagnosis includes benign tumors, primary liver malignancy, infection, and hematoma. Even in children with known cancer, all liver lesions are not metastases. One recent report describes a false positive liver and spleen sulfur colloid scan in 3 children with rhabdomyosarcoma and Wilms tumor.[1] These children develop focal defects on the liver and spleen scan within 10 days of starting chemotherapy. These defects resolve spontaneously and are believed to be artifacts caused, in some way, by the chemotherapy.

The optimum screening method for metastatic disease in the liver in children is not clearly identified. Many comparative studies have been done in adults and not children. My own strong belief is that at the present time CT scan is the method of choice. Liver and spleen scan is too insensitive and will miss many lesions either less than 2 cm in diameter or deeply located within the liver. On ultrasound, many small or moderate-sized metastatic lesions cannot be clearly differentiated from adjacent normal tissue. The best technique

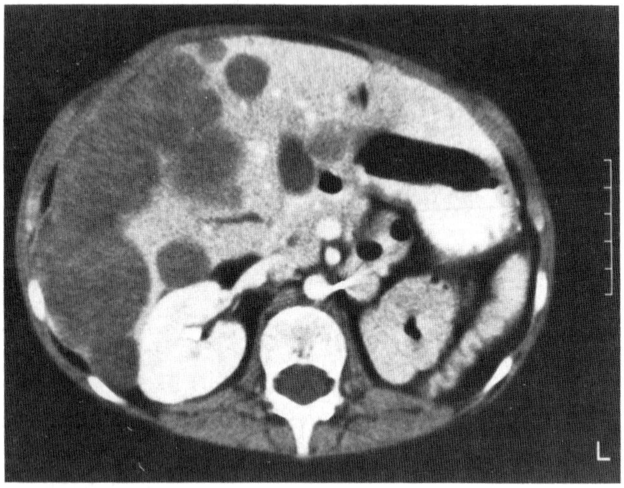

Figure 3-16. **Diagnosis: Metastases from Wilms tumor. CT image. There are multiple low-intensity metastatic nodules identified throughout the liver. There are no specific features that distinguish these metastases from a primary liver malignant tumor. (From Brody A. Metastatic Wilms tumor to the liver. Pediatr Radiol 1989; 19:337-338.)**

for performing the CT scan is not known. In one study in adults, it was reported that a bolus technique using a large volume of intravenous contrast showed more lesions than either a precontrast CT scan or CT scan performed with slow-drip infusion of contrast.[2] The reason for this is that some of the lesions will show rim enhancement only with a bolus technique, which enhances their visibility. My own preference is to utilize bolus injection of contrast in all patients and to perform dynamic 1 cm contiguous imaging slices through the entire liver. It is not known whether or not initial precontrast scanning through the liver will yield additional information. I suspect that any additional yield would be low.

There are some reports in adults that MR is more sensitive than CT for detection of liver metastases.[3-5] There is, however, conflicting data.[6] It is not surprising that different studies will provide different information when one considers the tremendously varied number of methods in which MR and CT scanning can be performed. One must caution also against transferring information from adult studies into the pediatric population. At the present time MR should be considered as having a significant potential for demonstrating metastatic disease of the liver in children. If only one study can be performed, CT should be done. Studies in children comparing CT and MR are needed. When considering performing MR, a large number of different pulse sequences can be utilized. There are many different claims as to which is the best pulse sequence.[4] At high field strengths T2 weighted images may be best, while at lower field strengths short TE, short TR, or STIR pulse sequences may be better.[3,4]

References

1. Abramson SJ, Barash FS, Seldin DW, et al. Transient focal liver scan defects in children receiving chemotherapy (pseudometastases). Radiology 1984;150:701–702.
2. Titelbaum DS, Burke DR, Meranze SG, et al. Fibrolamellar hepatocellular carcinoma: pitfalls in nonoperative diagnosis. Radiology 1988;167:25–30.
3. Reinig JW, Dwyer AJ, Miller DL, Liver metastases: detection with MR imaging at 0.5 and 1.5 T. Radiology 1989;170:149–153.
4. Paling MR, Abbitt PL, Mugler JP, et al. Liver metastases: optimization of MR imaging pulse sequences at 1.0 T. Radiology 1988;167:695–699.
5. Reinig JW, Dwyer AJ, Miller DL, et al. Liver metastasis detection: comparative sensitivities of MR imaging and CT scanning. Radiology 1987;162:43–47.
6. Chezmar JL, Rumancik WM, Megibow AJ, et al. Liver and abdominal screening in patients with cancer: CT versus MR imaging. Radiology 1988;168:43–47.

PANCREATIC TUMORS

Tumors of the pancreas are rare in children, and are much less common in children than in adults. In adults, a wide variety of different tumors are found. The classification of pancreatic tumors in adults is complicated. In children, it is fortunate that only a few tumor types are found and the classification is much simpler (Tables 3–7 and 3–8).

All pancreatic disease in children is uncommon, and pancreatic tumors are uncommon. In one study of 92 children with pancreatic disease, tumors were the etiology in only 10.[1] Of these 10 tumors, 5 were insulinomas, 2 rhabdomyosarcomas, 2 pancreatoblastomas, and 1 a cyst adenoma.

Reference

1. Vane DW, Grosfeld JL, West KW, et al. Pancreatic disorders in infancy and childhood: experience with 92 cases. J Pediatr Surg 1989;24:771–776.

TABLE 3-7
Classification of Pancreatic Tumors by Cell of Origin*[1]

Epithelial Cells	Nonepithelial Cells
Ductal	
Acinar	Sarcoma
Endocrine	Lymphoma

*Most adult tumors are adenocarcinoma, from ductal cells. Most pediatric tumors are pancreatoblastoma, from acinar cells. Papillary tumor, cell of origin unknown.

Reference

1. Kloppel G, Maillet B. Classification and staging of pancreatic nonendocrine tumors. Radiol Clin N Am 1989;27:105–119.

TABLE 3-8
Classification of Endocrine Tumors of Pancreas[1]

Name	Cell of Origin	Hormone Produced
Insulinoma	B cell	Insulin
Glucagonoma	Alpha-fetal cell	Glucagon
Zollinger Ellison	Unknown	Gastrin
Vipoma	PP cell	Active peptides
Somatostatinoma	D cell	Somatostatin

Reference
1. Dehner LP. Pediatric surgical pathology, 2nd ed. Baltimore: Williams & Wilkins, 1987:543–549.

PANCREATOBLASTOMA

Pancreatoblastoma is also called an infantile adenocarcinoma of the pancreas. This tumor can occur at any age in children,[1,2] but is most common in the age range of 1 to 8 years.[3,4] It can occur, however, in neonates, one case being reported in an infant of 3 weeks of age.[5] The tumors are most commonly located in the head of the pancreas. They are invariably large at the time of diagnosis (Figs. 3–17 and 3–18) and may be lobulated.[1–3] They

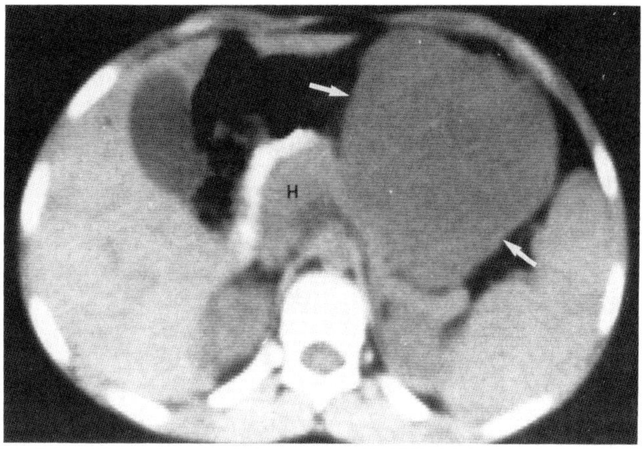

Figure 3-17. Diagnosis: Pancreatoblastoma.
CT. There is a very large well-defined homogeneous tumor *(arrows)* arising from body and tail of the pancreas. The head (*H*) of the pancreas appears normal.

Figure 3-18. Diagnosis: Pancreatoblastoma with calcified liver metastasis.
A, Barium study (prone). There is a very large soft-tissue mass indenting the lesser curve of the stomach.
B, CT scan of liver. There is a low-intensity metastatic lesion containing multiple areas of calcification.

A

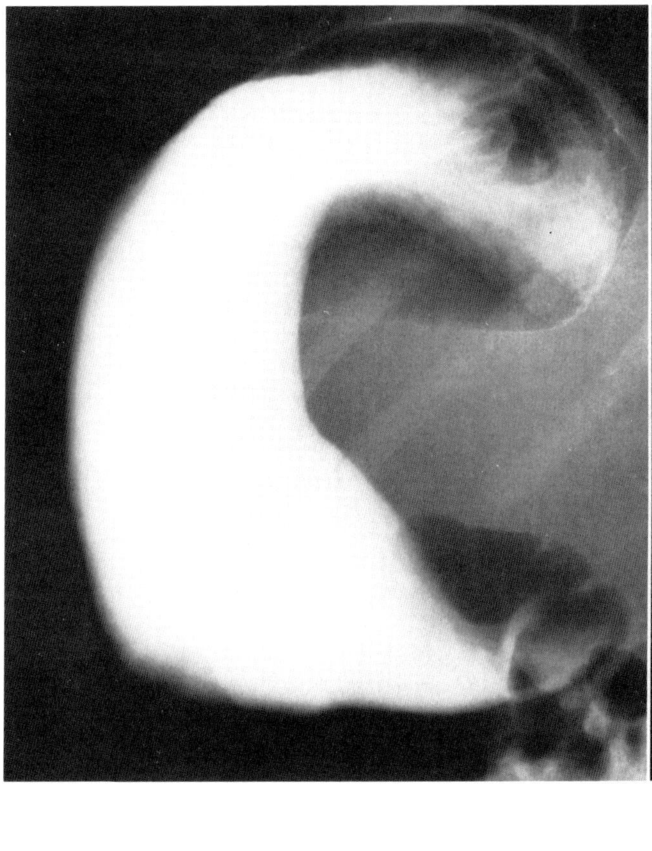

B

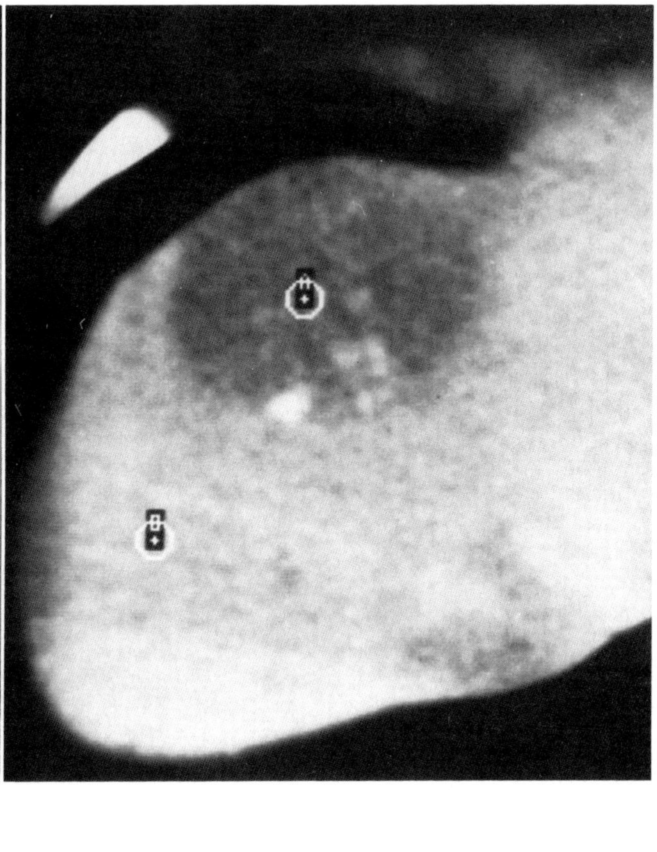

are well defined and well encapsulated.[2] (Fig. 3–17). Hemorrhage and necrosis in the tumors are common[3,4] and separate cystic areas may be identified.[1] Occasionally, these tumors may produce alpha-fetoprotein.[4]

Symptoms are nonspecific. An incidental large abdominal mass is probably the most common. One patient had an elevated alpha-fetoprotein serum concentration.[6]

Metastases can occur. They are most commonly to the liver and abdominal lymph nodes (see Fig. 3–18). Lung and brain metastases can also occur.[5] One case of bone metastases has been described.[6]

Imaging studies will identify a large mass in the region of the pancreas.[7] Abdominal radiograph or barium studies will show mass effect with displacement of adjacent loops of bowel. On ultrasound, the lesions are well defined. The solid areas are echogenic and the cystic areas of low echogenicity.[3] On CT scan, the tumors are well defined and of mixed attenuation.[3] The tumors are clearly in the region of the pancreas, but the precise origin from the pancreas itself may be difficult to determine confidently. Fine calcification can occur.[6,7]

The differential diagnosis is large and includes all retroperitoneal tumors.

Treatment is surgical resection whenever possible. In the absence of metastases, the prognosis is good. If metastic spread has occurred, prognosis is very poor.[3]

References

1. Dehner LP. Pediatric surgical pathology, 2nd ed. Baltimore: Williams & Wilkins, 1987:543–549.
2. Taxy JB. Adenocarcinoma of the pancreas in childhood. Cancer 1976;37:1508–1518.
3. Friedman AC, Edmonds PR. Rare pancreatic malignancies. Radiol Clin N Am 1989;27:177–190.
4. Kloppel G, Maillet B. Classification and staging of pancreatic nonendocrine tumors. Radiol Clin N Am 1989;27:105–119.
5. Robey G, Daneman A, Martin DJ. Pancreatic carcinoma in a neonate. Pediatr Radiol 1983;13:284–286.
6. Iseki M, Suzuki T, Koizumi Y, et al. Alpha-fetoprotein–producing pancreatoblastoma. A case report. Cancer 1986;57:1833–1835.
7. Grosfeld JL, Clatworthy HW, Hamoudi AB. Pancreatic malignancy in children. Arch Surg 1970;101:366–370.

PAPILLARY (Cystic) SOLID TUMOR

Papillary (cystic) solid tumor occurs almost entirely in young females,[1–4] the age range being from puberty to about 25 years.

Macroscopically, the tumors are large and well encapsulated. They are mixed, solid, and cystic, with a variable percentage of each component.[1,2] They are well defined and usually easily resected.

They are easily seen on ultrasound or CT. Both modalities show varying internal structure depending on the proportion of cysts to solid component. The cysts may frequently be irregular in outline and show some internal echoes because of hemorrhage into them.[2] Peripheral calcium may be identified.[2]

Differential diagnosis includes a pseudocyst of the pancreas.[5] In these patients, a history of trauma and inflammation of the pancreas is helpful. It should be remembered that in children the head of the pancreas is relatively larger and more bulky than in adults. This normal bulky appearance of the head of the pancreas should not be confused with tumor. In addition, an enlarged pancreatic head has been described in people with pancreas divisum.[6] In these patients, the dorsal and ventral ducts fail to fuse and the pancreatic head remains larger than normal.

Treatment of these tumors is resection. They are of low-grade malignancy. Metastases can rarely be identified, most commonly to the liver.[3]

References

1. Dehner LP. Pediatric surgical pathology, 2nd ed. Baltimore: Williams & Wilkins, 1987:543–549.
2. Friedman AC, Edmonds PR. Rare pancreatic malignancies. Radiol Clin N Am 1989;27:177–190.
3. Kloppel G, Maillet B. Classification and staging of pancreatic nonendocrine tumors. Radiol Clin N Am 1989;27:105–119.
4. Mathieu D, Guifui B, Valette PJ, et al. Pancreatic cystic neoplasms. Radiol Clin N Am 1989;27:163–176.
5. Pokorny WJ, Raffensperger JG, Harberg FJ. Pancreatic pseudocysts in children. Surg Gynecol Obstet 1980;151:182–184.
6. Soulen MC, Zerhouni EA, Fishman EK, et al. Enlargement of the pancreatic head in patients with pancreas divisum. Clin Imag 1989;13:51–57.

ENDOCRINE TUMORS

The classification of these tumors is given in Table 3–8. Glucagonomas almost never occur in children.

Of the other tumors, insulinoma is usually benign (90 percent), whereas the rest of the tumors are more likely to be malignant (all over 50 percent).[1]

Because of the hormones produced by these tumors (see Table 3–8), they often present with early symptoms and are, therefore, frequently very small at the time of initial diagnosis. This makes imaging identification of these tumors very difficult.

The symptoms from insulinoma are those of hypoglycemia. The child may present with fatigue, weight loss, and lethargy. Syncopal convulsions may occur. Gastrinomas will produce ulcers from increased secretion of gastric acid. The acid also inhibits enzyme function and damages small bowel mucosa so that diarrhea and malabsorption are also commonly found. The vipomas produce watery diarrhea and hypokalemia.

As mentioned previously, imaging of all of the endocrine tumors of the pancreas is difficult. There is no clear optimal imaging modality and unless the tumor is clearly identified by the first modality an approach using multiple modalities is advisable. In a particular patient, any of the modalities may miss the tumor. In addition, any modality may give a false positive result. It is easy to overread some of the images, particularly when the diagnosis is known from the clinical presentation and lab studies, and one has a very strong suspicion, therefore, for the presence of a tumor. Ultrasound should be performed with careful attention to detail. The patient should be studied using optimal resolution. The patient should be scanned in multiple positions, both with and without use of fluid in the stomach, to ensure that all areas of the pancreas are carefully and completely visualized. The success with ultrasound is improved with more widespread use of intraoperative ultrasound. CT should be performed using thin slices and also overlapping slices. The patient should always be given oral contrast. Scans should be performed both with and without utilization of intravenous contrast administration to ensure the best chance of identification of a tumor. The contrast scan should be performed in a dynamic mode following bolus injection of contrast. It may also be helpful to repeat the scans after a delay of 5 to 10 minutes. Intra-arterial injection of contrast may maximize tumor blush, but introduces an invasive component to the study and also provides streak artifacts from the catheter. Angiography needs subselective techniques to look for subtle vessel abnormality. Experience in interpretation of these studies is required.

Venous sampling using a percutaneous technique to place a catheter in the portal vein and its branches has been utilized.[2] This study is, however, not without problems. It is technically difficult, and the interpretation of data obtained may not be clear cut.[1,2]

Insulinomas are seen on ultrasound as well-defined round or oval lesions. They usually have decreased echoes compared to the normal pancreas. A slightly echogenic capsule may or may not be present. Lesions may be missed, because they are very small, isoechogenic with pancreas, or obscured by overlying structures. The CT appearance of insulinomas is that of a moderately well-defined focus of enhancement after contrast administration. This may be difficult to detect in tumors under 2 cm in size. Occasionally, tortuous vessels may be incorrectly diagnosed as tumor.

In patients with suspected pancreatic endocrine tumors, it is suggested that one start by performing both CT and ultrasound. If a clearly defined definite tumor is seen, surgery can be performed. If not, angiography and venous sampling should also be done. In many patients, even if all the imaging studies are negative, an exploratory laparotomy may still be performed. In this situation, intraoperative ultrasound should always be used.

The decision whether or not to perform an exploratory laparotomy, when no tumor is seen with imaging, is particularly difficult in patients with increased insulin secretion. This is because hyperinsulinemia is not always caused by a focal B cell tumor. It may, in some patients, be caused by diffuse hyperplasia of B cells and, in young children, to nesidioblastosis. This latter condition is caused by proliferation of neoeyelet cells derived from duct epithelium. These cells produce insulin. Treatment of this condition is subtotal pancreatectomy.

The role of MR imaging in evaluation of pancreatic tumors is unknown. In one study of 32 adult pancreatic tumors reported in 1989, MR was found to have no advantages over CT scanning.[3] The role of MR in children is completely unknown.

It is important to note that not all vipomas are pancreatic in origin. Secretion of active peptides can also be from neuroblastomas or pheochromocytomas. In children in whom the diagnosis of vipoma is suspected, imaging should include the entire sympathetic chain, if the pancreas is normal.

Other pancreatic tumors such as lymphoma and rhabdomyosarcoma are discussed in the sections dealing specifically with these tumor types.

> *Comment:* Endocrine pancreatic tumors may be very small and a very aggressive imaging approach is needed to identify them.

References

1. Rossi P, Allison DJ, Bezzi M, et al. Endocrine tumors of the pancreas. Radiol Clin N Am 1989;27:129–161.
2. Brunelle F, Negre V, Barth MO, et al. Pancreatic venous samplings in infants and children with primary hyperinsulinism. Pediatr Radiol 1989;19:100–103.
3. Steiner E, Stark DD, Hahn PF, et al. Imaging of pancreatic neoplasms: comparison of MR and CT. AJR 1989;152:487–491.

OTHER GASTROINTESTINAL TUMORS

SPLEEN

Tumors of the spleen are extremely rare. Malignant tumors include angiosarcoma, lymphoma,[1] and endovascular papillary angioendothelioma.[2] Benign tumors include lymphangioma, angioma, hamartoma, or cyst.[1] Apart from cysts, the appearance of most of the other tumors is fairly nonspecific. In addition, many of the lesions are difficult to identify on imaging. The poor performance of imaging in identification of involvement of the spleen with lymphoma is well known and is discussed in the section on lymphoma. On CT and ultrasound, many lesions have characteristics similar to normal spleen. Similarly, on MR, many lesions have long T1 and T2 relaxation times; the normal spleen also has a relatively long T1 and T2 relaxation time.[3] Tumors of the spleen are most likely to be identified with imaging if they are extremely large, if they contain areas of hemorrhage and necrosis within them, or if they are cystic.[3]

Insufficient malignant tumors of the spleen have been identified to permit many statements regarding comparative imaging, optimal therapy, or prognosis.

References

1. Sty JR, Wells RG. Other abdominal and pelvic masses in children. Semin Roentgenol 1988;23:216–231.
2. Katz JA, Mahoney DH, Shukla LW, et al. Endovascular papillary angioendothelioma in the spleen. Pediatr Pathol 1988;8:185–193.
3. Hahn PF, Weissleder R, Stark DD, et al. MR imaging of focal splenic tumors. AJR 1988;150:823–827.

ESOPHAGUS, STOMACH, AND INTESTINE

Tumors of the intestinal tract are extremely uncommon. In the stomach, the most common tumors are teratoma (especially in infants), leiomyosarcoma, rhabdomyosarcoma, myxosarcoma, fibrosarcoma, lymphomas, adenocarcinoma, and primitive neuroectodermal tumor.[1–3] There is one report of a hemangiopericytoma in a newborn. The child had hematemesis, and barium showed a fundal mass.[4] There is an association of gastric leiomyosarcoma with extra adrenal paragangliomas and lung hamartomas in young females.[5]

In the small bowel, lymphoma is the most common tumor. Other tumors that can be found include leiomyosarcoma, angiosarcoma, carcinoid tumor, and adenocarcinoma.[6]

In the colon, adenocarcinoma is the most common malignancy. Leiomyosarcoma and teratoma may also occur. Rhabdomyosarcoma, teratoma, and lymphoma of the bowel are discussed in chapters dealing specifically with these tumors.

References

1. Goto S, Ikeda K, Ishii E, et al. Carcinoma of the stomach in a 7 year old boy. Z Kinderchir 1984;39:137–140.
2. Dehner LP. Pediatric surgical pathology, 2nd ed. Balti more: Williams & Wilkins, 1987:334–432.
3. Mahour GH, Isaacs H, Chang L. Primary malignant tumors of the stomach in children. J Pediatr Surg 1980;15:603–608.
4. Lack EE. Leiomyosarcomas in childhood: a clinical and pathologic study of 10 cases. Pediatr Pathol 1986;6:181–197.
5. Knake JE, Gross MD. Extraadrenal paraganglioma, pulmonary chondroma, and gastric leiomyoblastoma: triad in young females. AJR 1979;132:448–451.
6. Tankel JW, Galasko CSB. Adencarcinoma of small bowel in 12 year old girl. J Roy Soc Med 1984;77:693–694.

INTESTINAL LEIOMYOSARCOMA

Leiomyosarcomas can occur in any site in the intestine. They may be quite large. They can occur at any age, but are most common under the age of 1 year. In one study of 15 patients, 9 were under 1 year and 6 were newborn.[1] In another review, 6 of 12 patients were newborn.[2] The mean age of 10 affected cases was 10 years.[3] Grossly, the tumors are a single mass that may project into the lumen.[4] They may encircle the bowel[5] (Fig. 3–19). The stomach is a common site.[3] In the stomach, it may be very difficult microscopically to differentiate leiomyoma from leiomyosarcoma,[4] and all of these tumors should be considered as potentially malignant. Metastases do occur. The liver is the most common site (Fig. 3–20). The lung is the next most common site. Microscopically, the tumors are very cellular and do not contain regions of hemorrhage or necrosis. Local invasion of adjacent loops of bowel may occur. Symptoms are variable. In one study, 6 of 8 newborns had obstruction and 3 of 8 had perforation.[5] Perforation, in the newborn, may cause meconium peritonitis.[2] In another literature review of 12 patients, 4 patients had perforation. Obstruction was the most common symptom.[2]

Imaging shows the presence of a mass related to the bowel. An insufficient number of children have been reported to permit any comparison between various imaging techniques. Barium studies may show ulceration, obstruction, or a mass lesion[6] (see Figs. 3–19 and 3–20). Ultrasound may show the mass, but ultrasound imaging may be hindered by the presence of bowel gas. CT will show a mass lesion closely related to the bowel (see Fig. 3–19). The utilization of adequate amounts of oral contrast is extremely important. There are no specific features to suggest the correct diagnosis, and the final diagnosis is made following surgery. In many children presenting with acute symptoms of obstruction or perforation, the diagnosis may be made initially at surgery without any imaging of the tumor being performed apart from an abdominal radiograph.

Treatment is wide surgical resection and the prognosis in children is very good[1] in the absence of metastases.[3]

References

1. Angerpointner TA, Weitz H, Haas RJ, et al. Intestinal leiomyosarcoma in childhood—case report and review of the literature. J Pediatr Surg 1981;16:491–495.
2. Nagaya M, Tsuda M, Ishiguro Y. Leiomyosarcoma of the transverse colon in a neonate: a rare cause of meconium peritonitis. J Pediatr Surg 1989;24:1177–1180.
3. Lack EE. Leiomyosarcomas in childhood: a clinical and pathologic study of 10 cases. Pediatr Pathol 1986;6:181–197.
4. Dehner LP. Pediatric surgical pathology, 2nd ed. Baltimore: Williams & Wilkins, 1987:334–432.

A B C

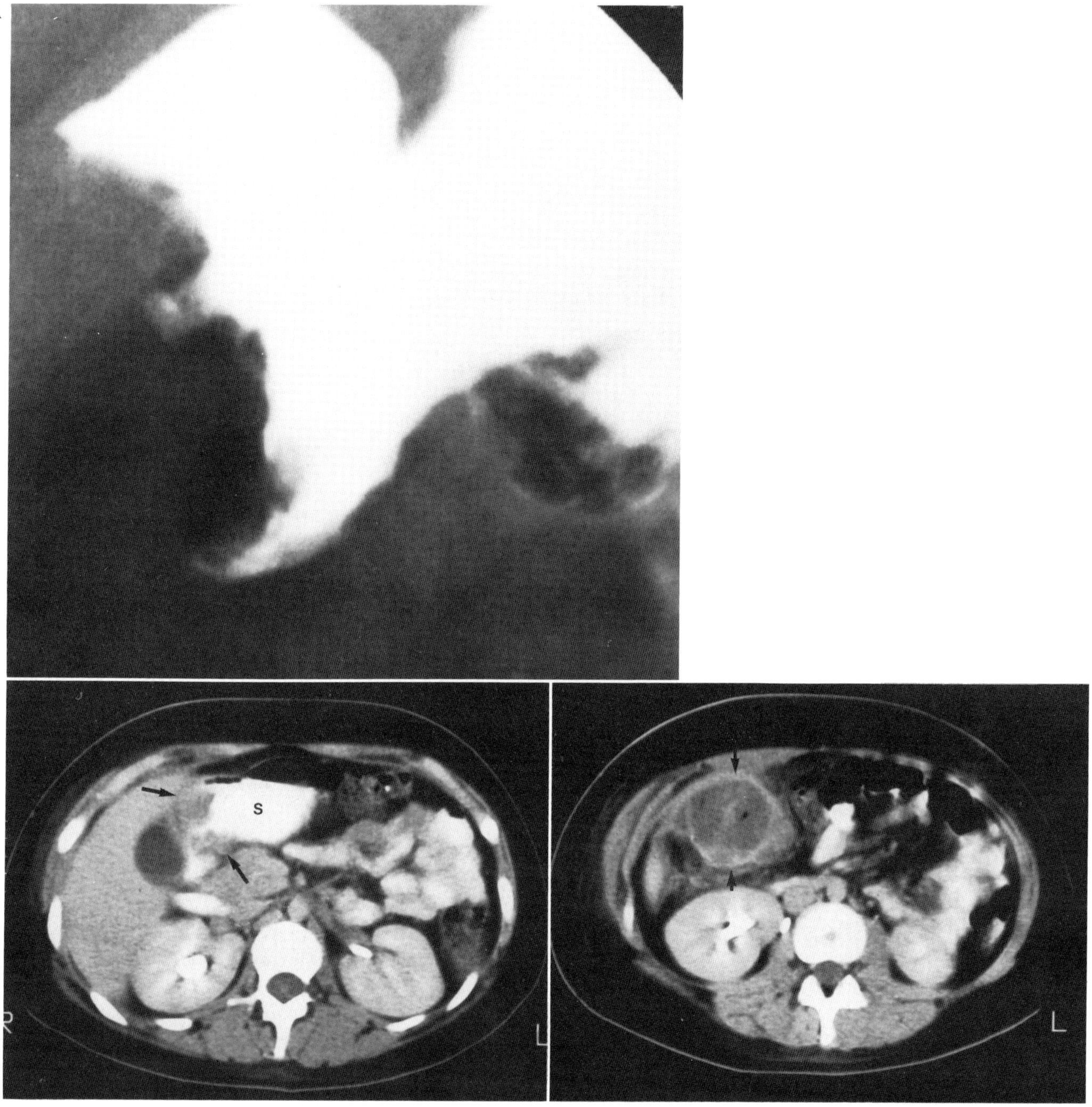

Figure 3–19. Diagnosis: Gastric leiomyosarcoma.
A, Barium study. There is a large mass obstructing the antrum. ***B,*** CT. Contrast is seen in the stomach (***S***). A mass *(arrows)* is seen causing almost complete obstruction to the antrum. ***C,*** CT image more inferior to ***B***. A large component of the tumor mass *(arrows)* is seen inferior to the gastric antrum.

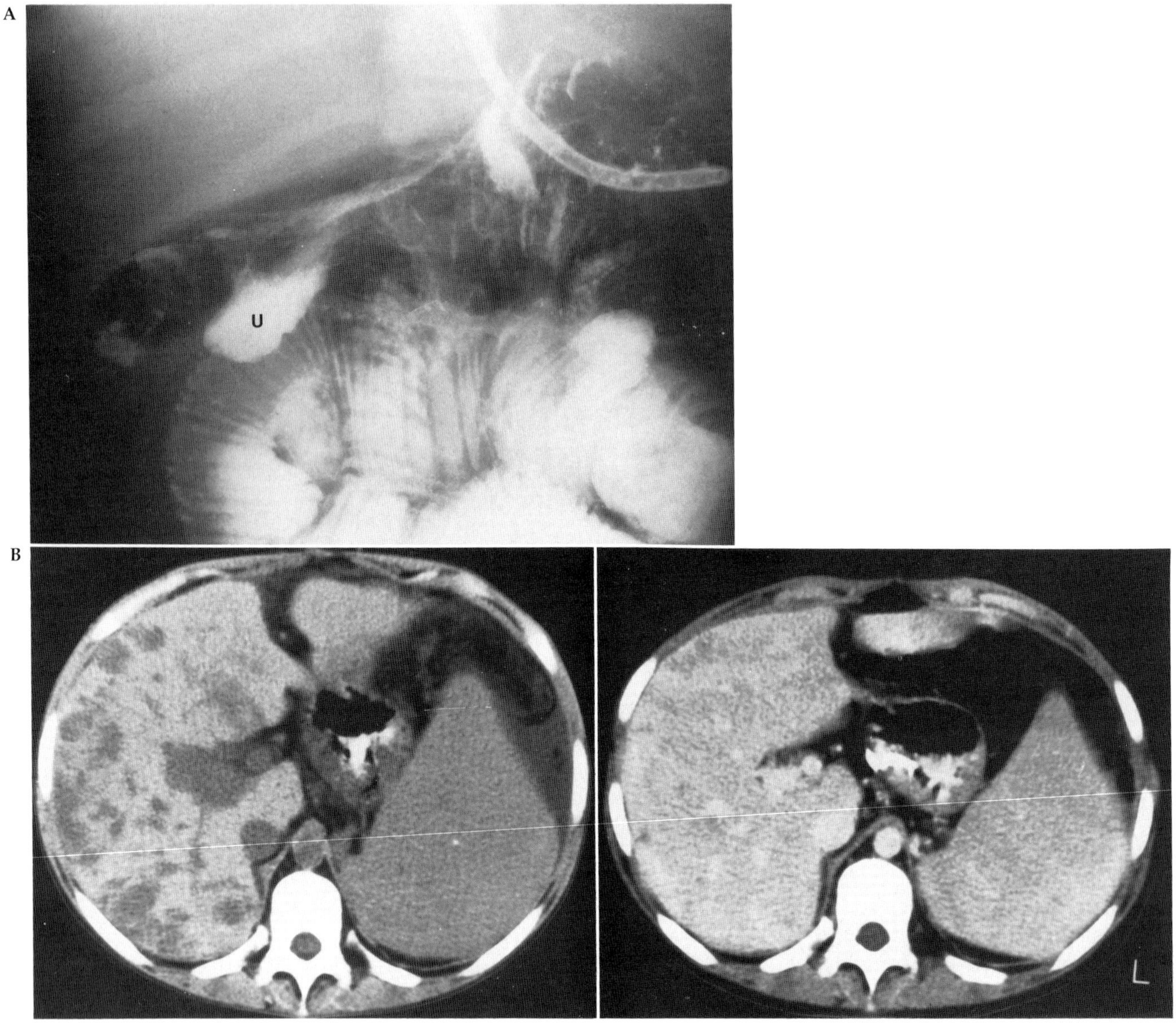

Figure 3–20. Diagnosis: Gastric leiomyosarcoma with liver metastases.
A, Barium study. There is a very large antral ulcer (*U*). ***B*** and ***C***, CT images obtained 5 years later without and with IV contrast. Multiple liver metastases are present. The lesions are much easier to visualize on the noncontrast enhanced scan.

5. Posen JA, Bar-Maor JA. Leiomyosarcoma of the colon in an infant. Cancer 1983;52:1458–1461.
6. Mahour GH, Isaacs H, Chang L. Primary malignant tumors of the stomach in children. J Pediatr Surg 1980;15:603–608.

INTESTINAL ADENOCARCINOMA

The vast majority of adenocarcinomas of the bowel in children occur in the colon and rectum, but they can occasionally occur at other sites (Fig. 3–21). Two cases have been described of adenocarcinoma in the stomach.[1] One patient developed an adenocarcinoma in the lower end of the esophagus 20 years after repair of esophageal atresia[2] (Fig. 3–22). Etiology in this patient was believed to be chronic reflux esophagitis. A literature review identified 15 cases of carcinoma of the stomach in children.[3] Adenocarcinoma was identified in the ileum in one 12-year-old child.[4] In the colon, most adenocarcinomas are spontaneous.[5] There is an increased incidence of adenocarcinoma in patients with ulcerative colitis or familial polyposis, but most of these people do not develop their tumors until they are outside the pediatric age range.[5,6] The risk of developing malignancy with colon polyps is high with familial adenomatous colonic polyps and with Gardner's syndrome. There is a small risk of carcinoma in Peutz-Jeghers syndrome, and an extremely low risk of malignancy with juvenile polyps.[5] Sites of metastasis include local lymph nodes, liver, and lung.[7]

Figure 3–21. **Diagnosis: Malignant gastric ulcer. Barium study. There is a large ulcer cavity, filled with barium, in the proximal part of the lesser curve of the stomach. Biopsy is required to make the final diagnosis. (From Hill R. Malignant gastroduodenal ulceration in children. Med J Pediatr Hematol/Oncol 1988; 10:109–111.)**

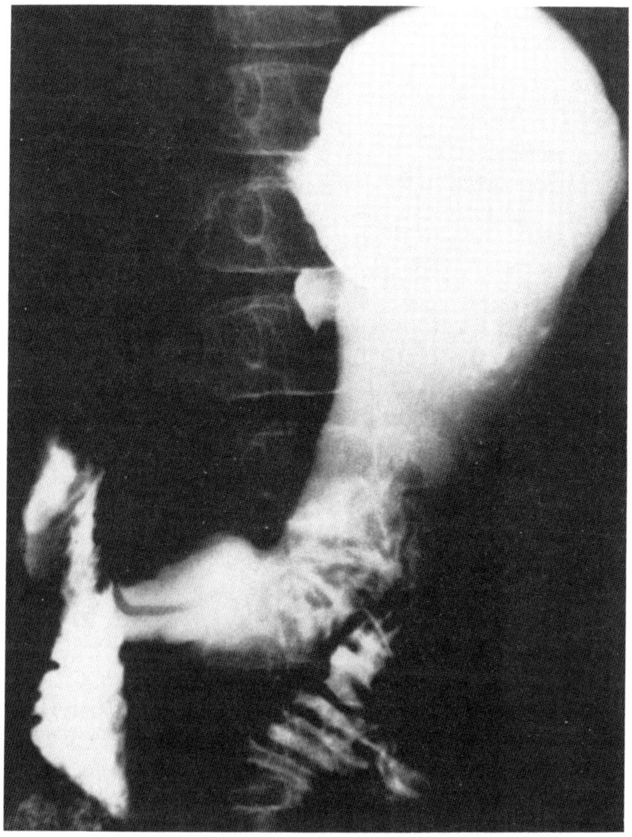

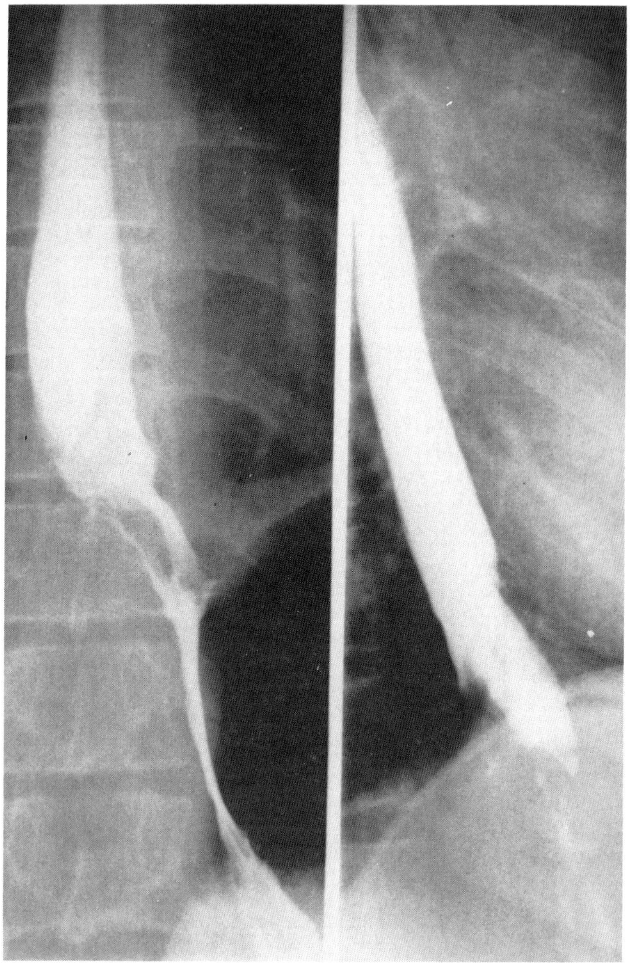

Figure 3–22. **Diagnosis: Adenocarcinoma of the esophagus. Barium study. There is a ragged intraluminal lesion seen in the lower esophagus. The lumen is narrowed and there is ulceration. (From Adzic KS, Fisher JH, Winter HS, et al. Esophageal adenocarcinoma 20 years after esophageal atresia repair. J Pediatr Surg 1989; 24:741–744.)**

Most children with adenocarcinoma of the colon are over the age of 10 years.[5] In a presentation of 11 patients and a literature review of an additional 212 patients, it was established that the rectosigmoid area was the most common location for these tumors.[8] Acute bowel obstruction is the most common symptom.[8] Other symptoms include hemorrhage, pain, intussusception, weight loss, or megacolon.[5,8]

A

B

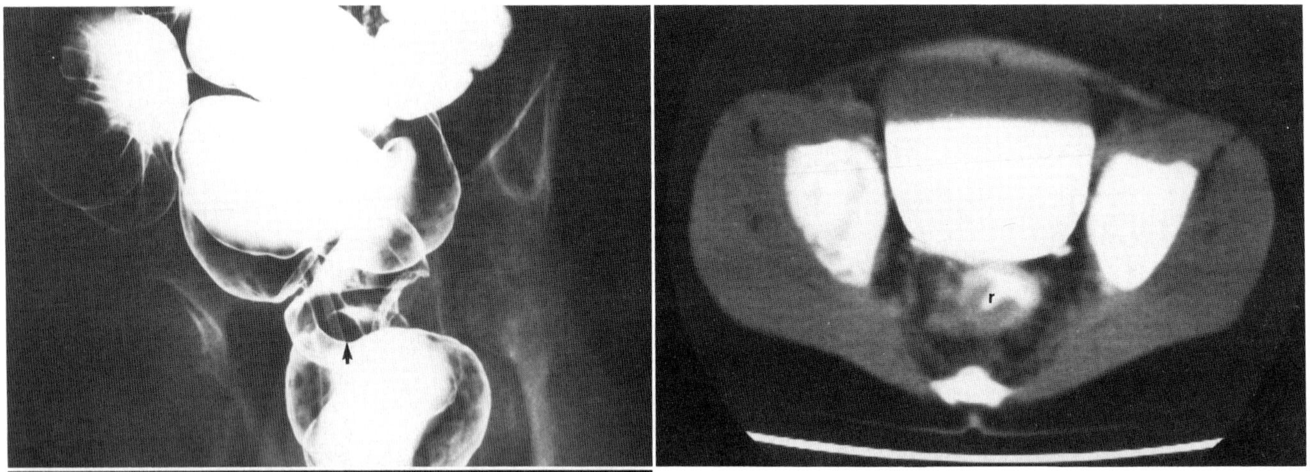

C

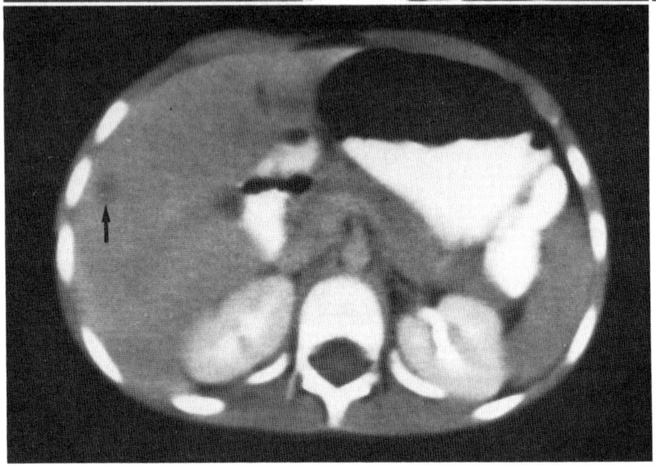

Figure 3–23. **Diagnosis: Adenocarcinoma of the rectum. *A*, There is a large polypoid mass lesion *(arrow)* in the rectum. *B*, CT. The tumor is causing marked narrowing of the lumen of the rectum (*R*). *C*, CT of liver. A low-intensity metastatic lesion is seen in the right lobe *(arrow).***

Figure 3–24. **Diagnosis: Adenocarcinoma of the rectum. Barium enema. There is a large mass lesion with ulceration *(arrow).* (From Torloni H. Colorectal adenocarcinoma in childhood and adolescence. Pediatr Radiol 1989; 19:504–508.)**

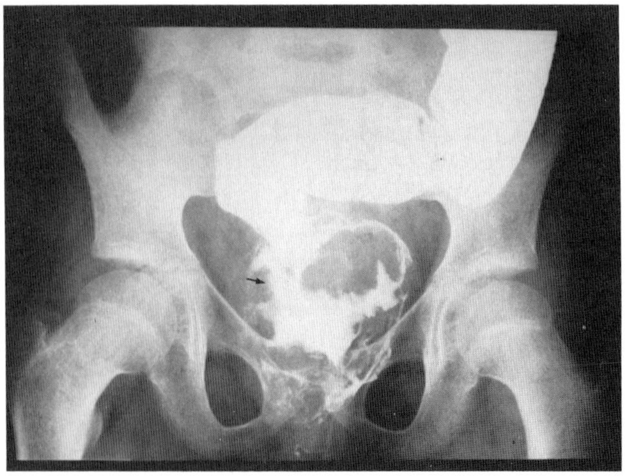

Histologically, the tumors are mostly mucinous (50 percent)[5]. Metastases occur to any site in the abdomen, lung, and brain.[8]

Macroscopically, the tumors tend to be an eccentric mass,[5,8] but they can encircle and constrict the bowel. The tumors, in up to 50 percent of patients, are diagnosed at the time of laparotomy.[8] This is because of the common presentation with acute symptoms. When imaging is performed, ultrasound usually shows a mass of low echoes. There may be areas of increased echogenicity from calcium or mucin.[6] Barium studies will show a mass lesion with possible ulceration (Figs. 3–23 and 3–24). Concentric narrowing of the bowel may be identified. CT shows similar findings with more accurate definition of the extent of the tumor beyond the wall of the bowel.

Treatment of these tumors is predominantly surgical. Compared to adults, the tumors are much more likely to be mucinous, inoperable at diagnosis, and to have a poor prognosis.[5,8] The differential diagnosis is large and includes other tumors such as leiomyosarcoma, teratoma, or rhabdomyosarcoma. Occasionally, a duplication cyst containing a large amount of hemorrhage may mimic a tumor. In the stomach, an inflammatory pseudotumor will mimic a malignancy.[9] These pseudotumors have the same pathology as pseudotumors in the lung. They are large mass lesions frequently containing hemorrhage and necrosis. On ultrasound, they are echogenic and on CT they are irregular, large, and may show loculated collections of air or contrast outside the stomach caused by perforation.

References

1. Angerpointer TA, Weitz H, Haas RJ, et al. Intestinal leiomyosarcoma in childhood—case report and review of the literature. J Pediatr Surg 1981;16:491–495.
2. Adzick NS, Fisher JH, Winter HS, et al. Esophageal adenocarcinoma 20 years after esophageal atresia repair. J Pediatr Surg 1989;24:741–744.
3. Goto S, Ikeda K, Ishii E, et al. Carcinoma of the stomach in a 7 year old boy. Z Kinderchir 1984;39:137–140.
4. Tankel JW, Galasko CSB. Adenocarcinoma of small bowel in a 12 year old girl. J Roy Soc Med 1984;77:693–694.
5. Dehner LP. Pediatric surgical pathology, 2nd ed. Baltimore: Williams & Wilkins, 1987:334–432.
6. King RM, Telander RL, Smithson WA, et al. primary mediastinal tumors in children. J Pediatr Surg 1982;17:512–520.
7. Mahour GH, Isaacs H, Chang L. Primary malignant tumors of the stomach in children. J Pediatr Surg 1980;15:603–608.
8. Lamego CMB, Torloni H. Colorectal adenocarcinoma in childhood and adolescent. Report of 11 cases and review of the literature. Pediatr Radiol 1989;19:504–508.
9. Maves CK, Johnson JF, Bove K, et al. Gastric inflammatory pseudotumor in children. Radiology 1989;173:381–383.

CARCINOID

Carcinoid tumors arise from neural crest tumors. They may be classified by their anatomic location of origin into three types[1]:

1. Foregut (including bronchus, stomach and, pancreas).
2. Midgut.
3. Hindgut.

In children, most carcinoid tumors occur in the appendix[2] and are usually not diagnosed preoperatively, with the children presenting as suspected appendicitis. In the appendix, the tumors are usually small. The tumor is much more common in females than in males and most children are in the age range of 8 to 15 years. The treatment is surgical resection and prognosis is excellent.

References

1. Hanson MW, Feldman JM, Blinder RA, et al. Carcinoid tumors: Iodine-131 MIBG scintigraphy. Radiology 1989; 172:699–703.
2. Jonsson T, Johannsson JH, Hallgrimsson JG. Carcinoid tumors of the appendix in children younger than 16 years. Acta Chir Scan 1989;155:113–116.

CHAPTER 4
GENITOURINARY TUMORS

WILMS TUMOR

Wilms tumor is truly intriguing from the radiologist's viewpoint. In the past 20 years, there have been dramatic changes in the therapy and prognosis of Wilms tumor, together with a fascinating unfolding of a subclassification of the pathology of this tumor and, most important, its correlation with prognosis. This tumor illustrates, perhaps better than any other tumor, the need for the radiologic approach to pediatric cancer to be flexible and to respond to the changing biology of Wilms tumor.

Epidemiology

Wilms tumor occurs with an incidence of 7.8 cases per million children under the age of 15 years each year.[1] This translates to approximately 450 new cases of Wilms tumor each year in the United States. There is no sex or race predilection.

Wilms tumor is a disease of young children. The age distribution at the time of initial presentation is given in Table 4–1. As can be seen, over 85 percent of children will present under the age of 6 years. The mean age of presentation is 3½ years.[2] Children with bilateral tumors and children in whom there is an association with a coexisting congenital disorder tend to present at a younger age.[1,3]

> *Comment:* Knowledge of the age of onset and knowledge of the age of presentation of Wilms tumor is particularly important when planning the duration of imaging screening for Wilms tumors in high-risk patients.

There are some genetic and familial associations of Wilms tumor. Some patients have been found to have a deletion of the P-13 part of chromosome 11[4]; there is an increased expression of the N myc oncogene in Wilms tumor; and there is a mild familial incidence.[5,6]

The occurrence of Wilms tumor is associated with a number of different congenital anomalies. Up to 12 percent of patients have some such association. These associations are important, since decisions need to be made as to which patients at increased risk for the development of Wilms tumor need to be routinely screened with imaging. Genitourinary anomalies, hemihypertrophy, and aniridia are the three most common anomalies having an increased incidence of Wilms tumor[7] (Table 4–2). Genitourinary anomalies are frequently hypospadias and cryptorchidism.[8,9] Genitourinary anomalies are common, and the incidence of Wilms tumor in these patients is low, so that it is not cer-

TABLE 4–1
Wilms Tumor: Age Distribution at Time of Diagnosis

Age (Years)	Percentage
<1	14
2	15
4	32
6	24
10	14
>10	1

TABLE 4–2
Incidence of the Three Most Common Associated Abnormalities in Patients with Wilms Tumor[1,2]

Abnormality	Percentage of Patients
Genitourinary anomalies	4.4
Hemihypertrophy	2.9
Aniridia	1.0

References
1. Belasco J, D'Angio GJ. Wilms' tumor. Ca-A Cancer J for Clinicians 1981;31:258–270.
2. Palmer N, Evans AE. The association of aniridia and Wilms' tumor: methods of surveillance and diagnosis. Med Pediatr Oncol 1983;11:73–75.

tain that every child with a congenital genitourinary anomaly should be screened for development of Wilms tumor. Hemihypertrophy is overgrowth of one side of the body. It is a very rare anomaly. Three percent of children with hemihypertrophy do develop Wilms tumor.[1,10–12] These children may develop the Wilms tumor on either side of the body[13]; they have no increased incidence of bilateral tumors[13]; and it is important to note that they also have an increased incidence of liver and adrenal cortical tumors.[1,14] Children with Beckwith syndrome (macroglossia, organomegaly, exomphalos, and sometimes hemihypertrophy) have a 10 percent chance of developing some tumor,[14,15] of which Wilms tumor is the most common. Aniridia may be hereditary or sporadic. Wilms tumor is only increased in children with bilateral sporadic aniridia, and these tumors are often bilateral.[1] Thirty-three percent of children with sporadic aniridia will develop Wilms tumor.[13] Other congenital anomalies associated with Wilms tumor include the Drash syndrome (male pseudohermaphrodite, glomerulonephritis)[8,9] Bloom syndrome (decreased growth, decreased immunity, facial telangiectasia),[16] imperforate anus and rectourethral fistula,[17] horseshoe kidney,[18,19] and trisomy 18.[20]

> *Comment:* Recognition of the association of Wilms tumor with certain congenital anomalies is important, as these children can be screened prospectively to facilitate early tumor diagnosis.

Wilms tumor occurs in both kidneys in up to 13 percent of patients[13,21] (Table 4–3). Bilateral tumors are most commonly synchronous[13] but can be metachronous (the second tumor is diagnosed later). Children at special risk for the development of bilateral tumors can be identified. These children tend to be younger,[1,3,13] have an increased incidence of associated congenital anomalies possibly as high as 60 percent,[1,8,13,22] more often have a history of familial Wilms tumors,[13] and almost invariably have the kidneys affected with nephroblastomatosis.[1] It is believed that the incidence of diagnosis of metachronous tumors is decreasing, probably because many subclinical metachronous tumors are being cured by chemotherapy without being clinically diagnosed.[11]

> *Comment:* Bilateral Wilms tumors occur. The opposite kidney must be observed for tumor development.

TABLE 4–3
Bilateral Wilms Tumor

Occurs in up to 12% of cases
Can be synchronous or metachronous
Younger age than unilateral Wilms
All have neprhogenic rests

References

1. Mesrobian H-GJ. Wilms tumor: past, present, future. J Urol 1988;140:231–238.
2. Ugarte N, Gonzalez-Crussi F, Hsueh W. Wilms' tumor: its morphology in patients under one year of age. Cancer 1981;48:346–353.
3. Wikstrom S, Parkkulainen KV, Louhimo I. Bilateral Wilms' tumor and secondary malignancies. J Pediatr Surg 1982;17:269–272.
4. Heideman RL, McGavran L, Waldstein G. Nephroblastomatosis and deletion of 11p. The potential etiologic relationship to subsequent Wilms' tumor. Am J Pediatr Hematol/Oncol 1986;8:231–234.
5. Shaw AP, Poirier V, Tyler S, et al. Expression of the N-myc oncogene in Wilms' tumour and related tissues. Oncogene 1988;3:143–149.
6. Cordero JF, Li FP, Holmes LB, et al. Wilms tumor in five cousins. Pediatrics 1980;66:716–719.
7. Belasco J, D'Angio GJ. Wilms' tumor. Ca-A Cancer J for Clinicians 1981;31:258–270.
8. Boechat MI, Kangarloo H. MR imaging in Drash Syndrome. J Comput Assist Tomogr 1988;12:405–408.
9. Goldman SM, Garfinkel DJ, Oh KS, et al. The Drash syndrome: male pseudohermaphroditism, nephritis, and Wilms tumor. Radiology 1981;141:87–91.
10. Hutson JM, Kent M, Ekert H, et al. The treatment of Wilms' tumor: results from Royal Children's Hospital, Melbourne, 1967–1977. J Pediatr Surg 1983;18:235–239.
11. Casale AJ, Flanigan RC, Moore PJ, et al. Survival in bilateral metachronous (asynchronous) Wilms tumors. J Urol 1982;128:766–769.
12. Tolchin D, Koenigsberg M, Santorineou M. Early detection of Wilms' tumor in a child with hemihypertrophy and ovarian cysts. Pediatrics 1982;70:135–136.
13. Bond JV. Bilateral Wilms' tumour: age at diagnosis, associated congenital anomalies, and possible pattern of inheritance. Lancet 1975;2:482–486.
14. Tank ES, Kay R. Neoplasms associated with hemihypertrophy, Beckwith-Wiedemann syndrome and aniridia. J Urol 1980;124:266–268.
15. Wojciechowski AH, Pritchard J. Beckwith-Wiedemann (exomphalos-macroglossia-gigantism-EMG) syndrome and malignant lymphoma. Eur J Pediatr 1981;137:317–321.
16. Cairney AEL, Andrews M, Greenberg M, et al. Wilms tumor in three patients with Bloom syndrome. J Pediatr 1987;111:414–417.
17. Early CK, Rosen D, Mirza M. The coexistence of Wilms' tumor and imperforate anus with rectourethral fistula. J Pediatr Surg 1981;16:756–757.
18. Gay BB, Dawes RK, Atkinson GO, et al. Wilms tumor in horseshoe kidneys: radiologic diagnosis. Radiology 1983;146:693–697.
19. Mesrobian H-GJ, Kelalis PP, Hrabovsky E, et al. Wilms tumor in horseshoe kidneys: a report from the National Wilms Tumor Study. J Urol 1985;133:1002–1003.
20. Karay J. Wilms' tumor in a 13-year-old girl with trisomy 18. Am J Dis Child 1981;135:665–666.
21. Ragab AH, Vietti TJ, Crist W, et al. Bilateral Wilms' tumor. A review. Cancer 1972;30:983–988.
22. Garrett RA, Donahue JR. Bilateral Wilms tumor. J Urol 1978;120:586–588.

Pathology

Wilms tumors are usually very large at the time of diagnosis. The mean weight of the whole specimen of tumor plus kidney was 572 gm in the NWTS-II study (the normal kidney weighs only 24 gm at birth and 100 gm at 3 years).[1] Only 65 of 390 tumors weighed less than 250 gm.[1] The large size of these tumors means that diagnosis is being made late. Grossly, these tumors are well defined, but they are friable and easy to tear, which may result in tumor spillage into the peritoneum during surgery. This is important, as it alters the tumor stage. On cut section, areas of hemorrhage and necrosis within the tumor are commonly identified.[2,3] There is no good correlation between the tumor size and the amount of necrosis identified.[4] The areas of necrosis may liquefy completely and therefore appear cystic on imaging studies. The tumors tend to arise peripherally in the kidney and spare the renal collecting system. This accounts for the relatively low incidence of gross hematuria clinically, and for the low incidence of nonfunction of the kidney on imaging studies. In horseshoe kidneys, the tumor can occur at any location, including the isthmus.[1] Isthmus lesions are easily missed on ultrasound and intravenous pyelography (IVP) studies.[5]

> *Comment:* The gross appearance and location of Wilms tumor explains many clinical and imaging findings.

Meticulous evaluation of tumor histology in over 2,000 patients enrolled in national Wilms tumor studies by Beckwith and other workers has yielded interesting information (Table 4–4). It is no longer adequate to make the diagnosis of Wilms tumor; an accurate identification of subtypes of histology must be made. The prognosis is directly related to this. Implications for imaging are that the various subtypes of Wilms tumor have distinct patterns of metastasis so that with knowledge of the histologic subtype, cost-effective follow-up imaging can be performed.

The classic Wilms is a triphasic tumor showing elements of primitive blastema, stroma, and epithelial cells.[6] All three cell lines do not have to be present to make the diagnosis of Wilms tumor.[6] Focal or diffuse areas of anaplasia may be present. These are much more common in patients over the age of 2 years.[6,7] Because Wilms tumor arises from primitive blastema, a variety of tissues not normally found in the kidney may be identified in Wilms tumor. This includes fat, muscle, and cartilage.[6] Some workers have used the term teratoid Wilms tumor to describe tumors in which an exceptionally large amount of some of the above tissues were present.[8–10] These probably do not represent a true subgroup of Wilms tumors, but it is of interest that in the six cases reported,[8–11] there was a very high incidence of bilateral tumors and of tumor involvement of the renal pelvis with obstructive hydronephrosis. Beckwith[6] stresses that none of these tumors should be called a true teratoma and says that a teratoma must be diagnosed only in the presence of formation of actual ectopic organs. Such tumors are extremely rare. Clear-cell sarcoma and rhabdoid tumor of the kidney have been included in many series as subgroups of Wilms tumor. The modern trend is to designate these as distinct tumors, and they are, therefore, discussed separately. It is very important, however, to note that in the National Wilms Tumor Studies I, II, and III, these tumors have been included and the term unfavorable histology is used to designate Wilms tumors with either anaplasia, a clear cell, or a rhabdoid histology.

TABLE 4–4
Histology of Wilms Tumors

- Arise from primitive metanephric blastema
- May contain tissues not normally found in the kidney
- Prognosis is very strongly related to histology
- Needle biopsy may miss focal areas of unfavorable histology
- Clear cell and rhabdoid tumors should no longer be considered Wilms tumors

> *Comment:* Knowledge of tumor histology is critical for planning imaging studies. Identification of nonrenal tissues, such as fat, in the tumor should not preclude the diagnosis of Wilms tumor.

Nephroblastomatosis is a term that can cause confusion. The development of the fetal kidney is normally complete by 36 weeks gestation, so that the kidneys of normal newborn infants do not contain any embryonal renal tissue.[12] Nephroblastomatosis refers to the presence of embryonal renal tissue in kidneys after birth (Fig. 4–1).[7] Many terms such as nephrogenic rests and persistent nodular blastema have been utilized to describe this phenomenon, but the term nephroblastomatosis is probably the most widely accepted. The importance of nephroblastomatosis is its association with Wilms tumor. It is seen in less than 1 percent of normal perinatal autopsies[7] but occurs in 25 to 40 percent of patients with unilateral Wilms tumor and almost 100 percent of patients with bilateral Wilms tumor.[13] The development of Wilms tumor in patients with previously identified nephroblastomatosis has been clearly defined.[14,15] Nephroblastomatosis is extremely prevalent in patients with hemihypertrophy.[16,17]

In a review of the subject in 1990, Beckwith[18] redefined the terminology of nephroblastomatosis. The suggested generic term for the persistent renal blastema is nephrogenic rests. These rests are now classified as focal perilobar, focal intralobar, or diffuse. Both the focal perilobar and intralobar types are found equally in kidneys resected with Wilms tumor. Their presence in such a resected kidney indicates the increased likelihood of subsequent development of a second tumor in the opposite kidney. Beckwith studied 282 kidneys with Wilms

A B

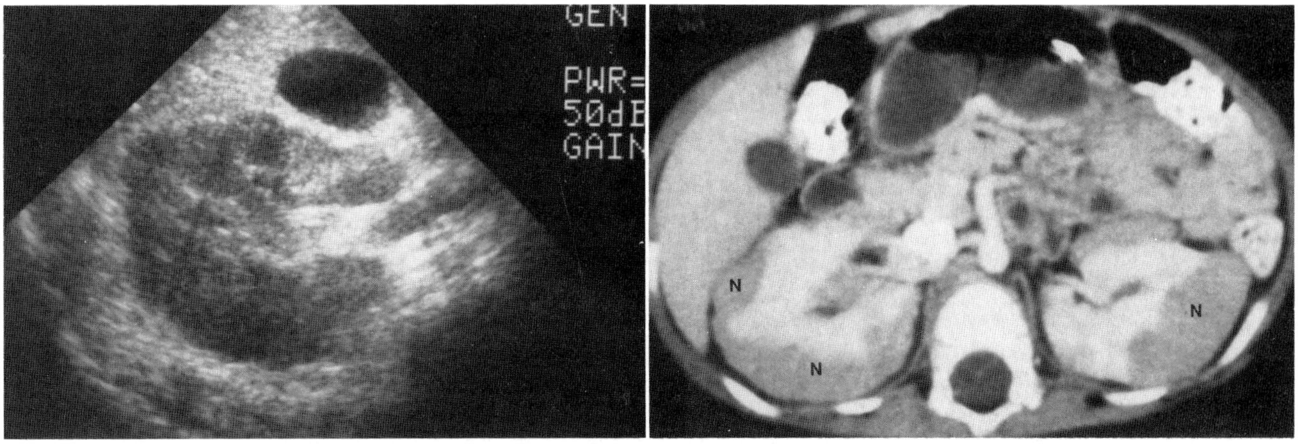

Figure 4–1. **Diagnosis: Diffuse nephrogenic rests (nephroblastomatosis).** ***A,*** **Ultrasound. The kidney is enlarged. Corticomedullary differentiation is lost. No clear focal lesions are identified. There are no specific diagnostic features to make the correct diagnosis.** ***B,*** **CT after intravenous contrast. The nephrogenic rests (*N*) appear as low-intensity regions distributed diffusely in the subcapsular regions of both kidneys. They enhance much less than the normal kidney tissue. (From Fernbach S. Fatty Wilms tumor stimulating teratoma. Pediatr Radio 1988;18:424–426.)**

tumor. Nephrogenic rests were definitely identified in 28 percent and were probably present in an additional 12 percent of these kidneys.[18] In normal kidneys obtained from infant postmortems, perilobar rests are seen in less than 1 percent and intralobar rests even less often. Beckwith suggested the term nephroblastomatosis be used to describe kidneys with multiple focal or diffuse nephrogenic rests. Beckwith further defines specific associations with nephrogenic rests. Intralobar rests are associated with tumors in younger patients, metachronous bilateral Wilms tumors, aniridia, and the Drash syndrome. Perilobar rests are associated with an increased incidence of synchronous bilateral Wilms tumors, hemihypertrophy, and Beckwith syndrome. Focal nephrogenic rests are usually fairly well defined and poorly vascular. Therefore, they do not enhance with intravenous contrast injection on CT scan. Diffuse nephroblastomatosis may cause massive kidney enlargement, with one reported case of kidney length of 22 cm in a 13-year-old child.[19] This age is unusual, since most children with diffuse bilateral nephroblastomatosis are usually under 1 year of age.[19] This disorder causes marked displacement of the calyces, and the appearance may be mistaken for polycystic renal disease on imaging.

Beckwith[18] concludes that the clinical implications of the findings of nephrogenic rests are:

1. Most rests do not develop into tumors, so that routine removal of focal large rests or routine chemotherapy, once rests have been identified, is not required.
2. Surgical exploration of the kidney cannot identify tumor development in nephrogenic rests. It also surveys only the surface of the kidney and cannot identify the presence of intralobar rests.
3. Imaging is the best and only way to follow patients with nephrogenic rests. Tumor is diagnosed by the identification of enlargement of a nephrogenic rest.
4. Because of the risk of developing subsequent additional Wilms tumors, kidney-saving surgery, rather than nephrectomy, may become more important in the management of children with Wilms tumors and nephrogenic rests.

> *Comment:* Recognition of nephrogenic rests is important because of the significant development of Wilms tumor in affected kidneys.

Multilocular cystic nephroma is a distinct entity, which must, however, be considered with Wilms tumor. This is a solitary well-defined renal mass composed of a number of well-defined cystic lesions. These lesions may be completely benign, may have partly differentiated blastema in their walls, or may have true triphasic Wilms histology tissue present.[20] They are discussed later in more detail. It is important to differentiate multilocular cystic nephroma from cystic degeneration and hemorrhagic necrosis occurring within a preexisting solid Wilms tumor. Differential features for multilocular cystic nephroma are given in Table 4–5.

Wilms tumor can spread locally via a variety of pathways. Penetration of the capsule is not uncommon, and as this may frequently only be microscopic it can be very difficult or impossible to identify by imaging. If the tumor penetrates the capsule completely, local invasion into the tail of pancreas, psoas muscle, diaphragm, splenic hilum, or porta hepatis can occur.[3] Preoperative identification of invasion of these tissues is helpful. Growth into the mesentery and bowel is extremely rare.[3] Within the kidney, growth into the calyces and renal pelvis is uncommon,[3] but growth into intrarenal vessels is common.

The tumor may also spread by contiguous growth into the renal vein and then into the inferior vena cava

TABLE 4–5
Differential Features of Multilocular Cystic Nephroma[1]

Multicystic Dysplastic Kidney	Multilocular Cystic Nephroma	Polycystic Kidney
Involves entire kidney	Well-defined single cluster of cysts	Diffuse distribution of cysts
No normal parenchyma	No renal parenchyma between cysts (rest of kidney is normal)	Have renal tissue between cysts
Other genitourinary anomalies	No associated anomalies	Associated cysts in other organs

Reference

1. Christ ML. Polycystic nephroblastoma. J Urol 1968;98:570–571.

(Table 4–6). Inferior vena caval extension of tumor was identified in 6 percent of 921,[15] 7 percent of 606,[3] and 4.1 percent of 1,865[21] patients. Three percent of these patients will have extension into the heart.[15] The tumor is usually localized within the right atrium but may extend through the tricuspid valve into the right ventricular outflow tract, causing obstruction. In these cases, tricuspid valve function is also abnormal. Growth through an atrial septal defect has also been described. Frequently unappreciated is the fact that tumor can invade into tributaries of the inferior vena cava, including the gonadal, adrenal, and hepatic veins. Such invasion has caused Budd Chiari syndrome.[22] Invasion can also occur into the renal vein of the opposite kidney.[23] Extension inferiorly, below the level of the renal veins, is not uncommon.[24] IVC extension can occur from either right- or left-sided tumors.[21] The tumor may invade the wall of the inferior vena cava,[21] which will make extraction difficult. Such invasion has not been identified preoperatively. The invading tumor very rarely causes occlusion of the inferior vena cava, so that clinical symptoms of caval extension of tumor are uncommon and heavy reliance is placed on imaging to identify this extension.

> *Comment:* Accurate imaging identification of local spread of Wilms tumor is very important, as it determines the surgical approach to the tumor. For example, identification of tumor in the right atrium would probably require cardiac by-pass surgery, while identification of retrohepatic caval tumor requires a combined thoracoabdominal rather than a simple abdominal approach.

Sites of metastatic spread of Wilms tumor are predictable and few, and knowledge of this greatly aids planning of imaging studies. Wilms tumors with favorable histology metastasize predominantly to the lung, sometimes to the liver, and extremely rarely to other sites. Of 236 stage IV NWTS patients between 1969 and 1983 who had metastases in either the lung or the liver, the liver alone was involved in 17 patients. Two hundred patients had metastases in the lung alone and the remaining 19 had lesions in both the liver and the lung.[25] Dural spread of Wilms tumor has been described.[26] It may or may not involve the adjacent bone, and the mechanism of spread may be direct or hematogenous. Bone metastases are seen only in patients with clear-cell histology tumors.[27] The rhabdoid tumors metastasize predominantly to the brain but can also metastasize to bone.[28] These two tumors are discussed in more detail separately. Spread to local lymph nodes in the hilum of the kidney and in the periaortic lymph node chain is quite common. Identification of enlargement of these lymph nodes does not, however, always indicate the presence of tumor, and histological confirmation is required in all cases.

TABLE 4–6
Inferior Vena Cava Spread of Wilms Tumor[1–3]

Approximately 6% of cases	
Can go below renal veins	
Can invade tributaries of renal veins	
Can invade wall of inferior vena cava	
Can extend to heart	
Superior level of extension	
Right atrium	21%
Retrohepatic inferior vena cava	18%
Infrahepatic inferior vena cava	61%

References

1. Ritchey ML, Kelalis PP, Breslow N, et al. Intracaval and atrial involvement with nephroblastoma: review of National Wilms Tumor Study–3. J Urol 1988;140:1113–1118.
2. Exelby PR. Retroperitoneal malignant tumors: Wilms' tumor and neuroblastoma. Surg Clin N Am 1981;61:1219–1227.
3. Mesrobian H-GJ. Wilms tumor: past, present, future. J Urol 1988;140:231–238.

Spread of tumor into the mediastinum, either by hematogenous metastases or direct invasion through the diaphragm, is recognized is some patients. Identification of mediastinal tumor frequently indicates a very poor prognosis.

Although early reports[29] considered the presence of tumor in the opposite kidney to be a metastasis, the overwhelming evidence and consensus at the present time is that tumor in the opposite kidney represents a second, independent primary tumor.[30]

> *Comment:* Imaging evaluation of Wilms tumors with favorable histology, for metastatic spread, can be confined to the chest and abdomen.

The staging of Wilms tumor depends on information provided by imaging, surgery, and histology. Note that the categorization into stage I, II, III, or IV does not depend on the presence or absence of favorable or unfavorable histology. The most current staging system is seen in Table 4–7. The most important change from previous staging systems is that the presence of any tumor in hilar or more distal lymph nodes automatically classifies the person as stage III. In earlier classifications, resection of hilar or periaortic lymph nodes with tumor resulted in stage II classification. With the present classification, surgery has the role of identifying local spread of tumor and also of selecting lymph nodes for histology (widespread lymph node dissection is not performed). Imaging guides the surgeon in detection of local tumor spread and potential involved lymph nodes and is the main method of identification of distant metastatic spread. Histology confirms the presence of tumor in biopsied material and is the only method for detection of microscopic tumor spread through the capsule (which indicates stage II). The stage at the time of diagnosis for the NWTS-II and NWTS-III studies is given in Table 4–8. Despite the fact that Wilms tumors are very large at the time of presentation, the number of patients with distant metastatic spread (stage IV) is small and represents only 12 percent of all cases.

> *Comment:* Radiology is important in tumor staging. It cannot be used alone, and surgical and histological confirmation of imaging findings are required. In patients with Wilms tumor, accurate staging is impossible unless surgery is performed prior to the administration of any chemotherapy or radiation therapy.

Extrarenal Wilms tumor does occur (Fig. 4–2). There are a number of well-documented cases of Wilms tumor arising outside the kidneys.[31–35] The histology and be-

TABLE 4–7
Staging of Wilms Tumor[1]

I. Tumor limited to kidney and completely excised. The surface of the renal capsule is intact. Tumor was not ruptured before or during removal. There is no residual tumor apparent beyond the margins of resection.
II. Tumor extends beyond the kidney but is completely removed. There is regional extension of the tumor, e.g., penetration through the outer surface of the renal capsule into perirenal soft tissues. Vessels outside the kidney substance are infiltrated or contain tumor thrombus. The tumor may have been biopsied or there has been local spillage of tumor confined to the flank. There is no residual tumor apparent at or beyond the margins of excision.
III. Residual nonhematogenous tumor confined to abdomen. Any one or more of the following occur:
   A. Lymph nodes on biopsy are found to be involved in the hilus, the periaortic chains, or beyond.
   B. There has been diffuse peritoneal contamination by tumor such as by spillage of tumor beyond the flank before or during surgery, or by tumor growth that has penetrated through the peritoneal surface.
   C. Implants are found on the peritoneal surfaces.
   D. The tumor extends beyond the surgical margins either microscopically or grossly.
   E. The tumor is not completely resectable because of local infiltration into vital structures.
IV. Hematogenous metastases. Deposits beyond stage III; e.g., lung, liver, bone, and brain.
V. Bilateral renal involvement at diagnosis. An attempt should be made to stage each side according to the above criteria on the basis of extent of disease before biopsy.

Reference
1. D'Angio GJ, Breslow N, Beckwith JB, et al. Treatment of Wilms' tumor: results of the third National Wilms' Tumor Study. Cancer 1989;64:349–360.

TABLE 4–8
Stage at Time of Diagnosis of Wilms Tumor[1,2]

Stage	NWTS-III*		Stage	NWTS-II†	
I	Favorable histology	43%	I	All histology	37%
II	Favorable histology	19%	II	All histology	31%
III	Favorable histology	19%	III	All histology	20%
IV	Favorable histology	8%	IV	All histology	12%
I–III	Unfavorable histology	9%			
IV	Unfavorable histology	2%			

*There were 1,439 patients; 10% were stage IV, including favorable and unfavorable histology.

†There were 513 patients; 11.9% had unfavorable histology.

References

1. D'Angio GJ, Breslow N, Beckwith JB, et al. Treatment of Wilms' tumor: results of the third National Wilms' Tumor Study. Cancer 1989;64:349–360.
2. D'Angio GJ, Evans A, Breslow N, et al. The treatment of Wilms' tumor: results of the second National Wilms' Tumor Study. Cancer 1981;47:2302–2311.

havior of these tumors is the same as that seen in Wilms tumors arising in the kidney. The mean age at diagnosis is 4½ years.[35] These tumors arise most commonly in the retroperitoneum, sometimes in the pelvis or inguinal areas, and very occasionally in the chest. They have been reported to have associated congenital anomalies such as horseshoe kidney.[33] They may invade local tissues.[32] Some reports give a high incidence of an associated teratoma, while others feel that this is extremely uncommon.[35,36] Primary Wilms tumor in the spinal canal, sometimes associated with diastematomyelia, has also been reported (Fig. 4–2).

> *Comment:* Extrarenal Wilms tumors are very rare. They should, however, be included in the differential diagnosis of a mass lesion, particularly in the retroperitoneum or inguinal areas.

Tumor markers for Wilms tumor have not been as well identified as with neuroblastoma and hepatoblastoma. Although some factors such as renin[37] may be elevated in the serum of patients with Wilms tumor, this is not a consistent or a specific finding. The absence of a tumor marker makes imaging even more important in follow-up of patients with Wilms tumors.

References

1. D'Angio GJ, Evans A, Breslow N, et al. The treatment of Wilms' tumor: results of the second National Wilms' Tumor Study. Cancer 1981;47:2302–2311.
2. Reiman TAH, Siegel MJ, Shackelford GD. Wilms tumor in children: abdominal CT and US evaluation. Radiology 1986;160:501–505.
3. Exelby PR. Retroperitoneal malignant tumors: Wilms' tumor and neuroblastoma. Surg Clin N Am 1981; 61:1219–1227.
4. Gates GF, Miller JH, Stanley P. Necrosis of Wilms tumor. J Urol 1980;123:916–920.
5. Gay BB, Dawes RK, Atkinson GO, et al. Wilms tumor in horseshoe kidneys: radiologic diagnosis. Radiology 1983;146:693–697.
6. Beckwith JB. Wilms' tumor and other renal tumors of childhood: a selective review from the National Wilms' Tumor Study Pathology Center. Hum Pathol 1983; 14:481–492.
7. Beckwith JB. Wilms tumor and other renal tumors of childhood: an update. J Urol 1986;136:320–333.
8. Fernandes ET, Parham DM, Ribeiro RC, et al. Teratoid Wilms' tumor: the St Jude experience. J Pediatr Surg 1988;23:1131–1134.
9. Variend S, Spicer RD, Mackinnon AE. Teratoid Wilms' tumor. Cancer 1984;53:1936–1942.
10. Fernbach SK, Donaldson JS, Gonzalez-Crussi F, et al. Fatty Wilms' tumor simulating teratoma; occurrence in a child with horseshoe kidney. Pediatr Radiol 1988; 18:424–426.
11. Parvey LS, Warner RM, Callihan TR, et al. CT demonstration of fat tissue in malignant renal neoplasms: atypical Wilms' tumors. J Comput Assist Tomogr 1981;5:851–854.
12. Heideman RL, Haase GM, Foley C, Nephroblastomatosis and Wilms' tumor. Clinical experience and management of seven patients. Cancer 1985;55:1446–1451.
13. Fernbach SK, Feinstein KA, Donaldson JS, et al. Nephroblastomatosis: comparison of CT with US and urography. Radiology 1988;166:153–156.
14. Rosenfield NS, Shimkin P, Berdon W, et al. Wilms tumor arising from spontaneously regressing nephroblastomatosis. AJR 1980;135:381–384.
15. Mesrobian H-GJ. Wilms tumor: past, present, future. J Urol 1988;140:231–238.
16. Fernbach SK, Feinstein KA, Donaldson JS, et al. Nephroblastomatosis: comparison of CT with US and urography. Radiology 1988;166:153–156.
17. Tank ES, Kay R. Neoplasms associated with hemihypertrophy, Beckwith-Wiedemann syndrome and aniridia. J Urol 1980;124:266–268.
18. Beckwith JB, Kiviat NB, Bonadio JF. Nephrogenic rests, nephroblastomatosis, and the pathogenesis of Wilms' tumor. Pediatr Pathol 1990;10:1–36.
19. Pichler E, Jurgenssen OA, Balzar E, et al. Massive bilateral

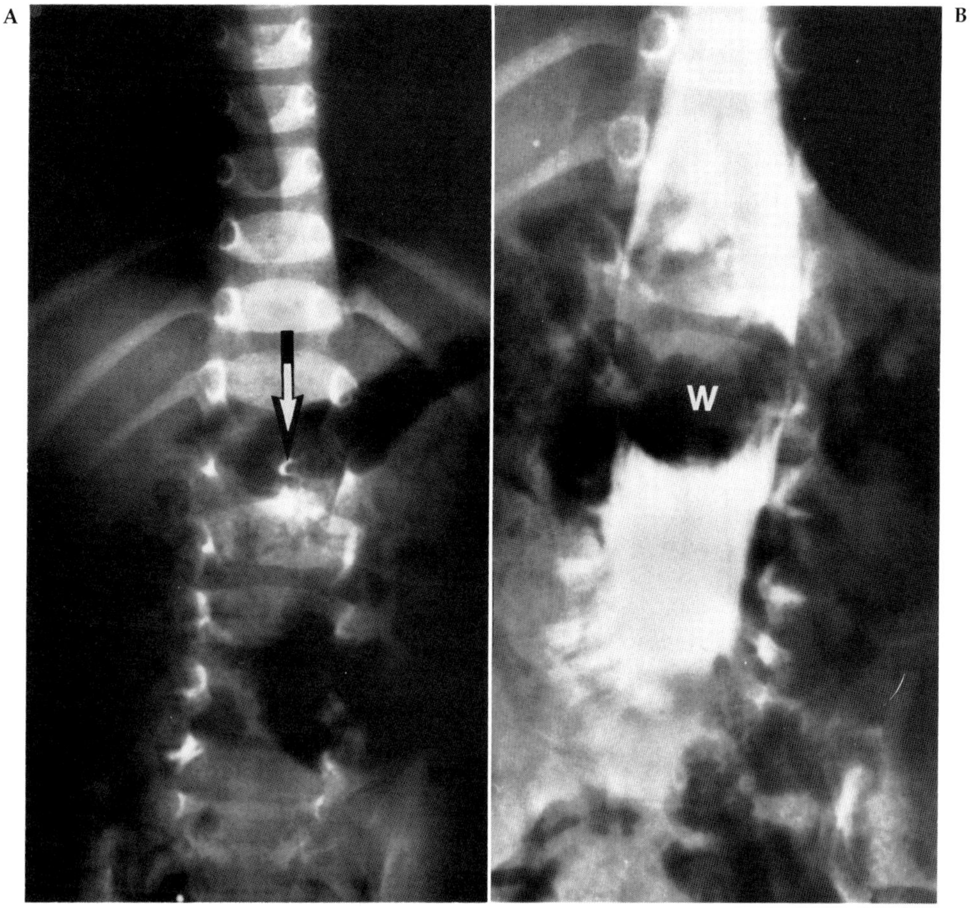

Figure 4-2. **Diagnosis: Nonrenal Wilms tumor. Primary tumor in the spinal canal. It is associated with diastematomyelia.**
***A*, Plain film radiograph. The spinal canal is widened. A bony spur *(arrow)* is caused by diastematomyelia. *B*, Myelogram. The Wilms tumor *(W)* is seen as a mass lesion lying within the widened spinal canal. This tumor cannot be differentiated from other intraspinal mass lesions.**

nephroblastomatosis in a 13-year-old girl. Eur J Pediatr 1982;138:231–236.
20. Andrews MJ, Askin FB, Fried FA, et al. Cystic partially differentiated nephroblastoma and polycystic Wilms tumor: a spectrum of related clinical and pathologic entities. J Urol 1983;129:577–581.
21. Ritchey ML, Kelalis PP, Breslow N, et al. Intracaval and atrial involvement with nephroblastoma: review of National Wilms Tumor Study-3. J Urol 1988;140:1113–1118.
22. Schraut WH, Chilcote RR. Metastatic Wilms' tumor causing acute hepatic-vein occlusion (Budd-Chiari syndrome). Gastroenterol 1985;88:576–579.
23. Slovis TL, Cushing B, Reilly BJ, et al. Wilms' tumor to the heart: clinical and radiographic evaluation. Am J Roentgenol 1978;131:263–266.
24. Luck SR, DeLeon S, Shkolnik A, et al. Intracardiac Wilms' tumor: diagnosis and management. J Pediatr Surg 1982;17:551–554.
25. Breslow NE, Churchill G, Nesmith B, et al. Cancer 1986;58:2501–2511.
26. Bever CT, Koenigsberger MR, Antunes JL, et al. Epidural metastasis by Wilms' tumor. Am J Dis Child 1981;135:644–646.
27. Lamego CMB, Zerbini MCN. Bone-metastasizing primary renal tumors in children. Radiology 1983;147:449–454.
28. Weeks DA, Beckwith JB, Mierau GW, et al. Rhabdoid tumor of kidney. A report of 111 cases from the National Wilms' tumor study pathology center. Am J Surg Pathol 1989;13:439–458.
29. Scott LS. Bilateral Wilms' tumour. Br J Surg 1955;42:513–517.
30. Casale AJ, Flanigan RC, Moore PJ, et al. Survival in bilateral metachronous (asynchronous) Wilms tumors. J Urol 1982;128:766–769.
31. Narashimharao KL, Marwaha RK, Kaushik MS, et al. Extrarenal Wilms' tumor. J Pediatr Surg 1989;24:212–214.
32. McCauley GK, Safaii H, Crowley CA, et al. Extrarenal Wilms' tumor. Am J Dis Child 1979;133:1174–1177.
33. Fernandes ET, Kumar M, Douglass EC, et al. Extrarenal Wilms' tumor. J Pediatr Surg 1989;24:483–485.
34. Fernbach SK, Naidich TP, McLone DG, et al. Computed tomography of primary intrathecal Wilms tumor with diastematomyelia. J Comput Assist Tomogr 1984;8:523–528.
35. Broecker RH, Caldamone AA, McWilliams NB, et al. Primary extrerenal Wilms' tumor in children. J Pediatr Surg 1989;24:1283–1288.

36. Adam YG, Rosen A, Oland J, et al. Extrarenal Wilms tumor. J Surg Oncol 1983;22:56–58.
37. Carachi R, Lindop GBM, Leckie BJ. Inactive renin: a tumor marker in nephroblastoma. J Pediatr Surg 1987;22:278–280.

Clinical Presentation

Patients with Wilms tumor are well and only occasionally present with systemic signs such as malaise, decreased appetite, and significant weight loss. Because of the lack of constitutional signs, the tumors grow to a large size and the most common presentation is the incidental finding of a palpable abdominal mass. This occurs in between 75 to 95 percent of patients.[1,2] Only 12 percent of patients[3] have metastatic spread at the time of initial presentation, and this explains the lack of symptoms in so many of these patients. Specific symptoms referable to the renal tract are also uncommon.[4] Microscopic hematuria may be detected in up to 25 percent of patients.[5] Gross hematuria is an indication of tumor invasion of the renal pelvis[6] or tumor occlusion of the renal vein.[7] The presence of gross hematuria therefore requires careful imaging attention to these sites of spread. In the NWTS-III, only 30 percent of children with inferior vena cava tumor had gross hematuria. Only 5 of 77 patients had other signs of vessel involvement. Two patients had a varicocele and 3 had signs of cardiac congestion.[8] Acute cardiac dysfunction can occur in those patients, with the tumor prolapsing through the tricuspid valve.[7] Hypertension can occur in patients with Wilms tumor,[9] which is caused by increased renin production by tumor cells and not by secondary compression of the renal vessels and ischemia by a large tumor. Hypertension is, therefore, independent of tumor size.

Comment: As most patients with Wilms tumor present with an incidental abdominal mass, the initial thrust of imaging focuses on the differential diagnosis of abdominal masses in children. Gross hematuria is uncommon and suggests renal sinus invasion or renal vein occlusion.

References

1. Andresen J, Steenskov V. Radiologic and prognostic aspects of Wilms' tumour. Acta Radiol Diag 1981;22:353–358.
2. Exelby PR. Retroperitoneal malignant tumors: Wilms' tumor and neuroblastoma. Surg Clin N Am 1981;61:1219–1227.
3. D'Angio GJ, Evans A, Breslow N, et al. The treatment of Wilms' tumor: results of the second National Wilms' Tumor Study. Cancer 1981;47:2302–2311.
4. Scott LS. Bilateral Wilms' tumour. Br J Surg 1955;42:513–517.
5. Exelby PR. Retroperitoneal malignant tumors: Wilms' tumor and neuroblastoma. Surg Clin N Am 1981;61:1219–1227.
6. Johnson KM, Horvath LJ, Gaisie G, et al. Wilms tumor occurring as a botryoid renal pelvicalyceal mass. Radiology 1987;163:385–386.
7. Slovis TL, Cushing B, Reilly BJ, et al. Wilms' tumor to the heart: clinical and radiographic evaluation. Am J Roentgenol 1978;131:263–266.
8. Ritchey ML, Kelalis PP, Breslow N, et al. Intracaval and atrial involvement with nephroblastoma: review of National Wilms Tumor Study–3. J Urol 1988;140:1113–1118.
9. Yokomori K, Hori T, Takemura T, et al. Demonstration of both primary and secondary reninism in renal tumors in children. J Pediatr Surg 1988;23:403–409.

Imaging Studies

IMAGING OF THE PRIMARY TUMOR

In the past 10 years, the methods for imaging of the primary Wilms tumor mass have undergone a major upheaval. Although computed tomography (CT) and possibly magnetic resonance imaging (MR) are now the primary methods for imaging the tumor mass, its appearance on other imaging modalities must be known and understood, as the tumor might be an incidental finding with any imaging modality.

The signs of a Wilms tumor on a plain abdominal radiograph are a bulging flank (75 percent), loss of outline of a kidney (66 percent), enlargement of a kidney (33 percent), displacement of bowel gas (50 percent), loss of the outline of the psoas muscle (33 percent), and abdominal calcification (10 percent[1]) (Fig. 4–3). All patients have more than one of these signs.

On intravenous urogram, Wilms tumor causes enlargement of the kidney. Approximately 75 percent of patients show normal excretion of contrast, 20 percent only a nephrogram or delayed filling of the collecting system, and 5 percent no excretion of contrast.[2] Nonfunction of the kidney is more likely to be identified in those patients with tumor obstructing the renal vein[3] or direct tumor invasion of the renal pelvis with obstruction.[4] Only very rarely will nonfunction be caused by complete replacement of an entire kidney by tumor. When function is present, the tumor mass is seen to displace and distort the calyces. In the NWTS-I study, intravenous pyelography misdiagnosed other lesions for Wilms tumors in about 5 percent of cases.[5] Note that complete nonfunction of a kidney with Wilms tumor is rare.[1,6]

Ultrasound can identify all but the smallest Wilms tumor. Unlike IVP, ultrasound does not rely purely on distortion of the collecting system or bulging of the renal contour to identify the tumor mass. The mass is usually well defined (Fig. 4–4). The peripheral margins of the lesion are well seen, but microscopic capsule invasion cannot be identified. The junction of the tumor with the adjacent normal renal tissue shows varying echogenicity or echolucency. Pathologic correlation shows that the hyperechogenic rim corresponds to the pseudocapsule and the adjacent hypoechogenic band to compressed normal renal tissue.[7,8] This interface between tumor and normal kidney is sharp in over 50 percent of patients,[6] but a less well-defined interface may also be found. Occasionally, the interface may be so well defined as to mimic an indented normal renal capsule, falsely suggesting the presence of an extrarenal tumor indenting a normal kidney.[8] There is some variation in reports of the internal echo pattern of Wilms tumors, probably reflecting differences in ultrasound equipment. Areas of liquid hemorrhage and areas of necrosis will appear as regions of low echogenicity, which may even appear cystic[6–8] (Fig. 4–4). Fat will usually be very echogenic (Fig. 4–4). The rest of the tumor has been reported as having heterogenous internal echoes,[8] varying homogenicity,[6] or a fairly even echogenicity apart from discrete foci of necrosis.[7] This report indicates correct blind differentiation of Wilms tumor from neuroblastoma in 23 of 26 cases on the basis of the even echogenicity of the Wilms tumor.[7] My own belief is that the internal echo pattern of the Wilms tumors is much more variable and that this pattern should not be much relied upon when attempting to differentiate Wilms tumors from other intrarenal or adjacent extrarenal solid mass lesions. Areas of focal echogenicity may be caused by blood clot or calcium, particularly if shadowing is present. In tumors not initially surgically resected, the development of anechoic areas within the tumor might indicate a favorable response to chemotherapy.[9]

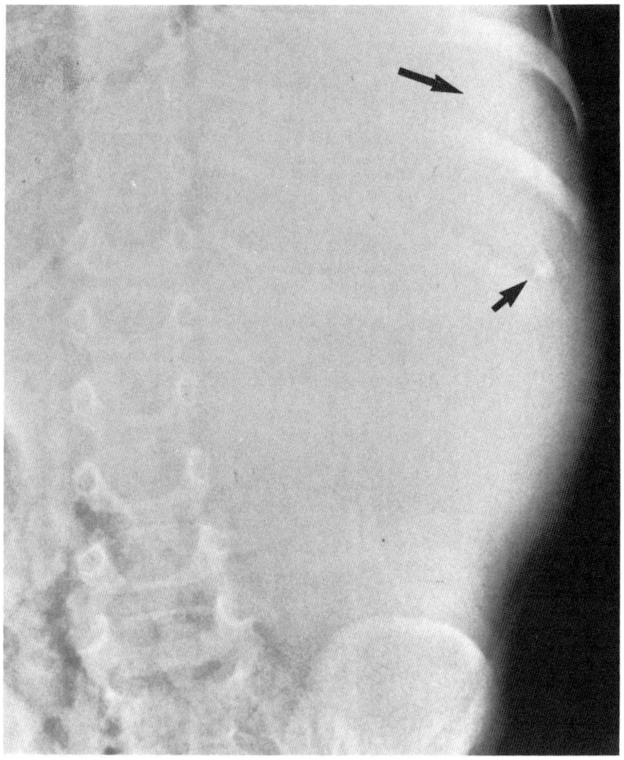

Figure 4-3. **Diagnosis: Wilms tumor with calcification. Plain film radiograph. There is a large mass lesion in the left side of the abdomen displacing bowel gas to the right. Speckled calcification *(arrows)* is identified in the tumor mass. This is an unusual finding in Wilms tumor.**

Wilms tumor is easy to diagnose with CT scan in over 90 percent of patients. Very small tumors can occasionally be missed with CT, and there is sometimes difficulty in the differential diagnosis of Wilms tumor from other tumors in the adjacent organs, particularly in neuroblastoma, especially when this tumor invades the kidney. CT cannot differentiate anaplasia from tumor with favorable histology and cannot separate clear-cell sarcoma and rhabdoid tumor of kidney from classic Wilms tumor. The tumors are seen as large, well-defined mass

Figure 4-4. **Diagnosis: Wilms tumor. CT and ultrasound findings. Identification of fat within the tumor. *A*, Ultrasound. The tumor has a large homogenous soft-tissue component (*1*) that is of fairly uniform echogenicity. Necrotic hemorrhagic areas are fluidlike and of low echogenicity (*2*). Fatty areas in the tumor are of strong echogenicity (*3*). *B*, CT. The tumor is again seen to have a soft-tissue component (*1*), necrotic hemorrhagic areas (*2*), and areas of fat (*3*). Normally functioning kidney tissue (*K*) surrounds the posterior aspect of the tumor. Note, incidentally, the isthmus (*I*) of a horsehoe kidney. (From Fernbach S. Nephroblastomatosis: comparison of CT with ultrasound and urography. Radiology 1988;166:153–156.)**

A

B

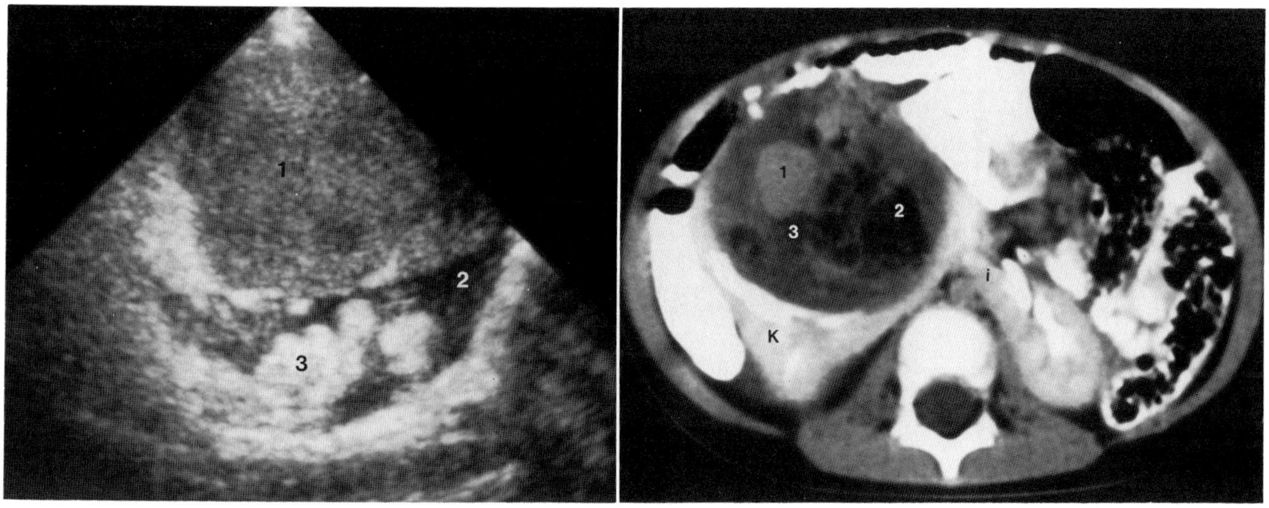

lesions of lower intensity than normal kidney tissue before contrast administration. Following contrast injection, there is mild enhancement of the tumor more marked at the margins than in central areas. Areas of hemorrhage and necrosis do not enhance. The adjacent normal renal tissue enhances more than the tumor mass (Figs. 4–5 and 4–6). There may be a very dense nephrogram from the residual normal tissue if the tumor is causing an element of obstruction.[10] Most tumors have a significant exophytic component projecting beyond the contour of the kidney (Fig. 4–7). Calcification is seen in between 7 to 13 percent of patients,[10,11] and areas of fat are recognized in up to 10 percent of patients[10,12] (Fig. 4–4). CT is poor for identification of subtle capsule penetration (Fig. 4–7) and cannot differentiate tumor from reactive lymphadenopathy (Figs. 4–8 and 4–9). CT can monitor response to chemotherapy (Fig. 4–10). CT may have difficulty in defining the interface between the tumor and liver (Fig. 4–11). It can define subcapsular bleeds (Fig. 4–12). Some of the CT features are summarized in Table 4–9.

MR, like CT and ultrasound, usually has no difficulty in identifying the presence of a renal mass. In 9 of 12

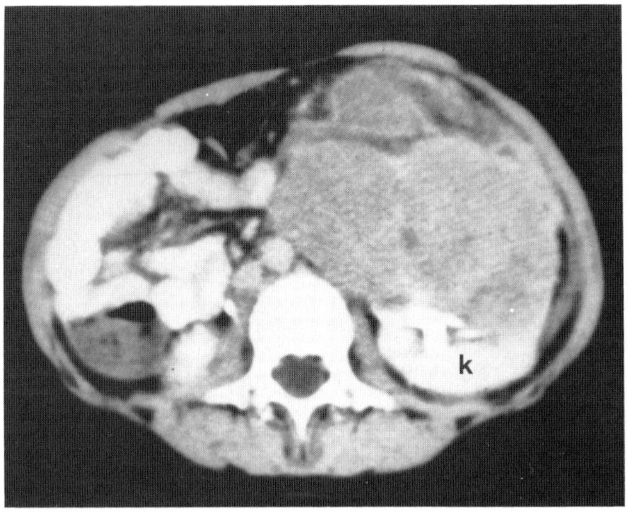

Figure 4-7. **Diagnosis: Wilms tumor. Typical CT appearance. Capsule penetration.**
CT. There is a large tumor mass involving the left kidney. It is seen as an exophytic lesion coming off the anterior part of the kidney. A large amount of normally functioning kidney tissue (*K*) is still present. The anterior margins of the mass are irregular and poorly defined, suggesting capsular penetration. Although this cannot be diagnosed with certainty, at surgery capsule penetration and invasion of the transverse colon mesentery was identified.

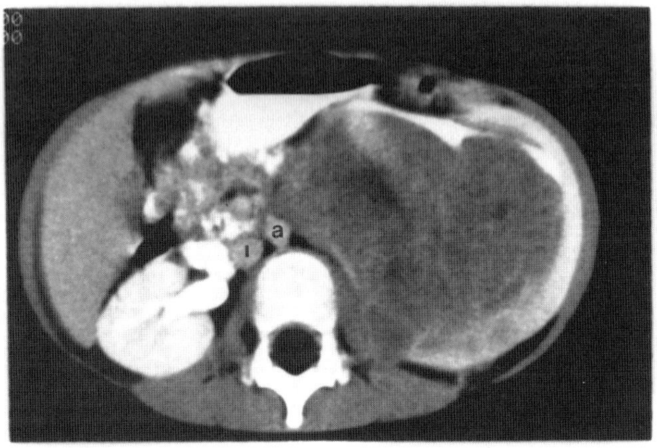

Figure 4-5. **Diagnosis: Wilms tumor: Classic appearance, stage I.**
There is a very large tumor of the left kidney. Functioning kidney tissue surrounds about half of the tumor. The tumor has a mixed internal structure owing to some areas of hemorrhage and necrosis. The aorta (*A*) and inferior vena cava (*I*) are displaced slightly to the right by the tumor but are not encased by it. No lymphadenopathy is identified.

Figure 4-6. **Diagnosis: Wilms tumor: Classic appearance, stage I.**
***A* and *B*, CT. There is a very large left renal mass. A small rim of functioning renal tissue can be identified. Large areas of hemorrhage and necrosis are seen as dark areas within the soft tissue intensity tumor mass.**

A

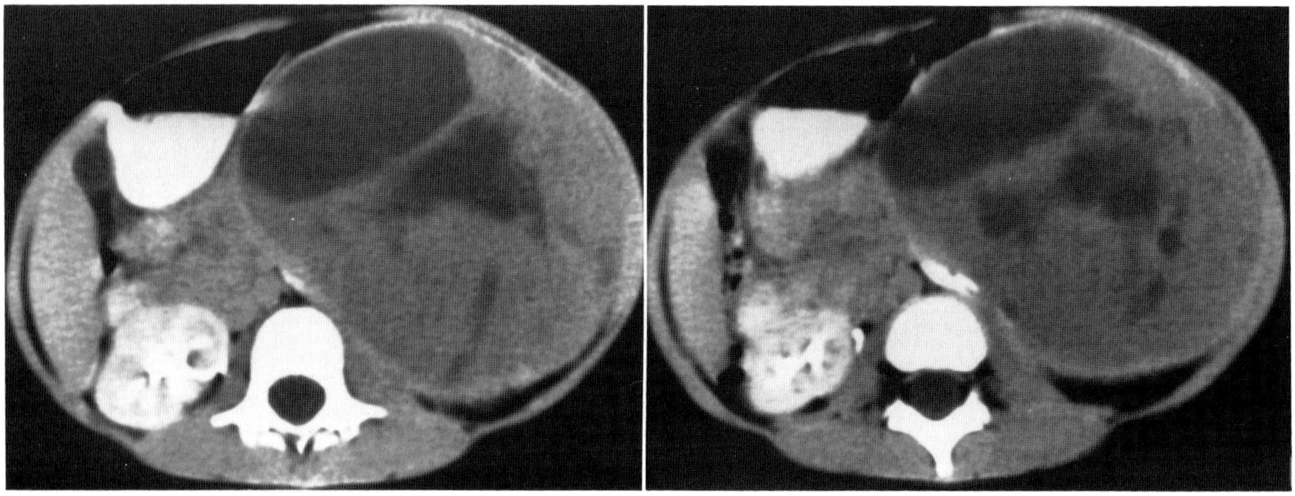

B

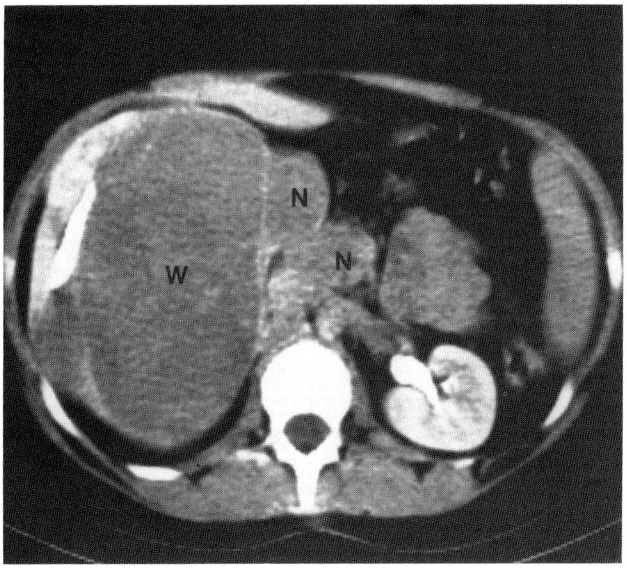

Figure 4-8. **Diagnosis: Wilms tumor with lymphadenopathy (nonmetastatic).**
CT. There is a large classic Wilms tumor (*W*) arising in the right kidney. Several enlarged lymph nodes (*N*) are seen. Histologically, these contained reactive hyperplasia and not tumor.

TABLE 4–9
CT Appearance of Wilms Tumor[1]

Appearance	Percentage of Tumors
Shape and margins	
Well-defined round or oval	87
Smooth margins	67
Crosses midline	29
Internal structure	
Nonhomogenous	87
Cystic necrosis	7
Calcium	7
Calyceal distortion	90
Hydronephrosis	40
Displacement of inferior vena cava or aorta	29
Encasement of inferior vena cava or aorta	0

Reference
1. Lowe RE, Cohen MD. Computed tomographic evaluation of Wilms tumor and neuroblastoma. RadioGraphics 1984;4:915–925.

patients,[13] tumor margins were smooth. Gross local extension and size of the tumor were accurately assessed by MR, but subtle capsule invasion could not be predicted.

MR signal intensity is highly variable because of necrosis and hemorrhage within the tumor.[13,14] The primary tumor tissue has signal intensity consistent with prolongation of T1 (Fig. 4–13) and T2 relaxation times; therefore, it has lower signal than normal kidney on T1 weighted pulse sequences and higher signal than normal kidney on T2 weighted pulse sequences.[15] The appearance of hemorrhage varies depending on the age of the blood[13,14] (Fig. 4–13).

Other imaging modalities have been utilized to evaluate Wilms tumor, but none are any longer recommended for the routine evaluation of these tumors. Retrograde pyelograms were performed, especially in patients with nonfunction on intravenous pyelography, to evaluate tumor extension into the renal pelvis.[1] CT, ultrasound, and MR now provide this information. Angiography used to be routinely performed in patients with renal tumors[1] but no longer has any routine role.

Figure 4-9. **Diagnosis: Wilms tumor with metastasis to local lymph nodes. CT missed microscopic capsular penetration and also renal vein invasion.**
***A* and *B*, CT. There is a very large left-sided Wilms tumor with multiple enlarged lymph nodes (*N*). These nodes contained tumor. The renal vein was not visualized. Capsular penetration cannot be clearly identified.**

A

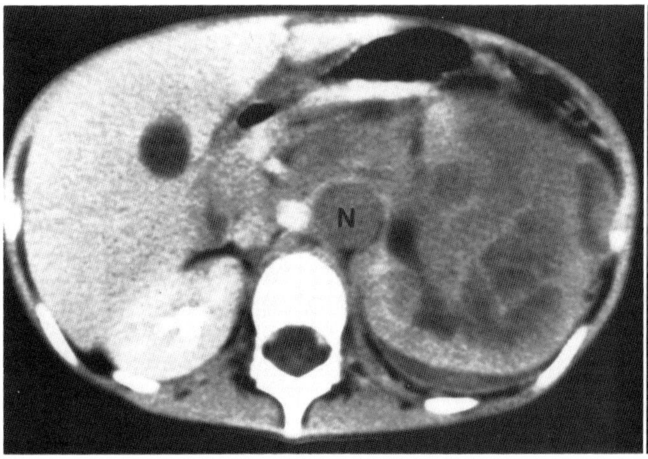

B

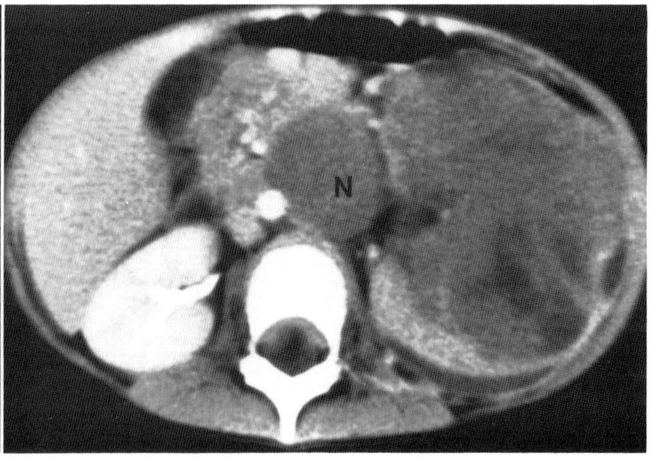

A

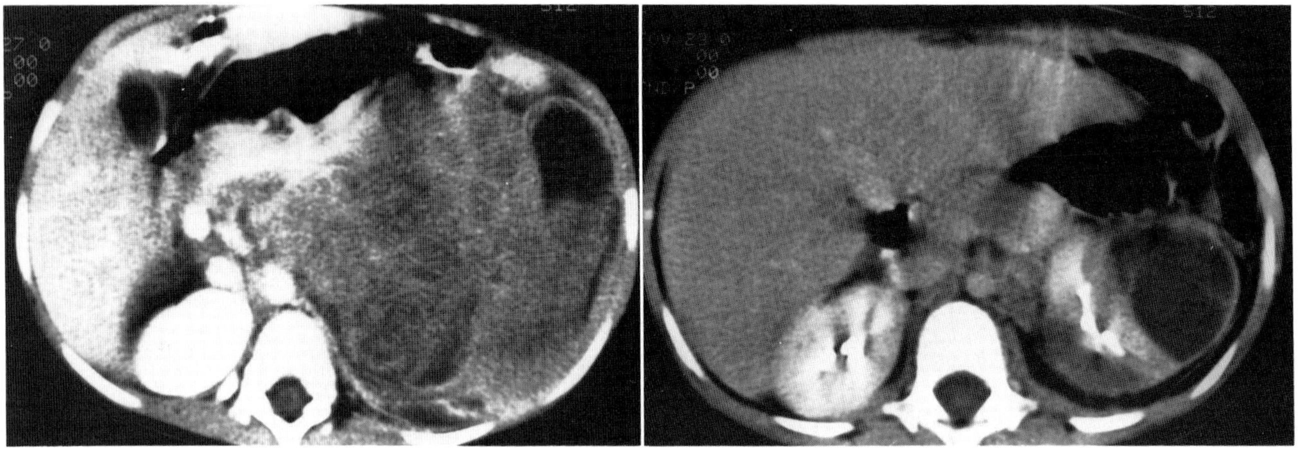

B

Figure 4-10. **Diagnosis: Wilms tumor. Utilization of CT to monitor chemotherapy.**
***A*, CT on initial presentation. There is a very large left renal tumor mass that was biopsied but could not be resected. *B*, Follow-up CT after chemotherapy. There is marked decrease in the size of the tumor, which was now easily resected.**

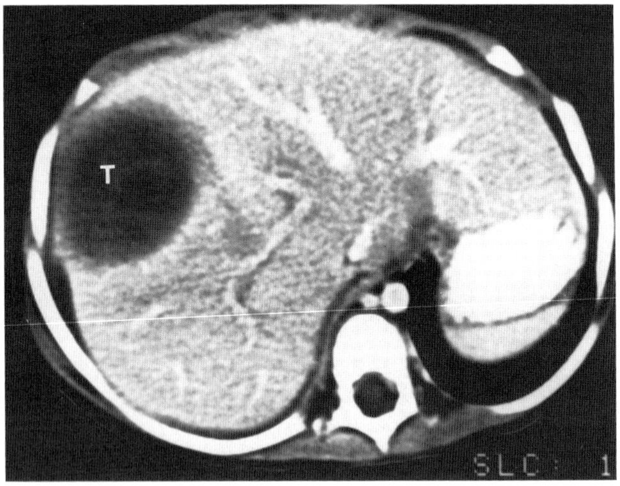

Figure 4-11. **Diagnosis: Wilms tumor. Differential diagnostic difficulties in the right upper quadrant.**
CT. This image is obtained through the superior part of a necrotic Wilms tumor. On this image, it is impossible to differentiate a primary hepatic tumor from an extrahepatic tumor. It is also impossible to differentiate between an extrahepatic tumor indenting the undersurface of the liver or invading the liver. At surgery this Wilms tumor had not invaded the liver. *T* = Tumor.

There is possibly still a role for angiography in the evaluation of partial nephrectomy for Wilms tumor in the second kidney[6] (in patients with bilateral tumors), but it is likely that MR and CT will provide equivalent and more information than angiography. Radioisotope images utilizing 99m technetium MDP (methylene diphosphonate) will show distortion of the normal uptake of the isotope in the kidney by Wilms tumor. Small tumors will be missed. Isotope uptake in the primary tumor mass can occasionally be detected.[16]

Which imaging modality should thus be performed on the primary Wilms tumor mass? There is good consensus that ultrasound should be utilized as the initial screening test for evaluation of any child with an abdominal mass. If the ultrasound reveals a solid tumor mass of the kidney, I would proceed directly to CT scan. CT studies have been demonstrated to be better than intravenous pyelography.[1] Apart from the identification of tumor within the inferior vena cava, CT is better than ultrasound for evaluation of Wilms tumor. In a study in 1986, CT was found to be better than ultrasound for the identification of necrosis, demonstration of the pseudocapsule, and for evaluation of local tumor spread.[17] CT is also better for the evaluation of nodal and liver spread of tumor in the abdomen. Unfortunately, there is still no universal agreement as to the role of CT in evaluation of Wilms tumor, with recommendations as recently as 1988 that intravenous pyelography and ultrasound alone should be used for the initial evaluation of Wilms tumor.[18] It is unfortunate that new technology is so slowly accepted. The role of MR is not yet known. It has promise of becoming perhaps the single modality to evaluate all the abdominal structures for local and metastatic spread of Wilms tumor.[13]

A study in 1985 indicated that imaging was poor for the preoperative identification of a horseshoe kidney in patients with Wilms tumors.[19] Few if any of these patients had had CT performed, and I suspect that the preoperative identification of the horseshoe kidney would no longer present a problem. This information is clearly important to the surgeon.

No modality has proven absolutely effective for demonstrating a second synchronous tumor in the opposite kidney. One reason is that these lesions are often quite small. There are no studies, however, in any large series of bilateral tumors, using state-of-the-art ultrasound, CT, or MR imaging equipment. I suspect that CT and MR should detect virtually all the tumors that are clinically palpated at the time of surgery and perhaps detect, in addition, some nonpalpable lesions.

A

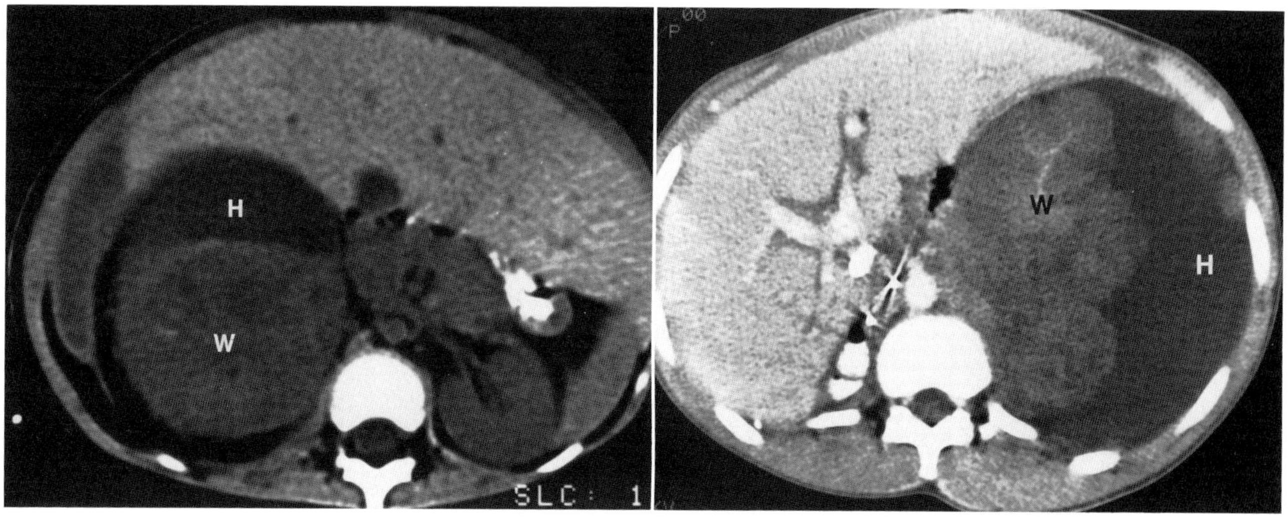

B

Figure 4–12. Diagnosis: Wilms tumor with subcapsular hemorrhage identified in two patients.
A, CT. There is a large right Wilms tumor (*W*) with a crescentic anterior subcapsular hematoma (*H*). ***B,*** The Wilms tumor (*W*) is on the left side in this patient. The hematoma (*H*) lies lateral to the main tumor mass.

A

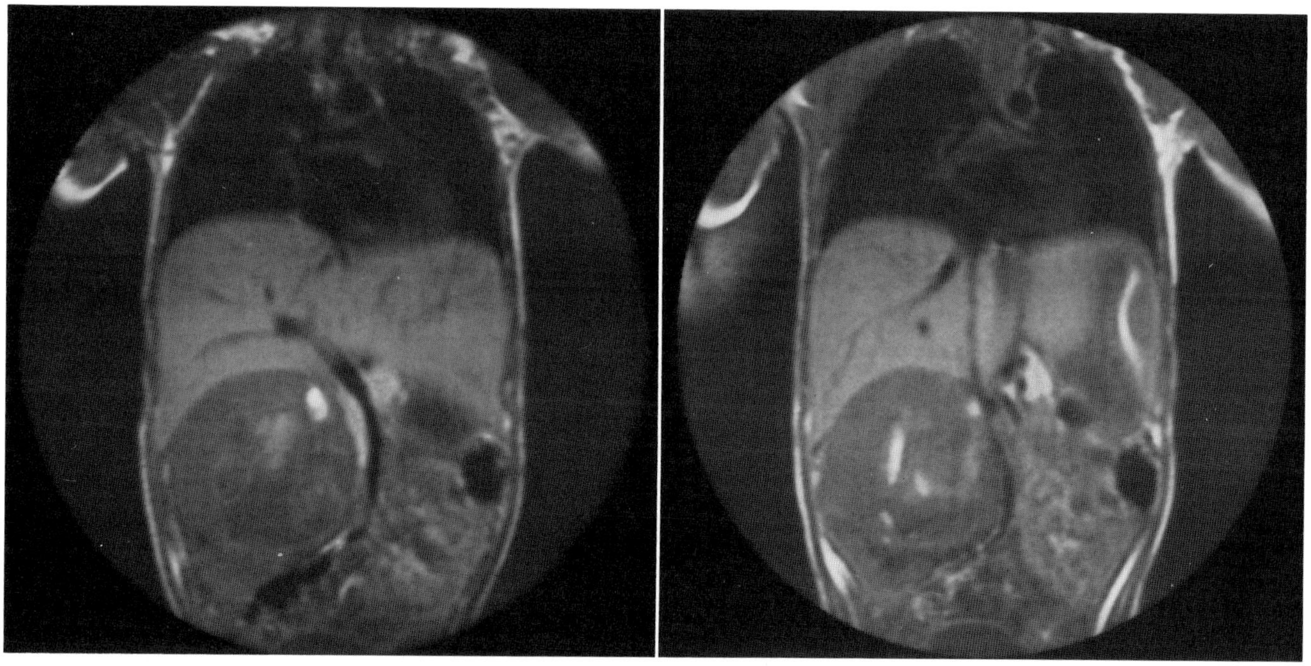

B

Figure 4–13. Diagnosis: Wilms tumor. MR appearance.
A and ***B,*** Coronal MR T1 weighted images. There is a large tumor that has arisen from the right kidney. Normal kidney is not identified on these slices. The tumor is predominantly of lower signal intensity than liver. Very bright areas within the tumor are caused by hemorrhage. Note the clear interface between the tumor and liver. Note good visualization of vessels displaced by tumor.

Comment: CT is the main investigative method for evaluation of the primary Wilms tumor mass. Ultrasound will in many cases have already been performed to differentiate a solid from cystic lesion and is excellent for identifying inferior vena cava tumor spread. In the future, MR may play a more dominant role. There is no place for the utilization of intravenous urogram, retrograde pyelogram, or routine angiogram.

TUMOR EXTENSION INTO THE RENAL VEIN, INFERIOR VENA CAVA, AND HEART

Identification of tumor in the cardiac chambers or the hepatic segment of the inferior vena cava must be accurately done prior to surgery, as it will greatly alter the surgical approach. Tumor extension into the renal vein or into the infrahepatic part of the inferior vena cava (Fig. 4–14) does not significantly alter the surgical ap-

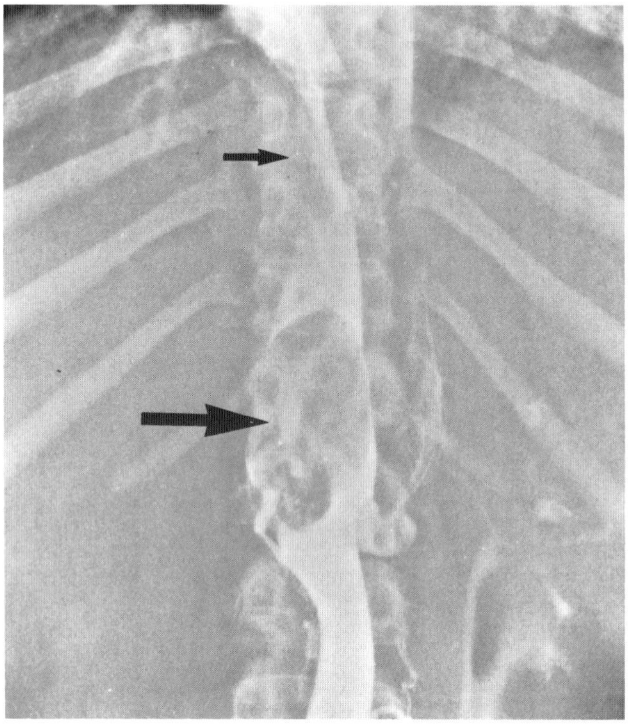

Figure 4–14. **Diagnosis: Inferior vena caval spread of Wilms tumor.**
Cavogram. A large tumor mass *(large arrow)* is seen in the inferior vena cava. It lies in the infrahepatic segment. Flow voids in the more superior part of the inferior vena cava *(small arrow)* should not be mistaken for tumor.

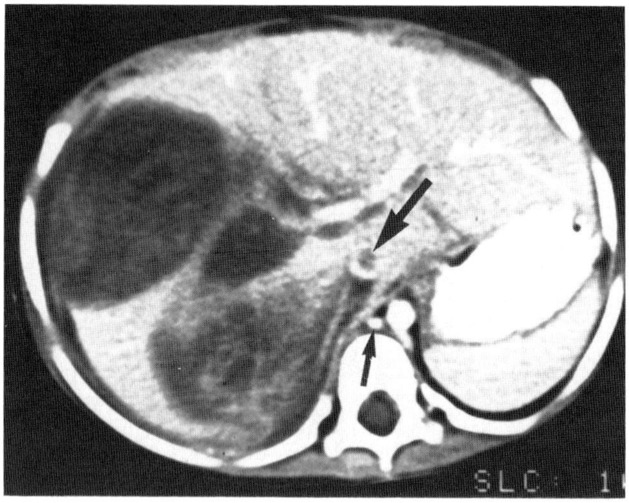

Figure 4–15. **Diagnosis: Wilms tumor. Tumor extension into the hepatic segment of the inferior vena cava.**
CT. A large necrotic right Wilms tumor is seen. A filling defect, caused by tumor, is seen in the inferior vena cava *(large arrow).* A dilated collateral azygos vein is identified *(small arrow).*

proach, but its identification prior to surgery is nonetheless helpful. As previously discussed, seldom do clinical findings suggest tumor extension into the inferior vena cava and, therefore, this tumor spread must be identified by imaging (Figs. 4–14 and 4–15).

Early attempts at identification of caval tumor were done using venography with injection of contrast for an intravenous pyelogram made into a vein in the foot rather than in the arm. By placing tourniquets around the legs a bolus of contrast could be seen flowing into the cava.[1] In one study of 34 patients in the 1970s, there were three false positive diagnoses and 11 equivocal studies,[20] indicating a poor efficacy for the study. The reasons for false results are streaming because of inflow of nonopacified blood from tributary veins, compression of the inferior vena cava by the tumor mass, layering of contrast within the vessel, diversion of contrast away from the inferior vena cava and into collateral vessels with raised pressure from straining, crying, or a Valsalva maneuver.[1] Foot venography is, therefore, no longer performed.

In the late 1970s,[21] ultrasound was able to demonstrate tumor spread into the atrium correctly in 2 patients. In a total of 14 patients, however, tumor spread into the inferior vena cava was identified in only 8.[22] Most investigators today would choose ultrasound (because of improved image quality) as their modality of choice for evaluation of the inferior vena cava for the presence of tumor. Most believe ultrasound to be extremely accurate, but no studies in the last 3 to 4 years in large numbers of patients prove this. In fact, the data from the NWTS-III study indicate that though ultrasound is better than CT it is by no means perfect.[23] The results of investigation of caval tumor in 77 patients are presented in Table 4–10. Ultrasound was accurate in only 54 percent of the patients but was better than CT.

Eighty-seven percent of patients had tumor correctly identified using catheter injection of contrast into the inferior vena cava. Disadvantages of this technique are that it is invasive and that it is not accurate in identifying the superior extent of tumor, which is the most important information required.

The MR results are not meaningful, because only 2 patients were studied. In another small study of 4 patients, MR was found to be better than CT or ultrasound for identification of tumor in the inferior vena cava and right side of the heart.[24]

Ultrasound was extremely accurate for identification of tumor extension into the right atrium. In fact, most of the tumor missed on ultrasound was in patients with tumor confined to the infrahepatic segment of the inferior vena cava. I suspect that in many of these cases the cava was displaced and possibly compressed so that it was not visualized. In summary, I believe that ultrasound should be the primary method utilized for evaluation of the inferior vena cava. It is at its best with tumor high in the cava or in the right atrium, and cardiac catheterization studies should seldom if ever be required. In reporting the results of an ultrasound study, I think it is important to give a separate report for the infrahepatic and hepatic segments of the inferior vena cava and the right atrium. For each segment the surgeon must be told whether or not the lumen of the cava was visualized and, if so, if tumor is present or not. I believe

TABLE 4–10
Accuracy of Imaging for Tumor Identification in the Inferior Vena Cava*

Modality	No. of Patients Studied	Positive Diagnosis Made No.	%
Ultrasound	56	33	54
CT	38	16	42
Inferior vena cava catheter injection of contrast	23	20	87
MR	2	2	100
Ultrasound for right atrial tumor	15	14	92

*Studies in 77 patients enrolled in NWTS-III, 1979–1987, with tumor at surgery.

that provided the lumen can be visualized errors with ultrasound will be extremely small.

In those patients in whom the inferior vena cava cannot be visualized either because of complete replacement with tumor or because of compression or marked displacement of the inferior vena cava, or because of overlying bowel gas other studies should be performed. In patients in whom only the intrahepatic segment of the inferior vena cava has not been visualized, the surgeon may elect to proceed with surgery without any other investigation. The surgeon will be armed with the knowledge of the possibility of tumor spread into the lower inferior vena cava, but his or her surgical approach will not be altered by the presence or absence of this tumor. If ultrasound fails to visualize the intrahepatic segment of the inferior vena cava, a venogram with catheterization of the inferior vena cava might be performed. Alternatively, one might attempt a CT scan with slow infusion of contrast through a vein in the foot. There are no studies reporting the success of this technique, but it is worth trying before a venogram. MR should also be tried.

The final role of MR remains to be determined. There are reports of successful identification of caval tumor with MR imaging.[13] Advantages of MR are its ability to image in the longitudinal planes, and this may facilitate identification of tumor. MR has the potential for replacing all other imaging modalities, but until such studies have been performed ultrasound remains the mainstay of inferior vena cava imaging. Occasionally, the tumor will invade the wall of the inferior vena cava. No reports of successful imaging of such invasion have been published.

EVALUATION FOR METASTASES ON INITIAL PRESENTATION

The pattern of metastatic spread of Wilms tumor and its associated clear-cell and rhabdoid tumors of the kidney is very predictable. Extensive imaging of all locations of possible metastatic spread from all three types of tumor should not be performed prior to surgery. Once the histology has been determined, imaging for metastatic spread can be performed, surveying only those anatomic areas to which the tumor is known to spread. Clear-cell sarcoma and rhabdoid tumor are discussed in a separate section. A classic Wilms tumor (Table 4–11) spreads almost entirely to regional abdominal lymph nodes (Figs. 4–9 and 4–16), the liver (Fig. 4–17), and lungs (Figs. 4–18, 4–19, and 4–20). In NWTS-I, metastatic disease was to the lung alone in 49 percent of patients. Only 18 percent of patients with metastatic disease had no lung involvement.[25] In the abdomen, CT is better than ultrasound for the detection of lymph node

Figure 4–16. **Diagnosis: Wilms tumor. Spread to retrocrural lymph nodes.**
Chest radiograph. Enlarged retrocrural lymph nodes are identified on the left side *(arrows)*. This is a somewhat unusual finding with Wilms tumor and is much more common with neuroblastoma.

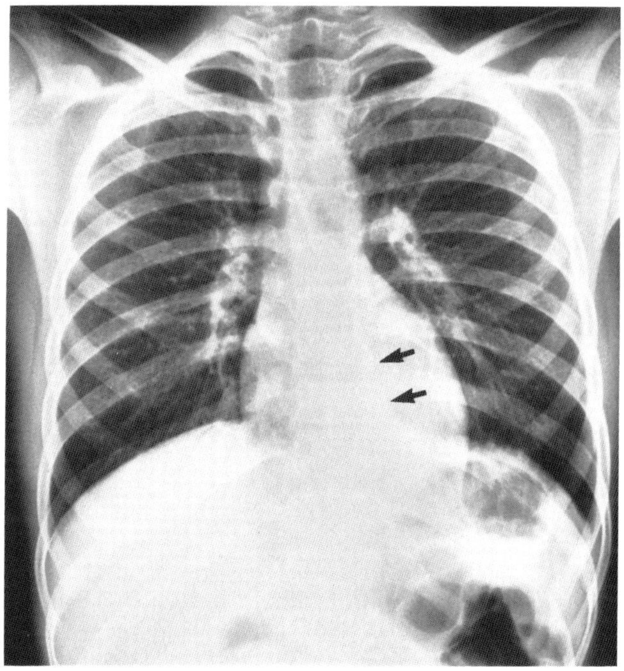

A B C

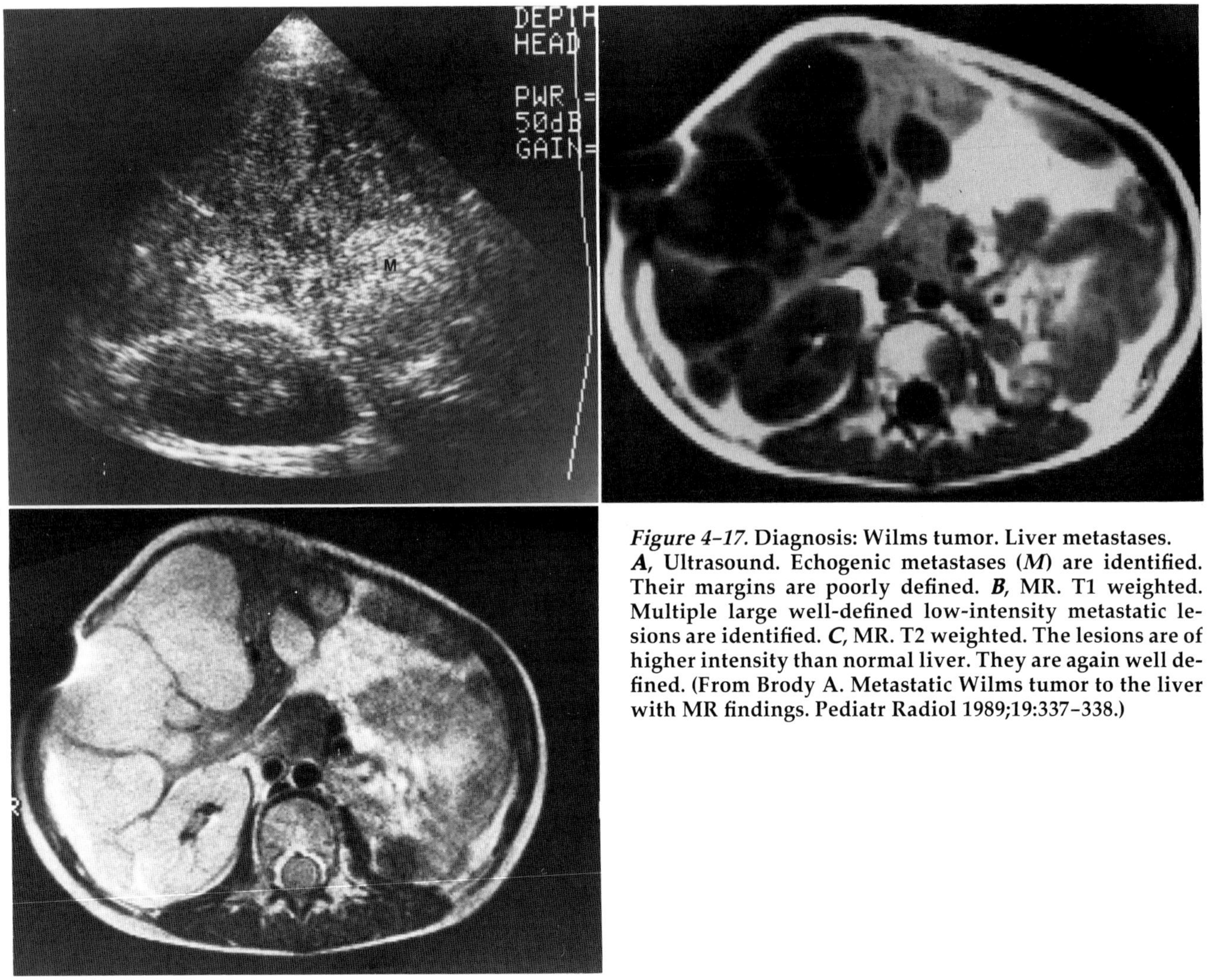

Figure 4–17. **Diagnosis: Wilms tumor. Liver metastases. *A,* Ultrasound. Echogenic metastases (*M*) are identified. Their margins are poorly defined. *B,* MR. T1 weighted. Multiple large well-defined low-intensity metastatic lesions are identified. *C,* MR. T2 weighted. The lesions are of higher intensity than normal liver. They are again well defined. (From Brody A. Metastatic Wilms tumor to the liver with MR findings. Pediatr Radiol 1989;19:337–338.)**

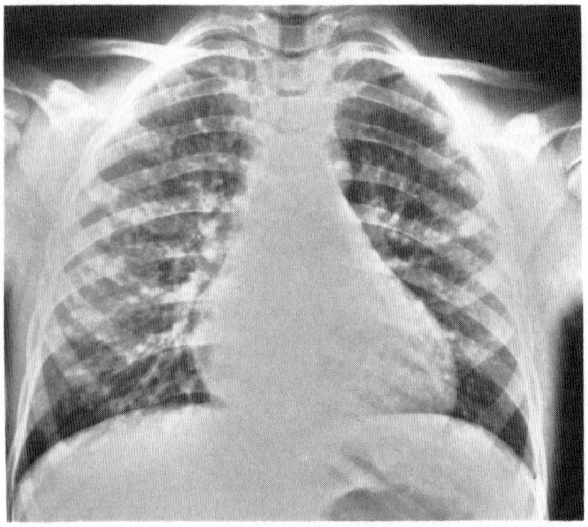

Figure 4–18. **Diagnosis: lung metastases from Wilms tumor. Chest radiograph. Multiple diffuse small nodular metastases are seen through both lung fields.**

and liver metastases,[6] and it is better than liver isotope scan for detection of liver metastases.[6,26]

I cannot agree with some workers[27] who believe that neither CT nor ultrasound of the liver should be performed to look for metastases because the yield is small. Imaging must be more sensitive than surgical palpation, except perhaps for the detection of small, superficial liver lesions. Examination of the liver at the time of surgery cannot detect deep-seated metastases. Lung me-

TABLE 4–11
Sites of Metastatic Spread of Classic Wilms Tumor

Abdominal lymph nodes
Liver
Lung
Rarely to mediastinum and chest wall

A B

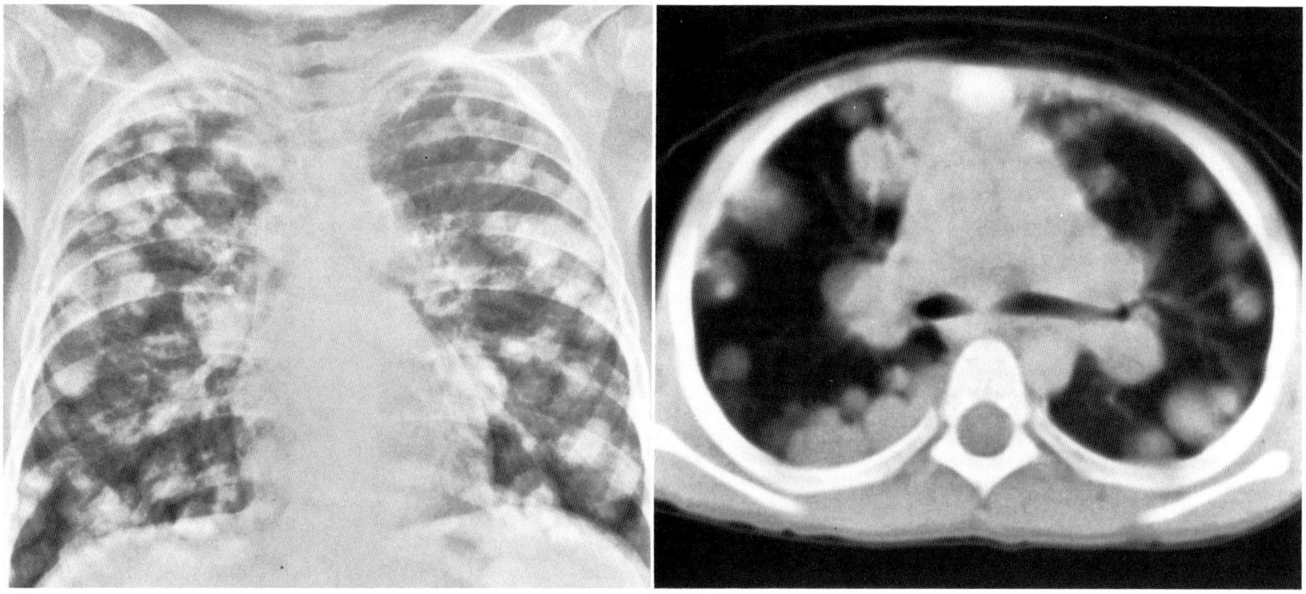

Figure 4–19. **Diagnosis: lung metastases from Wilms tumor.**
***A* and *B*, Chest radiograph and CT. Multiple medium and large metastatic nodules are identified throughout both lung fields.**

tastases should be sought with lung computed tomography. Initially, chest radiographs with whole lung tomography were performed. Since the introduction of CT scanning in the 1970s, there is overwhelming evidence of the superiority of CT for detection of lung lesions.

Some workers have argued that the small additional lesions detected by CT do not warrant the use of CT.[27] They feel that some of these lesions are benign and that the outcome and management of the patients are not affected by the detection of these lesions. This argument is fallacious. First, it could be argued that lung lesions detected on chest radiograph are just as likely to be benign as those detected on CT scan. Second, CT scan detects not only tiny lesions missed on radiograph but quite often will detect lesions as large as 2–3 cm in diameter originally missed on chest radiograph. As the chest radiograph and CT are often done simultaneously, I suspect that many lesions reported on chest radiograph were seen only with the aid of knowledge of the CT findings and that these lesions would have been missed if the chest radiograph had been reported without knowledge of the CT finding. Finally, in a study of 124 patients,[28] CT of the chest was positive in 11 children with negative chest radiographs. These 11 children were staged and treated ignoring the chest CT. One of these patients was stage IV because of liver metastases. The other 10 were staged as stage I, II, or III. Four of these latter children (40 percent) relapsed with metastases in the lung. This compares to only a 10 percent relapse for stage I, II, and III patients who had had an initial normal chest CT performed.

Conclusions from this study are that CT is more sensitive for the detection of lung nodules than chest radiograph and that the detection of these nodules is signifi-

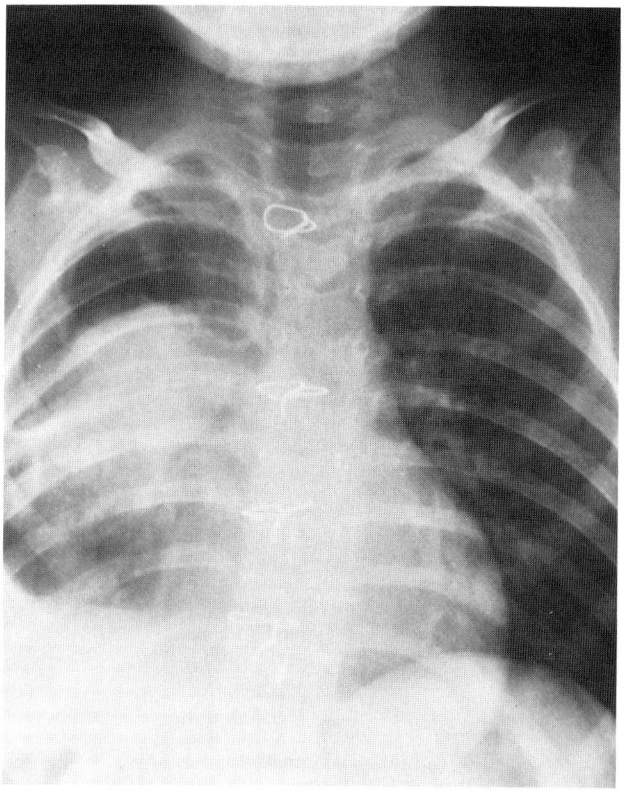

Figure 4–20. **Diagnosis: lung metastases from Wilms tumor. There is one very large metastatic lesion in the right lung.**

cant for patient's staging and prognosis. No imaging study is histologically specific and the fact that some nodules detected in the lung on CT will prove benign[29] is no reason not to perform the CT study. Multiple lung nodules can probably be assumed to be metastases. A single lung nodule should, in most cases, be biopsied to confirm the presence of tumor (particularly if the patient is not already known to be stage IV because of the presence of metastases in the liver).

The role of MR is as yet unknown. There is no evidence to suggest that it will have a significant role to play in the detection of lung metastases. A great deal of work on liver metastases in adults suggests superiority for MR when compared to CT, ultrasound, or liver isotope scanning. This area requires further evaluation in the pediatric patient and no recommendations can be made at this time.

> *Comment:* Surveillance for metastatic spread of Wilms tumor on initial presentation requires only a CT scan of the chest and a CT scan of the abdomen.

FOLLOW-UP OF PATIENTS FOR DETECTION OF LOCAL OR METASTATIC RECURRENCE

With Wilms tumor, the various National Wilms Tumor Studies provide a large amount of data that can be utilized in planning follow-up imaging of patients.

The incidence of relapse in Wilms tumor is in the range of 14 to 21 percent, with the most recent data from the NWTS-III being 14 percent (Table 4–12). Although relapse is more common in patients with unfavorable histology, it can occur in patients with any histology and with any original stage[30] (Table 4–13). Thus, even patients with stage I tumors with favorable histology require imaging surveillance for detection of metastatic spread.

The time of recurrence of the tumors is also well established. Seventy-three percent of recurrences will occur within the first year after diagnosis and 94 percent within the first 2 years[25,31] (Table 4–14). Few recurrences occur more than 2 years after diagnosis, and recurrences 5 or more years after diagnosis are exceedingly rare.[32] All this information means that imaging screening should be performed only during the first 2 years after initial diagnosis and that routine screening in asymptomatic patients after this time period is exceedingly unrewarding.

The site of metastatic spread of Wilms tumor is also well defined. In one study of 50 patients, lung metastases occurred in 18 percent and liver metastases in 12 percent.[33] In the absence of clear-cell or rhabdoid histology, recurrent or metastatic spread of Wilms tumor is virtually confined to chest and abdomen[30] (Table 4–15). The lung is the most common site of metastatic spread and is the only site in over 50 percent of patients.[30] The lung is also frequently involved in patients who have liver or abdominal nodal metastases or local tumor-bed recurrence.[30] The relationship of local tumor-bed recurrence to initial tumor stage is not known. The incidence of lung metastasis is higher in patients who have had inferior vena caval tumor, but this information cannot be utilized to select a subgroup of patients for lung follow-up screening, as lung metastases are common in patients who have not had inferior vena caval tumor.

The results of the NWTS-II study that were recently published provide some additional helpful information with regard to patterns of metastatic spread.[34] A total of 632 patients with unilateral tumor and no metastatic disease at the time of diagnosis were studied. One relapse was identified in 103 of the 632 patients. Sites in which relapse were detected were lung (86), abdomen (25), liver (17), bone (11), mediastinum and pleura (10), brain (6), epidural (4), and in individual cases in the soft tissues, eye, and heart. There was only minimal increased risk of metastasis if there was tumor in the inferior vena cava or extending into both renal veins. Operative spillage of tumor resulted in an increased incidence of local tumor recurrence. Unfavorable histology (anaplasia, rhabdoid, clear cell) or the presence of micrometastases in local lymph nodes resected at surgery were both associated with a significant likelihood of subsequent development of remote metastatic disease.

There are many published suggestions for routine follow-up screening of patients with Wilms tumor.[33,35] These studies suggest that CT is not particularly helpful. For example, in a series of 53 cases reported between 1978 and 1982, CT detected only 2 relapses not detected either clinically on chest radiograph or abdominal ultrasound. The quality of CT has improved dramatically since that time.

All the information given here indicates that imaging surveillance for Wilms tumor with classic histology should be confined to the chest and abdomen and that

TABLE 4–12
Incidence of Relapse in Wilms Tumor

17% of all stages relapsed (76 of 456 patients) NWTS-II[1]
21% of all stages relapsed (15 of 70 patients)[2]
14% of all stages relapsed (191 of 1439 patients) after complete remission NWTS-III[3]

References
1. Williams JA, Hammond E, Douglass EC, et al. The value of computerized tomography as a routine follow-up procedure for patients with Wilms' tumor. Med Pediatr Oncol 1984;12:221–223.
2. Hutson JM, Kent M, Ekert H, et al. The treatment of Wilms' tumor: results from Royal Children's Hospital, Melbourne, 1967–1977. J Pediatr Surg 1983;18:235–239.
3. D'Angio GJ, Breslow N, Beckwith JB, et al. Treatment of Wilms' tumor: results of the third National Wilms' Tumor Study. Cancer 1989;64:349–360.

TABLE 4–13
Relapse by Stage and Histology[1]

Stage, Histology	No. of Patients	Relapse No.	Relapse %
Stage I, favorable histology	607	46	8
Stage II, favorable histology	278	28	10
Stage III, favorable histology	275	53	19
Stage IV, favorable histology	120	19	16
All stages, unfavorable histology	130	37	28

Reference
1. D'Angio GJ, Breslow N, Beckwith JB, et al. Treatment of Wilms' tumor: results of the third National Wilms' Tumor Study. Cancer 1989;64:349–360.

it should also be confined to the first 2 years after initial diagnosis of the tumor. CT is the most appropriate imaging modality to use for the surveillance. The timing and frequency of the CT studies is to some extent arbitrary. Studies should obviously be performed on initial presentation. Studies should also be performed at the time that therapy is stopped and 6 months thereafter. The time of stopping of therapy will vary greatly, depending on local institutional protocols and also on the initial tumor stage. Studies should also be performed at any time that therapy is altered, if the patient presents with clinical symptoms suggestive of tumor spread or recurrence, or if relapse is detected in another site. Studies should be spaced so as not to be repeated more frequently than every 3 months, and one should probably aim to repeat the studies at least 3 times a year during the first 2 years after initial diagnosis. Following the 2 years, if no recurrence has occurred, all the data would suggest that no further imaging is required. Many institutions might feel more secure with an annaul chest radiograph for up to 5 or 10 years. I would have no objection to this, but remember that the yield will be extremely low.

In patients who fail to go into remission, or in patients with recurrent disease, CT should be utilized to follow the response of residual tumor to chemotherapy, radiation therapy, or both if surgical excision of the recurrent tumor had not been possible. If surgical excision of recurrent tumor is performed, a baseline CT scan should be done approximately 1 month after the surgery. If surgical excision has not been done, the frequency of follow-up CT scans should in most cases not exceed once every 3 months unless there is clinical deterioration and a change in therapy is contemplated.

Comment: Surveillance for metastases of Wilms tumor should be confined to the chest and abdomen.
The surveillance for metastases should be confined to the first 2 years after the diagnosis.
CT is the most appropriate modality for this surveillance.
Timing of follow-up imaging must not be rigid.

TABLE 4–14
Time of Relapse NWTS-I[1,2]

Time Period	Percentage
Within first 6 months after diagnosis	45
Within first year after diagnosis	73
During second year after diagnosis	21
More than 2 years after diagnosis	6

References
1. Williams JA, Hammond E, Douglass EC, et al. The value of computerized tomography as a routine follow-up procedure for patients with Wilms' tumor. Med Pediatr Oncol 1984;12:221–223.
2. Breslow NE, Palmer NF, Hill LR, et al. Wilms' tumor: prognostic factors for patients without metastases at diagnosis. Results of the National Wilms' Tumor Study. Cancer 1978;41:1577–1589.

SURVEILLANCE OF PATIENTS AT HIGH RISK OF DEVELOPING WILMS TUMOR

Patients with Wilms tumor in one kidney (particularly if nephroblastomatosis has been identified in this kidney) and patients with several well-defined congenital abnormalities and syndromes clearly have an increased risk of developing a Wilms tumor. Identification of this high-risk group of patients suggests that screening surveillance might be applied with a cost-effective benefit to the patient. The questions to be considered in the development of a screening program are summarized in Table 4–16. Clearly there are no easy answers to these questions.

It could be argued that no screening for Wilms tumors should be performed. In one study of 54 patients with Wilms tumor, 206 follow-up intravenous urograms were performed, all of which were normal. During screening 2 patients did develop Wilms tumors, both of whom presented with abnormal clinical findings.[33] There is other evidence that imaging will not di-

TABLE 4–15
Site of Relapse in 191 Patients in NWTS-III (All Histology)[1]

Site	No.	%
Lung alone	109	57
Liver or abdominal nodes (± lung)	49	18
Tumor bed (± other sites)	16	8
Other (mainly brain or bone)*	25	13
Second tumor in other kidney	8	4

*These patients had rhabdoid or clear-cell histology.

Reference
1. D'Angio GJ, Breslow N, Beckwith JB, et al. Treatment of Wilms' tumor: results of the third National Wilms' Tumor Study. Cancer 1989;64:349–360.

TABLE 4–16
Considerations in Screening High-Risk Patients for Wilms Tumor

Does screening permit early diagnosis and improve prognosis?
Does earlier diagnosis improve prognosis?
Which patients should be screened?
Which imaging modality should be used?
How frequently should imaging be done?
At what age can imaging be safely stopped?
What are the psychological effects of screening?

agnose early lesions, with small lesions being missed on ultrasound[15] and one-third of synchronous bilateral tumors, found at surgery, not being identified preoperatively on imaging.[36] The argument in favor of routine screening is, however, quite persuasive. Many of the reports of missed small lesions were done with old imaging equipment, and it is strongly felt that more modern equipment, though they will still miss tiny lesions, will be more effective. Although early studies showed no relationship between the size of the tumor and prognosis,[37] results in the NWTS-III clearly indicate an improved prognosis with early diagnosis, and this evidence is an overwhelming argument in favor of screening high-risk patients. This study identified a better prognosis, and reduction in local abdominal recurrence, in children whose initial specimen weight (tumor + kidney) was less than 250 g.[37] Above this specimen weight prognosis did not continue to worsen with further increase in specimen weight. The relationship of tumor weight to initial stage shows a significantly lower percentage of stage IV patients when the specimen weight is under 250 g (Table 4–17). One study[38] found that 6 patients with metachronous bilateral tumors had the second tumor present on initial intravenous pyelogram in retrospect. Missing the earlier diagnosis of the second tumor in these patients did not affect survival, as all 3 patients lived. Because of the very small number of patients in this study, however, one cannot attach significance to these findings.

TABLE 4–17
Relationship of Tumor Weight and Tumor Stage[1]

Specimen Weight (tumor + kidney)	Stage IV Patients
<250 g	3.9%
250–499 g	9.3%
500–999 g	15.9%
>1000 g	18.1%

Reference
1. Breslow NE, Churchill G, Nesmith B, Cancer 1986;58:2501–2511.

Information is required as to which patients should be screened. Clearly, the entire population cannot be routinely surveyed with imaging. A high-risk group of patients must be identified and some arbitrary cut-off point determined below which it will be decided that the cost-effective yield from screening is too low to justify it. Routine clinical screening has not been found to result in earlier detection of Wilms tumor.[39] During the 8-year period of this study, 313 patients were identified with Wilms tumor. Of these, 29 (9 percent) were diagnosed on routine physical examination (routine physical examination of the entire population had been carried out). Of these 29 children, seven were stage III or IV, which was the same percentage of stage III or IV patients as was seen in the Wilms tumor patients who were not diagnosed by routine clinical screening. It was concluded that routine clinical screening did not result in earlier diagnosis of tumor.

Sporadic aniridia is known to have an incidence of Wilms tumor of up to 33 percent.[40] This is the highest incidence in any high-risk group. In one study, ultrasound screening of 11 children with aniridia detected two Wilms tumors, one of which was as small as 2.5 cm in diameter.[41] This study indicates that screening can identify early tumors in high-risk patients. Patients with a risk of over 1 percent of developing Wilms tumor can arbitrarily be designated into a group that should be screened. Until further information is available, it is probably not unreasonable to recommend no screening for patients in whom the risk of development of Wilms tumor is less than 1 percent (Table 4–18).

The choice of modality for routine screening is ultrasound. Intravenous urogram has a lower sensitivity, and requires radiation and contrast injection. CT scan may perhaps be slightly more sensitive than ultrasound, although no large study provides evidence to support this. The radiation, cost, and contrast injection required for CT are all disadvantages. MR might in the future prove more sensitive than ultrasound for detection of small tumors, but again no comparative studies have been done. In any event, the cost and unavailability of MR for screening would preclude its use.

The frequency of repetition of the ultrasound studies is largely an arbitrary decision. There is a wide range of reported recommendations, none of which are based on any scientific studies. The cost, and psychological trauma to the patient, of performing studies more frequently than every 3 months suggests that the study should not be performed more frequently. On the other hand, annual screening may be too infrequent in view of the known potential for rapid growth of Wilms tumor.[42] The decision must be an individual one, but repetition time of between 3 and 6 months would seem most logical based on present knowledge. One study[43] suggested that Wilms tumor could grow just as rapidly in older children as in younger children, and if this is correct, the frequency of studies should not be decreased as the child grows older. One factor against a

TABLE 4-18
Recommendations for Screening Patients at "Risk" for Development of Wilms Tumor[1-3]

Low Risk (don't screen)	High Risk >1% (do screen)
General population	Sporadic aniridia
Family members or relatives	Hemihypertrophy
Incidental nephroblastomatosis (nephrogenic rests)	Beckwith syndrome
Genitourinary abnormality (except Drash syndrome)	Drash syndrome
Unilateral tumor without nephroblastomatosis (nephrogenic rests)	Unilateral tumor with nephroblastomatosis (nephrogenic rests)
	Nephroblastomatosis (nephrogenic rests) + congenital genitourinary anomalies

References
1. Gonzalez-Crussi F, Kidd JM, Hernandez RJ. Cystic nephroma: morphologic spectrum and implications. Urology 1982;20:88–95.
2. Bond JV. Bilateral Wilms' tumor: age at diagnosis, associated congenital anomalies, and possible pattern of inheritance. Lancet 1975;2:482–486.
3. Mesrobian H-GJ. Wilms tumor: past, present, future. J Urol 1988;140:231–238.

too-aggressive approach to study repetition is the fact that the vast majority of Wilms tumors that are not diagnosed through screening programs are very large at the time of diagnosis and yet the overall prognosis for Wilms tumor remains excellent.

Screening high-risk children for Wilms tumor can probably be stopped between the ages of 6 and 10 years and I would recommend stopping such screening closer to 6 than to 10 years. My reasons for this are as follows. Less than 1 percent of all Wilms tumors occur after the age of 10 years and less than 15 percent occur after the age of 6 years (see Table 4–1). Furthermore, the age of diagnosis of Wilms tumor in high-risk patients (those with congenital anomalies, nephroblastomatosis, or bilateral tumors) tends to be even younger than in patients without these risk factors. With regard to the small subgroup of patients who are being screened for development of a second metachronous tumor, several studies indicate that such a tumor can almost always be diagnosed within 2 years of the diagnosis of the first tumor,[33,44,45] and it may be possible to stop screening in these patients after 2 years.

IMAGING APPEARANCE OF NEPHROBLASTOMATOSIS (NEPHROGENIC RESTS)

There has not been a large number of reported studies on nephroblastomatosis. Nephroblastomatosis may be missed on imaging studies.[46,47] On intravenous pyelogram, focal nephroblastomatosis is seen as a nonspecific mass lesion with calyceal displacement. Diffuse nephroblastomatosis causes marked enlargement of both kidneys with significant distortion of the calyces. On ultrasound, nephroblastomatosis has been reported as having similar[46] or diminished echogenicity[48,49] when compared to normal kidneys. The definition of the margins of focal areas of nephroblastomatosis is variable. With diffuse nephroblastomatosis, ultrasound shows widespread decreased echogenicity and renal enlargement and can be confused with lymphoma, leukemia, or polycystic kidneys.[48] On CT scan, focal areas of nephroblastomatosis may be well defined. They enhance very poorly after intravenous contrast injection. CT of diffuse nephroblastomatosis shows enlarged kidneys with calyceal distortion.[48] CT is probably more sensitive than ultrasound for detection of small focal lesions.[49] It should be emphasized that the appearance of focal nephroblastomatosis is relatively nonspecific and cannot be clearly differentiated from a small Wilms tumor.

References
1. Cope JR, Roylance J, Gordon IRS. The radiological features of Wilms' tumour. Clin Radiol 1972;23:331–339.
2. Andresen J, Steenskov V. Radiologic and prognostic aspects of Wilms' tumour. Acta Radiol Diag 1981;22:353–358.
3. Ritchey ML, Kelalis PP, Breslow N, et al. Intracaval and atrial involvement with nephroblastoma: review of National Wilms Tumor Study-3. J Urol 1988;140:1113–1118.
4. Cremin BJ. Non-function in nephroblastoma (Wilms's tumour): a report on the excretory urography of nine cases. Clin Radiol 1979;30:197–201.
5. Ehrlich RM, Bloomberg SD, Gyepes MT, et al. Wilms tumor, misdiagnosed preoperatively: a review of 19 National Wilms Tumor Study I cases. J Urol 1979;122:790–794.
6. Cremin BJ. Wilms' tumour: ultrasound and changing concepts. Clin Radiol 1987;38:465–474.
7. Hartman DS, Sanders RC. Wilms' tumor versus neuroblastoma: usefulness of ultrasound in differentiation. J Ultrasound Med 1982;1:117–122.

8. Jaffe MH, White SJ, Silver TM, et al. Radiology 1981;140:147–152.
9. Shimizu H, Jaffe N, Eftekhari F. Massive Wilms' tumor: sonographic demonstration of therapeutic response without alteration in size. Pediatr Radiol 1987;17:493–494.
10. Fishman EK, Hartman DS, Goldman SM, et al. The CT appearance of Wilms tumor. J Comput Assist Tomogr 1983;7:659–665.
11. Lowe RE, Cohen MD. Computed tomographic evaluation of Wilms tumor and neuroblastoma. RadioGraphics 1984;4:915–925.
12. Parvey LS, Warner RM, Callihan TR, et al. CT demonstration of fat tissue in malignant renal neoplasms: atypical Wilms' tumors. J Comput Assist Tomogr 1981;5:851–854.
13. Belt TG, Cohen MD, Smith JA, et al. MRI of Wilms' tumor: promise as the primary imaging method. AJR 1986; 146:955–961.
14. Kangarloo H, Dietrich RB, Ehrlich RM, et al. Magnetic resonance imaging of Wilms tumor. Urology 1986;28:203–208.
15. Boechat MI, Kangarloo H. MR imaging in Drash Syndrome. J Comput Assist Tomogr 1988;12:405–408.
16. Siddiqui AR, Cohen M, Moran DP. Abdominal masses in children: multiorgan imaging with 99m Tc methylene diphosphonate. AJR 1982;139:35–38.
17. Reiman TAH, Siegel MJ, Shackelford GD. Wilms tumor in children: abdominal CT and US evaluation. Radiology 1986;160:501–505.
18. Nakayama DK, Ortega W, D'Angio GJ, et al. The nonopacified kidney with Wilms' tumor. J Pediatr Surg 1988;23:152–155.
19. Mesrobian H-GJ, Kelalis PP, Hrabovsky E, et al. Wilms tumor in horseshoe kidneys: a report from the National Wilms Tumor Study. J Urol 1985;133:1002–1003.
20. Mahboubi S, Rosenberg HK, D'Angio GJ. Should inferior venacavography be performed in management of children with Wilms' tumor? Clin Pediatr 1982;21:690–694.
21. Luck SR, DeLeon S, Shkolnik A, et al. Intracardiac Wilms' tumor: diagnosis and management. J Pediatr Surg 1982;17:551–554.
22. Ramirez EA, Guerra GM. Radionuclide angiography: as diagnostic method for Wilms' tumor with direct extension into the heart. Pediatr Radiol 1982;12:301–303.
23. Ritchey ML, Kelalis PP, Breslow N, et al. Intracaval and atrial involvement with nephroblastoma: review of National Wilms Tumor Study–3. J Urol 1988;140:1113–1118.
24. Weese DL, Applebaum H, Taber P. Mapping intravascular extension of Wilms' tumor with magnetic resonance imaging. J Pediatr Surg 1991;26:64–67.
25. Breslow NE, Palmer NF, Hill LR, et al. Wilms' tumor: prognostic factors for patients without metastases at diagnosis. Results of the National Wilms' Tumor Study. Cancer 1978;41:1577–1589.
26. Brasch RC, Randel SB, Bould RG. Follow-up of Wilms tumor: comparison of CT with other imaging procedures. AJR 1981;137:1005–1009.
27. D'Angio GJ, Beckwith JB, Breslow N, et al. Wilms' tumor (nephroblastoma, renal embryoma). In: Pizzo PA, Poplack DG, eds. Principles and practice of pediatric oncology. Philadelphia: JB Lippincott, 1989:583–606.
28. Williams JA, Douglass EC, Magill HL, et al. Significance of pulmonary computed tomography at diagnosis in Wilms' tumor. J Clin Oncol 1988;6:1144–1146.
29. Cohen M, Smith WL, Weetman R, et al. Pulmonary pseudometastases in children with malignant tumors. Radiology 1981;141:371–374.
30. D'Angio GJ, Breslow N, Beckwith JB, et al. Treatment of Wilms' tumor: results of the third National Wilms' Tumor Study. Cancer 1989;64:349–360.
31. Williams JA, Hammond E, Douglass EC, et al. The value of computerized tomography as a routine follow-up procedure for patients with Wilms' tumor. Med Pediatr Oncol 1984;12:221–223.
32. Kim TH, Zaatari GS, Baum ES, et al. Recurrence of Wilms tumor after apparent cure. J Pediatr 1985;107:44–49.
33. Cohen MD, Siddiqui A, Weetman R, et al. A rational approach to the radiological evaluation of children with Wilms tumor. Cancer 1982;50:887–892.
34. Breslow N, Churchill G, Beckwith JB, et al. Prognosis for Wilms' tumor patients with nonmetastatic disease at diagnosis—results of the second National Wilms' Tumor Study. J Clin Oncol 1985;3:521–531.
35. Kobrinsky NL, Talgoy M, Shuckett B, et al. Wilms' tumor. Pediatr Ann 1988;17:238–250.
36. Kelalis PP. Wilms tumor (editorial). J Urol 1986;135:989.
37. D'Angio GJ, Evans A, Breslow N, et al. The treatment of Wilms' tumor: results of the second National Wilms' Tumor Study. Cancer 1981;47:2302–2311.
38. Wasiljew BK, Besser A, Raffensperger J. Treatment of bilateral Wilms' tumors—a 22-yr experience. J Pediatr Surg 1982;17:265–268.
39. Gutjahr P. Wilms tumours diagnosed by routine physical examinations. Eur J Pediatr 1989;148:174.
40. Bond JV, Bilateral Wilms' tumour: age at diagnosis, associated congenital anomalies, and possible pattern of inheritance. Lancet 1975;2:482–486.
41. Friedman AL. Wilms' tumor detection in patients with sporadic aniridia. Successful use of ultrasound. AJDC 1986;140:173–174.
42. Azouz EM, Larson EJ, Patel J, et al. Beckwith Wiedemann syndrome development of nephroblastoma during the surveillance period. Pediatr Radiol 1990;20:550–552.
43. Grossman H. Observing the growth of Wilms' tumor. Radiology 1976;121:697–700.
44. Jafasia KH, Thurman WG, Pickett E, et al. Bilateral Wilms' tumors in children. J Pediatr 1964;65:371–376.
45. Ragab AH, Vietti TJ, Crist W, et al. Bilateral Wilms' tumor. A review. Cancer 1972;30:983–988.
46. Fernbach SK, Feinstein KA, Donaldson JS, et al. Nephroblastomatosis: comparison of CT with US and urography. Radiology 1988;166:153–156.
47. Cormier PJ, Donaldson JS, Gonzalez-Crussi F. Nephroblastomatosis: missed diagnosis. Radiology 1988; 169:737–738.
48. Franken EA, Yiu-Chiu V, Smith WL, et al. Nephroblastomatosis: clinicopathologic significance and imaging characteristics. AJR 1982;138:950–952.
49. Heideman RL, McGavran L, Waldstein G. Nephroblastomatosis and deletion of 11p. The potential etiologic relationship to subsequent Wilms' tumor. Am J Pediatr Hematol/Oncol 1986;8:231–234.

Differential Diagnosis

The major mass lesions in the differential diagnosis of Wilms tumor are listed in Table 4–19. These are all discussed in other sections, but it is important to note that the appearance of the lesion in the kidney is relatively

TABLE 4-19
Differential Diagnosis of Wilms Tumor

Rhabdoid tumor of kidney
Clear-cell sarcoma
Renal-cell carcinoma
Mesoblastic nephroma
Focal nephroblastomatosis
Lymphoma

nonspecific and final diagnosis depends upon histology. Knowledge of the patient's age is helpful. For example, a mass in a neonate is almost always a mesoblastic nephroma rather than a Wilms tumor. Other rare tumors to be considered in the differential diagnosis of Wilms tumor include angiolipoma, carcinoid tumor, rhabdomyosarcoma, stromal tumors, neurogenic tumors, mesenchymoma, and metastases. Nontumor conditions to be considered in the differential diagnosis include abscess and hematoma from trauma. In these situations, the history and clinical findings usually guide one to the correct diagnosis. Note should be made that patients with Wilms tumor can occasionally present following trauma, and any discrepancy between the size of the lesion identified on CT and the history should make one seriously consider the possibility of an underlying tumor.

The differential diagnosis of multilocular cystic nephroma with Wilms tumor has been presented in Table 4–5.

Local recurrence of Wilms tumor has no specific identifying features and may be mistaken for any other mass lesion in the region of the kidney. One patient with the incidental finding of a tumor (fibromatosis) in the colon wall was originally thought to have recurrent Wilms tumor.[1]

Comment: When one considers information provided from imaging, clinical evaluation, and laboratory studies, the preoperative diagnosis of Wilms tumor (apart from differentiating it from clear-cell and rhabdoid tumor) is usually fairly straightforward.

Reference

1. Mahboubi S, Meadows A, Chatten J. Fibrous lesion of the bowel complicating the management of bilateral Wilms' tumor. Pediatr Radiol 1981;11:49–51.

Therapy and Prognosis

Survival of Wilms tumor has increased from approximately 10 percent in 1920s to a modern-day 90 percent[1] (Table 4–20). The most recent survival data by tumor stage and histology for the NWTS-III is given in Table 4–21.

TABLE 4-20
Historical Wilms Tumor Survival[1]

Dates	Major Therapy Added	Approximate Survival (%)
1920s	Surgery	10
1940s	Radiation	50
1960s	Early chemotherapy	80
1980s	Modern chemotherapy	90

Reference

1. Belasco J, D'Angio GJ. Wilms' tumor. Ca-A Cancer J for Clinicians 1981;31:258–270.

TABLE 4-21
Wilms Tumor, 4-Year Survival[1]*

Stage, Histology	Percentage
Stage I, favorable histology	96
Stage II, favorable histology	92
Stage III, favorable histology	87
Stage IV	91
Stage IV, all histology + unfavorable histology stages I–III	73
Overall 127 of 1489 patients died	

*NWTS-III (1439 cases).

Reference

1. D'Angio GJ, Breslow N, Beckwith JB, et al. Treatment of Wilms' tumor: results of the third National Wilms' Tumor Study. Cancer 1989;64:349–360.

There are several points of interest to the radiologist. Patients with synchronous bilateral tumors have a prognosis almost as good as those patients with unilateral tumors.[2–5] The prognosis with metachronous tumors is not as good. This is possibly because with modern chemotherapy the only metachronous tumors that are being diagnosed are those of a more aggressive nature that have not responded to or not been controlled by the chemotherapy when they were too small to be diagnosed clinically or by imaging.[2] The finding on chest radiograph or chest CT of mediastinal or pleural tumor will often indicate a poor prognosis (Fig. 4–21). In one series, all eight patients with such spread died.[6] A specimen (kidney + tumor weight) of less than 250 g (i.e., early diagnosis) has a lower incidence of stage IV tumors[7] and a better prognosis.[8] The presence of tumor in the inferior vena cava does not adversely affect the prognosis when these patients are compared to other patients with the same stage but without inferior vena cava tumor.[3,9] Patients with inferior vena cava tumor are, however, more likely to have distant metastatic spread and, therefore, be stage IV.[7] Historically, patients with cardiac extension of tumor did very poorly. Recent NWTS data, however, showed that 11 of 14 patients with favorable histology and cardiac extension of

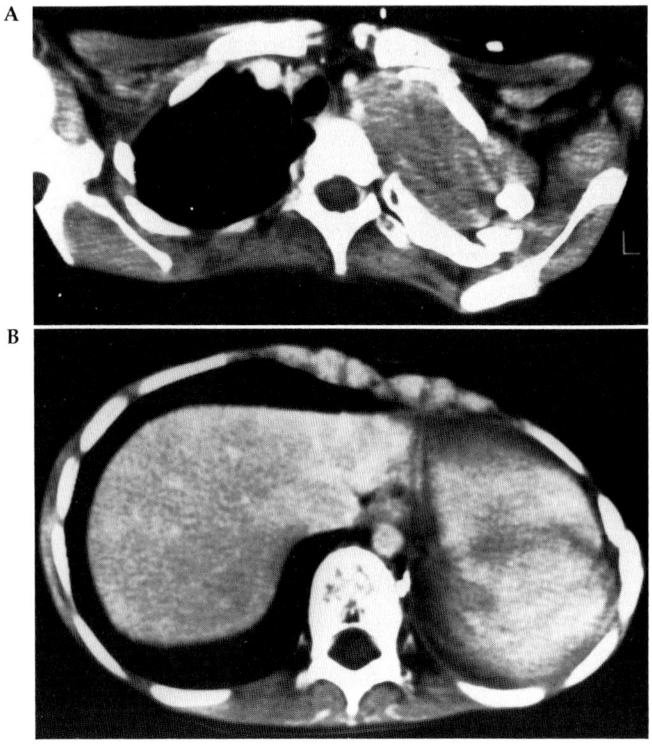

Figure 4-21. **Diagnosis: Wilms tumor. Pleural and mediastinal metastases. The left lung has previously been removed.**
***A* and *B*, CT. Solid tumor fills the visualized segments of the left hemithorax. The entire pleural space is occupied by tumor, which extends to the mediastinum.**

tumor survived.[5] This probably reflects the success of imaging in identifying cardiac tumor extension prior to the commencement of surgery.

Survival in patients who have relapsed is not nearly as good as in other patients with Wilms tumor. A study from the United Kingdom published in 1991 analyzed the results of 71 relapses in 381 patients with Wilms tumor. The overall survival was less than 50 percent. Prognosis was worst if the initial presentation was at stage III or IV, if there was unfavorable histology, or if the relapse was in a site other than the lung.[10]

The cause of death in large NWTS series is tumor in over 80 percent of cases and complications of therapy in the remainder.[11]

Comment: Overall survival in Wilms tumor is approaching 90%.

SURGERY

Apart from patients with extensive bilateral disease, surgery is the initial primary therapy employed for Wilms tumor.[12] The objective is complete resection of the primary tumor mass if at all possible. Imaging plays a vital role in guiding the surgical approach. In the NWTS-III study, only 133 of 2,496 patients were inoperable at the time of surgery.[11] It is not known in how many patients this determination was made prior to laparotomy. With modern imaging techniques it is hoped that the prediction of nonresectability can be made more accurately. In those patients in whom the tumor is initially deemed unresectable, reduction in size can be achieved with chemotherapy.[4] This has also been done using preoperative embolization.[13,14] Because chemotherapy is so successful and because of the invasive nature and risks of embolization, chemotherapy is preferred. After reduction in tumor size, surgery can be performed.

The objectives of surgery are summarized in Table 4–22, and imaging plays an important role in each of these. Other areas in which imaging will affect surgery are the identification of tumor invasion of the renal pelvis. Because of the risks of local spread of tumor into the ureter, the surgeon may elect to perform a radical rather than the conventional partial ureterectomy.[15,16] Imaging is important in guiding the surgeon to biopsy lymph nodes with possible tumor. This determination cannot be made accurately at surgery. In one study, the surgeon's evaluation of the lymph node compared to the histology revealed a 31 percent false negative and a 17 percent false positive result.[17]

The European approach to surgery in Wilms tumor is different from that in the United States.[5] Presurgical chemotherapy is routinely used, the rationale being to reduce tumor size, reduce tumor rupture at surgery, and, therefore, reduce the requirement for abdominal radiation therapy. The European Study Group also compared preoperative chemotherapy with preoperative chemotherapy combined with radiation therapy. They found there was no advantage to using radiotherapy in addition to chemotherapy as a means of reducing surgical rupture of tumor.[18] This approach of preoperative chemotherapy is not followed in the United States because of a 5 percent diagnostic error (other disorders misdiagnosed as Wilms tumor), the requirement of surgery for accurate tumor staging, and also because accurate histological subtyping cannot be performed following chemotherapy.

Bilateral tumors represent a special case.[16,19–22] The traditional approach has been to resect the larger tumor together with the kidney and then to attempt local resection of the second tumor either initially (if the tumor is very small) or at second-look surgery following che-

TABLE 4–22
Objective of Surgery for Which Imaging is Important

Resection of primary tumor
Biopsy of abnormal lymph nodes
Biopsy of possible tumor in opposite kidney
Biopsy of liver for possible metastases
Removal of tumor from inferior vena cava

motherapy. Unless there is a massive tumor with complete kidney destruction on one side, a more modern approach is to attempt kidney salvage surgery on both sides either before or after chemotherapy. Imaging is of vital importance in defining the preoperative extent of the tumor. CT should be performed in all cases. MR, particularly with its ability to image in multiple planes, will add useful additional information to the surgeon. In selected cases, the surgeon may require angiography to define the anatomy of the renal vessels and their relationship to the tumor; modern color Doppler ultrasound imaging has great potential for providing this information, but no data about its accuracy is available. CT, ultrasound, or MR can initially be used to follow the reduction in tumor volume in response to chemotherapy.

Liver metastases will be surgically excised wherever possible.

RADIATION THERAPY

Abdominal radiation is utilized only for patients with stage III disease and patients with stage IV disease in whom the primary tumor would not have been classified as stage I or II in the absence of metastases. Radiation is given to the tumor bed and across the midline for most patients requiring it. Whole abdomen radiation including pelvic radiation is utilized in those patients in whom there is peritoneal spread of tumor, gross residual disease following surgery, or diffuse spillage of tumor at surgery. These are surgical determinations and imaging has little role to play. In those patients in whom localized radiation is utilized, imaging is vitally important, as the radiation ports are determined by the extent of the tumor as defined on imaging prior to surgery. MR, with its ability to display tumor in the coronal plane, may prove of more help to the radiation oncologist than CT imaging.

Patients in whom any lung metastatic disease is identified are given radiation to both lung fields.

LUNG METASTASES

The demonstration of a lung nodule in a patient with known Wilms tumor cannot be assumed to be a metastasis. A variety of benign lesions, including histoplasmosis, round pneumonia, inflammatory pseudotumor, hamartoma, and radiation pneumonitis can mimic metastatic disease.[23] In most patients, therefore, metastatic disease should be confirmed by biopsy, which, provided the nodule is large enough, should be performed using percutaneous needle biopsy and not thoracotomy. Patients with diffuse nodules spread through both lungs can probably be safely assumed to have metastases, although in these patients needle biopsy should be particularly easy to perform. The presence of calcium within a lung nodule almost certainly indicates that it is benign, but care should be taken, because patients may have both histoplasmosis and metastatic disease at the same time.

> *Comment:* Prognosis in Wilms tumor is excellent.
> Imaging has an important role in guiding therapy.
> As therapy and prognosis change the questions asked of imaging must be altered.
> The presence of suspected metastatic disease must be histologically confirmed.

LATE EFFECTS

Long-term follow-up of patients with Wilms tumor is now being carried out. In a study published in 1991, 787 patients who were alive and without relapse more than 5 years after initial diagnosis of Wilms tumor were analyzed. Nineteen of the patients had developed other benign tumors, of which osteochondroma and bone exostoses were the most common. Five of the 787 patients had developed second malignant tumors. All 5 of these patients had received radiation therapy as part of their initial therapy.[24]

References

1. Belasco J, D'Angio GJ. Wilms' tumor. Ca-A Cancer J for Clinicians 1981;31:258–270.
2. Casale AJ, Flanigan RC, Moore PJ. Survival in bilateral metachronous (asynchronous) Wilms tumors. J Urol 1982;128:766–769.
3. Exelby PR. Retroperitoneal malignant tumors: Wilms' tumor and neuroblastoma. Surg Clin N Am 1981; 61:1219–1227.
4. Kelalis PP. Wilms tumor (editorial). J Urol 1986;135:989.
5. D'Angio GJ, Beckwith JB, Breslow N, et al. Wilms' tumor (nephroblastoma, renal embryoma). In: Pizzo PA, Poplack DG, eds. Principles and practice of pediatric oncology. Philadelphia: JB Lippincott, 1989:583–606.
6. Cushing BA, Watts FB, Brough AJ, et al. Significance of mediastinal metastatic disease in Wilms' tumor of favorable histology. Med Pediatr Oncol 1984;12:123–126.
7. Breslow NE, Churchill G, Nesmith B, et al. Cancer 1986;58:2501–2511.
8. D'Angio GJ, Evans A, Breslow N, et al. The treatment of Wilms' tumor: results of the second National Wilms' Tumor Study. Cancer 1981;47:2302–2311.
9. Ritchey ML, Kelalis PP, Breslow N, et al. Intracaval and atrial involvement with nephroblastoma: review of National Wilms Tumor Study-3. J Urol 1988;140:1113–1118.
10. Pinkerton GR, Groot-Loonen JJ, Morris-Jones PH, et al. Response rates in relapsed Wilms' tumor. Cancer 1991;67:567–571.
11. D'Angio GJ, Breslow N, Beckwith JB, et al. Treatment of Wilms' tumor: results of the third National Wilms' Tumor Study. Cancer 1989;64:349–360.
12. Kobrinsky NL, Talgoy M, Shuckett B, et al. Wilms' tumor. Pediatr Ann 1988;17:238–250.
13. Danis RK, Wolverson MK, Graviss ER, O'Connor DM, et al. Preoperative embolization of Wilms' tumors. Am J Dis Child 1979;133:503–506.
14. Harrison MR, de Lorimier AA, Boswell WO. Preoperative angiographic embolization for large hemorrhagic Wilms' tumor. J Pediatr Surg 1978;13:757–758.
15. Johnson KM, Horvath LJ, Gaisie G, et al. Wilms tumor occurring as a botryoid renal pelvicalyceal mass. Radiology 1987;163:385–386.

16. Mesrobian H-GJ. Wilms tumor: past, present, future. J Urol 1988;140:231–238.
17. Othersen HB, DeLorimer A, Hrabovsky E, et al. Surgical evaluation of lymph node metastases in Wilms' tumor. J Pediatr Surg 1990;25:330–331.
18. Lemerle J, Voute PA, Tournade MF. J Clin Oncol 1983;1:604–609.
19. Longaker MT, Harrison MR, Adzick NS, et al. Nephron-sparing approach to bilateral Wilms' tumor: in situ or ex vivo surgery and radiation therapy. J Pediatr Surg 1990;25:411–414.
20. Martin LW, Kloecker RJ. Bilateral nephroblastoma (Wilms' tumor). Pediatrics 1961;28:101–106.
21. Wasiljew BK, Besser A, Raffensperger J. Treatment of bilateral Wilms' tumors—a 22-yr experience. J Pediatr Surg 1982;17:265–268.
22. Pumberger W, Wurnig P. Surgical treatment of bilateral Wilms' tumours with special reference to second operations in metachronous disease. Prog Pediatr Surg 1989;23:96–103.
23. Cohen M, Smith WL, Weetman R, et al. Pulmonary pseudometastases in children with malignant tumors. Radiology 1981;141:371–374.
24. Evans AE, Norkool P, Evans I, et al. Late effects of treatment of Wilms' tumor. A report from the National Wilms' Tumor Study Group. Cancer 1991;67:331–336.

OTHER RENAL TUMORS

CLEAR-CELL SARCOMA

This tumor is often included with Wilms tumor as a variant or subgroup. It has several features that distinguish it from classic Wilms tumor (Table 4–23).

Epidemiology

Clear-cell sarcomas represent about 4 percent of renal pediatric tumors.[1] In large series of patients with Wilms tumor, it has been reported as occurring in 2 of 39 cases,[2] 9 of 123 cases,[3] 50 of 1,439 cases,[4] and 13 of 358 cases.[5] The age of onset has been reported as being similar to conventional classic Wilms tumor[6] or slightly younger than classic Wilms tumor.[9]

TABLE 4–23
Features Differentiating Clear-Cell Sarcoma of the Kidney from Classic Wilms Tumor

Worse prognosis
Bone metastasis
Never bilateral
Can be partly cystic
No capsule

Pathology

Grossly, the tumors are large single renal masses. They are never multicentric and never bilateral.[1] Cystic spaces may be present and the tumors may mimic multilocular cystic nephroma.[8] The tumor lacks a capsule or pseudocapsule and infiltrates into adjacent normal renal tissue.[1] As with classic Wilms tumor, metastases can occur in the lung. The tumors are, however, distinguished by the very high incidence of bone metastases. In one study, 42 percent of patients had bone metastases[1] and in another literature review, bone metastases were identified in up to 76 percent of patients.[9] The bone metastases are frequently multiple and extensive[9] and can involve all sites except the hands and feet.[10] These tumors will also occasionally metastasize to unusual sites such as the tonsil, pancreas, and adrenal gland.[11] Lymph node metastases can occur.

Imaging Studies

On imaging, large focal masses are seen within the kidney. On ultrasound, they are moderately well defined and predominantly echogenic. Cystic areas will be of low echogenicity. CT shows mixed intensity with the focal tumor mass (Fig. 4–22). There are no specific features, on imaging of the primary tumor, to differentiate these tumors from conventional classic Wilms tumor.[9]

The appearance of the bone metastases varies. They can be lytic, permeative, or sclerotic. There are no specific diagnostic features of the metastases.[10]

From a radiographic point of view the important features in this tumor are the high incidence of bone metastases and the late development of metastases in some patients. Routine bone scanning is not performed preoperatively in patients with suspected Wilms tumor. In those patients in whom histology identifies a clear-cell sarcoma, bone scan should be routinely performed to look for metastases. This should be continued for several years.

Therapy and Prognosis

Treatment is surgical resection and chemotherapy. The prognosis is relatively poor. Even with patients initially thought to be stage I, the recurrence rate is high.[6,8] This indicates that micrometastases must frequently be present at the time of diagnosis. The onset of development of metastatic disease can be significantly delayed. In one series of 13 patients, metastases occurred more than 2 years after diagnosis in 5 patients. Survival in the NWTS-I and NWTS-II studies was 52 percent and in 50 patients in the NWTS-III study, there was a 75 percent 4-year survival.[4]

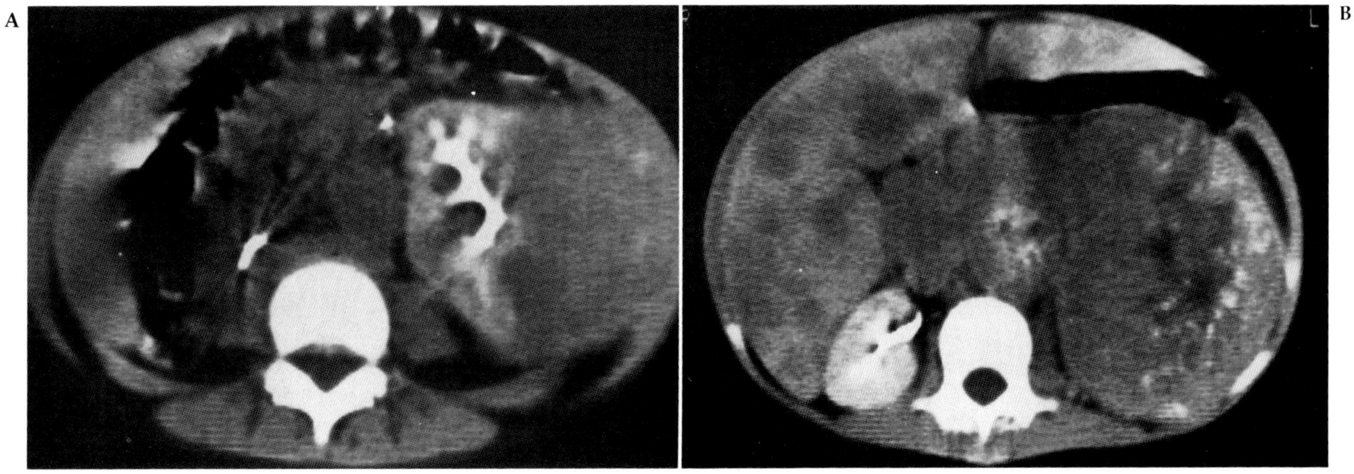

Figure 4-22. **Diagnosis: Clear-cell sarcoma of the kidney with liver metastases. *A,* CT. Soft-tissue tumor mass is seen arising from the lateral aspect of the kidney. *B,* CT. Several centimeters above the previous image. The tumor mass has expanded superiorly and is very large. There is patchy irregular enhancement. Extensive low-intensity metastases to the liver are seen. There are no specific features differentiating this tumor from classic Wilms tumor.**

> *Comment:* Clear-cell sarcoma of the kidney is distinguished from classic Wilms tumor by having a worse prognosis and a high likelihood of metastasizing to bone.

References

1. Beckwith JB. Wilms' tumor and other renal tumors of childhood: a selective review from the National Wilms' Tumor Study Pathology Center. Hum Pathol 1983;14:481–492.
2. Levick RK, Steiner GM. Skeletal survey in Wilms' tumour assessment. Ann Radiol 1983;26:235–236.
3. Morgan E, Kidd JM. Undifferentiated sarcoma of the kidney. A tumor of childhood with histopathologic and clinical characteristics distinct from Wilms' tumor. Cancer 1978;42:1916–1921.
4. D'Angio GJ, Breslow N, Beckwith JB, et al. Treatment of Wilms' tumor: results of the third National Wilms' Tumor Study. Cancer 1989;64:349–360.
5. Marsden HB, Lawler W. Bone-metastasizing renal tumour of childhood. Br J Cancer 1978;38:437–440.
6. D'Angio GJ, Beckwith JB, Breslow N, et al. Wilms' tumor (nephroblastoma, renal embryoma). In: Pizzo PA, Poplack DG, eds. Principles and practice of pediatric oncology. Philadelphia: JB Lippincott, 1989:583–606.
7. Gonzalez-Crussi F, Baum ES. Renal sarcomas of childhood. A clinicopathologic and ultrastructural study. Cancer 1983;51:898–912.
8. Beckwith JB. Wilms tumor and other renal tumors of childhood: an update. J Urol 1986;136:320–329.
9. Kagan RA, Steckel RJ. Clear cell sarcoma of the kidney: a renal tumor of childhood that metastasizes to bone. AJR 1986;146:64–66.
10. Lamego CMB, Zerbini MCN. Bone-metastasizing primary renal tumors in children. Radiology 1983;147:449–454.
11. Movassaghi N, Leikin S, Chandra R. Wilms' tumor metastasis to uncommon sites. J Pediatr 1974;84:416–417.

RHABDOID TUMOR OF THE KIDNEY

Rhabdoid tumor was once included with Wilms tumor as a subgroup, but it is now recommended that it be considered a separate, distinct tumor type. Some of the features distinguishing it from Wilms tumor are summarized in Table 4–24.

Epidemiology

Rhabdoid tumor occurs in young infants. The median age in two studies was 11 months and 13 months.[1,2] It is extremely rare over the age of 5, but can occur in the neonatal period.[1]

TABLE 4–24
Features Differentiating Rhabdoid Tumor of the Kidney from Classic Wilms Tumor

Metastases to brain
Very poor prognosis
Hypercalcemia
Not bilateral
Younger patients
Origin in center of kidney
Second primary brain tumors occur
No identifiable high-risk clinical syndrome

Rhabdoid tumor is uncommon, occurring in 31 of 1,439 patients enrolled in National Wilms Tumor Study–III.[3] There is no association of rhabdoid tumor with any of the high-risk tumors that have been identified with classic Wilms tumor. There is no increased incidence of nephroblastomatosis in patients with rhabdoid tumor.[1] The tumors are slightly more common in boys than girls.

Pathology

Grossly, these tumors are often large. In 111 patients, the mean diameter of tumor plus kidney was 9 cm. They usually arise in the central portion of the kidney compared to Wilms tumors, which are more frequently peripheral. The tumors spread throughout the kidney, destroying most of the renal tissue. Hilar and renal vein invasion are common.[1] Microscopically, the tumors have a distinctive pathological picture and can be diagnosed from needle biopsy.[4]

Metastatic spread is extremely common. The lung and liver, as with classic Wilms tumor, are the most common sites of metastatic spread.[5] Rhabdoid tumor does, however, show several distinctive patterns of metastases. Metastatic spread to brain is common.[1,6] The brain metastases in 7 patients were found in any location, with the cerebrum the most common site.[1] Like clear-cell sarcoma, but unlike classic Wilms tumor, bone metastases can occur with rhabdoid tumor.[1]

A unique finding with rhabdoid tumor is the association of second primary tumors in the brain.[1,6,7] In one series of 111 patients with rhabdoid tumor, 13.5 percent developed an associated primary brain tumor. These tumors were all midline, mostly in the posterior fossa or just above the tent. They occurred either before, at the same time, or after the diagnosis of the renal rhabdoid tumor. The most common brain tumor was medulloblastoma, with primitive neuroectodermal tumor being the second most common. In another study of 6 patients with associated primary brain tumors, 3 had medulloblastomas, 1 a primitive neuroectodermal tumor, 1 an astrocytoma, and 1 a pinealoblastoma.[7] All children in this study were under the age of 2 years and both the brain and renal tumors were diagnosed within 4 months of each other in each patient.[7]

Clinical Presentation

The clinical features are the large abdominal mass, which grows quickly. A striking finding in rhabdoid tumor, which never occurs in Wilms tumor, is the appearance of hypercalcemia caused by the tumor's producing either parahormone or prostaglandin E. In one study, this was present in 6 patients,[6] in another study in 4 patients,[1] and in another study 1 of 2 cases.[8]

Imaging Studies

Imaging evaluation of rhabdoid tumors shows a very large tumor mass in the kidney (Fig. 4–23). In most patients, the tumors have similar appearance to classic Wilms tumor and differentiation cannot be made. In 2 patients, both CT and ultrasound showed an unusual feature that might be suggestive of rhabdoid tumor.[5] Both of these patients had large subcapsular fluid collections with thickening of the renal capsule and tumor nodules identified adjacent to the capsule. Another study reports subcapsular fluid in 1 of 2 cases.[8]

From an imaging viewpoint most of these patients cannot be differentiated from classic Wilms tumor prior to nephrectomy and histology. Occasionally, presentation with metastatic disease in an unusual site may suggest the correct diagnosis prior to nephrectomy. Once the diagnosis has been established, widespread screening for metastatic disease should be performed. This should include chest and abdominal CT scans, bone scan and head CT or MR, even in the absence of symptoms.

Therapy and Prognosis

The prognosis of rhabdoid tumor is poor. Metastatic spread at diagnosis is common. Following resection of tumor, local recurrence is not infrequent,[1] occurring in 9 of 111 patients. In one study of 21 patients, 19 died[2]; in another study, mortality was 90 percent.[9] Of 111 patients with rhabdoid tumor 80 percent died.[1] In 31 patients with rhabdoid tumor of the kidney enrolled in the National Wilms Tumor Study-III, 4-year survival was only 25 percent.[3]

References
1. Weeks DA, Beckwith JB, Mierau GW, et al. Rhabdoid tumor of kidney. A report of 111 cases from the National Wilms' Tumor Study Pathology Center. Am J Surg Pathol 1989;13:439–458.
2. Beckwith JB. Wilms' tumor and other renal tumors of childhood: a selective review from the National Wilms' Tumor Study Pathology Center. Hum Pathol 1983;14:481–492.
3. D'Angio GJ, Breslow N, Beckwith JB, Treatment of Wilms' tumor: results of the third National Wilms' Tumor Study. Cancer 1989;64:349–360.
4. Beckwith JB. Wilms tumor and other renal tumors of childhood: an update. J Urol 1986;136:320–329.
5. Sisler CL, Siegel MJ. Malignant rhabdoid tumor of the kidney: radiologic features. Radiology 1989;172:211–216.
6. Cormier PJ, Donaldson JS, Gonzalez-Crussi F. Nephroblastomatosis: missed diagnosis. Radiology 1988;169:737–738.
7. Bonnin JM, Rubinstein LJ, Palmer NF, et al. The association of embryonal tumors originating in the kidney and in the brain. A report of seven cases. Cancer 1984;54:2137–2146.
8. Eftekhari F, Erly WK, Jaffe N. Malignant rhabdoid tumor of the kidney: imaging features in two cases. Pediatr Radiol 1991;21:39–42.
9. Gonzalez-Crussi F, Kidd JM, Hernandez RJ. Cystic nephroma: morphologic spectrum and implications. Urology 1982;20:88–95.

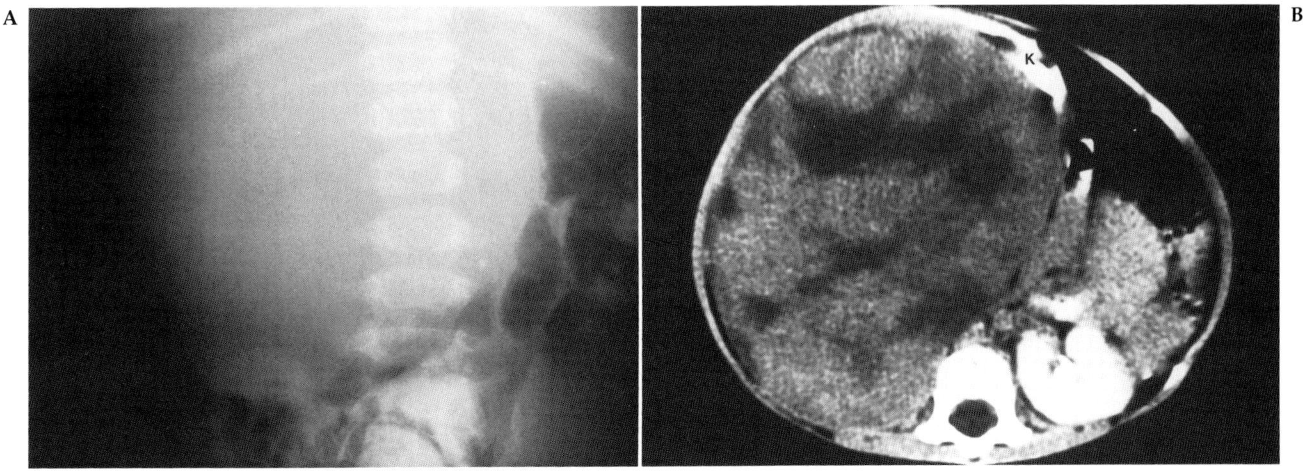

Figure 4–23. **Diagnosis: Rhabdoid tumor of the kidney.**
***A*, Plain film radiograph. There is a very large right upper quadrant mass displacing bowel loops inferiorly and to the left. *B*, CT scan. Once again a large right upper quadrant mass is identified. Low-intensity areas within it represent hemorrhage or necrosis. A small rim of functioning kidney tissue (*K*) is seen anteriorly. This tumor cannot be differentiated from a classic Wilms tumor.**

RENAL CELL CARCINOMA

Epidemiology

Renal cell carcinoma is very common in adults but is a rare tumor in children. It occurs at an older age than Wilms tumor, with the mean age in three series of 44 patients being 10, 11, and 12 years.[1,2] The incidence of the tumor is equal in boys and girls.[1–4] Reported associations include tuberosclerosis[1] and von Hippel-Lindau syndrome.[3]

Pathology

Grossly, the tumors tend to be much smaller than Wilms tumor at the time of diagnosis.[1,3] Calcification is more common than in Wilms tumor, occurring in up to 25 percent of patients.[2] The calcification tends to be denser and more homogenous than in Wilms tumor. Calcification can also be seen in metastatic disease in local lymph nodes. Some of the features that help to differentiate renal cell carcinoma from Wilms are summarized in Table 4–25. Renal cell carcinoma, in the teenage group, tends to be bilateral much more commonly than Wilms tumor.[5] Bilateral Wilms tumors occur in very young children. The tumor spreads by local invasion. In one study, the capsule was penetrated in 4 of 17 patients[1] and in another, 7 of 8 patients had either capsular invasion or local lymph node involvement.[6] Lymph node metastases were found in 9 of 17 patients.[1] Metastases can also occur to liver, lung, and bone. The staging of renal cell carcinoma in children is the same as in adults (Table 4–26). In 17 patients, the stage at diagnosis was stage I (6), stage II (4), stage III (4), and stage

TABLE 4–25
Features that May Help Differentiation of Renal Cell Carcinoma and Wilms Tumor[1–3]

Renal cell carcinoma
- Smaller at the time of diagnosis
- Calcification more common and more homogenous
- Older children
- Hematuria is more common

References
1. Chan HSL, Daneman A, Gribbin M, et al. Renal cell carcinoma in the first two decades of life. Pediatr Radiol 1983;13:324–328.
2. Hartman DS, Davis CJ, Madewell JE, et al. Primary malignant renal tumors in the second decade of life: Wilms tumor versus renal cell carcinoma. J Urol 1982;127:888–891.
3. Lack EE, Cassady JR, Sallan SE. Renal cell carcinoma in childhood and adolescence: a clinical and pathological study of 17 cases. J Urol 1985;133:822–828.

TABLE 4–26
Staging of Renal Cell Carcinoma[1]

I, confined to kidney
II, extension into perirenal tissues
III, extension into renal vein or local nodes
IV, invasion of adjacent organs (except adrenal) or distant metastases

Reference
1. Mancini AF, Paloucci G. Renal cell carcinoma in childhood. Med Pediatr Oncol 1989;17:53–57.

IV (3). In another study, 80 percent of patients were reported as being stage I.[7]

Clinical Presentation

Symptoms of renal cell carcinoma are relatively nonspecific and include pain, hematuria, or a palpable mass.[1–3,6] Hematuria is much more common than with Wilms tumor and may sometimes be the presenting sign after incidental minor trauma.[6] In these patients, it is important not to misdiagnose the tumor as a hematoma in the kidney.

Imaging Studies

On imaging studies, renal cell carcinoma is identified quite easily as a mass lesion. It can be seen with urography, CT, ultrasound, or MR. Intravenous pyelography shows a nonspecific mass lesion.[2] On ultrasound, the lesions are predominantly complex echogenic masses[1] and on CT, they are well-defined nonhomogenous masses with varying enhancement[1] (Fig. 4–24). Angiography identifies masses of varying vascularity with no specific features.[1] In general terms, it is not possible to differentiate renal cell carcinoma from Wilms tumor by imaging in the majority of patients. In a study comparing 56 teenagers with Wilms tumor with 52 teenagers with renal cell carcinoma, factors favoring a diagnosis of renal cell carcinoma were the presence of a relatively small mass, calcification within the mass, or nodal metastases (Fig. 4–24), bone metastasis, or bilateral tumors.

Imaging studies should include ultrasound of the inferior vena cava, CT of the chest and abdomen, and a technetium 99m bone scan. Angiography or urography are not required.

Differential Diagnosis

Differential diagnosis includes any renal mass lesion, including Wilms tumor, lymphoma, and angiomyolipoma.

Therapy and Prognosis

Treatment is mainly surgical resection together with chemotherapy and radiation therapy. Reported survival varies; in reported series, 9 of 17 patients,[1] 6 of 17 patients,[2] and 1 of 8 patients died.[6] It is important to remember that all these series include patients treated with different modalities over many years.

> *Comment:* Renal cell carcinoma does occur in children. The children are older than those with Wilms tumor.

References

1. Chan HSL, Daneman A, Gribbin M. Renal cell carcinoma in the first two decades of life. Pediatr Radiol 1983;13:324–328.
2. Lack EE, Cassady JR, Sallan SE. Renal cell carcinoma in childhood and adolescence: a clinical and pathological study of 17 cases. J Urol 1985;133:822–828.
3. Hartman DS, Davis CJ, Madewell JE. Primary malignant renal tumors in the second decade of life: Wilms tumor versus renal cell carcinoma. J Urol 1982;127:888–894.
4. Leuschner I, Harms D, Schmidt D. Renal cell carcinoma in children: histology, immunohistochemistry, and follow-up of 10 cases. Medical Pediatr Oncol 1991;19:33–41.
5. Kirks DR, Kaufman RA. Function within mesoblastic nephroma: imaging—pathologic correlation. Pediatr Radiol 1989;19:136–139.
6. Cassady JR, Filler R, Jaffe N, et al. Carcinoma of the kidney in children. Radiology 1974;112:691–693.
7. Mancini AF, Paloucci G. Renal cell carcinoma in childhood. Med Pediatr Oncol 1989;17:53–57.

Figure 4-24. **Diagnosis: Renal cell carcinoma.**
A, **CT. There is a moderate-sized mass in the right kidney *(arrowheads).* The very dense areas within the mass was shown on plain film radiograph to be calcium. *B*, CT. Heavily calcified metastatic lesions to retrocrural lymph nodes are identified *(arrowheads).* The relatively small size of this tumor and the heavy calcification suggest renal cell carcinoma rather than Wilms tumor as the diagnosis.**

A

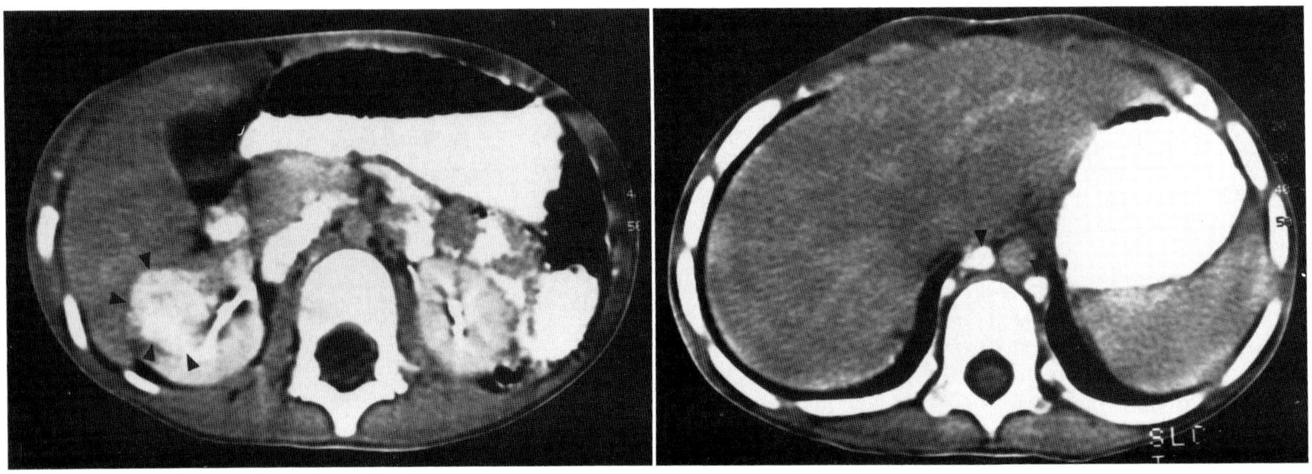

B

MULTILOCULAR CYSTIC NEPHROMA

Multilocular cystic nephroma is a disorder that causes much confusion and debate. The first issue to consider is whether these lesions are congenital malformations or true tumors. As they can grow in size, and have the potential for metastases, they should definitely be considered a tumor and not a congenital malformation. The next issue is to determine whether the tumor is benign or malignant. Although the vast majority of multilocular cystic nephromas are benign, these tumors can contain areas of microscopic or macroscopic nephroblastoma and can occasionally metastasize. They should, therefore, be considered as predominantly benign lesions with occasional propensity for malignancy. They are, moreover, unusual tumors in that even when malignant they are not particularly aggressive.

Epidemiology

Multilocular cystic nephroma occurs either in very young children or in adults.[12] In children, 75 percent of these tumors are found in males[1] and most of the children are in the age range between 3 months and 4 years.[1] In fact over 90 percent of these tumors present under the age of 2 years.[2]

Pathology

Grossly, multilocular cystic nephroma is a large well-defined focal renal tumor. The criteria for diagnosis are summarized in Tables 4–5 and 4–27. These tumors are never bilateral and never multifocal.[3] They involve only part of the kidney and, therefore, can easily be differentiated from multicystic dysplastic kidney.[1] A thick capsule is usually present.[2] The cysts vary considerably in size. They can be very small or very large. They do not communicate either with each other or with the collecting system[1,2,4–8] and this feature helps differentiate them from other cystic disorders such as polycystic kidney. They have definite growth potential, and while they usually grow slowly,[2] rapid growth was seen in 2 infants on sequential imaging studies.[9] The remaining part of the kidney containing the multilocular cystic nephroma functions normally. The tumors can prolapse or herniate into the renal pelvis and cause partial or complete obstruction. This was identified in one-third of cases in one study.[2]

Microscopically, the cysts are lined by epithelium, which is helpful to differentiate them from other cystic disorders.[1,2,4] The septa contain stromal tissue. Mature nephrons are not present within the septa[4] and this is also helpful in differentiating from some other cystic kidney disorders. Areas of metanephric blastema[3] or definite nephroblastoma (Wilms tumor) may be identified in the septa between the cysts.[1,6–8] In one study, microscopic nephroblastoma was identified in the septal stroma in 6 of 30 children under the age of 2.[2] Very occasionally, macroscopic nodules of nephroblastoma may be identified.[10,11]

TABLE 4–27
Criteria for Diagnosis of Multilocular Cystic Nephroma

Single unilateral renal mass
Multilocular and cystic
No communication between cysts or with collecting system
Cysts lined by epithelium
No functioning or normal renal tissue in septa between cysts
Involves only part of a kidney

Clinical Presentation

Symptoms of multilocular cystic nephroma are entirely nonspecific. The most common presentation is a finding of an incidental mass lesion.[2] There are frequently no other symptoms.

Imaging Studies

On imaging studies, multilocular cystic nephroma is easily identified as a mass lesion (Figs. 4–25, 4–26, and 4–27). Intravenous urography will identify a mass but will not characterize it as cystic. Some obstruction of collecting system will be identified in up to one-third of patients. Ultrasound will identify a large well-defined cystic mass with septa (Figs. 4–25 and 4–27). The cysts are multiple. The cysts may all be sharply defined (Fig. 4–27) or in some patients less well defined, creating the appearance of a more nonspecific complex mass lesion. The cysts may appear not well defined either, because they are multiple and very tiny and may or may not contain hemorrhage, causing some internal echoes and also loss of sharpness of definition of their margins. In one study, only about one-half of 17 patients had sharply defined clear cysts.

On CT scan, the lesions are also well identified (see Fig. 4–25). The cysts are seen to vary in size. As with ultrasound the cyst walls may sometimes be very irregular, and hemorrhage may be present within the cysts. Thickening and irregularity of the septa may suggest a tumor.[13] Thick myxomatous material may be present in the septal walls, which may also lead to lack of sharp definition.[2] Calcification may occasionally be seen in a curvilinear pattern, although in one study it was not identified in any of 34 patients.[2] Some confusion exists in that enhancement of the septa has been reported fol-

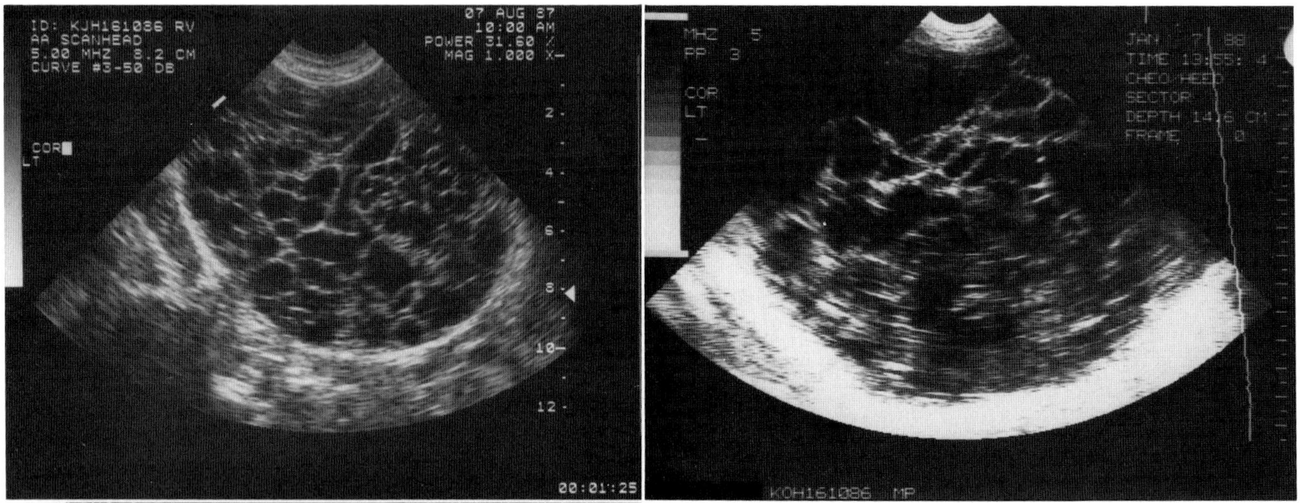

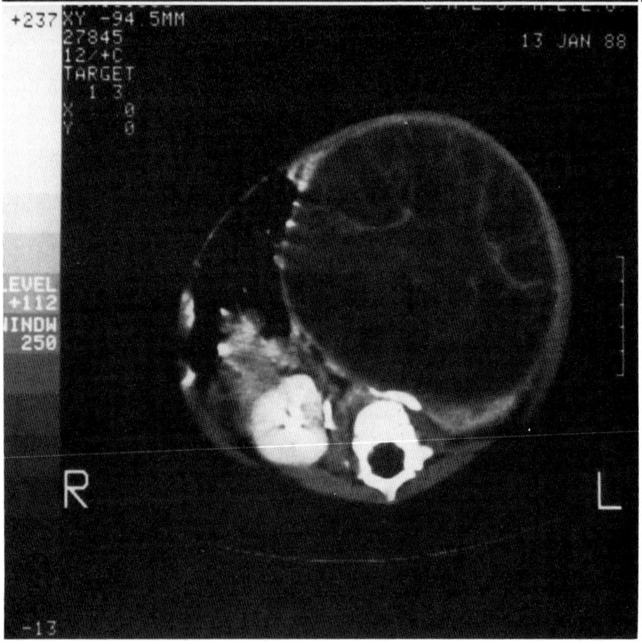

Figure 4-25. Diagnosis: Multilocular cystic nephroma. ***A*** and ***B***, Ultrasound. Large multilocular cyst is seen. Four months later (***B***) some cysts have enlarged. ***C***, CT. Shows a large cystic mass with compression of residual functioning tissue. (From Thijssen A. Multilocular cystic nephroma. J Urol 1989;142:346–348.)

Figure 4-26. Diagnosis: Multilocular cystic nephroma.
A, MR, T1 weighted. Serous (hypointense) and hemorrhagic fluid is present in a complex cystic mass.
B, MR, T2 weighted. There is bright signal from serous and very bright signal from hemorrhagic fluid.
(From Dickengill A, Benson M, Sanders L, et al. MRI of multilocular cystic nephroma. Urol Radiol 1988;10:95–99.)

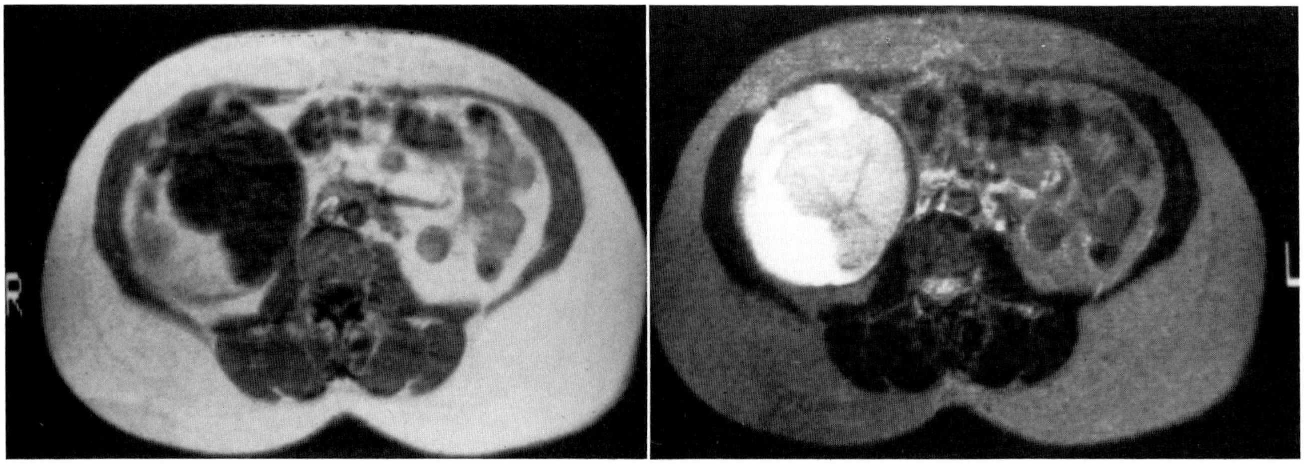

A

B

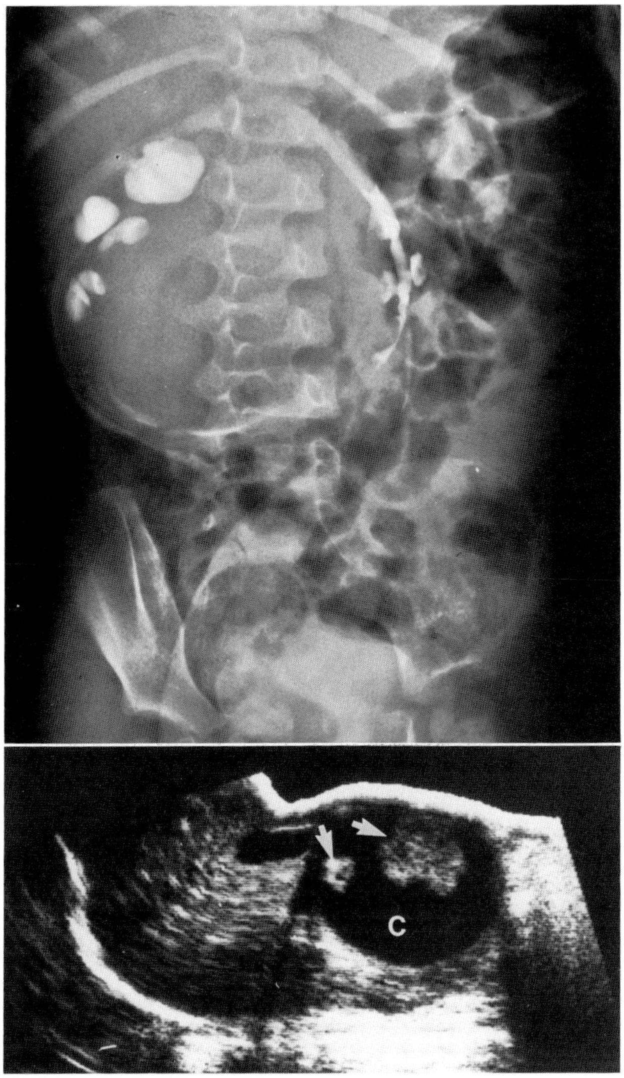

Figure 4-27. **Diagnosis: Horseshoe kidney with multilocular cystic nephroma and nodular Wilms tumor.**
***A*, Intravenous urogram. There is a large soft-tissue mass in the central and right side of this horseshoe kidney. There is moderate obstruction to the collecting system of the right kidney with hydronephrosis. *B*, Ultrasound. The mass is predominantly composed of well-defined cysts (*C*) and well-defined soft-tissue nodules *(arrows)* that project into the cysts. Histologically these were Wilms tumor.**

lowing bolus injection of intravenous contrast,[2] but this is surprising in view of the fact that mature renal tissue is not believed to be present in the septa. At this stage it is important to note that some variations in the criteria for diagnosis of multilocular cystic nephroma, described in Table 4–27, have been reported in various studies.

Angiography will show a renal mass lesion with no specific features. There may be an initial blush, and vascularity may be increased or decreased depending on the proportion of septal tissue present.[2] Nuclear medicine isotope studies show no function from the region of the cystic nephroma.[2]

Differential Diagnosis

The differential diagnosis is large. Multicystic dysplastic kidney can be differentiated because it involves the entire kidney and no function is identified in the kidney. Adult polycystic kidney, particularly if unilateral, may cause confusion.[14] The cysts in this lesion are less well defined, communication with the collecting system occurs, and function is seen in the tissue between the individual cysts.[14]

Therapy and Prognosis

The treatment of multilocular cystic nephroma is resection and at the present time nephrectomy is usually performed.[2] I suspect that with the ability of modern imaging to define the total extent of these lesions better in the future we may see a push for more conservative partial nephrectomy. The tumors do require resection, first, because of their ability to grow, and second, because of the potential for malignancy. There is some confusion regarding the use of chemotherapy. Obviously, if no nephroblastoma is identified, no chemotherapy is required. Even in those patients with microscopic nephroblastoma, it would seem that no treatment other than surgery is required.[2] If macroscopic nephroblastoma with or without metastases is identified, the lesions are usually treated as Wilms tumors. The prognosis for most reported series is excellent. Metastases are very uncommon, being reported in only 4 of 55 patients in one study.[2] Metastases are especially uncommon if only microscopic nephroblastoma is identified in the tumor.

Comment: Multilocular cystic nephroma is a poorly understood entity. Its importance is that in a small number of cases it behaves like a true malignant Wilms tumor.

References

1. Garrett A, Carty H, Pilling D. Multilocular cystic nephroma: report of three cases. Clin Radiol 1987;38:55–57.
2. Madewell JE, Goldman SM, Davis CJ, et al. Multilocular cystic nephroma: a radiographic-pathologic correlation of 58 patients. Radiology 1983;146:309–321.
3. Carlson DH, Carlson D, Simon H. Benign multilocal cystic nephroma. AJR 1987;131:621–625.
4. Boggs LK, Kimmelstiel P. Benign multilocular cystic nephroma: report of two cases of so-called multilocular cyst of the kidney. J Urol 1956;76:530–541.
5. Donaldson JS, Shkolnik A. Pediatric renal masses. Semin Roentgenol 1988;23:194–204.
6. Andrews MJ, Askin FB, Fried FA, et al. Cystic partially differentiated nephroblastoma and polycystic Wilms tumor: A spectrum of related clinical and pathologic entities. J Urol 1983; 129:577–581.
7. Boggs LK, Kimmelstiel P. Benign multilocular cystic nephroma: report of two cases of so-called multilocular cyst of the kidney. J Urol 1956;76:530–534.
8. Christ ML. Polycystic nephroblastoma. J Urol 1968; 98:570–571.
9. Thijssen AM, Carpenter B, Jiminez C, et al. Multilocular cyst (multilocular cystic nephroma) of the kidney: a report

of 2 cases with an unusual mode of presentation. J Urol 1989;142:346–348.
10. Gonzalez-Crussi F, Kidd JM, Hernandez RJ. Cystic nephroma: morphologic spectrum and implications. Urology 1982;20:88–95.
11. Datnow B, Daniel WW. Polycystic nephroblastoma. JAMA 1976;236:2528–2530.
12. Richards DG, Stafford AJ, DeMaria JE. Asymptomatic abdominal mass in a child. BJR 1987;60:775–776.
13. Kirks DR, Kaufman RA, Babcock DS. Renal neoplasms in infants and children. Semin Roentgenol 1987;22:292–302.
14. Strand WR, Rushton HG, Markle BM, et al. Autosomal dominant polycystic kidney disease in infants: asymmetric disease mimicking a unilateral renal mass. J Urol 1989;141:1151–1153.

MESOBLASTIC NEPHROMA

Mesoblastic nephroma is another renal tumor that causes much debate and confusion. There is universal agreement that it is a tumor, but there is disagreement regarding its malignant potential. At the present time it should be considered as a predominantly benign renal tumor but one that does have malignant cystic nephroma.

Epidemiology

Mesoblastic nephroma has been reported as having an equal sex incidence[1,2] or having a male dominance.[3] It is a tumor of young children but can occasionally occur in older children.[2] In 57 patients, the mean age at presentation was 3 months.[3] The tumor is often present at birth, being congenital in 9 of 11 patients in one study.[4]

The etiology of mesoblastic nephroma is not known. In a large study of 51 patients, a slight increase in the incidence of congenital anomalies, anywhere in the body, was identified.[3]

Pathology

Grossly, these tumors can be large, replacing over 60 percent of the normal kidney in a high percentage of patients.[2] They are characterized by the absence of a capsule, by the absence of sharp margins, and by local infiltration.[1,2] This local invasion will commonly penetrate through the capsule and the perirenal fascia[2] and there may occasionally be invasion of adjacent organs such as the pancreas or colon.[3] Hemorrhage and necrosis within these tumors are rare, in contrast to Wilms tumor.[4] Tiny cysts caused by trapped urine within the tumor mass may occasionally be seen.[2] Microscopically, there are a number of very important features. The tumors are composed predominantly of mature spindle cells.[5] They have a remarkable infiltrative growth pattern and invasion of adjacent tissues, seen microscopically, is always much greater than that predicted from the gross examination of the tumor.[6] This is important in that an unwary surgeon will frequently not excise the tumor adequately unless he or she is aware of the invading potential of this tumor. Functioning nephrons may be trapped within the tumor[2,7] and may, therefore, cause function within the tumor mass on imaging studies. A specific subgroup of patients have a unique histology, which has been termed cellular mesoblastic nephroma.[6,8] These tumors are densely cellular and have a very high number of cells showing active mitosis.[6] These cellular mesoblastic nephromas are potentially more aggressive, and the implications of this finding is discussed further in regard to patient management. Important histologic features of mesoblastic nephroma are summarized in Table 4–28.

Clinical Presentation

In most patients, the only symptom is the incidental finding of an abdominal mass.[1–3,8] This is usually detected on routine physical examination after birth. In one study of 51 patients, an abdominal mass was detected in 48.[3] These tumors can, however, present in other ways and it is important to include them in differential diagnosis. First, mesoblastic nephroma can produce renin[9] and the children may, therefore, present with hypertension. Second, these tumors may produce prostaglandin or parathyroid hormone (Wilms tumor never does this), causing hypercalcemia.[5,10–11] Finally, one patient has been reported presenting as congestive cardiac failure from a large arteriovenous shunt within a proven mesoblastic nephroma.[12] It is thus seen that mesoblastic nephroma can present in a variety of unusual ways.

Imaging Studies

On imaging studies, a mass lesion is easily identified (Fig. 4–28). A mass was seen on the abdominal radio-

TABLE 4–28
Important Histologic Features of Mesoblastic Nephroma

Finding	Implication
Very infiltrative growth pattern	Imaging and gross evaluation at surgery do not reveal entire tumor
Nephrons trapped in tumor	Function, within the tumor mass, is seen on imaging
Subgroup of patients with very "cellular" histology	Increased malignant potential

graph in 18 of 20 patients with mesoblastic nephroma.[3] Intravenous urogram shows a mass lesion. Hydronephrosis is uncommon, being identified in 3 of 17 patients.[2] The tumors are unusual in that occasionally some function may be identified within the tumor. One patient has been described with focal entrapment of urine within a small cyst in the tumor.[7] On ultrasound studies, a mass lesion is seen in the kidney (Fig. 4–28). The echo pattern is probably variable but has been described as being of relatively low echogenicity in some patients.[2] Renal isotope scans will show a mass lesion. In one patient, uptake of DTPA technetium 99m was identified in a tumor.[14] CT scan will show a mass lesion. It may falsely appear well defined on CT imaging (Fig. 4–28), but it should be borne in mind that extensive infiltration beyond the margins identified on CT scan is usually present. Contrast excretion within the mass has been identified on CT scan.[13]

Figure 4-28. **Diagnosis: Mesoblastic nephroma. Age 3 months.**
***A*, Ultrasound. There is a large mass lesion *(arrows)* arising from the anterior aspect of the right kidney (*K*). *B*, CT. This again shows the tumor *(arrows)* arising from the anterior aspect of the right kidney (*K*). The apparent sharp margin between the tumor and kidney is false, as extensive tumor infiltration through this margin existed.**

A

B

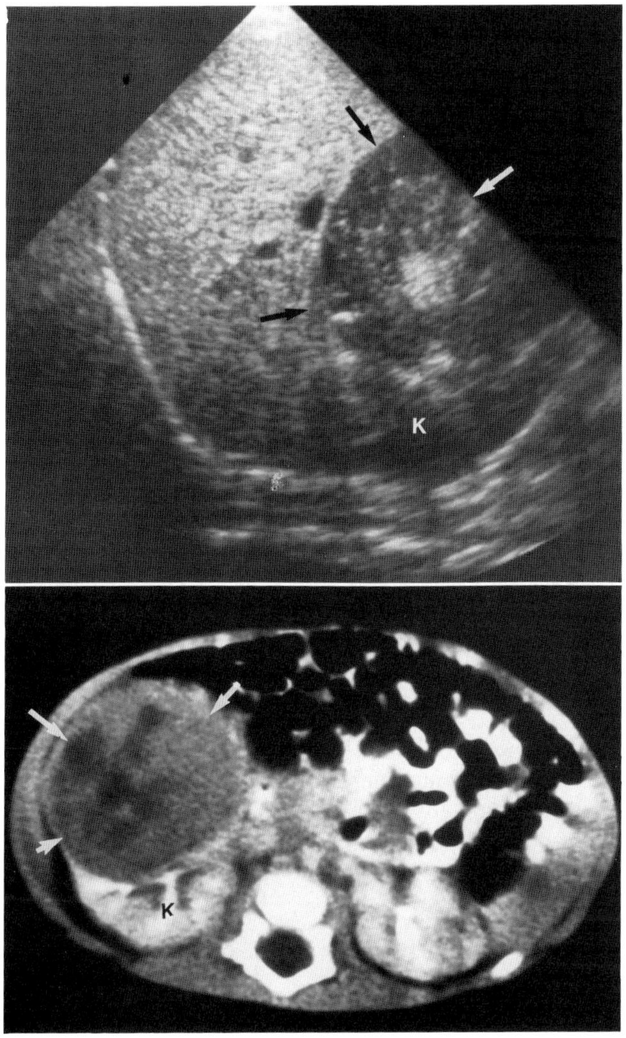

Therapy and Prognosis

At the present time nephrectomy is recommended for all patients with mesoblastic nephroma. Wide margins need to be carefully achieved because of the infiltrating ability of this tumor. There is considerable debate regarding the need for further therapy. With conventional histology it has been said that metastases never occur[4] and that no further therapy is required, tiny amounts of microscopic residual resolving spontaneously. In those patients with the cellular subtype of histology, local recurrence or metastases may occur. In a report of 3 patients, together with a literature review of 38 patients, it was identified that 7 patients had local recurrence and 2 had lung metastases.[8] The mean time to recurrence was 7 months and 3 of these 7 patients apparently died.[8]

There does appear to be a difference in the behavior of children with cellular mesoblastic nephroma, depending on the age at diagnosis. In those children in whom the tumor is resected under the age of 3 months, metastatic disease, local recurrence, or both would appear to be much less likely than in children over the age of 3 months.[6] It would seem, from a review of the literature, that all children with cellular mesoblastic nephroma under the age of 3 months should also be treated only with surgical resection and follow-up, and that chemotherapy and radiation therapy be reserved for patients over 3 months of age with extensive local invasion, perhaps of adjacent organs, the presence of metastatic disease, and the presence of recurrent disease following initial resection.[2,3,6] The role of imaging becomes particularly important in evaluating these children for metastatic disease and particularly for local recurrence. For this reason it is probably important to obtain a baseline CT scan within a few weeks after surgery. Several workers have cautioned against the use of unnecessary chemotherapy and radiation therapy because of the potential toxicity, particularly in infants under the age of 1 year.[2]

The prognosis of mesoblastic nephroma is excellent in most patients. In the literature review,[8] 3 patients out of 41 were reported to have died. Many of these may have been from a long time ago and with more aggressive modern surgery the death rate may be lower. The largest reported series of mesoblastic nephroma is of 51 patients reported by the Children's Cancer Study Group.[3] In these children, complete resection was achieved in only 43 of 51 patients; 23 of the 51 patients had only surgery. This report included patients up to about 1980 and at that time the remaining patients had combinations of chemotherapy and radiation therapy. The overall survival was excellent, with 50 of 51 patients surviving. The only death was caused by overwhelming infection complicating chemotherapy.[3]

Comment: Imaging is important in mesoblastic nephroma. As surgery is the primary method of treatment imaging should define the local invasion of the tumor as accurately as possible prior to surgery. Imaging is also important in following up these patients for local recurrence. Imaging cannot differentiate between conventional histology and the potentially more aggressive cellular history.

References

1. Gerber A, Gold JH, Bustamante S, et al. Congenital mesoblastic nephroma. J Pediatr Surg 1981;16:758–759.
2. Hartman DS, Lesar MSL, Madewell JE, et al. Mesoblastic nephroma: radiologic-pathologic correlation of 20 cases. AJR 1981;136:69–74.
3. Howell CG, Othersen HB, Kiviat NE. Therapy and outcome in 51 children with mesoblastic nephroma: a report of the national Wilms' tumor study. J Pediatr Surg 1982;17:826–831.
4. Snyder HM, Lack EE, Chetty-Baktavizian A. Congenital mesoblastic nephroma: relationship of other renal tumors of infancy. J Urol 1981;126:513–515.
5. Vido L, Carli M, Rizzoni G, et al. Congenital mesoblastic nephroma with hypercalcemia. Am J Pediatr Hematol/Oncol 1986;8:149–152.
6. Beckwith JB. Wilms tumor and other renal tumors of childhood: an update. J Urol 1986;136:320–329.
7. McAlister WH, Siegel MJ, Askin F, et al. Congenital mesoblastic nephroma. Radiology 1979;132:356.
8. Gormley TS, Skoog SJ, Jones RV, et al. Cellular congenital mesoblastic nephroma: what are the options. J Urol 1989;142:479–483.
9. Malone PS, Duffy PG, Ransley PG, et al. Congenital mesoblastic nephroma, renin production, and hypertension. J Pediatr Surg 1989;24:599–600.
10. Woolfield NF, Abbott GD, McRae CU. A mesoblastic nephroma with hypercalcaemia. Aust Paediatr J 1988; 24:309–310.
11. Jayabose S, Iqbal K, Newman L, et al. Hypercalcemia in childhood renal tumors. Cancer 1988;61:788–791.
12. King N. Congenital mesoblastic nephroma. Am J Dis Child 1978;132:1139–1140.
13. Kirks DR, Kaufman RA. Function within mesoblastic nephroma: imaging—pathologic correlation. Pediatr Radiol 1989;19:136–139.

ANGIOMYOLIPOMA

Angiomyolipoma is a benign and not a malignant lesion. It is, however, included because disease may be identified in lymph nodes and associated malignancy can occur.[1]

Angiomyolipoma is found in between 50 to 80 percent of patients with tuberosclerosis; 50 percent of patients with angiomyolipoma have tuberosclerosis. Macroscopically, these tumors are frequently multiple and bilateral and vary in size. They can be small. Microscopically, the tumors contain blood vessels, mature smooth muscle, and mature fat.

The patients may have no symptoms, the tumors being identified on routine screening in patients with known tuberosclerosis. The most troublesome symptom is hematuria, which can be persistent and require embolization or even rarely nephrectomy.

Diagnosis is easily made on the finding of multiple renal tumors in patients with known tuberosclerosis. A characteristic finding is the appearance of fat within the tumor. The fat can usually be characterized easily with either CT or MR scanning. Some difficulties may occur with MR, particularly if hemorrhage has occurred into the tumor. Ultrasound is not good for characterization of fat. It is important that fat may occasionally be identified within Wilms tumor.

Enlarged nymph nodes may be identified in patients with angiomyolipoma. In a report of 3 cases, together with a review of 8 additional cases from the literature, angiomyolipoma of the kidney was associated with angiomyolipoma in local and regional lymph nodes.[1] This was believed to represent the multicentric, multifocal nature of this tumor and is not evidence of malignancy or metastases. Angiomyolipoma may, however, occasionally be associated with renal cell carcinoma in the same kidney.[2] Rapid growth or change in the appearance of a kidney with known angiomyolipoma should raise the possibility of the presence of associated renal cell carcinoma.

Reference

1. Taylor RS, Joseph DB, Kohaut EC. Renal angiomyolipoma associated with lymph node involvement and renal cell carcinoma in patients with tuberous sclerosis. J Urol 1989;141:930-932.

PROSTATIC CARCINOMA

Prostatic carcinoma is extremely rare in children. One tumor in a boy of 11 years of age together with 15 cases from the literature were reviewed.[1] The tumors present as prostatic masses that cause difficulty in micturition and urine retention. Of the reported patients, 4 were under the age of 5 years and 10 were over the age of 10 years. Metastatic disease was common. Bone metastases were seen in 6 patients, being lytic in 5 and blastic in 1. Metastases were also identified in liver, lymph nodes, and lung and occasionally an unusual site such as pancreas, spleen, and testes.

Microscopically, all the prostatic carcinomas in children are undifferentiated. The prognosis is extremely poor and 15 of the 16 patients reviewed died within a year of diagnosis.[1]

Reference

1. Shimada H, Misugi K, Sasaki Y. Carcinoma of the prostate in childhood and adolescence: report of a case and review of the literature. Cancer 1980;46:2534–2452.

CHAPTER 5
RETICULOENDOTHELIAL TUMORS

LYMPHOMA

Comment: Pediatric lymphomas are completely different from adult lymphomas.

Lymphoma is an extremely important malignancy in childhood. The clinical, pathological, and imaging features of both Hodgkin and non-Hodgkin lymphoma in children are completely different from those in adults, and it is, therefore, extremely important not to transfer results from studies done in the adult population to children. Unfortunately, a large amount of the published information with regard to lymphoma is from the adult population. Some children are frequently included in large adult series, but the distinguishing features between children and adults are often not emphasized. Hodgkin disease and non-Hodgkin lymphoma are distinct and separate disorders with many differences. Some of these differences are summarized in Table 5–1.

Epidemiology

Lymphoma occurs with an incidence of about 9 cases per annum per million children under the age of 15 years.[1] If all children are considered, Hodgkin disease is slightly more common than non-Hodgkin lymphoma. Non-Hodgkin lymphoma is much more likely than Hodgkin disease to occur in very young children. In children under the age of 10, non-Hodgkin lymphoma is more common than Hodgkin disease. The incidence of non-Hodgkin lymphoma is moderately evenly distributed throughout childhood, except for the large-cell type, which tends to occur only in older children.[2] Non-

TABLE 5–1
Comparison of Hodgkin Disease and Non-Hodgkin Lymphoma[1]

Feature	Hodgkin	Non-Hodgkin
Age	Mostly >10 yrs	Any age in children
Stage at diagnosis	Mostly localized	Commonly widespread
Constitutional symptoms	Alter prognosis	Don't affect prognosis
CNS involvement	Rare	Occurrence increasing with AIDS
Mediastinal involvement	Most common with nodular sclerosing	Most common with lymphoblastic
Gastrointestinal involvement	Rare	Occurs
Abdominal nodes	Can be small or large, mesenteric rare	Usually enlarged, mesenteric common
Bone	Rare	Occurs
Marrow	Rare	Common

Reference

1. Dehner LP. Non-Hodgkin's lymphomas and malignant histiocytosis in children. Semin Oncol 1977;4:273–286.

Hodgkin lymphoma can occur in very young infants, with one case being reported in a child of 3 weeks of age.[3] Hodgkin disease in childhood has a peak in late teenage years, overlapping into young adulthood.[4] There is a later peak in older adults.

Non-Hodgkin lymphoma is much more common in boys than in girls.[1,2] The reported sex distribution of Hodgkin disease in children will vary by study.[4–6] This is because the sex incidence varies with age. In very young children, Hodgkin disease is more common in males than in females, whereas in older children the sex incidence is more equal.[4]

There are a number of factors associated with the occurrence of Hodgkin disease and non-Hodgkin lymphoma. Both disorders have an increased incidence in patients with suppressed immune systems,[4,5] including ataxia-telangiectasia, posttransplantation immune suppression, Wiskott Aldrich syndrome, and AIDS.[1,7] In addition, there is an increased incidence of Hodgkin disease in some families with some specific HLA antigens and, rarely, with Gaucher's disease.[5,8] Non-Hodgkin lymphoma has an increased incidence in patients after bone marrow transplantation.[9] There is a very high incidence in children under the age of 15 years with ataxia-telangiectasia.[10] There is a significant increase in non-Hodgkin lymphoma in patients with Crohn's disease, ulcerative colitis, or celiac disease[11]; it is rarely reported associated with Down syndrome.[3] One child developed T cell lymphoma 14 years after Wilms tumor.[12]

> *Comment:* Non-Hodgkin lymphoma occurs at any age. Hodgkin disease occurs in older children.

References

1. Magrath IT. Malignant non-Hodgkin's lymphomas. In: Pizzo PA, Poplack DG, eds. Principles and practice of pediatric oncology. Philadelphia: JB Lippincott, 1989:415–455.
2. Kjeldsberg CR, Wilson JF, Berard CW. Non-Hodgkin's lymphoma in children. Hum Pathol 1983;14:612–627.
3. Lorenzana AN, Schorin MA. Non-Hodgkin's lymphoma in a neonate with Down's syndrome. Am J Pediatr Hematol/Oncol 1989;11:186–190.
4. Leventhal BG, Donaldson SS. Hodgkin's disease. In: Pizzo PA, Poplack DG, eds. Principles and practice of pediatric oncology. Philadelphia: JB Lippincott, 1989:457–476.
5. Desforges JF, Rutherford CJ, Piro A. Hodgkin's disease. New Engl J Med 1979:301:1212–1222.
6. Makepeace AR, Maclennan KA, Hudson GV, et al. Hodgkin's disease in childhood: the British National Lymphoma Investigation Experience (BNLI Report No 27). Clin Radiol 1987;38:7–11.
7. Lynch MA, Cho KC, Jeffrey RB, et al. CT of peritoneal lymphomatosis. AJR 1988;152:713–715.
8. Goodman S. Case report: nodular sclerosing Hodgkin's disease in association with Gaucher's disease. Clin Radiol 1988;39:326–327.
9. Day DL, Shapiro RS, Yueh N, et al. B-cell lymphoproliferative disorders in children after bone marrow transplantation: radiologic manifestations. Radiology 1987; 162:807–810.
10. Levine C, Vrlenich L. Renal lymphoma in ataxis-telangiectasia: CT contribution. J Comput Assist Tomogr 1989;13:537–539.
11. Brady LW, Asbell SO. Malignant lymphoma of the gastrointestinal tract. Radiology 1980;137:291–298.
12. Coppes MJ, Byard R, Stringer DA, et al. T-cell lymphoma and mature nephroblastoma after synchronous bilateral Wilms' tumor. Cancer 1991;67:337–341.

Pathology

Lymphomas arise from the constituent cells of the immune system. The precise cell of origin in Hodgkin disease is not known. In order for the diagnosis of Hodgkin disease to be made, the characteristic Reed-Sternberg cell must be identified in children.[1,2] Non-Hodgkin lymphomas arise mainly from lymphocyte precursors in the marrow and thymus. This is unlike adult patients in whom non-Hodgkin lymphoma arises predominantly from mature immunocompetent lymphoid cells.[3] This difference in part explains the marked difference in the histological types of non-Hodgkin lymphoma found in adults and children.[4] Histologically, it may be difficult if not impossible to differentiate non-Hodgkin lymphoma from lymphocytic leukemia. Microscopically, the cells are identical.[3,5] Leukemia involves predominantly the bone marrow and blood, but can involve other tissues. Non-Hodgkin lymphoma predominantly involves tissues other than bone marrow, but bone marrow can be involved. In patients in whom the differentiation between leukemia and non-Hodgkin lymphoma is difficult, a somewhat arbitrary differentiating factor is utilized. This is the percentage of blast cells present in the bone marrow. The presence of more than 25 percent of blast cells in the bone marrow will usually be accepted as a diagnosis of acute lymphocyte leukemia rather than non-Hodgkin lymphoma.[3]

HISTOLOGIC CLASSIFICATION OF LYMPHOMA

The histologic classification of Hodgkin disease is the same in children as it is in adults. The tumors are divided into four groups: lymphocyte predominant, nodular sclerosing, mixed cellularity, and lymphocyte depleted (Table 5–2).[6] The distribution of patients between the four histologic types is summarized in Table 5–2. As can be seen from the table there is some variation in reported incidence of each histologic type between different series. Other studies not included in Table 5–2 report even more imbalance between the histologic subtypes. For example, in one study from the United Kingdom, 88 percent of 68 children were reported as being nodular sclerosing Hodgkin disease.[7] Several conclusions about Hodgkin disease can be drawn from Table 5–2.

1. Lymphocyte depleted is very rare in children.
2. Nodular sclerosing and mixed cellularity are the most common types, although the ratios may vary.

TABLE 5-2
Histologic Classification of Hodgkin Disease in Children*

	% Distribution			% Distribution by Age			
	Children of All Ages			<10 yrs		11–15 yrs	
Ref No.	(1)	(2)	(3)	(4)	(5)	(4)	(6)
No. Children	46	?	651	65	?	126	?
Lymphocyte predominant	9%	11%	10–28%	17%	18%	10%	13%
Nodular sclerosing	67%	65%	12–65%	45%	38%	72%	70%
Mixed cellularity	21%	18%	2–53%	32%	38%	13%	13%
Lymphocyte depleted	3%	1%	1–12%	0	2%	2%	1%
Unclassified	–	5%					

*Summary of 6 series of patients.

References

1. Baccarani M, Bosi A, Papa G. Second malignancy in patients treated for Hodgkin's disease. Cancer 1980;46:1735–1740.
2. Castellino RA. Hodgkin disease: practical concepts for the diagnostic radiologist. Radiology 1986;159:305–310.
3. Dehner LP. Pediatric surgical pathology, 2nd ed. Baltimore: Williams & Wilkins, 1987:822–837.
4. Leventhal BG, Donaldson SS. Hodgkin's disease. In: Pizzo PA, Poplack DG, eds. Principles and practice of pediatric oncology. Philadelphia: JB Lippincott, 1989:457–476.
5. Parker BR, Castellino RA, Kaplan HS. Pediatric Hodgkin's disease. I. Radiographic evaluation. Cancer 1976; 37:2430–2435.
6. Patel PJ, Bahakim HM, Kolawole TM. Renal sonography in childhood lymphoma. Urol Int 1990;45:34–37.

3. Part of the difference among different studies is that age is a factor in the histologic type. Nodular sclerosing is more common in older children than in children under the age of 10.

In addition to the information presented in Table 5–2, it should also be noted that lymphocyte depleted Hodgkin disease is particularly common in children with immune deficiency, being present in up to 33 percent of these children.[8] The histologic classification of Hodgkin disease is extremely important, because prognosis is directly related to the cell type.

The histologic classification of non-Hodgkin lymphoma is much more complicated. Unfortunately, an overwhelming number of classification systems have been described,[3] with confusion compounded by the fact that the same term means different things in different classification systems. At least 6 or 7 well-recognized classification systems exist.[9,10] These were consolidated in the working formulation published in 1982[11,12] and revised in 1990.[13] Compared to adults, pediatric non-Hodgkin lymphoma is very different.[4,9] The pediatric lymphomas are predominantly extranodal, high grade, rapidly growing, and more frequently leukemic.[5] The classification of pediatric non-Hodgkin lymphoma is much simpler than adult non-Hodgkin lymphoma, with all of the pediatric tumors falling into a few of the very many subgroups described in the working formulation.[11,13] Those subgroups into which the pediatric non-Hodgkin lymphomas fall are summarized in Table 5–3. As can be seen from Table 5–3, lymphoblastic and small cell tumors are by far the most common. The cell of origin is described in the table. As can also be seen from Table 5–3, almost all pediatric non-Hodgkin lymphomas are high grade (aggressive).[4] The immunoblastic type, although uncommon in the general population, is the most common pediatric non-Hodgkin lymphoma in children with depressed immunity.[4]

STAGING

The staging system for Hodgkin disease is presented in Table 5–4, and the distribution between stages at diagnosis is presented in Table 5–5. Non-Hodgkin lymphoma is often assumed to be diffuse at the time of diagnosis and specific staging is not always utilized. One suggested staging system from St. Jude's is presented in Table 5–6.

DISEASE DISTRIBUTION

The distribution of disease with non-Hodgkin lymphoma is widespread in over 75 percent of cases.[14] The distribution varies depending on the histology. The major anatomic areas that are involved, for each histologic type, are summarized in Table 5–7, which gives the primary site of disease on initial presentation. As can be seen, a wide variety of different locations may be affected. The distribution of disease on initial presentation in 40 children in the United States with Burkitt's lymphoma is given in Table 5–8.[15] This disease occurs most commonly in the abdomen and also affects the neck, occasionally thoracic lymph nodes, bone, and other sites. The reported incidence of renal disease in non-Hodgkin lymphoma is probably much lower than truly occurs, because the kidneys frequently are not imaged. In addition to the sites presented in Table 5–8, children in the United States with Burkitt's disease may also have involvement of the central nervous system or bone marrow.[16]

TABLE 5–3
Histologic Classification of Pediatric Non-Hodgkin Lymphoma

	Incidence			Cell of Origin	Histologic Grade
Ref. No.	(1)	(2)	(3)		
Lymphoblastic	30%	30–50%	35%	T cell	High
Small noncleaved	50%	20–40%	40–50%	B cell	High
Burkitt					
non-Burkitt					
Large Cell					
Immunoblastic	10%	<10%	10–15%	T or B cell	High
Cleaved	10%	<10%	10–15%	B cell	Intermediate
Noncleaved	10%	<10%	10–15%	B cell	Intermediate

References
1. Magrath IT. Malignant non-Hodgkin's lymphomas. In: Pizzo PA, Poplack DG, eds. Principles and practice of pediatric oncology. Philadelphia: JB Lippincott, 1989:415–455.
2. Dehner LP. Pediatric surgical pathology, 2nd ed. Baltimore: Williams & Wilkins, 1987:822–837.
3. Kjeldsberg CR, Wilson JF, Berard CW. Non-Hodgkin's lymphoma in children. Hum Pathol 1983;14:612–627.

TABLE 5–4
Ann Arbor Staging Classification of Hodgkin Disease

Stage	Criteria
I	Involvement of a single lymph node region
II	Involvement of two or more lymph node regions on the same side of the diaphragm (II) or localized involvement of an extralymphatic organ or site and of one or more lymph node regions on the same side of the diaphragm (IIE)
III	Involvement of lymph node regions on both sides of the diaphragm (III), which may also be accompanied by involvement of the spleen (IIIS) or by localized involvement of an extralymphatic organ or site (IIIE) or both (IIISE)
IV	Diffuse or disseminated involvement of one or more extralymphatic organs or tissues, with or without associated lymph node involvement

Note: E = extralymphatic site, S = splenic involvement. The absence or presence of fever, night sweats, and unexplained loss of 10 percent or more of body weight in the 6 months prior to diagnosis are denoted by the suffix letters A or B, respectively.

TABLE 5–5
Hodgkin Disease in Children: Stage at Diagnosis (350 Children)[1]

Stage	Percentage
I	22
II	41
III	28
IV	10

Reference
1. Leventhal BG, Donaldson SS. Hodgkin's disease. In: Pizzo PA, Poplack DG, eds. Principles and practice of pediatric oncology. Philadelphia: JB Lippincott, 1989:457–476.

Subdiaphragmatic involvement in Hodgkin disease at the time of diagnosis varies depending on histology (Table 5–9). Of children with mixed cellularity 80 percent (8 of 10) had subdiaphragmatic involvement compared to 37 percent (11 of 30) of children with nodular sclerosing Hodgkins.

Many points regarding the distribution of lymphoma have an important radiologic implication. These points are summarized in Tables 5–10 and 5–11.

Comment: A thorough knowledge of the pathologic behavior of Hodgkin disease and non-Hodgkin lymphoma is mandatory if logic is to be applied to imaging strategies.

References
1. Castellino RA. Hodgkin disease: Practical concepts for the diagnostic radiologist. Radiology 1986;159:305–310.
2. Leventhal BG, Donaldson SS. Hodgkin's disease. In: Pizzo PA, Poplack DG, eds. Principles and practice of pediatric oncology. Philadelphia: JB Lippincott, 1989:457–476.
3. Magrath IT. Malignant non-Hodgkin's lymphomas. In: Pizzo PA, Poplack DG, eds. Principles and practice of pe-

TABLE 5–6

St. Jude Staging System for Non-Hodgkin's Lymphoma[1]

Stage	Criteria
I	A single tumor (extranodal) or single anatomic site (nodal), excluding mediastinum or abdomen
II	A single tumor (extranodal) with regional node involvement
	Two or more nodal sites on the same side of the diaphragm
	Two single (extranodal) tumors with or without regional node involvement on the same side of the diaphragm
	A primary gastrointestinal tract tumor, usually ileocecal, with or without associated mesenteric nodes
III	Two single tumors (extranodal) on opposite sides of the diaphragm
	Two or more nodal areas above and below the diaphragm
	All primary intrathoracic tumors (mediastinal, pleural, thymic)
	All extensive primary intra-abdominal disease
	All paraspinal or epidural tumors, regardless of other tumor site(s)
IV	Any of the above with initial central nervous system (CNS) or bone marrow involvement

Reference

1. Link MP, Donaldson SS, Berard CW, et al. Results of treatment of childhood localized non-Hodgkin's lymphoma with combination chemotherapy with or without radiotherapy. New Engl J Med 1990;322:1169–1174.

diatric oncology. Philadelphia: JB Lippincott, 1989:415–455.

4. Dehner LP. Pediatric surgical pathology, 2nd ed. Baltimore: Williams & Wilkins, 1987:822–837.
5. Kjeldsberg CR, Wilson JF, Berard CW. Non-Hodgkin's lymphoma in children. Hum Pathol 1983;14:612–627.
6. Banks PM. The pathology of Hodgkin's disease. Semin Oncol 1990;17:683–695.
7. Makepeace AR, Maclennan KA, Hudson GV, et al. Hodgkin's disease in childhood: the British National Lymphoma Investigation Experience (BNLI Report No 27). Clin Radiol 1987;38:7–11.
8. Robison LL, Stoker V, Frizzera G, et al. Hodgkin's disease in pediatric patients with naturally occurring immunodeficiency. Am J Pediatr Hematol/Oncol 1987;9:189–192.
9. Hait WN, Farber L, Cadman E. Non-Hodgkin's lymphoma for the nononcologist. JAMA 1985;253:1431–1435.
10. Wang Y. Classification of non-Hodgkin's lymphoma. AJR 1986;147:205–208.
11. Williams D. The lymphomas: introduction. Semin Oncol 1990;17:1–2.
12. The Non-Hodgkin's Lymphoma Pathologic Classification Project. National Cancer Institute sponsored study of classifications of non-Hodgkin's lymphomas. Cancer 1982;49:2112–2135.
13. Burke JS. The histopathologic classification of non-Hodgkin's lymphomas: ambiguities in the working formulation and two newly reported categories. Semin Oncol 1990;17:3–10.
14. Smith SD, Rubin CM, Horvath A, et al. Non-Hodgkin's lymphoma in children. Semin Oncol 1990;17:113–119.
15. Dunnick NR, Reaman GH, Head GL, et al. Radiographic manifestations of Burkitt's lymphoma in American patients. AJR 1979;132:1–6.
16. Rivera-Luna R, Martinez-Guerra G, Borrego-Roman R. Burkitt's lymphoma. Experience at the Instituto Nacional de Pediatria, Mexico City. Am J Pediatr Hematol/Oncol 1986;8:183–190.

Clinical Presentation

Non-Hodgkin lymphoma has a very broad spectrum of clinical presentation, reflecting its widespread distribution through the body (Table 5–12). Abdominal disease may cause pain. Weight loss is very common. Nausea, vomiting, and diarrhea can occur; there may be intestinal bleeding; and intussusception can cause bowel obstruction.[1,2] Large masses may cause intrinsic bowel obstruction or obstruction to urine outflow.[2] In the chest, signs of tracheal or superior vena cava obstruction

TABLE 5–7

Non-Hodgkin Lymphoma: Primary Site of Disease by Histology[1]

	No.	Mediastinal Nodes	Other Nodes	Abdomen	Other Site
Lymphoblastic	136	46%	20%	6%	28%
Small cell					
Burkitt's	86	0	10%	54%	36%
Non-Burkitt's	104	4%	16%	50%	30%
Large cell	66	14%	29%	23%	34%

Reference

1. Kjeldsberg CR, Wilson JF, Berard CW. Non-Hodgkin's lymphoma in children. Hum Pathol 1983;14:612–627.

TABLE 5-8
Distribution of Disease on Initial Presentation in 40 Children in the U.S. with Burkitt's Lymphoma[1]

Presentation	Percentage of Children
Abdominal mass	70
Enlarged nodes in neck or pharynx	25
Pleural effusion	22
Mediastinal or hilar nodes	7
Bone	10
Renal	5

Reference
1. Dunnick NR, Reaman GH, Head GL, et al. Radiographic manifestations of Burkitt's lymphoma in American patients. AJR 1979;132:1–6.

caused by compression may be found. Less common symptoms include bone pain, abnormal central nervous system signs, neck masses, dysphagia, and nasal obstruction. Systemic signs such as fever, anorexia, and weight loss are not uncommon.[1,3]

Two acute emergencies may occur in patients with non-Hodgkin lymphoma. The radiologist has a role in suggesting the likelihood of occurrence of these problems. The first emergency is caused by tracheal or superior vena cava obstruction from tumor. The potential for this should be identified on plain film radiographs, CT scan, or both. Problems are particularly likely to occur during anesthesia (for biopsy or tumor excision) and, if there is significant tracheal compression identified, the anesthetist should be aware of this. In some patients, the clinician may elect to give a small dose of radiation therapy to shrink the tumor prior to anesthesia. The second emergency is the tumor lysis syndrome. This may be suggested by the presence of a very large mass lesion, especially if serial studies are available that show rapid growth. This syndrome is the result of the accumulation of breakdown products such as urate, potassium, and phosphate. These products accumulate prior to therapy but their accumulation is accentuated once chemotherapy is commenced. The phosphate and potassium may cause severe metabolic abnormalities and even death. High concentrations of urate result in urate deposition in the kidney and acute renal failure. The likelihood of renal problems is obviously increased if renal function is impaired. Imaging might suggest this either by demonstrating diffuse renal involvement with lymphoma or secondary involvement owing to urinary tract obstruction from an extrinsic lymphoma mass.

The most common presentation of Hodgkin disease is an enlarged, painless lymph node in the neck (see Table 5–12).[4] About 20 to 30 percent of patients have systemic symptoms of fever, weight loss, or night sweating (see Table 5–4).[4]

References
1. Brady LW, Asbell SO. Malignant lymphoma of the gastrointestinal tract. Radiology 1980;137:291–298.
2. Rivera-Luna R, Martinez-Guerra G, Borrego-Roman R, et al. Burkitt's lymphoma. Experience at the Instituto Nacional de Pediatria, Mexico City. Am J Pediatr Hematol/Oncol 1986;8:183–190.
3. Smith SD, Rubin CM, Horvath A, et al. Non-Hodgkin's lymphoma in children. Semin Oncol 1990;17:113–119.
4. Donaldson SS. Hodgkin's disease in children. Semin Oncol 1990;17:736–748.

Imaging Studies

Imaging is important for the diagnosis and management of patients with both Hodgkin disease and non-Hodgkin lymphoma (see Table 5–12).[1] It is perhaps more important for Hodgkin disease, because therapy and prognosis are very dependent on the location and distribution of disease. Non-Hodgkin lymphoma, by contrast, is assumed to be a disseminated disease process at

TABLE 5-9
Subdiaphragmatic Involvement at Staging Laparotomy by Histologic Subtype in 46 Children with Newly Diagnosed Hodgkin Disease[1]

Histology	No. of Patients	No. with Subdiaphragmatic Involvement	Site of Subdiaphragmatic Involvement: Spleen Only	Spleen + Lymph Node	Lymph Node Only
Lymphocyte predominant	4	1	0	1	0
Nodular sclerosing	30	11	4	4	3
Mixed cellularity	10	8	2	4	2
Lymphocyte depleted	2	1	1	0	0
Total	46	21	7	9	5

Reference
1. Baker L, Parker BR, Donaldson SS, et al. Staging of Hodgkin disease in children: comparison of CT and lymphography with laparotomy. AJR 1990;154:1251–1255.

TABLE 5-10
Notes on Distribution of Non-Hodgkin Lymphoma at the Time of Presentation*

Over 75 percent of children have disseminated disease[1]
Mediastinum and hilar node involvement is most common with lymphoblastic lymphoma[2]
Pleural effusions do not indicate the presence of pleural disease but can be secondary to ascites or lymphatic drainage obstruction
Large cell lymphoma is the least likely type to involve the central nervous system or bone marrow. It is the most likely type to involve bone cortex[3]
Small cell lymphoma is very rare in bone[4]
The central nervous system is an uncommon site of involvement at initial presentation. The likelihood of central nervous system involvement increases if the bone marrow is abnormal[5]
Bowel lymphoma in children is most likely to involve the ileocecal region[6]
The omentum may be involved in lymphoma, particularly Burkitt's lymphoma
Bone involvement may be focal or diffuse
Renal involvement occurred in 12 percent of 99 children with non-Hodgkin lymphoma.[7] The true incidence is probably higher
Renal involvement may be unilateral or bilateral, diffuse or focal[7]
Lymphoma in children following bone marrow transplantation or in children with AIDS is likely to be very aggressive and involve unusual sites such as the bone marrow, skin, peritoneum, liver, and lung[8,9]
Relapse in patients with non-Hodgkin lymphoma usually occurs relatively early but occasionally can occur more than 2 years after initial presentation. Relapse can occur at the sites of initial tumor or in other locations
It is important at this stage to note that lymphomas are among the most rapidly growing tumors. This applies particularly to the non-Hodgkin lymphomas and especially to Burkitt's lymphoma. Burkitt's tumor is the fastest-growing human tumor, with a potential doubling time of less than 24 hours[10]

*These have important imaging implications.

References
1. Smith SD, Rubin CM, Horvath A, et al. Non-Hodgkin's lymphoma in children. Semin Oncol 1990;17:113–119.
2. Bragg DG, Colby TV, Ward JH. New concepts in the non-Hodgkin lymphomas: radiologic implications. Radiology 1986;159:289–304.
3. Dehner LP. Pediatric surgical pathology, 2nd ed. Baltimore: Williams & Wilkins, 1987:822–837.
4. Spjut HJ, Ayala AG. Skeletal tumors in children and adolescents. Hum Pathol 1983;14:628–642.
5. Magrath IT. Malignant non-Hodgkin's lymphomas. In: Pizzo PA, Poplack DG, eds. Principles and practice of pediatric oncology. Philadelphia: JB Lippincott, 1989:415–455.
6. Brady LW, Asbell SO. Malignant lymphoma of the gastrointestinal tract. Radiology 1980;137:291–298.
7. Goodman P, Raval B. Omental cakes in American Burkitt lymphoma computed tomography demonstration. Clin Imag 1989;13:117–118.
8. Lynch MA, Cho KC, Jeffrey RB, et al. CT of peritoneal lymphomatosis. AJR 1988;152:713–715.
9. Day DL, Shapiro RS, Yueh N. B-cell lymphoproliferative disorders in children after bone marrow transplantation: radiologic manifestations. Radiology 1987;162:807–810.
10. Kjeldsberg CR, Wilson JF, Berard CW. Non-Hodgkin's lymphoma in children. Hum Pathol 1983;14:612–627.

the time of diagnosis, regardless of the actual anatomical sites demonstrated by imaging. The unnecessary use of imaging in evaluation of children with cancer is no better illustrated than with the lymphomas. Many studies that were traditionally performed in the evaluation of lymphoma should no longer be performed, either because they have extremely low yield, because the information provided is of little clinical significance, or because this information is readily available from other imaging studies. As is seen from the following discussion, there are some imaging studies it is easy to recommend, others it is easy to recommend against using, and others (such as MR of the chest and abdomen, CT of the abdomen, gallium scanning) for which use is very debatable. Table 5–13 summarizes low-yield studies.

Some dogmatic statements regarding recommendations for studies to perform on the initial presentation of children with Hodgkin disease or non-Hodgkin lymphoma can be made (Tables 5–14 and 5–15). These recommendations suggest studies that have an acceptably high positive yield, and those that define the extent of disease to enable accurate staging to be performed. Studies that yield positive results, that do not impact on treatment, and that are in areas in which it is not desired to monitor response to therapy are no longer included.

There is general agreement on the importance of imaging for staging Hodgkin disease and this importance increases as fewer staging laparotomies are done. If non-Hodgkin lymphoma is assumed to be a diffuse disease, imaging staging is less important. There are, however, severe inconsistencies in the literature. A 1990 study bases therapy on stage of non-Hodgkin lymphoma, but recommends *no* routine imaging of the central nervous system (MR) or bone marrow (sulfur colloid) to exclude disease in these areas.[2] It is much more difficult to find a scientific basis for recommendation of

TABLE 5–11

Notes on the Distribution of Hodgkin Disease on Initial Presentation*

Unlike non-Hodgkin lymphoma, Hodgkin disease is much more likely to be confined to and involve lymph nodes (see Table 5–10)

Hodgkin disease invariably involves lymph nodes at the time of presentation. Disease outside the lymph nodes may or may not be present

Hodgkin disease is rarely diffuse at the time of presentation. The disease spreads in an orderly fashion from one involved area to adjacent contiguous areas. The thoracic duct provides a route of spread from the chest to the abdomen

85% of children have involvement of intrathoracic lymph nodes. A child with nonthoracic adenopathy with no involvement in the chest is unlikely to have Hodgkin disease

In the thorax, paratracheal lymph node involvement is the most common. Hilar node involvement occurs in 25 percent, subcarinal in 22 percent, and posterior mediastinal node in 5 percent of patients[1,2]

Mediastinal node involvement is more likely with nodular sclerosing Hodgkin than with any other cell type[3]

Hilar node involvement without mediastinal node involvement is extremely rare. Therefore, isolated hilar adenopathy is unlikely to be Hodgkin disease[4]

The mediastinal and hilar lymph nodes displace rather than constrict adjacent blood vessels, trachea, and bronchi[1]

The lung may be involved in up to 10 percent of patients with Hodgkin disease at the time of diagnosis.[1,2,5] If the lung is involved, it is more likely to be because of direct invasion from adjacent lymph nodes than a separate discrete focus of tumor. This may, however, occur[5]

Lung involvement with Hodgkin disease is extremely unusual in the absence of lymphadenopathy.[6] In all age groups, only 15 cases of primary lung Hodgkin disease have been described[6]

Pleural effusion is only likely to be malignant if pleural nodules can be identified.[1] Pericardial involvement occurs in about 5 percent of patients. A pericardial effusion is always an indication of pericardial tumor[1]

The spleen is the most common site of non-nodal involvement. If disease is identified in other non-nodal locations, the spleen is invariably involved as well

The liver is never involved unless the spleen is involved.[1]

Other sites of involvement on presentation with Hodgkin disease are rare. The gastrointestinal and genitourinary tracts can occasionally be involved.[1] Bone involvement at the time of diagnosis is extremely unusual and when present is more likely to be caused by invasion from adjacent lymph nodes than by primary bone disease.[1] Bone involvement is more likely with mixed cellularity or lymphocyte depleted tumors[7]

The likelihood of subdiaphragmatic involvement with Hodgkin disease is very much dependent on tumor histology and is much more common with mixed cellularity than with nodular sclerosing disease (see Table 5–9)

Relapse with Hodgkin disease can be in any location or at the site of the original primary tumor. Involvement beyond lymph nodes is much more likely at relapse than on initial presentation. For example, in 15 of 68 patients with stage I to III Hodgkin disease who relapsed, the relapse sites were lung (4), nodes (4), bone (3), breast (1), and other (3).[8] Relapse is not uncommon, occurring in 94 of 197 patients between 1961 and 1985 in one large series[9]

*These have important imaging implications.

References

1. Castellino RA. Hodgkin disease: practical concepts for the diagnostic radiologist. Radiology 1986;159:305–310.
2. Dehner LP. Pediatric surgical pathology, 2nd ed. Baltimore: Williams & Wilkins, 1987:822–837.
3. Bragg DG, Colby TV, Ward JH. New concepts in the non-Hodgkin lymphomas: radiologic implications. Radiology 1986;159:289–304.
4. Roskos RR, Evans RC, Gilchrist GS, et al. Prognostic significance of mediastinal mass in childhood Hodgkin's disease. Cancer Treat Rep 1982;66:961–968.
5. Kolygin BA, Vesnin AG. Hodgkin's disease in children: clinico-roentgenologic features of the lesion in the chest. Pediatr Radiol 1976;4:144–148.
6. Yousem SA, Weiss LM, Colby TV. Primary pulmonary Hodgkin's disease: a clinicopathologic study of 15 cases. Cancer 1986;57:1217–1224.
7. Braunstein EM. Hodgkin disease of bone: radiographic correlation with the histological classification. Radiology 1980;137:643–646.
8. Mauch PM, Weinstein H, Botnick L, et al. An evaluation of long-term survival and treatment complications in children with Hodgkin's disease. Cancer 1983;51:925–932.
9. Chang PJ, Parker BR, Donaldson SS, et al. Dynamic probabilistic model for determination of optimal timing of surveillance chest radiography in pediatric Hodgkin disease. Radiology 1989;173:71–75.

studies to do for follow-up and how frequently to perform these studies. The information regarding patterns and rates of relapse is perhaps not known as well as it might be. Also the impact of finding recurrent disease slightly earlier, for example with a chest CT rather than a chest radiograph, is not known. Although some guidelines for follow-up studies may be given, these must be modified in the light of existing and future protocols being utilized and also as more information of relapse patterns becomes available. This whole area is very complex, as evidenced by one recent report presenting a theoretical statistical model to optimize follow-up studies in children with lymphoma. This report is very complex but does, for example, suggest that chest radiographs are done too frequently in the follow-up of children with lymphoma.[3] Another study illustrates inconsistencies and lack of logical use of imaging for follow-up of 66 children with lymphoma (Table 5–16).[4]

TABLE 5-12

Clinical and Radiographic Sites of Lymphoma on Initial Presentation[1]

Site	Hodgkin Disease	Non-Hodgkin Lymphoma
Clinical		
Neck nodes	24	8
Groin nodes	3	2
Axillary nodes	1	1
Abdomen	1	5
Tonsil	0	5
Bone pain	0	2
Radiographic		
Mediastinal or hilar nodes	23	14
Lung or pleura	2	6
Bone	1	5
Pharynx	1	
Abdominal mass or nodes	9	12
Liver	0	3
Intussusception	0	1
Total No. of Patients	36	30

Reference
1. Cohen MD, Siddiqui A, Weetman R, et al. Hodgkin disease and non-Hodgkin lymphomas in children: utilization of radiological modalities. Radiology 1986;158:499–505.

TABLE 5-13

Low-Yield Studies for Investigation of Hodgkin Lymphoma on Initial Presentation

Study	No. Done	No. Positive
Skeletal survey	61[1]	1
	27[2]	3
	68[1]	1
Intravenous urogram	66[3]	0
	25[2]	2
	40[1]	0
Cavogram	24[3]	2 (displaced)
Upper GI barium study	17[3]	0
Liver spleen scan	98[2]	1
Marrow isotope scan	51[2]	5
Bone isotope scan	16[2]	2

References
1. Parker BR, Castellino RA, Kaplan HS. Pediatric Hodgkin's disease. I. Radiographic evaluation. Cancer 1976;37:2430–2435.
2. Cohen MD, Siddiqui A, Weetman R, et al. Hodgkin disease and non-Hodgkin lymphomas in children: utilization of radiological modalities. Radiology 1986; 158:499–505.
3. Linden A, Zankovich R, Theissen P, et al. Malignant lymphoma: bone marrow imaging versus biopsy. Radiology 1989;173:335–339.

TABLE 5-14

Recommended Studies for Initial Evaluation of Non-Hodgkin Lymphoma[1,2]

	Study	Comment
Do:	Chest CT	May not greatly alter therapy
	Abdominal CT	
	CT of other sites of clinically delectable primary disease	e.g., head and neck
	Upper GI or barium enema	Only do in the presence of clinical symptoms or plain film radiographic signs of bowel disease[2]
	Bone radiograph	Only for areas of positive symptoms
	Bone isotope scan	Selected cases only—may be helpful in a child with apparent localized abdominal tumor
Don't Do:	Skeletal survey	
	Bone isotope scan (routinely)	
	Intravenous urogram	
	Liver spleen scan	
	Barium studies (routinely)	
Controversial:	Gallium	Probably not needed
Unknown Role:	Magnetic resonance	
	Sulfur colloid bone marrow scan	

References
1. Moormeier JA, Williams SF, Golomb HM. The staging of non-Hodgkin's lymphomas. Semin Oncol 1990;17:43–50.
2. Castellino RA, Bellani FF, Gasparini M, et al. Radiographic findings in previously untreated children with non-Hodgkin's lymphoma. Radiology 1975;117:657–663.

TABLE 5–15
Recommended Studies for Initial Evaluation of Hodgkin Lymphoma

	Study	Comment
Do:	Chest radiograph	
	Chest CT	
	Abdominal CT	
	CT of other clinical sites of disease	e.g., neck
	Bone radiograph	Only of regions of + clinical symptoms
Don't do:	Skeletal survey	
	Bone isotope scan	
	Intravenous urogram	
	Barium studies	
	Liver spleen scan	
Controversial:	Lymphangiogram	My personal opinion is not to do this study
	Gallium scan	My personal opinion is not to do this study routinely. It is helpful for selected problems
Unknown role:	Magnetic resonance	

IMAGING BY MODALITY

Chest Radiograph. This should be done in all patients on initial presentation and routinely on follow-up. Both Hodgkin and non-Hodgkin lymphoma frequently involve the thorax. The chest radiograph provides excellent information about disease in the mediastinum, lungs, pleura, and some bone (Figs. 5–1 and 5–2). Evaluation of the lungs is also important for detection of many therapy complications.

Whole Lung Tomography. This study provides intermediate information about the lungs, hila, and mediastinum, between that of chest radiograph and chest CT. It is time-consuming, expensive, there is a high radiation dose, and it should, therefore, no longer be performed. The yield from linear chest tomography is high (over 40 percent),[4] but the information provided is already known from chest radiograph and chest CT.

Chest CT. This is an important study, providing information about the presence and distribution of disease in the mediastinum, lungs, pleura and pericardium, chest wall, and bone (see Figs. 5–1 and 5–2). It will alter treatment in a significant number of patients.[5] It should be performed

- on all patients on presentation
- regularly (every few months) to follow response of known disease to treatment
- to further evaluate any recurrence or other new abnormality detected on chest radiograph at any other time
- to obtain a baseline at the conclusion of therapy
- at times when major changes in therapy are contemplated

At other times, chest radiograph is probably adequate for evaluation of the thorax.

There are no special factors regarding technique of chest CT apart from the fact that a large, good bolus of contrast is needed, together with dynamic scanning, to maximize visualization of mediastinal vessels. CT is extremely good for identification of abnormality and definition of extent of disease. As is discussed later, it may not be particularly good for differentiation of residual tumor from fibrosis or for the differential diagnosis of pulmonary abnormality developing on therapy. On initial presentation, chest CT in 11 patients provided information, compared to chest radiograph, that altered stage in 3 children.[4] Seventeen CT scans in children with non-Hodgkin lymphoma revealed more abnormality than chest radiograph in 9 cases.

Abdominal CT. Abdominal CT is a relatively sensitive method for evaluation of abdominal disease, but it has problems. In Hodgkin disease, it will consistently miss abnormality in the liver, spleen, and small lymph nodes, when compared to laparotomy.[4] In one study, laparotomy provided more information than CT in 4 of 15 patients.[4] In addition to the errors, the overall yield of positive results from Hodgkin disease is low.[4] The importance of performing abdominal CT is that the finding of positive disease has a significant impact on patient management, particularly if the presence of disease can be confirmed by needle biopsy rather than laparotomy. Second, it is important to have a baseline normal study prior to initiation of therapy.

For follow-up, CT scans of the abdomen should probably be done only to monitor known tumor but not in patients in whom no abdominal disease was present at diagnosis. It may be advisable to obtain a baseline normal study at the time of conclusion of therapy, although it may be argued that this is not necessary in the absence of any symptoms. In non-Hodgkin lymphoma, the positive yield in the abdomen is slightly higher than with Hodgkin disease. Affected lymph nodes tend to be larger than with Hodgkin disease and more readily identified on CT scan. In addition, CT scan may identify disease in the liver, spleen, and kidneys. Lymphoma involving primarily the bowel may also be identified. Many of these patients may, however, present with an acute abdomen and have the tumor resected prior to performing any imaging.

Although the CT yield in non-Hodgkin lymphoma[4] is slightly higher than with Hodgkin disease, the impact on therapy is perhaps less, since most patients with non-Hodgkin lymphoma are treated as if disseminated disease is present at the time of diagnosis. As with Hodgkin disease, CT abdominal scan is recommended in all patients on initial presentation and for follow-up in patients in whom abdominal disease is identified. If no abdominal disease is identified on initial presenta-

TABLE 5-16

Lymphoma in 66 Children: Percentage of Patients Still Alive Who Were Studied at Varying Intervals after Initial Presentation[1]

	0	6 mo	1 yr	2 yr	3 yr	4 yr	5 yr
Chest radiograph							
NHL	100	100	90	100	90	100	100
HD	100	100	96	96	100	93	100
Chest CT							
NHL	43	21	25	13	10		
HD	44	34	25	28	29	29	
Chest tomography							
NHL	9	4		7			
HD	28	25	18	12	5		
Abdominal CT							
NHL	80	25	30	26	20	17	
HD	64	50	36	52	29	7	
Excretory urography							
NHL	43	4	5				
HD	33	3	7	16	5		
Skeletal survey							
NHL	60	14	30	40	50	16	
HD	44	3	11	7	14		
Liver spleen scan							
NHL	66	50	40	40	20	33	
HD	75	31	57	64	52	14	
Gallium scan							
NHL	43	29	10	20	20	16	25
HD	69	34	71	68	33	7	
Marrow scan							
NHL	46	25	25	33	2	16	
HD	61	16	35	10	24		
Bone scan							
NHL	56	21	25	40	30	16	
HD	17	6	14	12			

NHL = non-Hodgkin lymphoma; HD = Hodgkin disease.

Reference

1. Cohen MD, Siddiqui A, Weetman R, et al. Hodgkin disease and non-Hodgkin lymphomas in children: utilization of radiological modalities. Radiology 1986;158:499–505.

tion, routine follow-up CT scans are not required. Again, as with Hodgkin disease, it may be worthwhile to perform a baseline repeat CT scan at the time therapy is stopped.

Barium Studies. The bowel is virtually never involved on presentation in Hodgkin disease. In non-Hodgkin lymphoma, the bowel may be involved, but the overwhelming evidence suggests that in all patients with bowel involvement clinical symptoms are present. Therefore, barium studies are recommended for patients with possible non-Hodgkin lymphoma in whom there are signs and symptoms suggesting bowel disease. Barium studies are not recommended for routine screening in either Hodgkin disease or non-Hodgkin lymphoma.

Liver/Spleen Scan. The yield and sensitivity of liver/spleen scan is low and this study is not recommended for lymphoma in children.

Bone Isotope Scan. Bone disease on initial presentation with Hodgkin disease is extremely rare and routine isotope scans are not recommended. In non-Hodgkin lymphoma, bone involvement is more common but the impact of positive findings on therapy is slight. Bone scanning is, therefore, not recommended for routine evaluation.

Bone Marrow Scanning. As with bone scanning, this will identify disease in a number of patients with non-Hodgkin lymphoma but the impact on therapy is minimal and the study is at the present time not recommended for routine use.

Intravenous Urography. The yield in Hodgkin disease is minimal. Kidneys may be involved in non-Hodgkin lymphoma but as with bone isotope and bone marrow scan, the impact of positive findings on therapy is minimal. In addition, the kidneys will be studied on a CT scan of the abdomen. Therefore, this study should not be done.

Gallium Scanning. Gallium was once widely used for the evaluation of lymphoma, fell into some disrepute, and is now perhaps undergoing a slight resurgence in

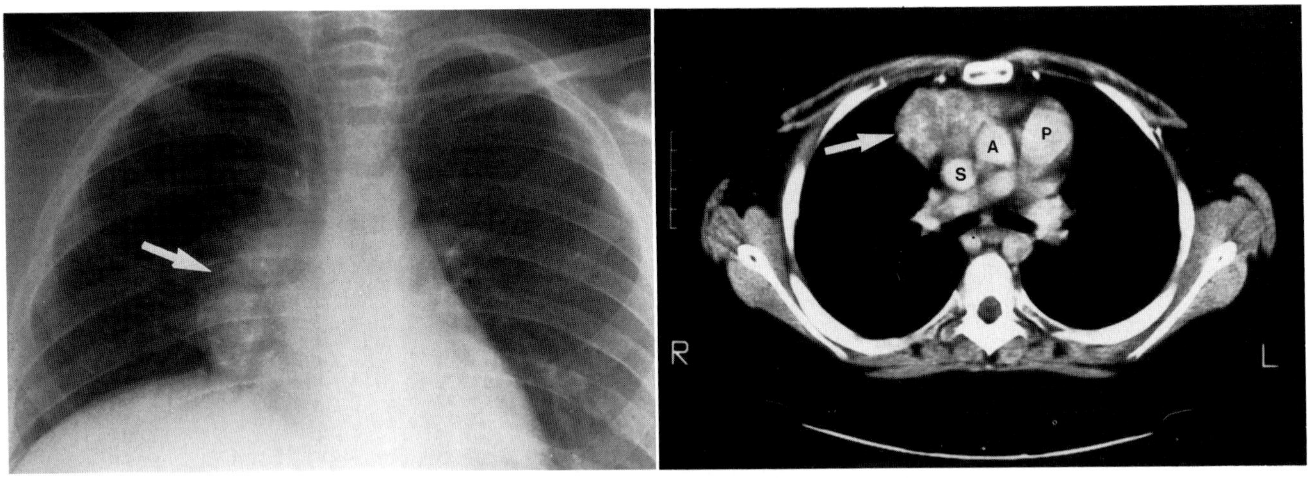

Figure 5–1. **Diagnosis: Hodgkin disease.**
***A*, Chest radiograph. Right-sided lymphadenopathy is identified *(arrow)*. The chest radiograph cannot identify the precise location of the adenopathy. It does, however, show elevation of the right hemidiaphragm presumably caused by to phrenic nerve paralysis from infiltration of the nerve by the tumor. *B*, CT. At the level of the main pulmonary artery (*P*), extensive anterior mediastinal lymphadenopathy *(arrow)* is identified. *A* = Ascending aorta; *S* = superior vena cava.**

popularity.[6] The disadvantages with gallium are that it is not uniformly sensitive, being worse for detection of disease in the abdomen than in the chest or pelvis.[7] In addition, uptake of gallium varies with tumor histology, all disease is never detected with gallium, and false positive results occur (e.g., infection). Another disadvantage with gallium is that it is time consuming, with results not available for a couple of days.[7,8] Recent studies, utilizing higher doses of isotope, better imaging gamma cameras, and SPECT (single photon emission computed tomography)[6,7,9] have improved sensitivity of gallium studies. There is still, however, no clear-cut evidence that gallium scanning provides additional information over that provided by CT scan for routine clinical use.

The main use for gallium scanning may be to help differentiate residual tumor from fibrosis in children with residual soft-tissue masses following therapy[8,10] (Fig. 5–3). It may also be useful when results of CT imaging are somewhat equivocal with regard to the presence or absence of disease.[9] Recent reports suggest that gallium might also be helpful in following therapy. In patients with mediastinal Hodgkin disease, evaluation with gallium, after initial chemotherapy, was very helpful in predicting outcome. The patients were all gallium positive at commencement of therapy. Those patients in whom gallium scan became negative had an excellent outcome, whereas those in whom the gallium scan stayed positive had a poor outcome.[11]

Ultrasound. Although ultrasound can identify disease in the mediastinum, pleura, pericardium, liver, spleen, abdominal nodes, and bowel, it suffers from the problems of some degree of complete anatomical coverage being obscured by gas or bone and also by decreased sensitivity compared to other imaging studies.

Although ultrasound may be performed for specific indications in some patients, I do not believe that it has any routine role in the evaluation of lymphoma in children.

Lymphangiography. This is a controversial study that is presently performed in very few centers. Proponents of lymphangiography cite accuracy, sensitivity, and specificity of over 90 percent in very large series of patients.[12] In an adult study, lymphangiography was more sensitive than CT for nodal disease detection.[13] This study was, however, retrospective and because dates of enrollment are not given many CT studies may have been done on old, out-of-date equipment. There is no doubt that lymphangiography can detect Hodgkin disease in lymph nodes in the abdomen that are not enlarged and, therefore, not detectable on CT scan. Because the contrast persists in the nodes for very many months, follow-up abdominal radiographs can also be utilized to monitor shrinkage of affected lymph nodes following lymphangiography. Opponents of lymphangiography correctly point out that it is technically somewhat difficult to perform (especially in children) and, even more important, is difficult to interpret. Many other studies cite much lower accuracy rates than 90 percent for lymphangiography. Lymphangiography can only detect disease in retroperitoneal and not mesenteric or splenic hilar lymph nodes. It obviously provides no information about the liver or spleen. Lymphangiography will still miss disease detected at laparotomy and, therefore, cannot be used to avoid laparotomy. For these reasons most centers no longer perform lymphangiography, and I do not predict a resurgence in its popularity.

MR Imaging. MR imaging can detect disease in lymphoma in children. It is particularly sensitive for detection of disease in the mediastinum, the main advantages being its ability to image in multiple planes and also the easy identification of blood vessels (Fig. 5–4). The co-

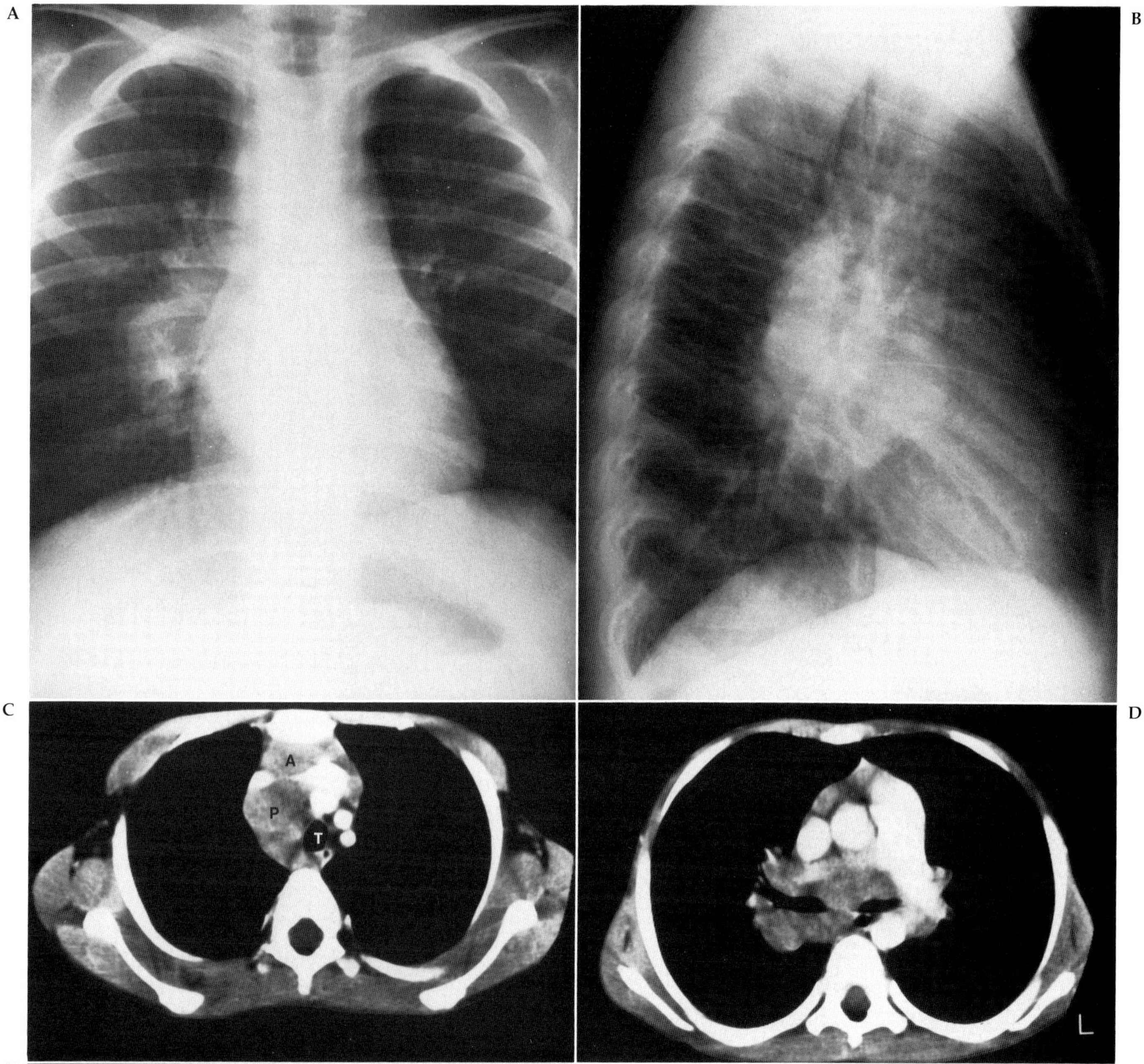

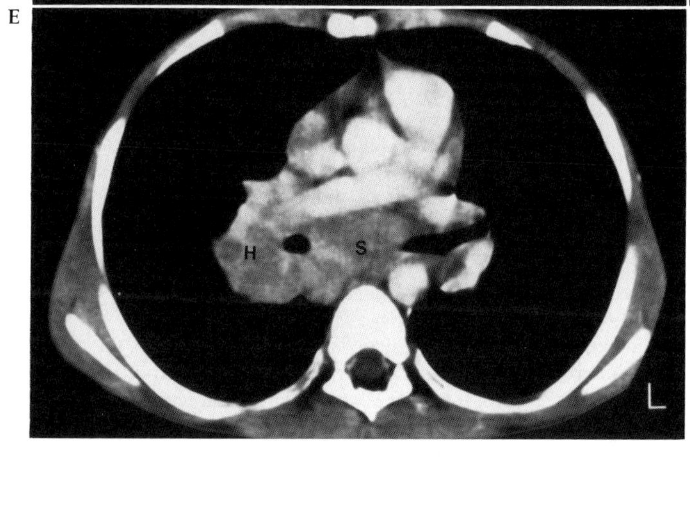

Figure 5–2. Diagnosis: Hodgkin disease with extensive hilar and mediastinal lymphadenopathy.
A and ***B***, PA and lateral chest radiographs. There is marked hilar lymphadenopathy on the right side. Paratracheal adenopathy on the right side is displacing the trachea to the left but does not appear to be causing significant narrowing of the tracheal lumen. ***C***, ***D***, and ***E***, CT at the level of the mid thoracic trachea, carina, and immediately below the carina. Extensive lymphadenopathy is identified involving the anterior (*A*) mediastinum, right paratracheal (*P*) lymph node, subcarinal (*S*) lymph nodes, and hilar (*H*) lymph nodes. The trachea (*T*) is slightly flattened but not significantly narrowed.

A B C D

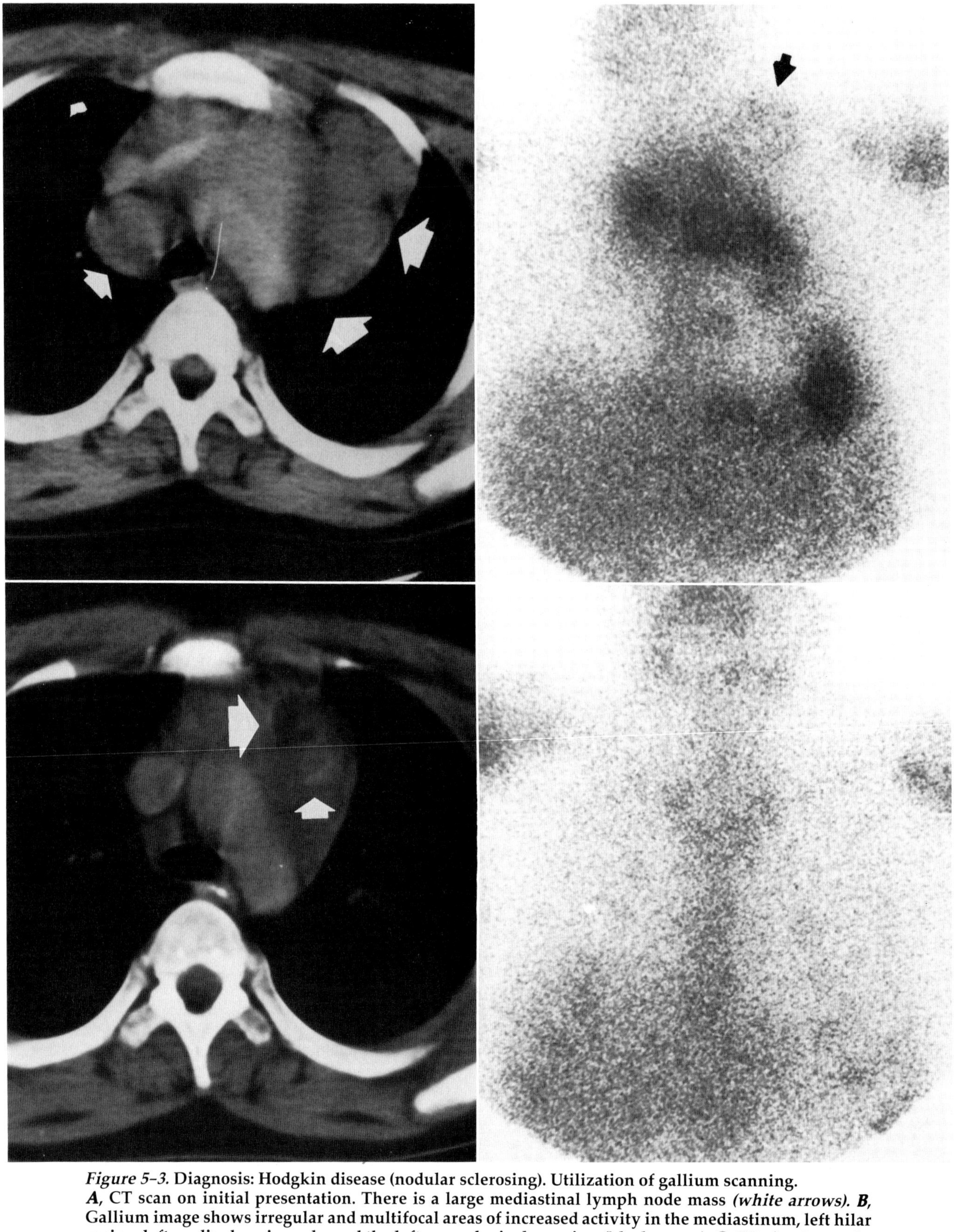

Figure 5-3. Diagnosis: Hodgkin disease (nodular sclerosing). Utilization of gallium scanning. ***A***, CT scan on initial presentation. There is a large mediastinal lymph node mass *(white arrows)*. ***B***, Gallium image shows irregular and multifocal areas of increased activity in the mediastinum, left hilar region, left cardiophrenic angle, and the left supraclavicular region *(black arrow)*. ***C***, CT after 2 months of chemotherapy. A residual, smaller mass lesion is still identified in the mediastinum *(arrows)*. ***D***, Gallium scan at the same time reveals no abnormal uptake of isotope and apparent complete resolution of the lesion, suggesting that no active disease is still present. The tissue was not biopsied, but the patient was alive and well 14 months later. (From Drossman SR. Lymphoma of the mediastinum and neck. Evaluation with gallium 67 imaging and CT correlation. Radiology 1990;174:171–175.)

A B C

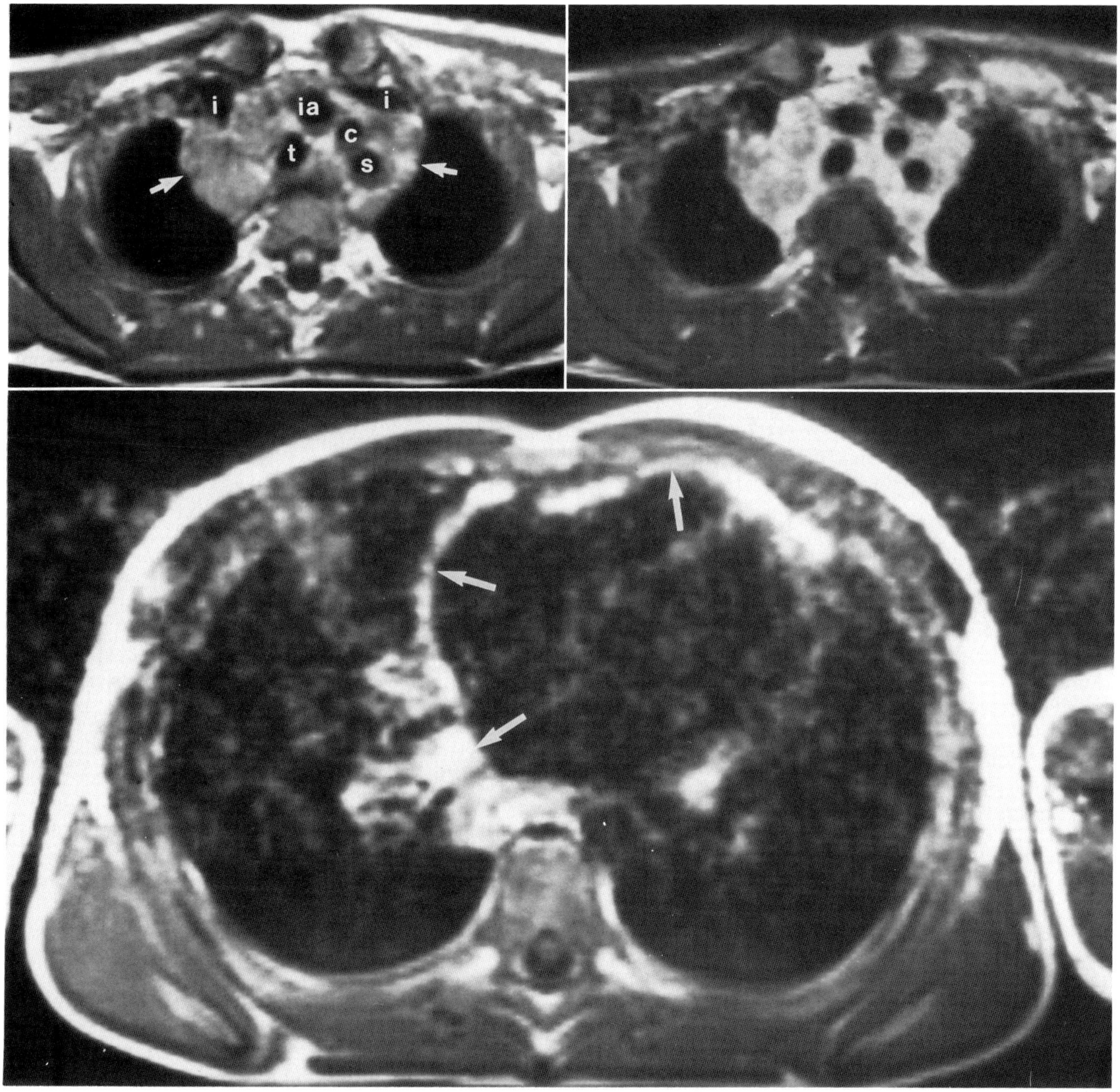

Figure 5-4. Diagnosis: Hodgkin disease. Mediastinal and pericardial involvement. MR findings. ***A,*** Axial MR T1 weighted image. There is extensive lymphadenopathy involving the anterior and mid mediastinum on both sides *(arrows).* The abnormality is of intermediate signal intensity. Note the excellent visualization of blood vessels without the need for utilization of contrast. *I* = Innominate veins; *IA* = innominate artery; *C* = left common carotid artery; *S* = subclavian artery; *T* = trachea. ***B,*** T1 weighted image at the same level, obtained following intravenous injection of gadolinium-DTPA. There has been fairly widespread enhancement of all of the tumor. ***C,*** T1 weighted image after intravenous gadolinium-DTPA. Level of heart. There is extensive enhancement of tumor in the pericardium *(arrows).* Note the advantage of gadolinium-DTPA. On T1 weighted images without gadolinium-DTPA, or on T2 weighted images, it might prove difficult to differentiate the tumor from pericardial effusion. Note that on the right side the tumor extends into the adjacent mediastinum.

ronal plane is helpful for differentiating a normal thymus from lymphadenopathy in the chest. In the abdomen, MR can identify disease in the liver, spleen, and lymph nodes. There is, however, no evidence to suggest that it is more accurate than CT or other imaging for the identification of such disease, and it is certainly not sensitive enough to avoid the requirement for laparotomy in some patients. The precise role of MR in children with lymphoma is not known. At the present time, studies should continue to be performed for research interests, but no routine clinical role can or should be recommended. In selected clinical indications, however, MR will obviously have a significant role, e.g., in evaluation of a child with clinical central nervous system symptoms and suspected central nervous system lymphoma and evaluation of a child with focal bone pain with a normal radiograph.

Experimental techniques An experimental technique using iodine-labeled monoclonal antibody to Reed Sternberg cells has been studied in 6 patients, including 2 children. This technique was able to identify pathology within lymph nodes, bone, spleen, and liver and has a possible future role in staging of Hodgkin disease—especially identification of splenic disease—and in the evaluation of residual mass lesions.[14] Another experimental technique is the use of MR spectroscopy, and early work found that changes occur in the spectrum obtained from non-Hodgkin lymphoma involved nodes in response to therapy.[15]

IMAGING BY ANATOMIC SITE

Mediastinum and Chest. Involvement of the chest with non-Hodgkin lymphoma is common, but less frequent than with Hodgkin lymphoma. In one large study of children with Hodgkin disease,[16] the chest radiograph was abnormal in 36 percent of those under the age of 10 years and 77 percent of those over the age of 10 years. This reflects the difference in the prevalence of the various histologic subtypes depending on age. CT will show even more abnormality than chest radiograph. In both types of lymphoma, the detection of pericardial fluid almost always indicates pericardial tumor (Fig. 5–5). Pleural effusion, however, may be present without the presence of pleural tumor. In Hodgkin disease, the most common abnormality is mediastinal lymphadenopathy with or without hilar lymphadenopathy (Fig. 5–5). Hilar lymphadenopathy without mediastinal adenopathy is very rare, being present in only 2 of 105 children.[16] In another study of 60 children, a mediastinal mass was present in two-thirds at the time of diagnosis.[17] The most likely histology with a mediastinal mass is nodular sclerosing.[17] Evaluation of the extent of disease by imaging is important in the staging of Hodgkin disease (Fig. 5–6 and 5–7).

In many studies, bulky tumor is defined as mediastinal tumor with maximal width on a chest radiograph greater than one-third of the chest diameter at the level of the diaphragm.[18] With modern CT techniques I believe that this definition will quickly fall from favor, since CT is capable of giving much more accurate estimations of tumor extent together with calculation of approximate tumor volume. When comparing CT of the chest with chest radiograph, CT was positive in 10 percent of times when the chest radiograph was negative.[18] In another study, it was estimated that 44 percent of recurrences of disease would have been missed if only chest radiograph and not chest CT had been performed.[19] CT is better than chest radiograph for detection of recurrence not only in the mediastinum but also in the lung.[19] In another study of 107 adults, CT demonstrated a total of 194 new sites of disease and disproved disease in 24 sites of suspected abnormality on chest radiograph.[20] CT will alter staging in a significant number of patients[20] (see Fig. 5–6). The actual number of patients depends on the therapeutic protocol being utilized. CT will frequently alter the planned radiation field.[21]

Chest imaging must look carefully at the degree of tracheobronchial compression[22] (Fig. 5–8). This is frequently ignored, but if carefully looked for, may be seen in up to 50 percent of children with Hodgkin disease.[22] In one study of 20 children, the tracheobronchial lumen was decreased by at least one-third of the diameter in 5 cases. Recently 6 patients were reported with life-threatening airway obstruction from Hodgkin disease compressing the airway.[23] This compression of the airway is important to detect, especially prior to anesthesia.

The thymus may frequently be involved with lymphoma.[24] In one study in adults, it was enlarged in 30 percent, probably because of tumor.[25] The thymus is never involved with Hodgkin disease in the absence of mediastinal lymphadenopathy.[25] The size of the thymus will vary with age. In most patients, thymic disease can readily be diagnosed by looking for an alteration in the shape and contour of the gland together with a loss of normal homogeneity.[26] Gallium scanning is not helpful for detection of thymic disease, as it may frequently be falsely positive[27] (Fig. 5–9). This is particularly true in younger children. Thymic enlargement is not always caused by tumor. Enlargement of the thymus is commonly seen as a rebound phenomenon after cessation of chemotherapy (Fig. 5–9). This is an important event and should not be mistaken for tumor recurrence. In addition, thymic cysts have been reported occurring following therapy of Hodgkin disease.[28] These cysts are seen on CT scan varying in size from tiny to very large (Fig. 5–10). They are of water density with thin walls and are well defined. Occasionally, hemorrhage into the cyst may be seen.[28] Although initially reported as occurring after chemotherapy, there is now good evidence that the cysts are present prior to the commencement of therapy, either as an associated abnormality or as a result of the presence of Hodgkin disease in the thymus. In one 14-year-old, multiple large cysts were seen in the thymus prior to the start of therapy for Hodgkin disease. In another study of 3 patients, cysts were present

A B

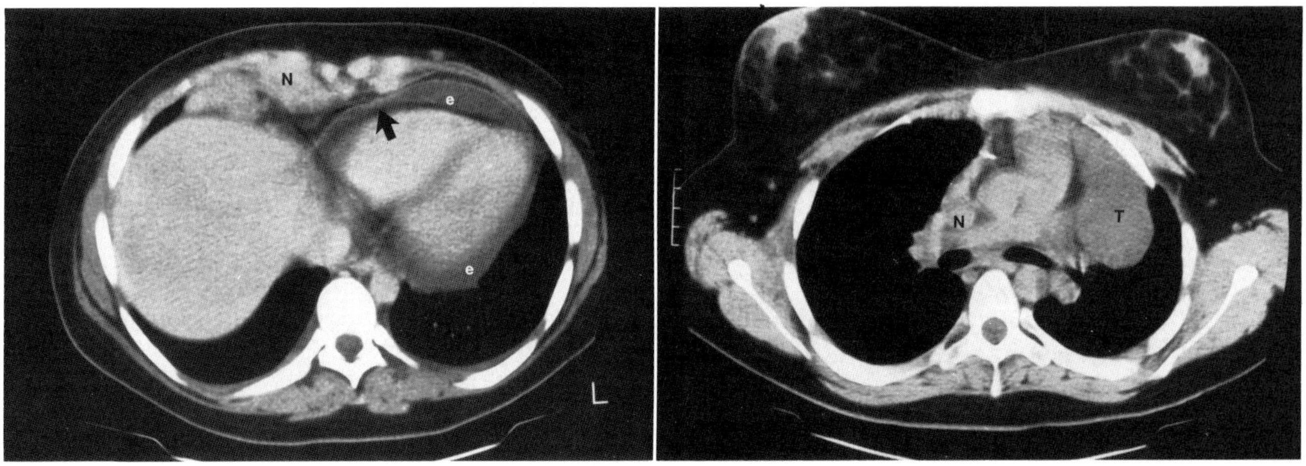

Figure 5–5. Diagnosis: Hodgkin disease with pericardial involvement.
A and ***B***, CT images. There is thickening of the pericardium *(arrows)* because of tumor infiltration. A large pericardial effusion (*E*) is identified. Note that pericardial disease does not occur in the absence of mediastinal lymph node tumor. Extensive tumor is identified in the mediastinal lymph nodes (*N*). Tumor is also seen in the thymus (*T*).

A B C

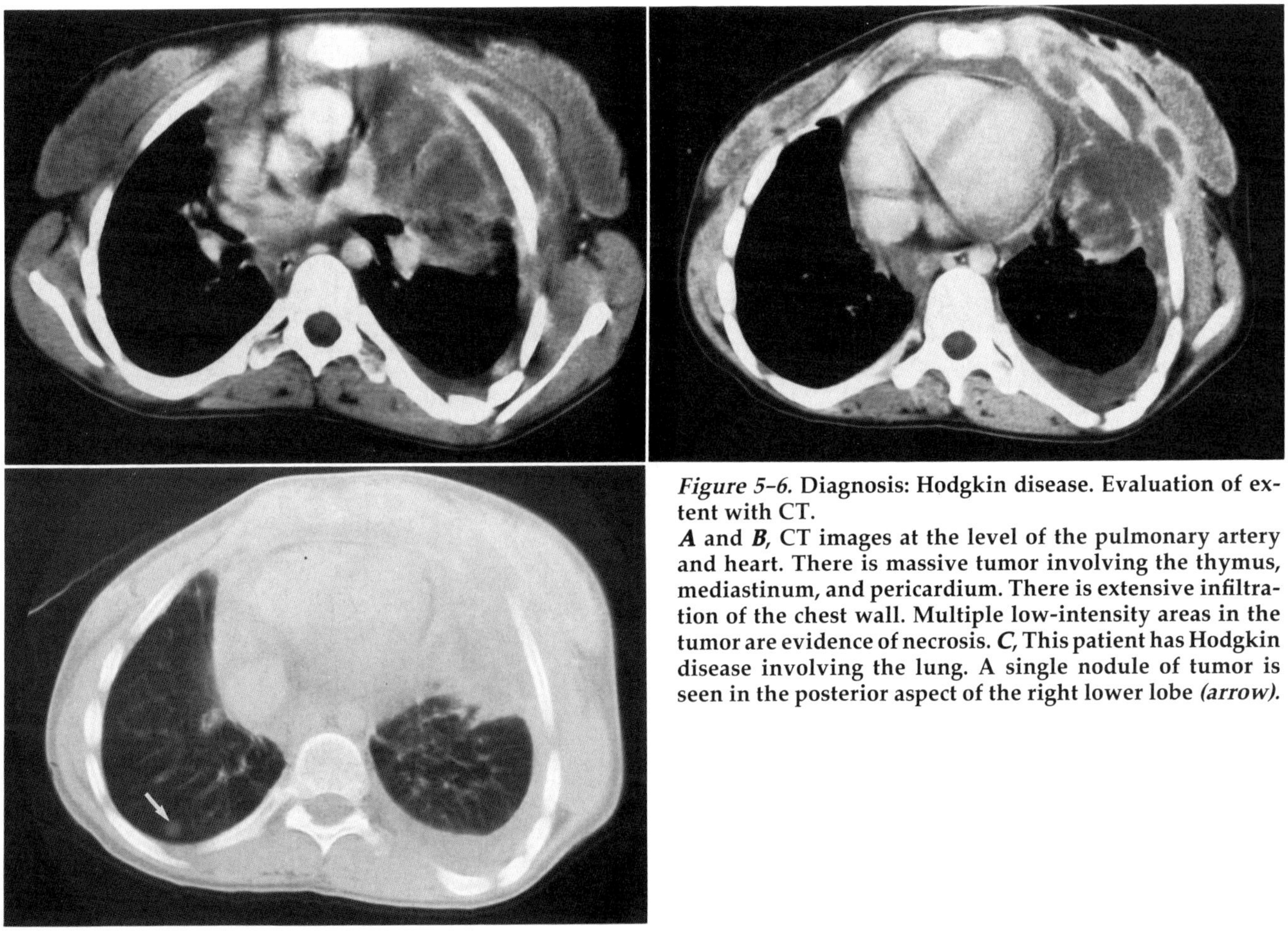

Figure 5–6. Diagnosis: Hodgkin disease. Evaluation of extent with CT.
A and ***B***, CT images at the level of the pulmonary artery and heart. There is massive tumor involving the thymus, mediastinum, and pericardium. There is extensive infiltration of the chest wall. Multiple low-intensity areas in the tumor are evidence of necrosis. ***C***, This patient has Hodgkin disease involving the lung. A single nodule of tumor is seen in the posterior aspect of the right lower lobe *(arrow).*

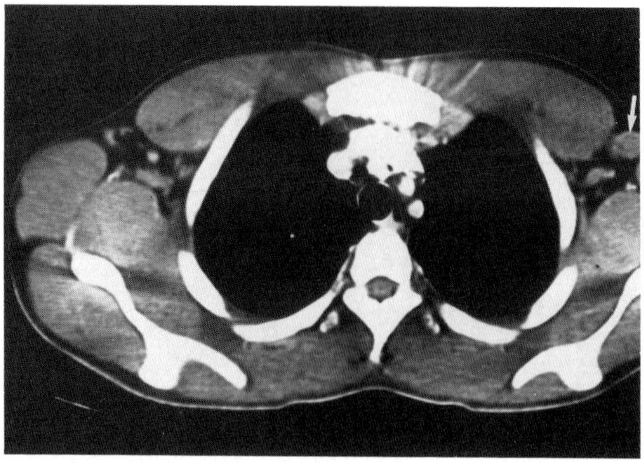

Figure 5-7. **Diagnosis: Hodgkin disease. Evaluation of tumor extent with CT. Tumor is seen in an enlarged axillary lymph node *(arrow).***

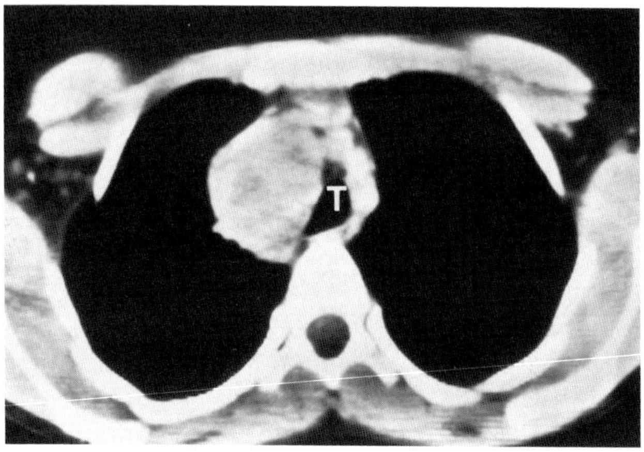

Figure 5-8. **Diagnosis: Tracheal compression by Hodgkin disease.**
CT. A large right paratracheal node mass compresses the trachea (*T*) and narrows the airway.

prior to the start of chemotherapy. With therapy the tumor resolved but the cysts persisted.[28,29]

Imaging should also be utilized to follow response of mediastinal tumor to therapy. In one study between 1969 and 1979 of 72 patients, half of the patients had achieved complete remission by 3 months and all by 11 months. The rate of regression is, therefore, rapid. Follow-up imaging studies should be planned accordingly. In this study, the relapse rate was not found to be related to the rate of regression of tumor.[20]

MR imaging has been utilized to evaluate response to therapy. In 18 patients, reduction in T2 relaxation time was identified with therapy.[31] At the present time the role of MR is still experimental and further work regarding changes in relaxation times and spectroscopy, as early predictors of response to therapy, needs to be done.

Calcification has been reported in one case of anterior mediastinal lymphoma.[32] For practical purposes, however, it is not believed that calcification occurs in involved lymph nodes with lymphoma, especially prior to treatment. Incidental calcification may be associated with lymphoma (Fig. 5–11). For example, patients with preexisting histoplasmosis and calcified lymph nodes may subsequently develop a lymphoma. Thus, although calcification does not occur in lymph nodes involved with lymphoma, the presence of calcification in the affected region should not be taken as a sign excluding lymphoma.

Liver and Spleen. The appearance on imaging of Hodgkin disease and non-Hodgkin lymphoma is similar and the histology cannot be predicted from the imaging appearance. In most cases, there is diffuse involvement of liver or spleen with tiny areas of tumor (Fig. 5–12). Occasionally, more focal, larger areas of tumor may be seen (Figs. 5–13 and 5–14). When evaluating patients for splenic disease, the possibility of congenital anomalies must be borne in mind and images interpreted accordingly. For example, one patient with Hodgkin disease and polysplenia has been described.[33] All imaging modalities are very poor for identification of lymphoma in the liver or spleen. Detection of hepatomegaly or splenomegaly does not correlate well with the presence of disease, with a large number of false positive and false negative results. One study conflicts with this statement, showing that CT measurement of three diameters of the spleen, and calculation of a splenic index for size, predicted spleen involvement with Hodgkin disease in 91 percent of 35 adults.[35] Despite this study, it is not recommended that organ size be utilized as a criterion for tumor involvement. Compared to laparotomy or postmortem, all imaging misses a significant amount of tumor. This is perhaps not surprising, as one study of 16 patients with splenic disease showed that on histology 88 percent of all identified nodules were less than 5 mm in diameter.[36]

On ultrasound, lymphoma in the liver and spleen has a very varied appearance.[37] The most common finding appears to be decrease in echoes.[37–40] There may be homogenous or more focal involvement. The lesions are usually diffuse and poorly defined,[37,38] but sometimes can be focal.[38] Mixed patterns of echogenicity are common and focal areas of increased echogenicity or target lesions were seen in 13 percent of 443 patients.[40] As previously mentioned, the overall accuracy of ultrasound for detection of disease in liver and spleen is low. New experimental techniques aimed at improving sensitivity include utilization of highly filtered ultrasound beams and correlation of amplitude of the beam with the presence of tumor.[39] It is not known if these techniques will have routine clinical application.

CT is probably better than ultrasound for identification of splenic disease. It is still poor, with varying detection rates, but an overall sensitivity of probably no more than 40 percent.[36] CT scanning may show an increase in size of the liver or spleen. There are problems in definition of organomegaly and, as mentioned above, a large number of false results.[36,41]

MR has been reported as being no better than CT[36] or showing the disease in more spleens than CT.[42] MR still

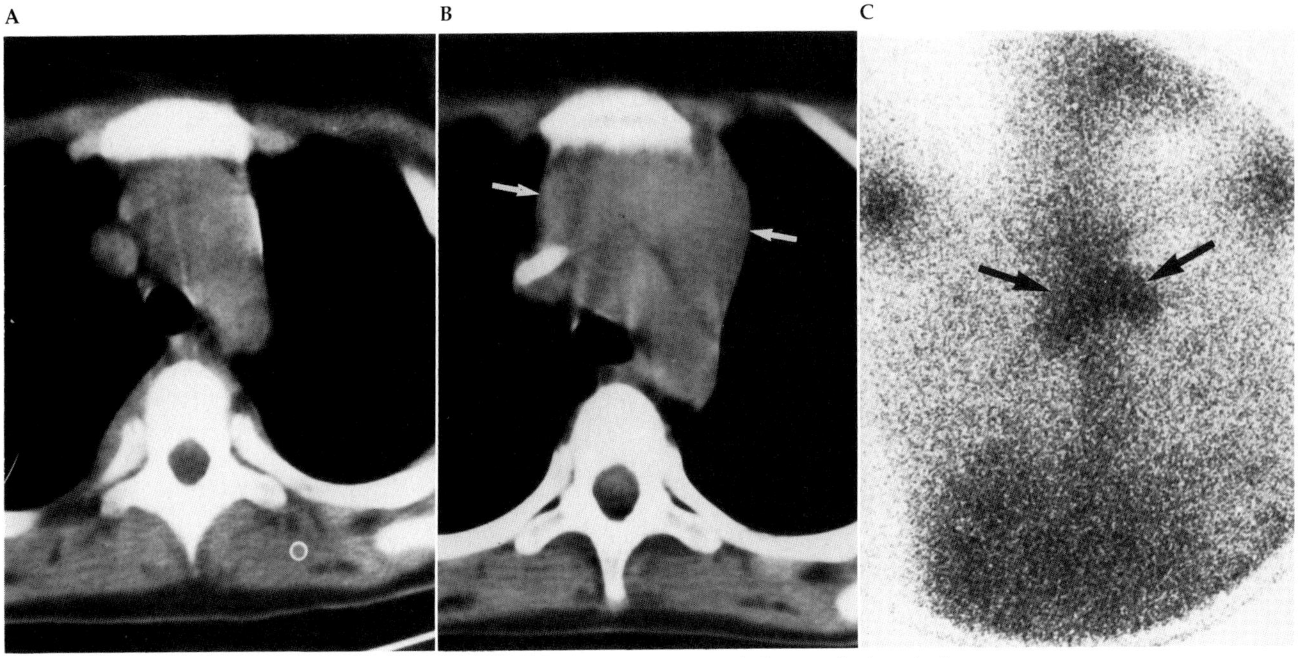

Figure 5-9. **Diagnosis: Burkitt's lymphoma. Rebound thymic hyperplasia mimics tumor recurrence. *A*, CT. On initial presentation the thymus appeared normal. *B* and *C*, CT and gallium images. The CT shows enlargement of the thymus *(arrows)*. Gallium images show uptake of gallium in the thymus *(arrows)*. This was rebound thymic hyperplasia and not tumor recurrence. (From Drossman SR. Lymphoma of the mediastinum and neck. Evaluation with gallium 67 imaging and CT correlation. Radiology 1990;174:171–175.)**

misses disease when compared to laparotomy or postmortem. MR imaging has potential for better demonstration of disease in the liver and spleen. In an early study in 1984, it missed disease in 12 of 13 patients with known non-Hodgkin lymphoma of the liver.[43] More recent studies have shown improved sensitivity,[42] but there is no doubt that MR still misses disease. Lymphoma tissue has a T1 and T2 relaxation time similar to normal spleen,[44] and tumor is best identified on T2 weighted images as a mottled appearance in the organ

Figure 5-10. **Diagnosis: Hodgkin disease. Thymic cysts mimic tumor recurrence. *A*, Chest radiograph after chemotherapy. This radiograph showed large bilateral mediastinal masses. *B*, CT. A large cystic (*C*) mass is seen on both sides of the mediastinum. These masses are thymic cysts and not recurrent tumor.**

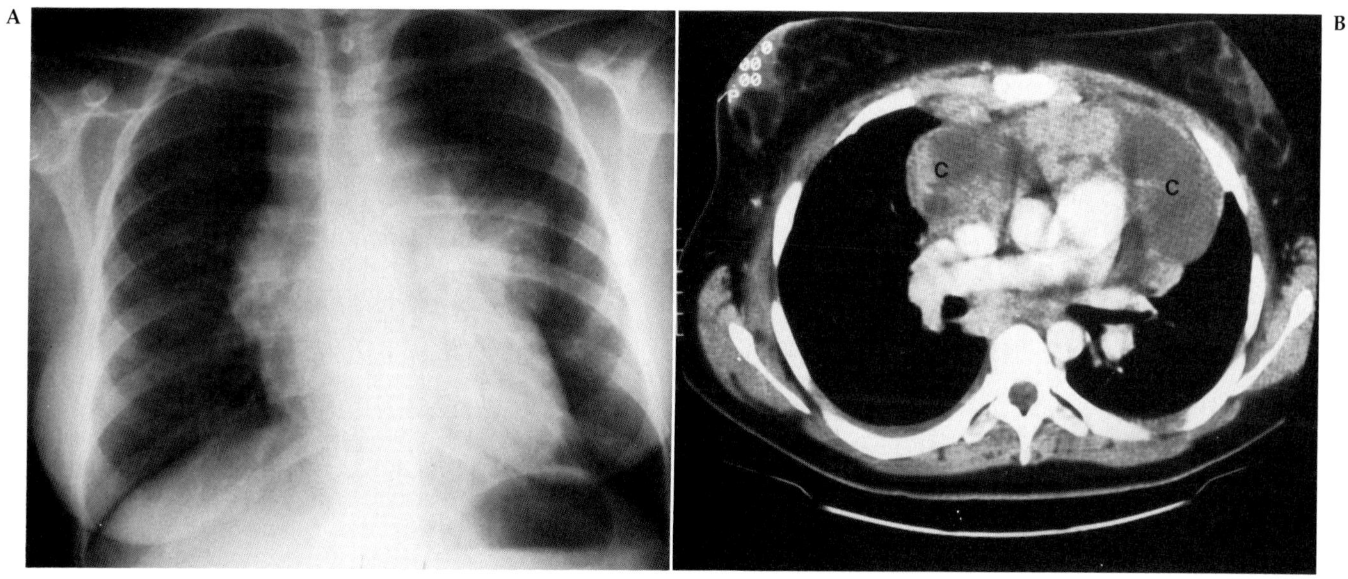

A B

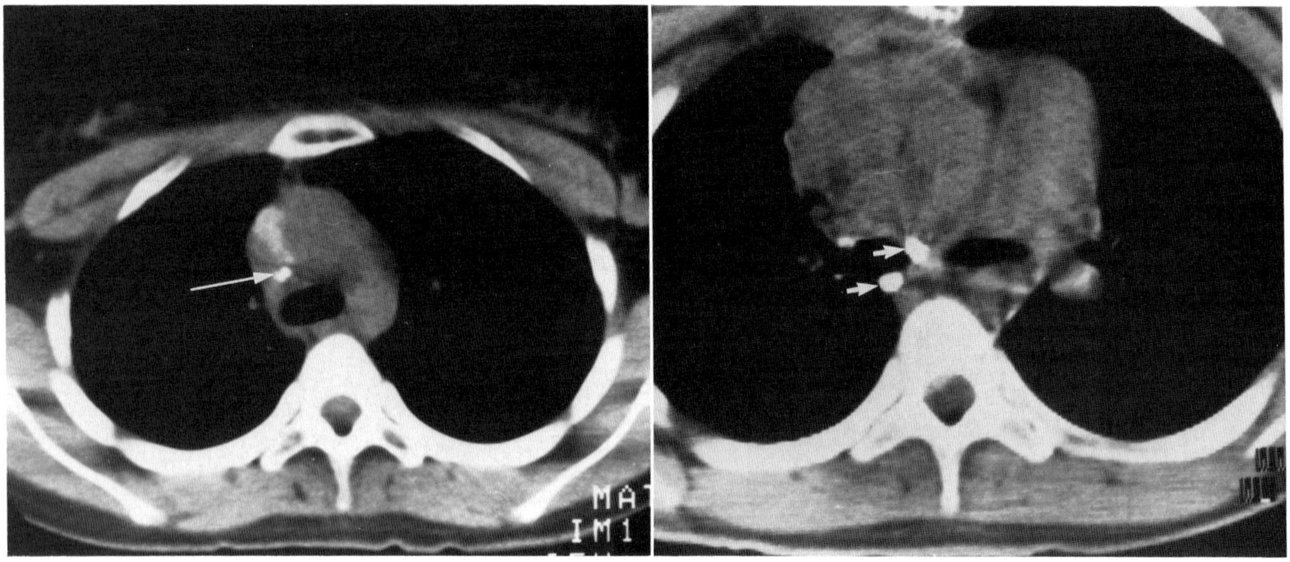

Figure 5-11. **Diagnosis: Hodgkin disease with calcification.**
A **and** ***B,*** **Extensive tumor is seen in the mediastinum, sternum, and adjacent soft tissues. Calcification** ***(arrows)*** **is noted in multiple lymph nodes. In this newly diagnosed patient, I believe that this is incidental preexisting calcification (e.g., from prior histoplasma infection) and not calcification in tumor. Because of calcification, tumor should not be excluded from the differential diagnosis. Tumor can develop in patients who have previously had mediastinal histoplasma infection.**

because of the presence of associated fibrosis, hemorrhage, edema, or necrosis[42,44] (see Fig. 5–13). In the absence of these secondary features, the tumor may be very difficult to identify, especially when diffuse. Ferrite has been used experimentally to attempt to identify splenic disease. Ferrite is normally taken up by macrophages in the spleen. It reduces signal intensity on T2 weighted images. In a few patients with severe disease, signal intensity from involved spleens was much higher than in normal controls. This was caused either by macrophage suppression by tumor or replacement of macrophages by tumor cells.[45]

Figure 5-12. **Diagnosis: B cell non-Hodgkin lymphoma in a child with prior leukemia and AIDS. Diffuse liver tumor infiltration.**
CT. There is enlargement of the liver. Widespread low-intensity liver parenchyma is the result of diffuse tumor infiltration. No focal masses are identified.

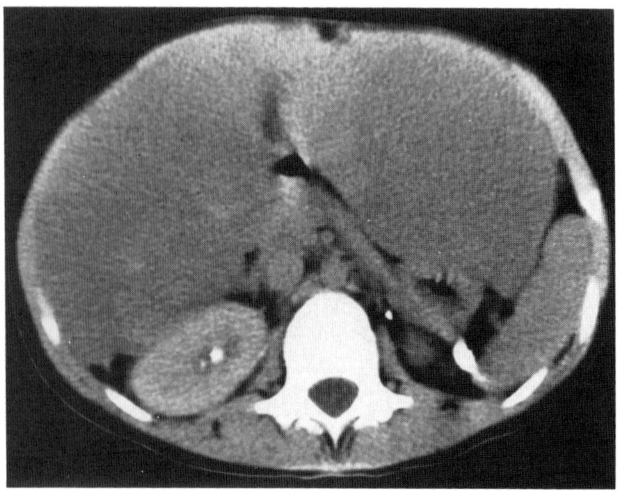

Bowel and Mesentery. Involvement of the bowel and mesentery is almost always caused by non-Hodgkin lymphoma and is extremely rare with Hodgkin disease. Imaging may identify some or all of the pathological findings of mucosal destruction, lumen narrowing, focal or nodular mass lesions, edema, and prominence of the valvulae, focal aneurysmal bowel dilatation, broad-based ulcers, intussusception (Fig. 5–15), omental or peritoneal seeding, ascites, bowel wall thickening, or, rarely, a rectal polyp[46–49] (Figs. 5–16 and 5–17). Barium studies may show displacement of bowel loops from mass lesions, mucosal ulceration, strictures, ulceration, or obstruction[47] (Fig. 5–17). On ultrasound studies, the serosa and mucosa are usually seen as lines of high echoes. A tumor in the bowel wall has very low echoes and is seen separating the high echo lines from the serosa and mucosa.[50] The echoes may be so diminished as to make the tumor mass appear anechoic.[51] A second rim of low echoes may be seen from fluid lying within the lumen of the bowel.[50]

Abdominal radiograph findings are nonspecific. The most common findings are displaced loops of bowel or obstruction.[52] CT requires excellent opacification of bowel loops with an oral contrast agent. In addition to identification of the tumor in the bowel wall, additional disease in abdominal lymph nodes, liver, or spleen may also be identified. Mass lesions may be large, particularly with Burkitt's lymphoma (see Fig. 5–15). With Burkitt's lymphoma the omentum may be involved. CT will show omental cakes lying between the bowel and the anterior abdominal wall, with loss of normal fat planes.[53] In many patients, the tumor will initially be

A B C

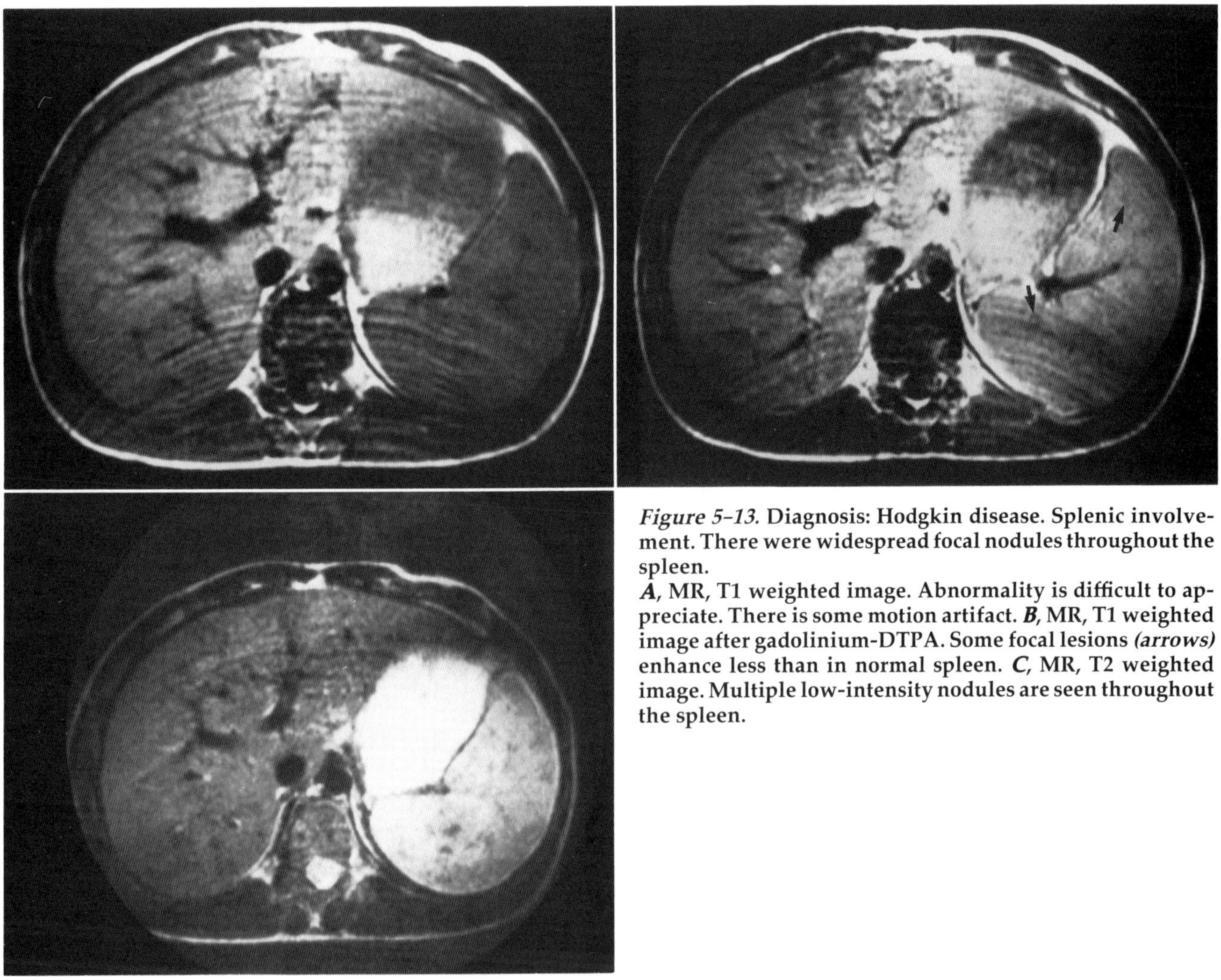

Figure 5-13. **Diagnosis: Hodgkin disease. Splenic involvement. There were widespread focal nodules throughout the spleen.**
***A*, MR, T1 weighted image. Abnormality is difficult to appreciate. There is some motion artifact. *B*, MR, T1 weighted image after gadolinium-DTPA. Some focal lesions *(arrows)* enhance less than in normal spleen. *C*, MR, T2 weighted image. Multiple low-intensity nodules are seen throughout the spleen.**

Figure 5-14. **Diagnosis: Burkitt's lymphoma. Focal liver tumor.**
CT after intravenous contrast. Multiple moderately well-defined low-intensity tumor nodules are identified *(arrows)*. The findings are nonspecific.

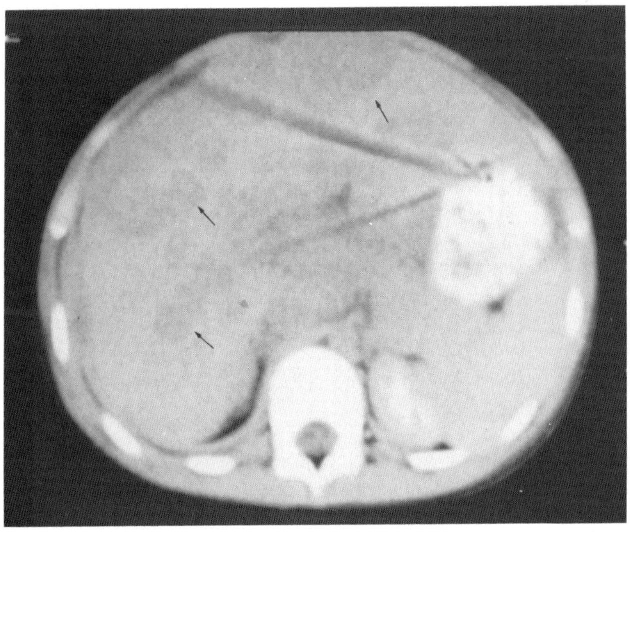

surgically resected. If not, CT is the best modality for evaluating treatment response. Reduction in size may occur dramatically with chemotherapy.[54]

Bowel involvement with Hodgkin disease is usually caused by direct invasion from adjacent involved lymph nodes. This occurred, for example, in one 9-year-old boy, causing ulceration in the lesser curve of the stomach.[55]

The differential diagnosis of bowel lymphoma includes other tumors, inflammation, Henoch Schonlein purpura, hemolytic uremic syndrome, and bowel edema with inflammation, such as Crohn's disease, histoplasmosis, giardia, and tuberculosis. The diagnosis of lymphoma is suggested by other clinical findings and in some cases identification of disease in other locations.[49]

Pancreas. The pancreas can occasionally be involved with non-Hodgkin lymphoma (Figs. 5–16 and 5–18).

Bone. Bone cortical involvement is present at diagnosis in up to 20 percent with non-Hodgkin lymphoma. It is very rare with Hodgkin disease, occurring in less than 1 percent of patients.[56] The incidence of bone cortical abnormality with lymphoma is not related to the presence or absence of disease in bone marrow. Cortical

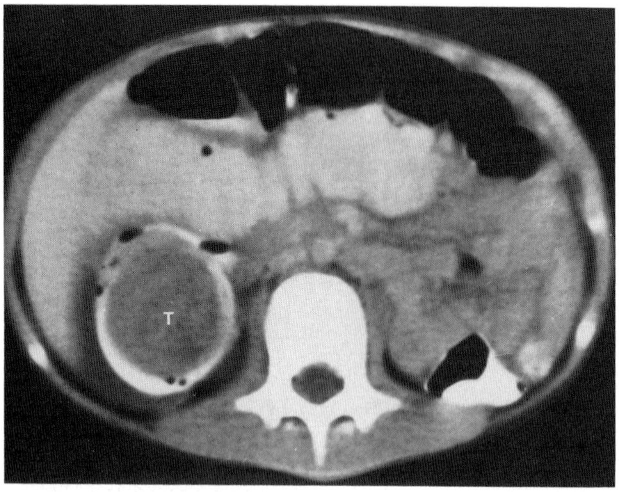

Figure 5-15. **Diagnosis: Non-Hodgkin lymphoma presenting with intussusception.**
CT. The intussuscepting tumor mass (*T*) is seen in the ascending colon. Orally administered contrast is seen as a white rim surrounding the tumor mass.

involvement may occasionally be the primary site of disease with non-Hodgkin lymphoma, with no abnormality detected in other organ systems.[56,57] Primary bone involvement usually affects one bone and only occasionally are there widespread lytic lesions in many bones.[58] Bone involvement as part of widespread non-Hodgkin lymphoma is most likely to affect multiple bones.[59,60] Distribution of disease is predominantly axial with non-Hodgkin lymphoma (75 to 80 percent of lesions)[56,60,61] and variable with Hodgkin disease, with about half of the lesions being axial.[60] For detection of bone cortical abnormality MDP technetium 99m bone scan is the most sensitive imaging modality, followed by gallium scanning and skeletal survey.[52,60,61] Symptoms from bone lymphoma are described as being present seldom[60] or often.[56] The most common symptom is pain.[62]

The appearance of bone lesions with lymphoma is very varied and lymphoma may mimic almost any bone disease.[63] The lesions are most likely to be lytic[62] (Fig. 5-19), but can be sclerotic.[64] There is a marked variation.

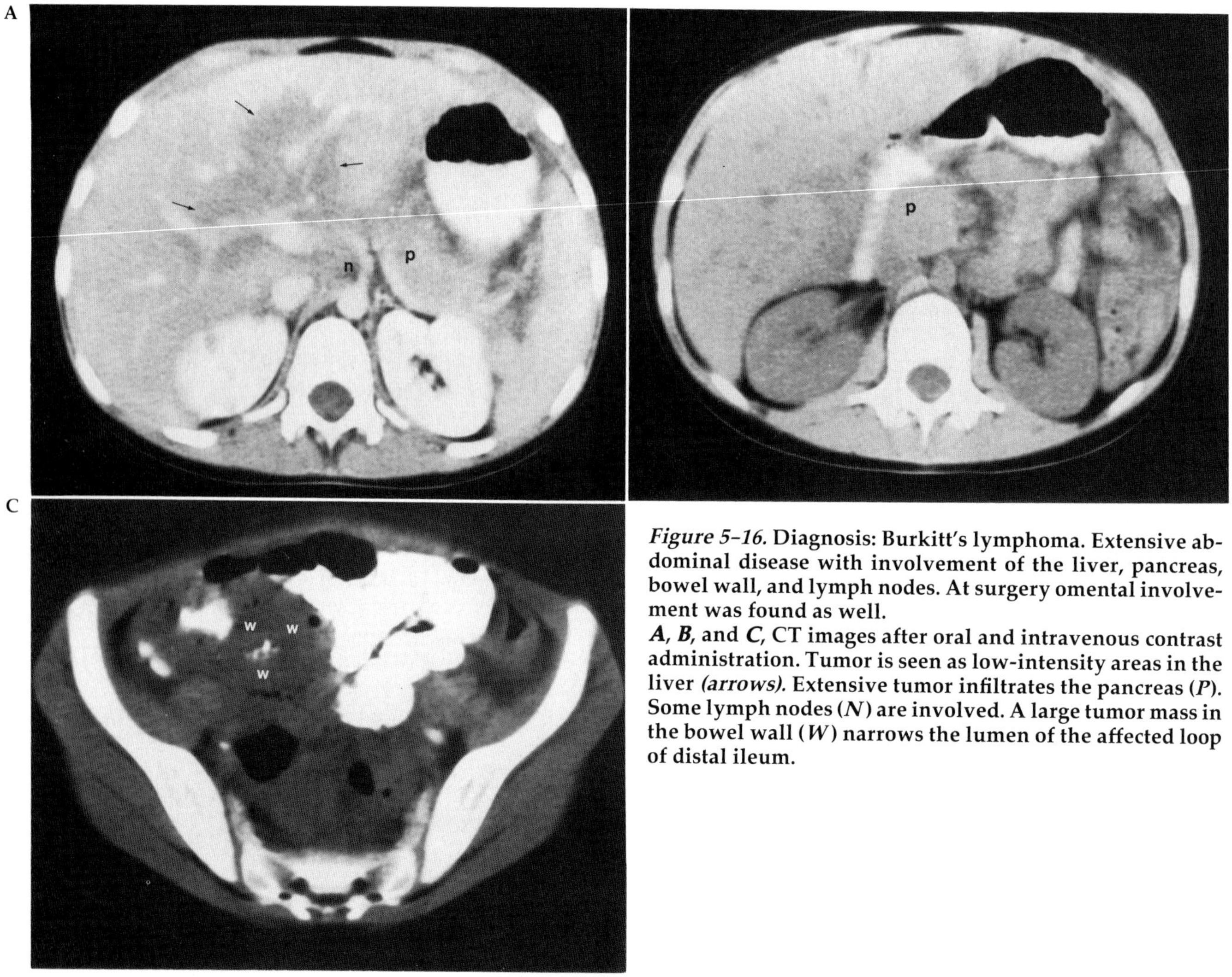

Figure 5-16. **Diagnosis: Burkitt's lymphoma. Extensive abdominal disease with involvement of the liver, pancreas, bowel wall, and lymph nodes. At surgery omental involvement was found as well.**
***A, B,* and *C,* CT images after oral and intravenous contrast administration. Tumor is seen as low-intensity areas in the liver *(arrows).* Extensive tumor infiltrates the pancreas (*P*). Some lymph nodes (*N*) are involved. A large tumor mass in the bowel wall (*W*) narrows the lumen of the affected loop of distal ileum.**

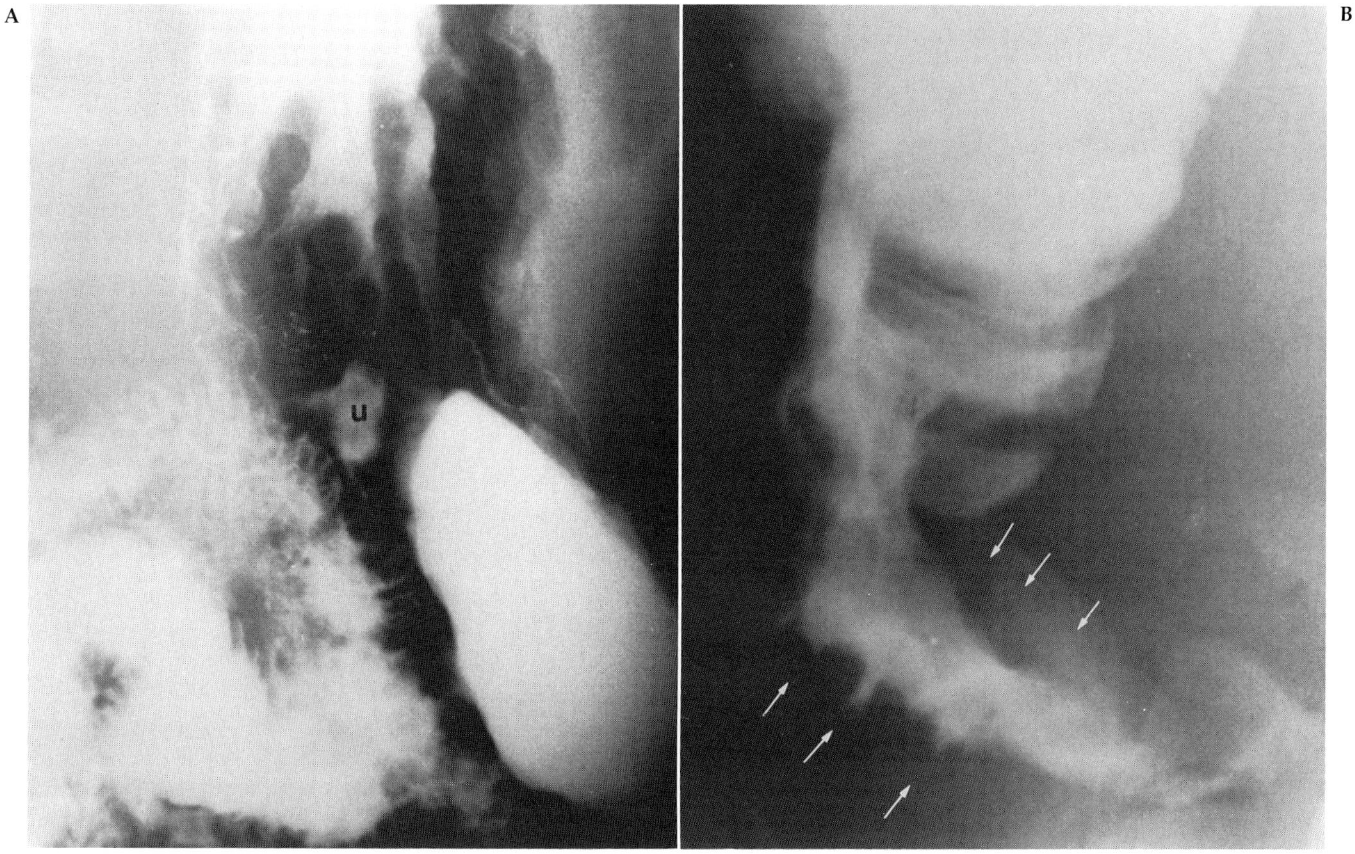

Figure 5-17. **Diagnosis: Multifocal bowel Burkitt's lymphoma.**
***A*, Barium study. Stomach. There is diffuse thickening of mucosal folds. A large tumor ulcer (*U*) is identified. *B*, Barium study. Terminal ileum. The bowel is markedly narrowed and ulcerated as a result of extensive tumor in the wall *(arrows)*.**

The appearance in one series was lytic (12), blastic (5), and mixed (6),[63] and in another series permeative (18), and mixed sclerotic (8).[61] Lytic areas may be well defined or permeative[65] (Fig. 5-20). Pathologic fractures can occur (Figs. 5-20 and 5-21). With healing, increased sclerosis is seen in the lesion. Soft-tissue involvement may occur,[62] being described in 10 of 23 patients.[63] Periosteal reaction is varied but is more likely to be present when there is soft-tissue involvement.[63] In Hodgkin disease, bone involvement can be the result of direct invasion from adjacent soft-tissue tumor (Figs. 5-22 and 5-23).

Bone Marrow. Bone marrow involvement is common with non-Hodgkin lymphoma. Traditionally, iliac bone marrow biopsy has been utilized to detect bone marrow disease. This study gives false negative results. For example, it is known that performing bilateral iliac biopsies will increase the yield by between 10 and 40 percent.[66] It is not surprising that focal sampling of bone marrow will give false negative results. One study attempted to correlate iliac biopsy with sulfur colloid marrow scan and MR of the pelvis and femurs in 107 patients with leukemia and lymphoma.[66,67] MR is sensitive for detection of abnormality, but very nonspecific[68,69] (Fig. 5-24). In the study,[66] imaging could miss pathol-

Figure 5-18. **Diagnosis: Burkitt's lymphoma. Pancreatic involvement.**
The pancreas (*P*) is markedly enlarged with a lobulated contour. The entire gland is affected. (Note: kidneys are also involved.)

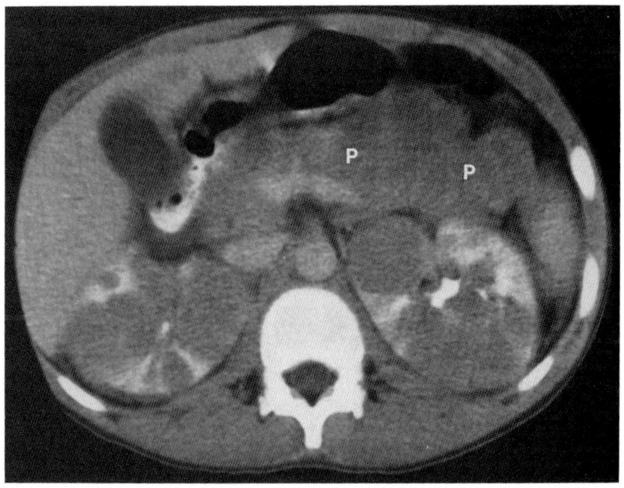

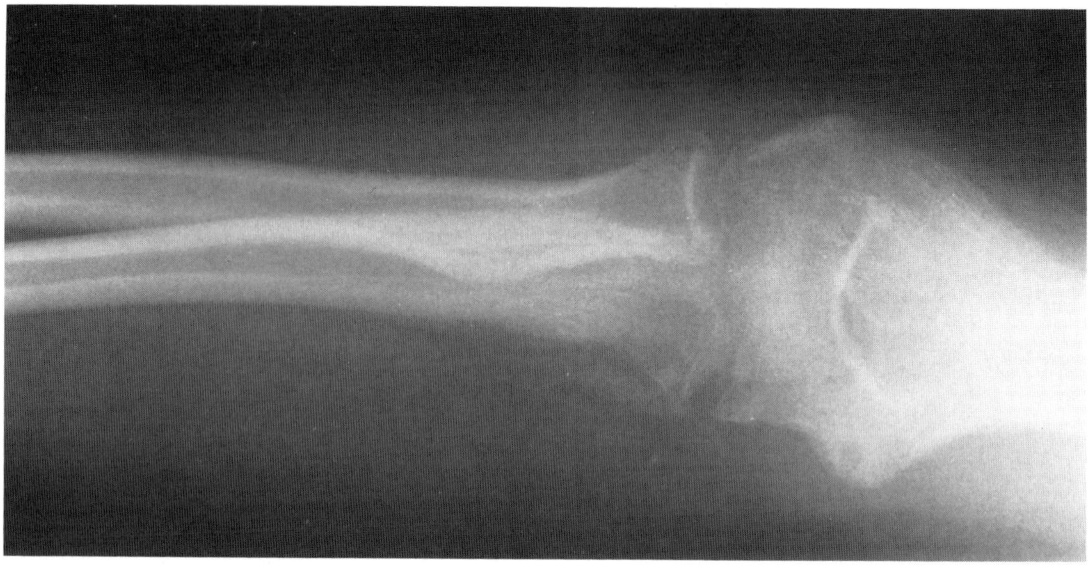

Figure 5-19. **Diagnosis: Non-Hodgkin lymphoma of bone. Immunoblastic type. This was the only site of detected disease. The patient presented with pain.**
Radiograph of elbow. There is a lesion in the proximal ulna. It is predominantly lytic with cortical destruction.

ogy when the biopsy was positive and the biopsy could be negative when imaging studies were positive. The results suggest that imaging may have a useful role to play in detection of marrow abnormality, but one difficulty with the study was that there was no standard by which to determine the final result. This is particularly true in patients in whom imaging was positive but iliac marrow biopsy was negative.

Central Nervous System. This can be involved with lymphoma (Figs. 5–25, 5–26, and 5–27). In one study in adults, lesions were described as being multiple in 38 percent and being isointense or hyperintense prior to contrast and showing homogenous enhancement following intravenous contrast.[36] In another patient, MR was excellent for identifying early cord compression from lymphoma.[70]

Figure 5-20. **Diagnosis: Non-Hodgkin lymphoma. Small-cell histology. Primary spine tumor.**
***A,* Lateral neck radiograph. The fifth cervical vertebra is abnormal. There is extensive patchy destruction with loss of vertebral height. The superior/anterior cortical margin is almost completely destroyed.**
B,* CT at the same level. Extensive mottled destruction of the vertebral body is seen *(arrow).

A

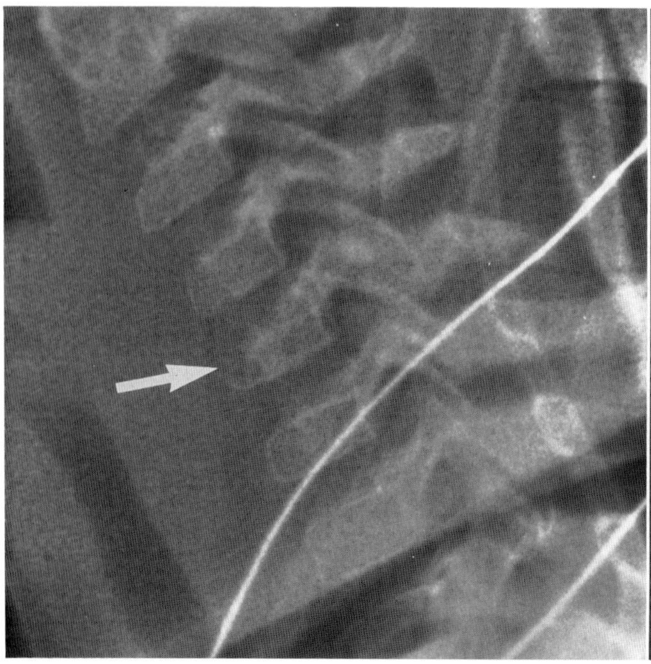

B

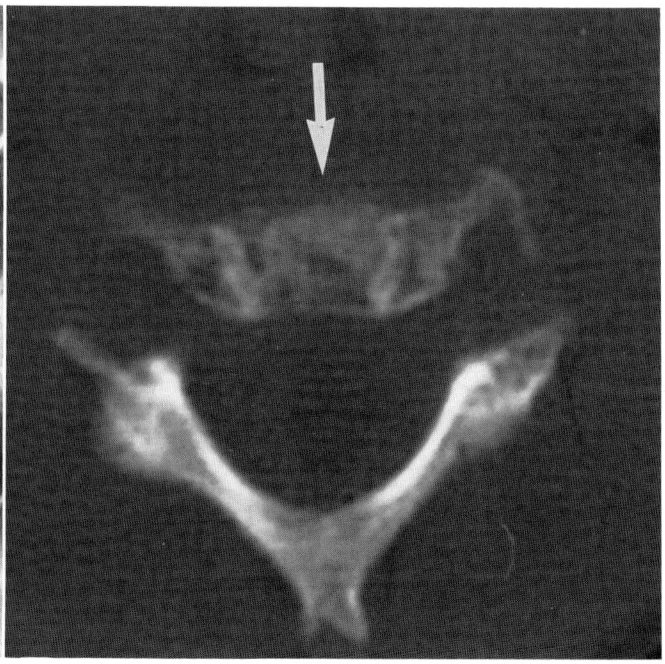

A B C

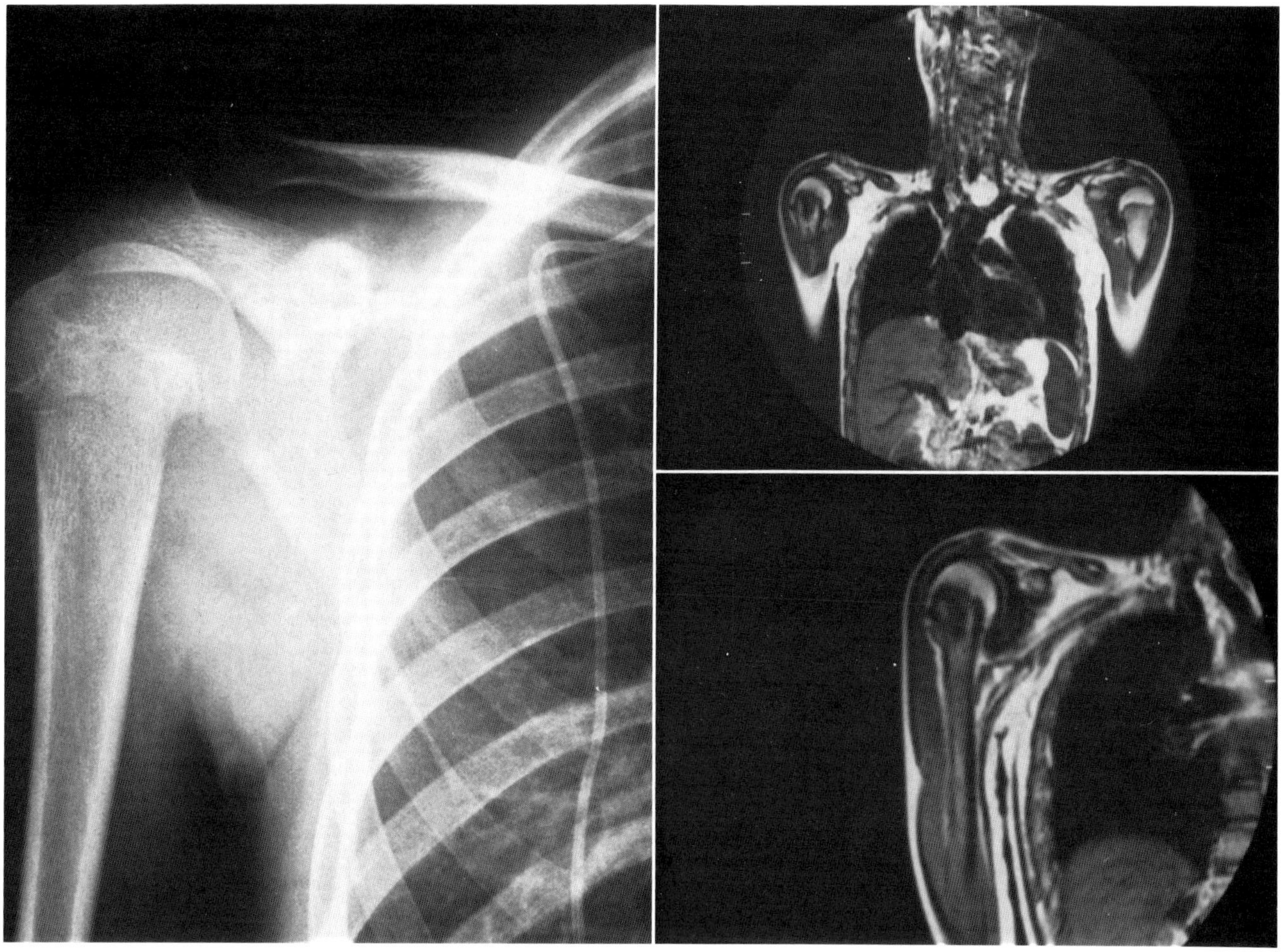

Figure 5-21. Diagnosis: Burkitt's lymphoma. Pathological fracture through proximal humerus. ***A***, ***B***, and ***C***, Plain film radiograph, T1 weighted and spin density MR images. All images show the pathological fracture through the proximal humerus. Image ***C*** shows patchy low signal through most of the marrow of the visualized humerus probably representing tumor extension but possibly caused by edema from the fracture.

Figure 5-22. Diagnosis: Hodgkin disease. Bone involvement from direct tumor invasion.
CT. There is mediastinal disease. The tumor extends into the soft tissues of the anterior chest wall and invades the sternum. The sternum is expanded and shows mottled diffuse destruction.

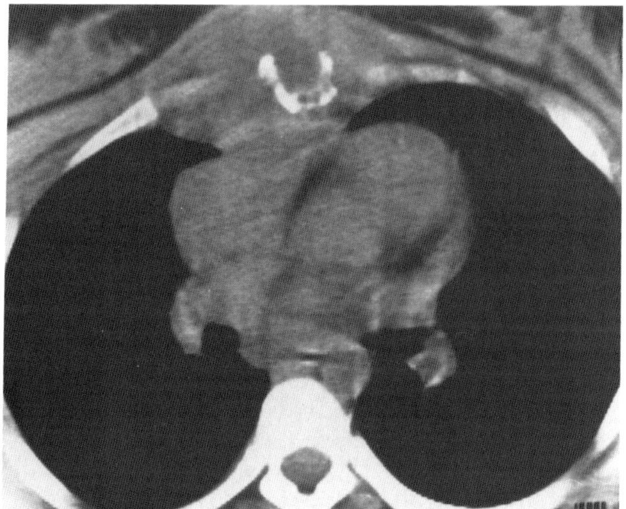

Figure 5-23. Diagnosis: Hodgkin disease. Bone involvement caused by direct invasion by tumor.
There is extensive tumor of the anterior mediastinum and adjacent soft tissues of the chest wall. The tumor has invaded an adjacent rib *(arrow)* causing destruction and a periosteal reaction. Note also the pleural effusions.

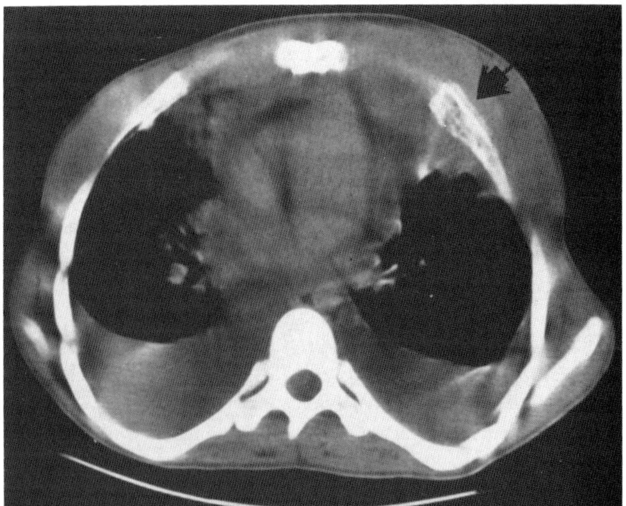

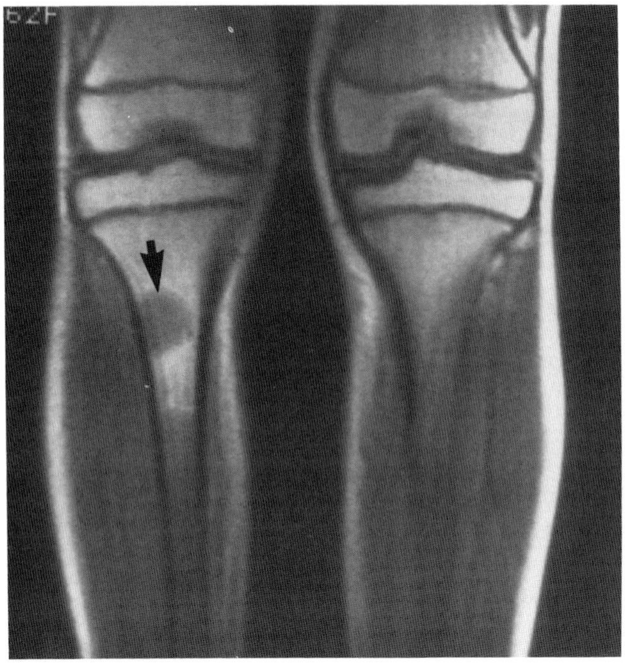

Figure 5-24. **Diagnosis: Burkitt's lymphoma. MR findings. The child presented with bone pain.**
Coronal spin density MR image. There is a well-defined focal low-intensity metastatic lesion *(arrow)* in the proximal metaphysis of the right tibia. MR is very sensitive for detection of this disease but the appearance is relatively nonspecific.

Genitourinary System. Involvement is extremely rare with Hodgkin disease but not uncommon with non-Hodgkin lymphoma. In the kidneys, one may identify hydronephrosis caused by secondary urinary obstruction from enlarged lymph nodes, a persistent nephrogram and poor renal function from urate nephropathy, or direct involvement with tumor.[71] Tumor involvement may cause diffuse uniform nephromegaly, which may be bilateral or unilateral. Single or multiple focal mass lesions may also be identified.[54,71–75] With diffuse renal involvement, all modalities show the enlarged kidney (Fig. 5–28). On IVP or CT, the collecting system is seen to be stretched. Lymphoma lesions in the kidney are usually of low echogenicity on ultrasound[71,74] (Figs. 5–29 and 5–30), but increased echoes can be seen.[74] Ultrasound may not be as good as other modalities for showing lesions (Fig. 5–28). CT scanning of focal lesions identifies masses that are usually well defined (Fig. 5–30). Enhancement of the lesion is usually less than normal kidney[73] (Fig. 5–30). In one patient, a dense contrast rim around the mass was seen on a delayed CT scan at 12 hours. This was believed to be caused by urine stasis in tubules surrounding the tumor.[73] While most lymphoma focal masses are well defined, they have been described as being poorly defined.[71] Renal function, even with diffuse extensive infiltration with non-Hodgkin lymphoma, is usually well preserved in the absence of obstruction or urate nephropathy. The appearance of renal involvement is nonspecific. The differential diagnosis of diffuse renal abnormalities includes leukemia and congenital abnormalities (duplex, cystic kidney). Differential diagnosis of focal lesions include all inflammatory, congenital, and tumor masses of the kidney.

Testicular involvement with lymphoma can also occur[76] and this can involve the testis or spermatic cord[76,77] (Fig. 5–31). On ultrasound, the echoes of the affected testis or cord are low.[73,77] There is usually associated disease present elsewhere in the body.

Lung. Lung involvement can occur in lymphoma. It is more common with Hodgkin disease[78,79] (Fig. 5–32). There is usually involvement of hilar nodes, although very rarely has primary lung Hodgkin disease been described.[79] The lung may be involved by contiguous invasion from adjacent lymph nodes.[78] Lung abnormality may be seen as single or multiple nodules, a reticular nodular infiltrate, or an area of consolidation.[79] Cavitation may occasionally occur.[33,78,79] In patients with follow-up for Hodgkin disease, biopsy of a new lung lesion may be helpful.

Abdominal Lymph Nodes. The detection of lymphoma in abdominal lymph nodes is especially important in Hodgkin disease. While lymph node involvement can commonly occur in non-Hodgkin lymphoma, the detection of subtle disease is not as important as in Hodgkin disease, where it is crucial for staging. On imaging, Hodgkin disease and non-Hodgkin lymphoma cannot be differentiated from each other.

On ultrasound, the diagnosis of abnormality is made by demonstration of enlarged lymph nodes almost invariably with fairly characteristic, very low echoes. On CT scan, diagnosis is made by demonstration of enlarged lymph nodes (Figs. 5–33 and 5–34). Precise definition of lymph node enlargement is not possible, but in general, in children, tumor should not be diagnosed or suspected in lymph nodes under about 1 cm in diameter. If nodes larger than this are identified, tumor should be suspected. The appearance is, however, nonspecific, and enlargement from inflammation or infection cannot be differentiated from lymphoma. As previously discussed, the reported accuracy of lymphangiography is very variable, being reported as low as 70 percent.[80] It is believed that more false positive results occur in children[81] than adults.

With regard to Hodgkin disease in the abdomen, there is uniform agreement that laparotomy is more sensitive than any imaging modality for detection of lymph node disease. Unfortunately, surgery has always been taken as the standard, and while surgery *and* histology should not yield false positive results, the false negative information provided by surgery is completely unknown. It may be higher than is generally recognized, bearing in mind that the surgeon may have difficulty in visualizing all abdominal lymph nodes and that the surgeon cannot differentiate affected from nonaffected lymph nodes. It is quite possible that surgery will miss tumor, particularly in lymph nodes that are not enlarged. There is some disagreement about the relative frequency of sites of positive abdominal lymph nodes in Hodgkin disease. Positive nodes are common in all retroperitoneal sites,[82] but are very unusual in the mesen-

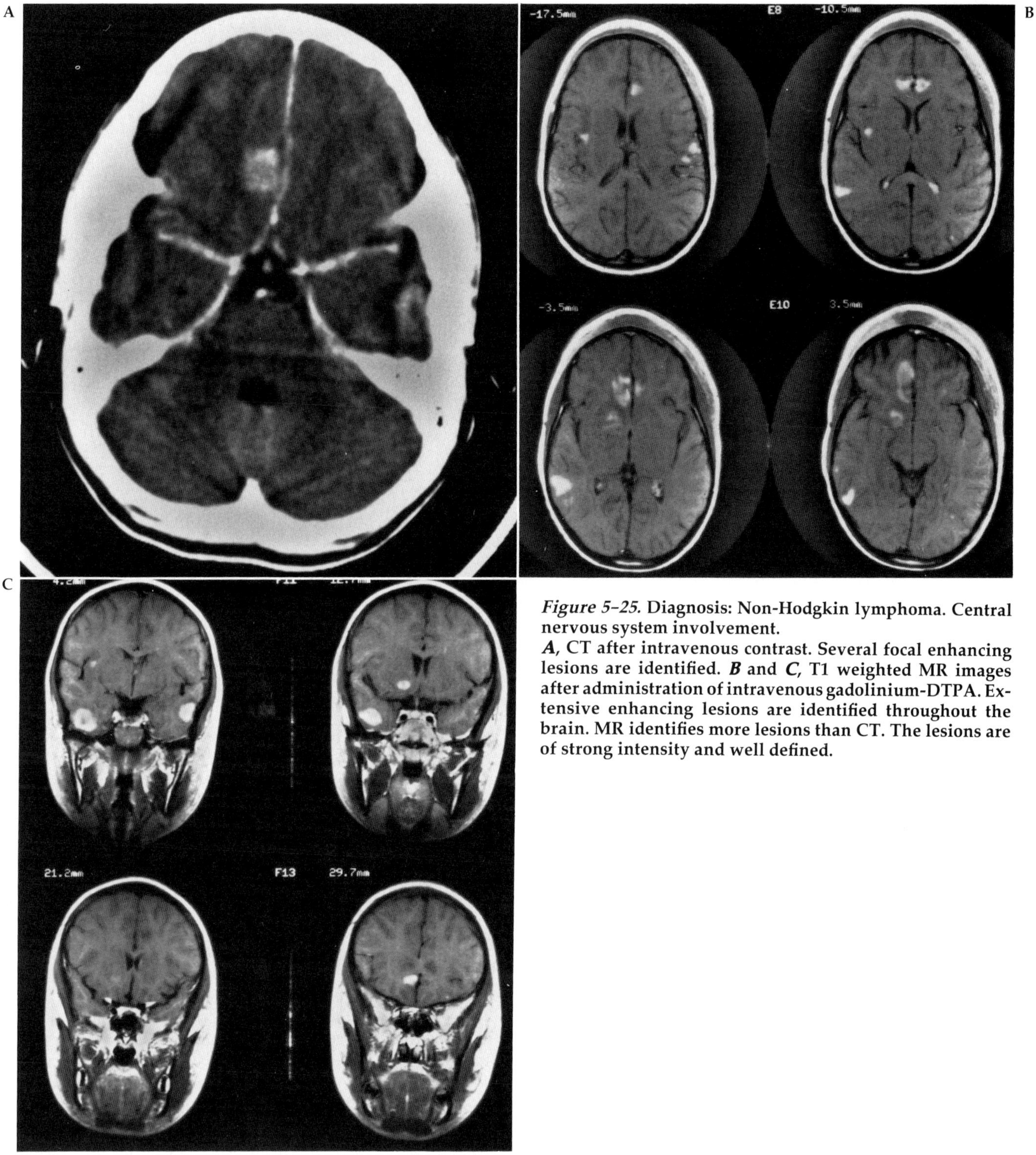

Figure 5–25. **Diagnosis: Non-Hodgkin lymphoma. Central nervous system involvement.**
***A*, CT after intravenous contrast. Several focal enhancing lesions are identified. *B* and *C*, T1 weighted MR images after administration of intravenous gadolinium-DTPA. Extensive enhancing lesions are identified throughout the brain. MR identifies more lesions than CT. The lesions are of strong intensity and well defined.**

teric lymph nodes. In one study, the splenic hilar nodes were reported as being the most common site, being positive in 10 of 16 children,[36] while in another study, the celiac group of nodes were reported as being the most common, followed by splenic, hilar, and periaortic nodes.[84] Even though imaging cannot identify all disease, its role is important, particularly with the reduction in the number of staging laparotomies performed in recent years. (This is discussed in more detail later.)

Head and Neck. Hodgkin disease in the neck is common. It involves the cervical lymph nodes (Figs. 5–35 and 5–36). Non-Hodgkin lymphoma can also occur in cervical lymph nodes, but is common in other sites in the head and neck as well, including salivary glands and

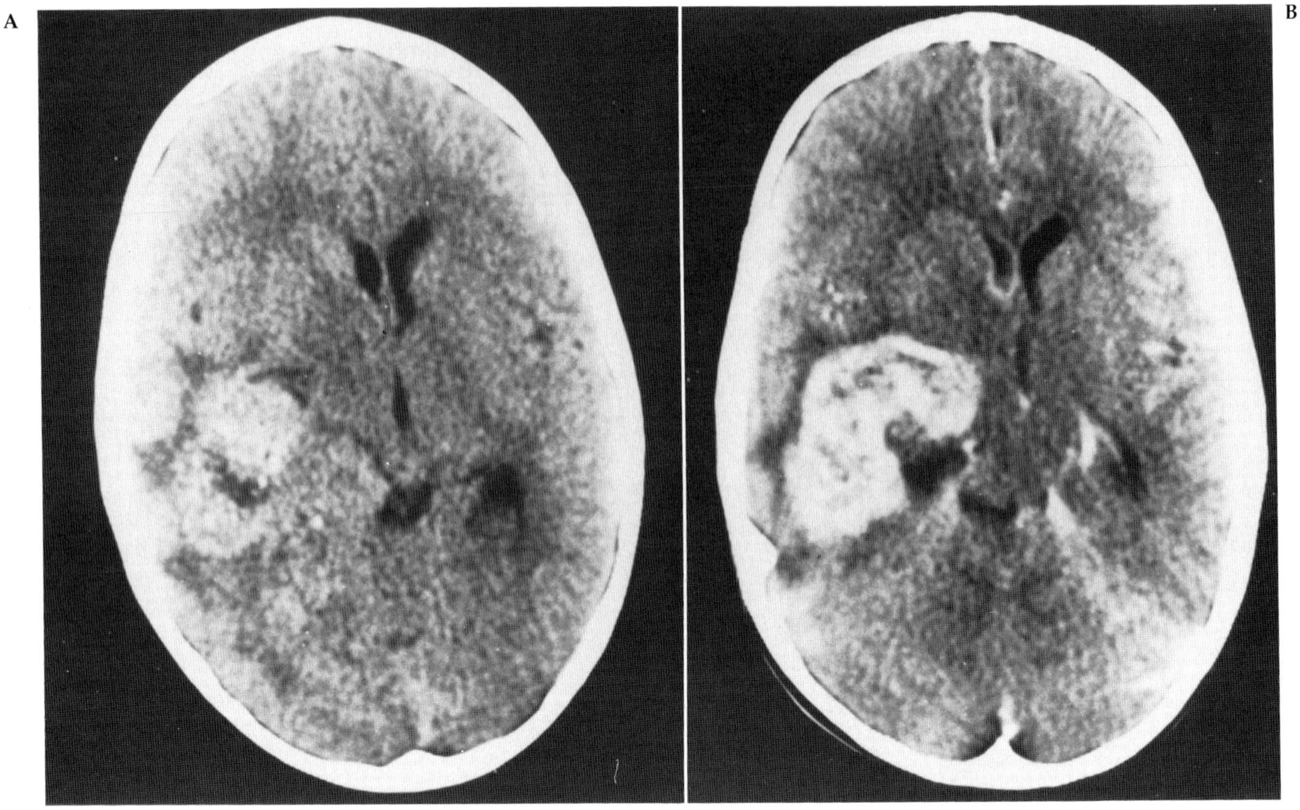

Figure 5-26. Diagnosis: Small cell lymphoma with central nervous system involvement. ***A***, CT without contrast. There is a right parietotemporal mass lesion with calcification, some surrounding edema, and mass effect with displacement of the midline structures to the opposite side. ***B***, CT after intravenous contrast. There is extensive enhancement of the tumor mass. (From Egelhoff JC, Beatty EC. Primary B cell lymphoma of the CNS in an infant. Pediatr Radiol 1989;19:204–205.)

Figure 5-27. Diagnosis: B cell non-Hodgkin lymphoma. Central nervous system involvement. This patient had received a prior bone marrow transplantation.
T2 weighted MR image. Extensive tumor abnormality is seen in the brain. (From Day D. B cell lymphoproliferative disorders in children. Radiology 1987;162:807–810.)

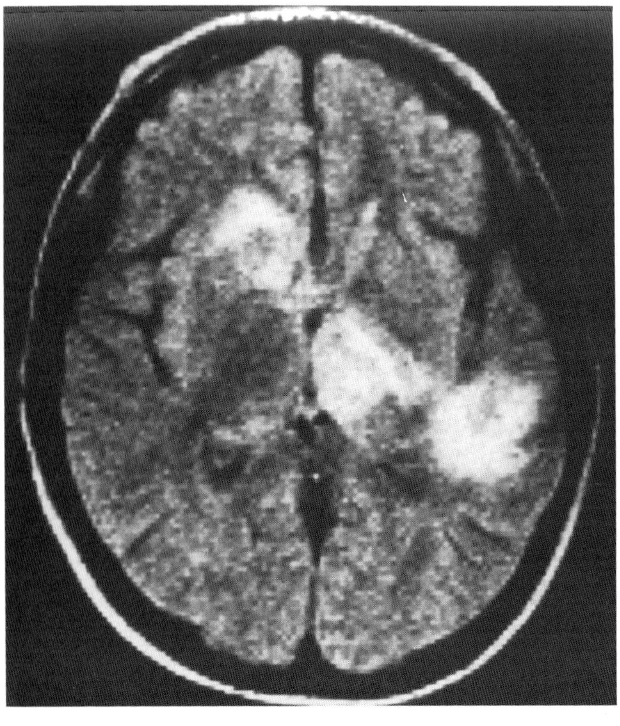

non-nodal lymphatic tissue such as tonsil and adenoids[85] (Fig. 5–37). Non-Hodgkin lymphoma is also common in the nose, orbit, and sinuses and, in these locations, is frequently infiltrating, causing bone destruction[85] (Fig. 5–38). CT and MR are the most useful tests for defining the extent of disease in these locations. Often, however, particularly in the tonsils and adenoids, the tumor is discovered as an incidental finding following surgery, before imaging has been performed.

SPECIAL IMAGING PROBLEMS

Residual Mass after Therapy. With the development of more effective chemotherapy and radiation therapy for lymphoma, a perplexing problem is finding a residual soft-tissue mass in the location of a pretreatment larger region of tumor. The differential diagnosis lies between residual tumor that is active and a fibrotic lesion not containing tumor. The finding of a residual mass is important, because in a large study of patients with Hodgkin disease, relapse was found to be twice as common in patients with a residual mass at the end of treatment compared to those patients without any residual soft-tissue mass.[86] Donaldson (1990), however, does not believe that residual mediastinal widening indicates persistent active disease or an increased risk of relapse.[1]

I am not certain that one should accept this statement. Residual mediastinal widening, in 10 of 72 patients, was associated with an increased relapse rate

A

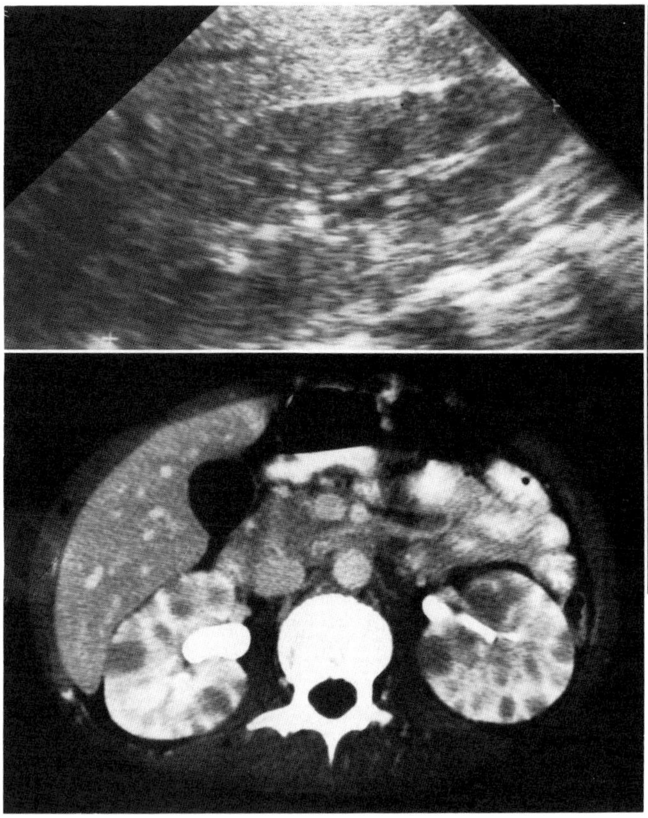

B

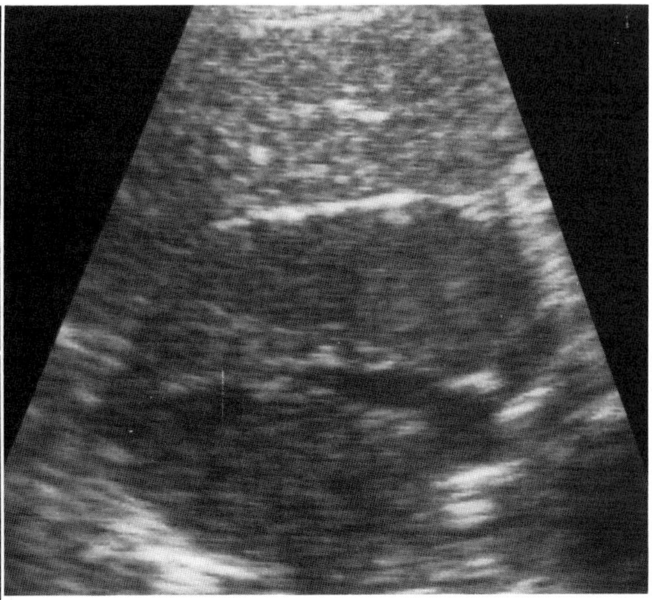

C

Figure 5-28. **Diagnosis: Non-Hodgkin lymphoma. Renal involvement.**
***A* and *B*, Longitudinal and transverse ultrasound. The kidney is enlarged. Internal echo pattern is abnormal, with loss of corticomedullary differentiation. Discrete nodules of tumor are not clearly defined. *C*, CT after intravenous contrast obtained on the same day. The kidneys are diffusely enlarged. Widespread focal nodules of lower intensity than normal kidney are fairly sharply defined. (From Weinberger E. Renal involvement in children with lymphoma: comparison of CT with sonography. AJR 1990;155:347–349.)**

compared to patients with no residual, even when this residual mass was initially stable.[30]

The three options after detection of a residual mass are to perform immediate biopsy, to wait and observe the behavior of the mass with time, or to attempt to utilize imaging to differentiate benign from malignant tissue. While surgery is definitive, it is obviously desirable to avoid this if possible. Imaging has not proved very effective in differentiating benign from malignant tissue, and in the absence of surgery, the best method of making this distinction is by repeating studies over a period of several months. Stability with time is the best method for excluding tumor.[5] The yield from surgery may be low. In 41 patients with Hodgkin disease, a residual mass after initial therapy was identified in 20. Surgery revealed active tumor in only 6 of these 20 patients.[87] In other series, laparotomy identified no tumor in 4 children with residual masses,[88] and thoracotomy no tumor in 3 children with residual masses.[89] In the mediastinum, residual masses may be caused by thymic cysts.

CT, ultrasound, or MR might be helpful in identifying fluid in the cysts, indicating the correct diagnosis. Theoretically, MR should be helpful in differentiating tumor from fibrosis. Fibrotic tissue should be of low signal intensity on T1 and T2 weighted images, whereas tumor should show increase in signal intensity on T2 weighted images. This simplistic statement, however, cannot always hold true. Tiny foci of tumor within a large mass of fibrotic tissue may be missed. In addition, strong signal intensity on T2 weighted images is not

Figure 5-29. **Diagnosis: Non-Hodgkin lymphoma. Renal involvement.**
Ultrasound. In this patient, the tumor appears of well-defined focal low echogenicity nodules *(arrows)*. (From Patel PJ. Renal sonography in childhood lymphoma. Urologic Inv 1990;45:34–37.)

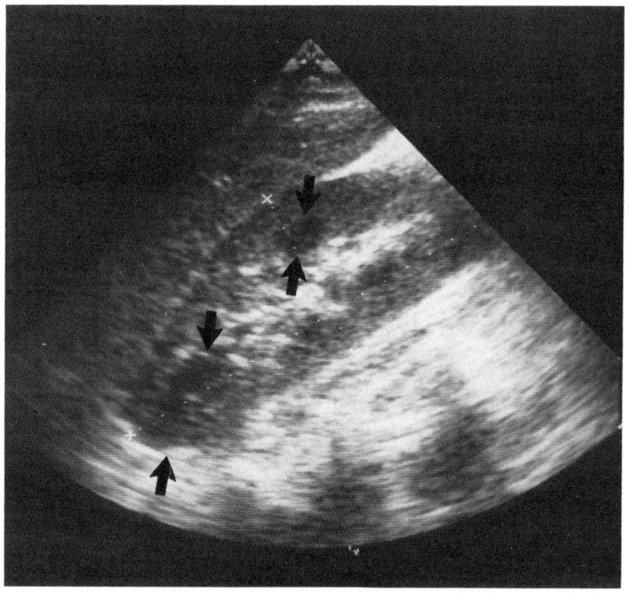

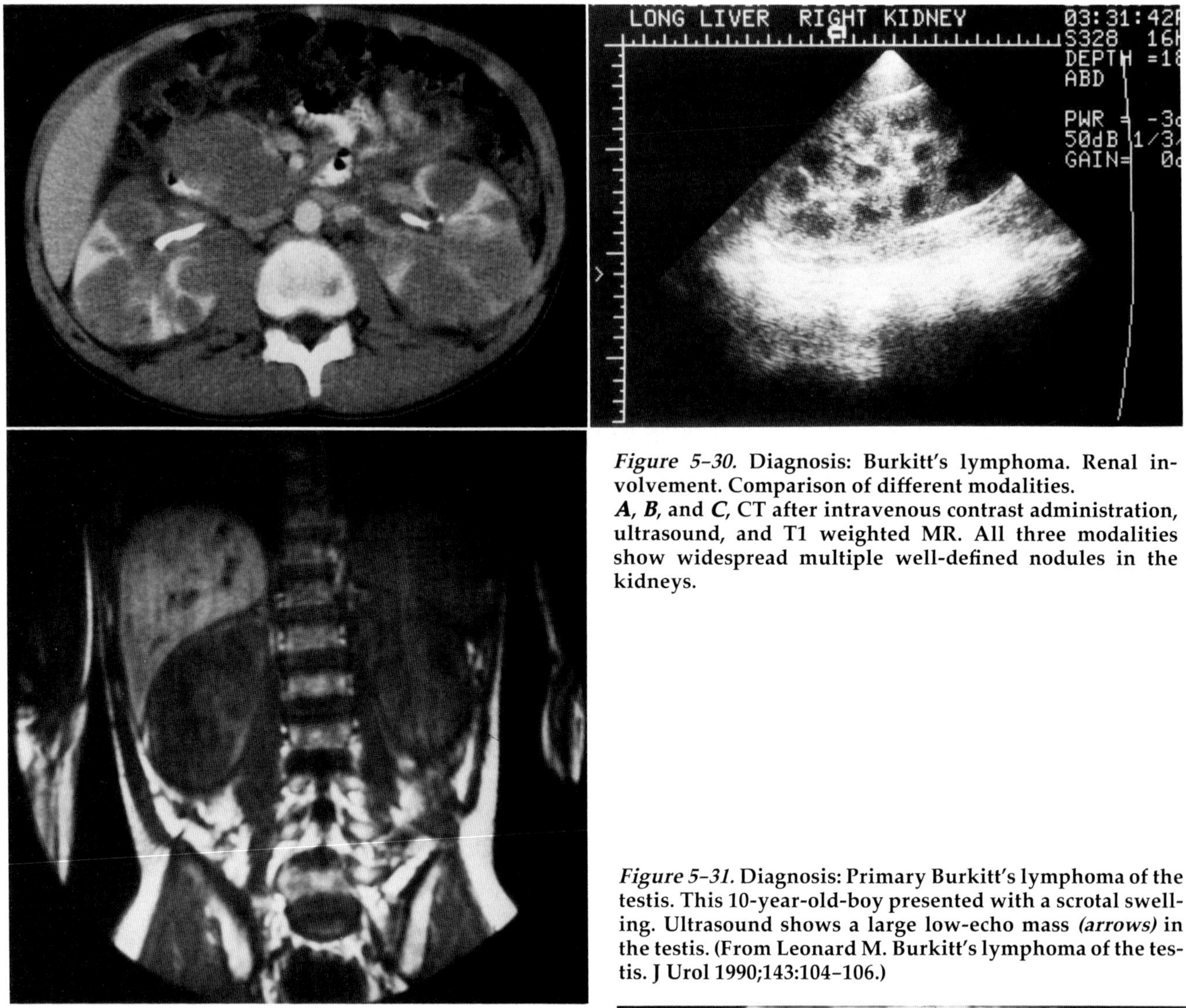

Figure 5–30. **Diagnosis: Burkitt's lymphoma. Renal involvement. Comparison of different modalities.**
***A, B,* and *C,* CT after intravenous contrast administration, ultrasound, and T1 weighted MR. All three modalities show widespread multiple well-defined nodules in the kidneys.**

Figure 5–31. **Diagnosis: Primary Burkitt's lymphoma of the testis. This 10-year-old-boy presented with a scrotal swelling. Ultrasound shows a large low-echo mass *(arrows)* in the testis. (From Leonard M. Burkitt's lymphoma of the testis. J Urol 1990;143:104–106.)**

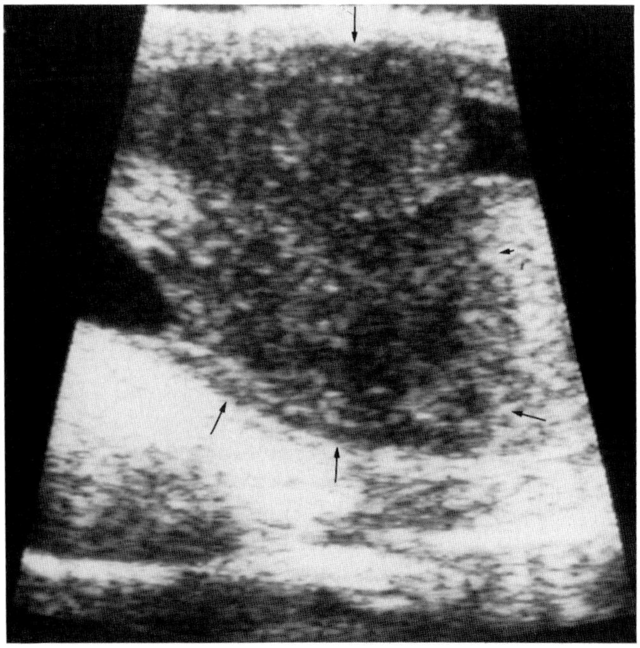

specific for tumor and can be found with inflammation or infection. One MR study suggests that fibrous residual tissue seen after chemotherapy was in fact present as a fibrous component of the primary tumor, persisting with resolution of the more cellular part of the tumor.[31] This study suggested that these tumors, prior to therapy, have less intense signal on T2 weighted images than more homogeneously cellular tumors and that the likelihood of fibrotic residual can be predicted from the pretherapy MR images.[31] Another study suggests that in a residual mass of low signal intensity on T2 weighted images, a change with follow-up from low to high signal intensity on T2 weighted images should be a definite indication for biopsy.[90] It has been suggested that gadolinium-DTPA may prove to be helpful in differentiating tumor from fibrosis.[10] Bear in mind that inflammation can cause false positive results[89] and that gadolinium-DTPA will miss a few tumor cells in a predominantly fibrotic mass. My own recommendation is to take a somewhat conservative approach to the pres-

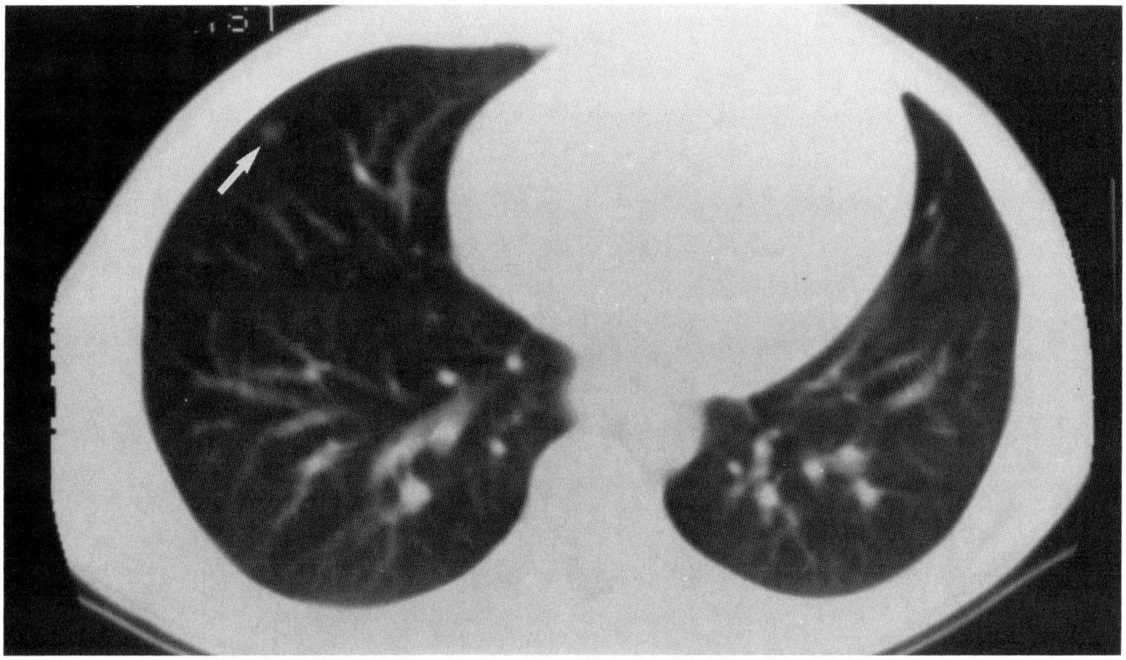

Figure 5-32. Diagnosis: Nodular sclerosing Hodgkin disease. Lung involvement. CT. A focal area of involvement is seen in the middle lobe *(arrow).*

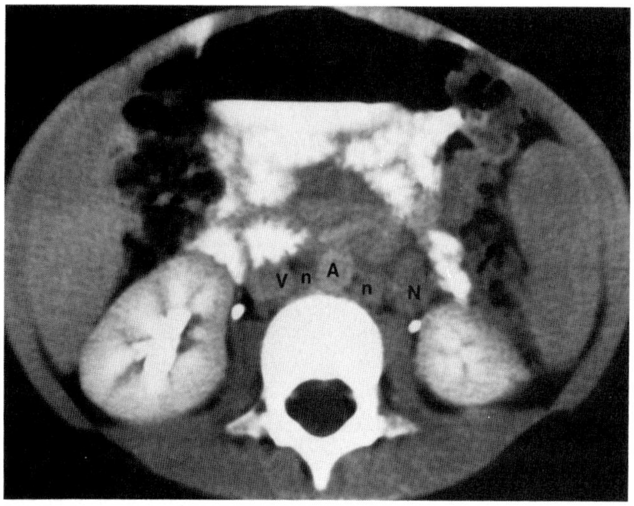

Figure 5-33. Diagnosis: Hodgkin disease. Retroperitoneal lymphadenopathy.
Multiple enlarged lymph nodes (*N*) are identified. *A* = aorta; *V* = vena cava.

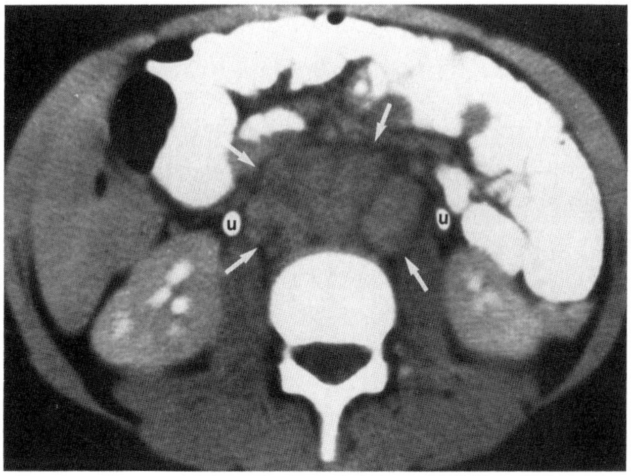

Figure 5-34. Diagnosis: Nodular sclerosing Hodgkin disease. Retroperitoneal lymph node enlargement.
CT after intravenous contrast. A mass of retroperitoneal nodes *(arrows)* is identified. A bolus of contrast has passed so that it is not possible to differentiate vessels from nodes. Both ureters (*U*) are displaced anterolaterally. They are not obstructed.

ence of residual soft-tissue masses, utilizing the presence or absence of change with time as the major guide for intervention and biopsy.

In addition to residual tumor masses, new abnormalities developing in patients after initial remission must also be evaluated. In one large series of 197 children with Hodgkin disease, relapse occurred in 94.[91] Relapse can occur at any site. When it occurs in the mediastinum, it must be differentiated from rebound hyperplasia of the thymus. MR imaging in the coronal plane may be particularly helpful in differentiating normal thymus from recurrent tumor.

All patients with new abnormality or residual abnormality must be carefully followed because of the increased risk of tumor being present.

STAGING LAPAROTOMY

This procedure is now fairly rapidly passing out of favor. The indications for performing a staging laparotomy in Hodgkin disease are outlined in Table 5-17. Laparotomy will detect disease not identifiable by im-

A

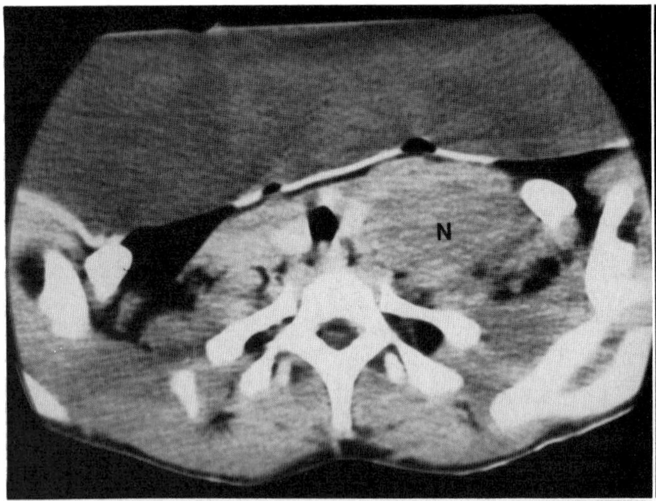

B

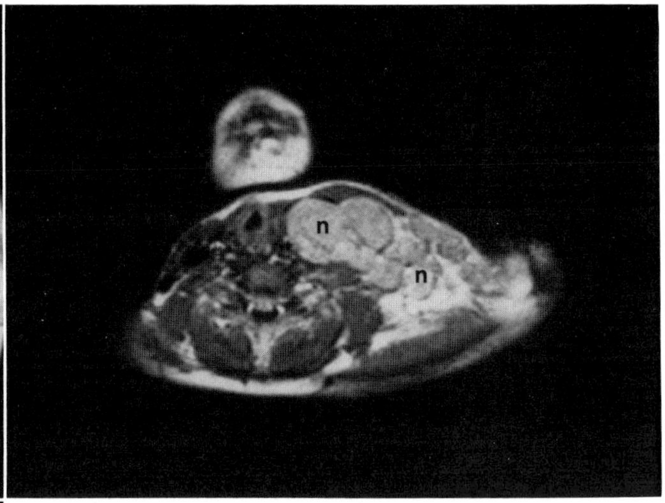

C

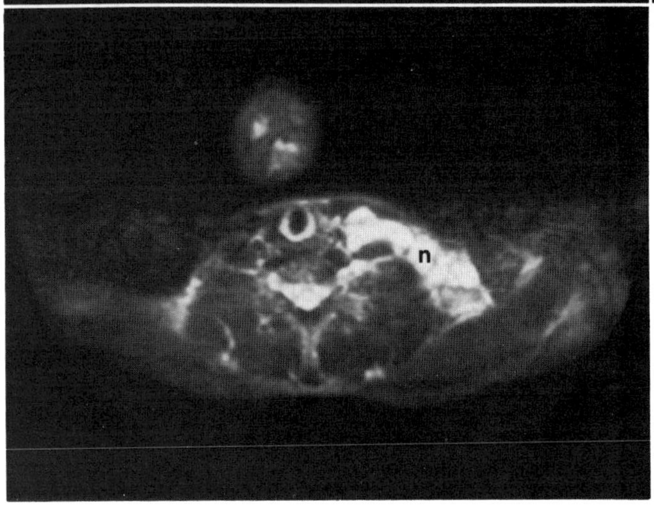

Figure 5–35. Diagnosis: Hodgkin disease. Cervical lymphadenopathy with displacement of the trachea.
A, CT. A large node mass of enlarged lymph nodes (*N*) seen in the lower left neck. ***B***, MR, T1 weighted image. The node mass (*N*) is again seen. The individual nodes are better defined than on the CT image. The nodes are of slightly greater intensity than normal muscle. ***C***, MR, T2 weighted image. There is increase in signal intensity in the diseased lymph nodes (*N*), which now appear extremely bright.

Figure 5–37. Diagnosis: Non-Hodgkin lymphoma of the parotid gland (*P*).
CT. The left parotid gland is diffusely enlarged and of similar intensity to muscle. There is diffuse infiltration with lymphoma.

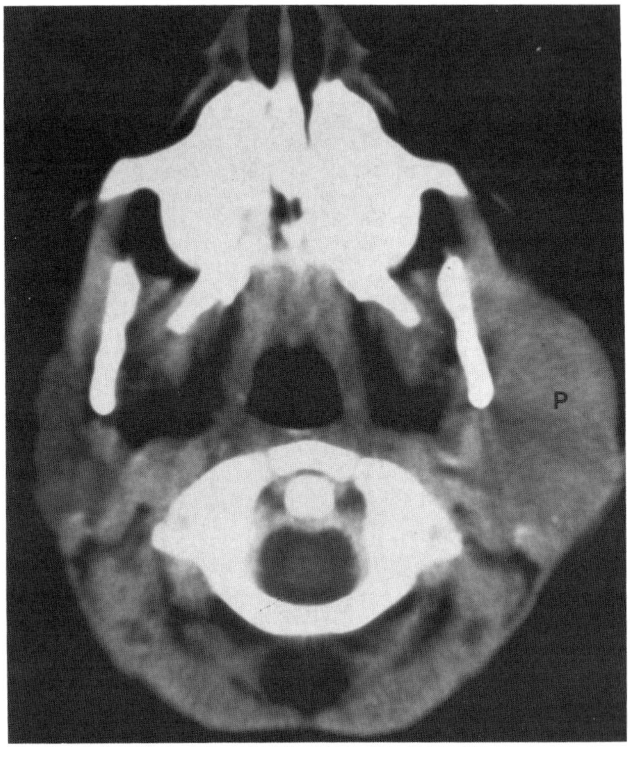

Figure 5–36. Diagnosis: Hodgkin disease. Cervical and mediastinal lymphadenopathy.
CT at the level of the thoracic inlet. Enlarged lymph nodes (*N*) extend from the neck around the clavicle into the superior mediastinum.

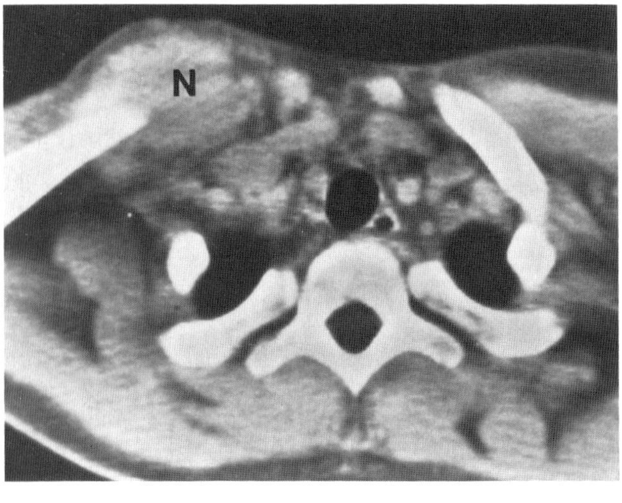

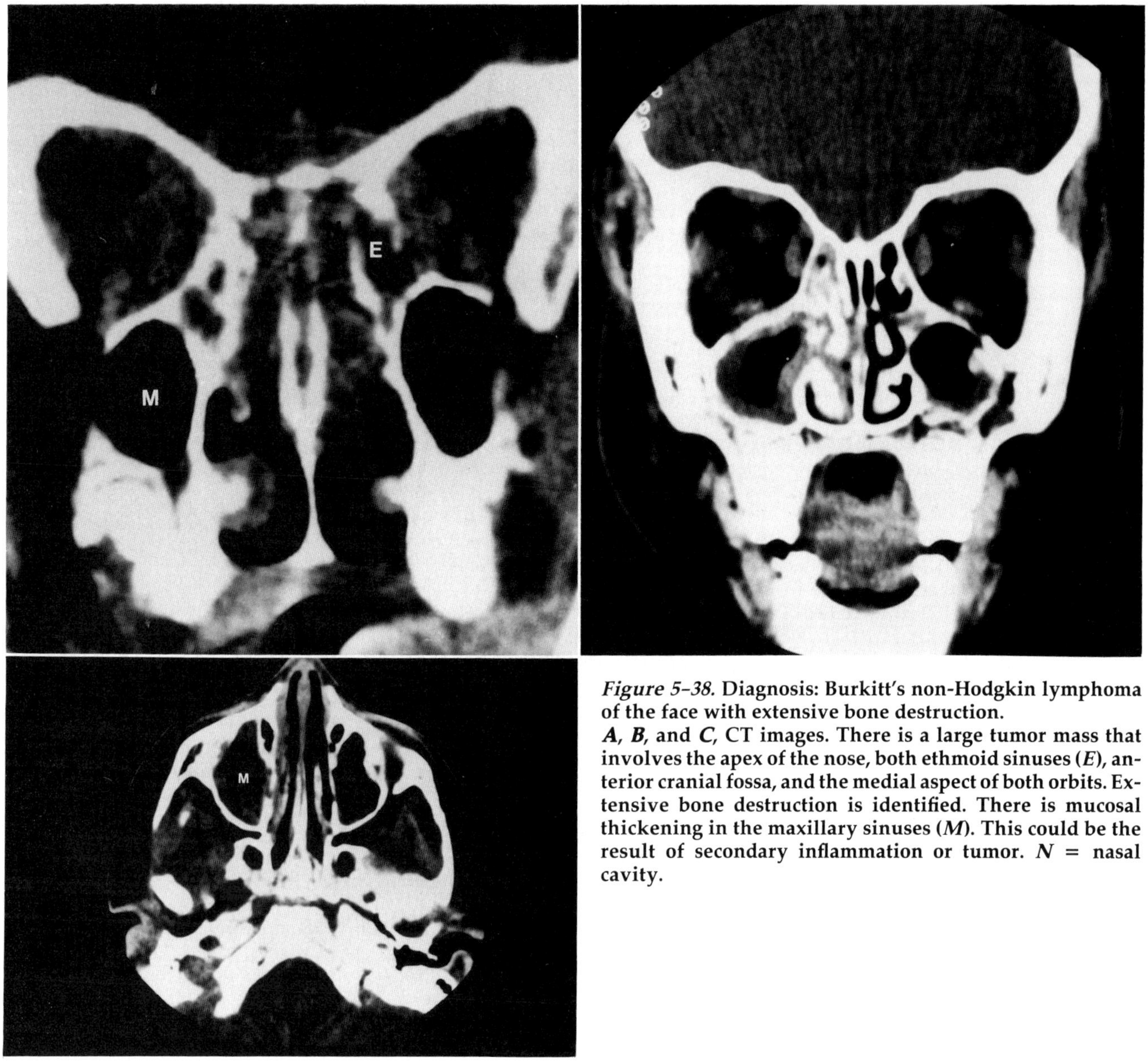

Figure 5–38. **Diagnosis: Burkitt's non-Hodgkin lymphoma of the face with extensive bone destruction.**
***A, B,* and *C,* CT images. There is a large tumor mass that involves the apex of the nose, both ethmoid sinuses (*E*), anterior cranial fossa, and the medial aspect of both orbits. Extensive bone destruction is identified. There is mucosal thickening in the maxillary sinuses (*M*). This could be the result of secondary inflammation or tumor. *N* = nasal cavity.**

aging in a significant number of patients and, therefore, alter staging. The reasons against performing a staging laparotomy are also outlined in Table 5–17. The most important factor explaining the falling enthusiasm for laparotomy is a changing philosophy in patient treatment, with many more patients receiving chemotherapy.[1] Because of this, although laparotomy may alter stage, its impact on the therapy in an individual patient is becoming very small. Even if errors are made by not performing a laparotomy, the rescue and long-term survival following relapse are now excellent with modern therapy.

References

1. Donaldson SS. Hodgkin's disease in children. Semin Oncol 1990;17:736–748.
2. Link MP, Donaldson SS, Berard CW, et al. Results of treatment of childhood localized non-Hodgkin's lymphoma with combination chemotherapy with or without radiotherapy. New Engl J Med 1990;322:1169–1174.
3. Chang PJ, Parker BR, Donaldson SS, et al. Dynamic probabilistic model for determination of optimal timing of surveillance chest radiography in pediatric Hodgkin disease. Radiology 1989;173:71–75.
4. Cohen MD, Siddiqui A, Weetman R, et al. Hodgkin disease and non-Hodgkin lymphomas in children: utilization of radiological modalities. Radiology 1986;158:499–505.
5. Castellino RA. Hodgkin disease: practical concepts for the diagnostic radiologist. Radiology 1986;159:305–310.
6. Tumeh SS, Rosenthal DS, Kaplan WD. Lymphoma: evaluation with Ga-67 SPECT. Radiology 1987;164:111–114.
7. Drossman SR, Schiff RG, Kronfeld GD, et al. Lymphoma of the mediastinum and neck: evaluation with Ga-67 imaging and CT correlation. Radiology 1990;174:171–175.
8. Moormeier JA, Williams SF, Golomb HM. The staging of non-Hodgkin's lymphomas. Semin Oncol 1990;17:43–50.

TABLE 5–17
Staging Laparotomy for Hodgkin Disease

Reasons For Doing Laparotomy
High incidence of finding tumor missed by imaging[1]
Alters stage in large number of children (30 to 40 percent of cases)[2–4]
Will alter decision regarding use of chemotherapy in many cases
Will alter radiation fields in many cases[1]
Yield is very high in selected groups of patients (e.g., 80 percent for mixed cellularity)[1,5]
Splenic disease is very poorly diagnosed by imaging and its presence cannot be inferred even if splenic hilar nodes are enlarged[6]
Splenectomy decreases the amount of body requiring radiation[3]
Reasons Against Doing Laparotomy
Mortality—although uncommon, it occurs[3]
Increased infection, because of splenectomy[3]
Cost
Even if initial stage is wrong, prognosis and recovery after relapse are excellent
Slight increased risk of second tumor after splenectomy (e.g., non-Hodgkin lymphoma, leukemia)[7]
With more children getting chemotherapy, even if laparotomy alters stage it may not alter treatment (e.g., with many protocols all stage II, III, and IV and all children with B symptoms now get chemotherapy). Previously, many children were given radiation therapy alone for stage I, II, or IIIA disease[3]
Surgical and pathology sampling can still miss disease and be false negative[4]

References
1. Baker L, Parker BR, Donaldson SS, et al. Staging of Hodgkin disease in children: comparison of CT and lymphography with laparotomy. AJR 1990;154:1251–1255.
2. Blackledge G, Best JJK, Crowther D, et al. Computed tomography (CT) in the staging of patients with Hodgkin's disease: a report on 136 patients. Clin Radiol 1980;31:143–147.
3. Desforges JF, Rutherford CJ, Piro A. Hodgkin's disease. New Engl J Med 1979:301:1212–1222.
4. Coon WW, Dabich L, Votaw ML. Indications for and morbidity associated with operative staging in patients with lymphoma. Am J Surg 1982;143:178–182.
5. Hoppe RT. The contemporary management of Hodgkin disease. Radiology 1988;169:297–304.
6. Moormeier JA, Williams SF, Golomb HM. The staging of non-Hodgkin's lymphomas. Semin Oncol 1990;17:43–50.
7. Meadows AT, Obringer AC, Marrero O, et al. Second malignant neoplasms following childhood Hodgkin's disease: treatment and splenectomy as risk factors. Med Pediatr Oncol 1989;17:477–484.

9. Rossleigh MA, Murray IPC, Mackey DWJ. Pediatric solid tumors: evaluation by gallium-67 SPECT studies. J Nucl Med 1990;31:168–172.
10. Zollars LE, Nagel JS, Tumeh SS. Three cases demonstrating the role of gallium scanning in relapsing Hodgkin's disease and non-Hodgkin lymphoma. J Nucl Med 1987;28:1611–1615.
11. Wylie BR, Southee AE, Joshua DE, et al. Gallium scanning in the management of mediastinal Hodgkin's disease. Eur J Haematol 1989;42:344–347.
12. Marglin S, Castellino R. Lymphographic accuracy in 632 consecutive, previously untreated cases of Hodgkin disease and non-Hodgkin lymphoma. Radiology 1981;140:351–353.
13. Mansfield CM, Fabian C, Jones S, et al. Comparison of lymphangiography and computed tomography scanning in evaluating abdominal disease in stages III and IV Hodgkin's disease. Cancer 1990;66:2295–2299.
14. Carde P, Pfeundschuh M, da Costa L. Radiolabeled monoclonal antibodies against Reed-Sternberg cells for in vivo imaging of Hodgkin's disease by immunoscintigraphy. Recent Results in Cancer Research 1989;117:101–111.
15. Bryant DJ, Bydder GM, Case HA, et al. Use of phosphorus-31 MR spectroscopy to monitor response to chemotherapy in non-Hodgkin lymphoma. J Comput Assist Tomogr 1988;12:770–774.
16. Parker BR, Castellino RA, Kaplan HS. Pediatric Hodgkin's disease. I. Radiographic evaluation. Cancer 1976;37:2430–2435.
17. Roskos RR, Evans RC, Gilchrist GS, et al. Prognostic significance of mediastinal mass in childhood Hodgkin's disease. Cancer Treat Rep 1982;66:961–968.
18. Hoppe RT. The contemporary management of Hodgkin disease. Radiology 1988;169:297–304.
19. Heron CW, Husband JE, Williams MP, et al. The value of thoracic computed tomography in the detection of recurrent Hodgkin's disease. Br J Radiol 1988;61:567–572.

20. Hopper KD, Diehl LF, Lesar M. Hodgkin disease: clinical utility of CT in initial staging and treatment. Radiology 1988;169:17–22.
21. Jochelson MS. Planning mantle radiation therapy in patients with Hodgkin disease: role of gallium-67 scintigraphy. AJR 1988;151:1229–1231.
22. Mandell GA, Lantieri R, Goodman LR. Tracheobronchial compression in Hodgkin lymphoma in children. AJR 1982;139:1167–1170.
23. Jeffrey GM, Mead GM, Whitehouse JMA. Life-threatening airway obstruction at the presentation of Hodgkin's disease. Cancer 1991;67:506–510.
24. Banks PM. The pathology of Hodgkin's disease. Semin Oncol 1990;17:683–695.
25. Heron CW, Husband JE, Williams MP. Hodgkin disease: CT of the thymus. Radiology 1988;167:647–651.
26. St. Amour TE, Siegel MJ, Glazer HS, et al. CT appearance of the normal and abnormal thymus in childhood. J Comput Assist Tomogr 1987;11:645–650.
27. Hibi S, Todo S, Imashuku S. Thymic localization of gallium-67 in pediatric patients with lymphoid and nonlymphoid tumors. J Nucl Med 1987;28:293–297.
28. Lindfors KK, Meyer JE, Dedrick CG. Thymic cysts in mediastinal Hodgkin disease. Radiology 1985;156:37–41.
29. Nogues A, Tovar JA, Sunol M, et al. Hodgkin's disease of the thymus: a rare mediastinal cystic mass. J Pediatr Surg 1987;22:996–997.
30. North LB, Fuller LM, Sullivan-Halley JA, et al. Regression of mediastinal Hodgkin disease after therapy: evaluation of time interval. Radiology 1987;164:599–602.
31. Nyman RS, Rehn SM, Glimelius BLG, et al. Residual mediastinal masses in Hodgkin disease: prediction of size with MR imaging. Radiology 1989;170:435–440.
32. Wycoco D, Raval B. An unusual presentation of mediastinal Hodgkin's lymphoma on computed tomography. CT 1983;7:187–188.
33. Costello P, Mauch P. Radiographic features of recurrent intrathoracic Hodgkin's disease following radiation therapy. AJR 1979;133:201–206.
34. Curran JG, Ryan MJ. Hodgkin's disease in a patient with polysplenia. Br J Radiol 1987;60:929–931.
35. Sanders LM, Botet JF, Straus DJ. CT of primary lymphoma of the liver. AJR 1989;152:973–976.
36. Baker L, Parker BR, Donaldson SS, et al. Staging of Hodgkin disease in children: comparison of CT and lymphography with laparotomy. AJR 1990;154:1251–1255.
37. Carroll BA, Ta HN. The ultrasonic appearance of extranodal abdominal lymphoma. Radiology 1980;136:419–425.
38. Sekiya T, Meller ST, Cosgrove DO, et al. Ultrasonography of Hodgkins disease in the liver and spleen. Clin Radiol 1982;33:635–639.
39. Friedman PA, Sommer FG, Chen H-S, et al. Characterization of splenic structure in Hodgkin disease by using narrow-band filtration of backscattered ultrasound. AJR 1989;152:1197–1203.
40. Ginaldi S, Bernardino ME, Jing G-S, et al. Ultrasonographic patterns of hepatic lymphoma. Radiology 1980;136:427–431.
41. Carroll BA. Ultrasound of lymphoma. Semin Ultrasound 1982;3:114–123.
42. Nyman R, Rehn S, Glimelius B, et al. Magnetic resonance imaging, chest radiography, computed tomography and ultrasonography in malignant lymphoma. Acta Radiol 1987;28:253–262.
43. Weinreb JC, Brateman L, Maravilla KR. Magnetic resonance imaging of hepatic lymphoma. AJR 1984;143:1211–1214.
44. Nyman R, Rhen S, Ericsson A, et al. An attempt to characterize malignant lymphoma in spleen, liver and lymph nodes with magnetic resonance imaging. Acta Radiol 1987;28:527–533.
45. Weissleder R, Elizondo G, Stark DD, et al. The diagnosis of splenic lymphoma by MR imaging: value of superparamagnetic iron oxide. AJR 1989;152:175–180.
46. Pais RC, Hammami A, Kim H. Non-Hodgkin's lymphoma presenting as a rectal polyp in a child. J Pediatr Surg 1990;25:1280–1282.
47. Gourtsoyiannis NC, Nolan DJ. Lymphoma of the small intestine: radiological appearances. Clin Radiol 1988;39:639–645.
48. Lynch MA, Cho KC, Jeffrey RB, et al. CT of peritoneal lymphomatosis. AJR 1988;152:713–715.
49. Siegel MJ, Evans SJ, Balfe DM. Small bowel disease in children: diagnosis with CT. Radiology 1988;169:127–130.
50. Sener RN, Alper H, Demirci A, et al. A different sonographic "pseudokidney" appearance detected with intestinal lymphoma: "hydronephrotic-pseudokidney." J Clin Ultrasound 1989;17:209–212.
51. Miller JH, Hindman BW, Lam AHK. Ultrasound in the evaluation of small bowel lymphoma in children. Radiology 1980;135:409–414.
52. Martin DJ, Ash JM. Diagnostic radiology in non-Hodgkins lymphoma. Semin Oncol 1977;4:297–309.
53. Goodman P, Raval B. Omental cakes in American Burkitt lymphoma computed tomography demonstration. Clin Imag 1989;13:117–118.
54. Krudy AG, Dunnick NR, Magrath IT, et al. CT of American Burkitt lymphoma. AJR 1981;136:747–754.
55. Catto-Smith A, Forbes D, Willoughby M, et al. Malignant gastroduodenal ulceration in childhood. Am J Pediatr Hematol/Oncol 1988;10:109–111.
56. Parker BR, Margin S, Castellino RA. Skeletal manifestations of leukemia, Hodgkin disease, and non-Hodgkin lymphoma. Semin Roentgenol 1980;15:302–315.
57. The Non-Hodgkin's Lymphoma Pathologic Classification Project. National Cancer Institute sponsored study of classifications of non-Hodgkin's lymphomas. Cancer 1982;49:2112–2135.
58. Vanel D, Bayle C, Hartmann O, et al. Radiological study of two disseminated malignant non-Hodgkin lymphomas affecting only the bones in children. Skeletal Radiol 1982;9:83–87.
59. Newcomer LN, Silverstein MB. Bone involvement in Hodgkin's disease. Cancer 1982;49:338–342.
60. Orzel JA, Sawaf NW, Richardson ML. Lymphoma of the skeleton: scintigraphic evaluation. AJR 1988;150:1095–1099.
61. Braunstein EM, White SJ. Non-Hodgkin lymphoma of bone. Radiology 1980;135:59–63.
62. Coppes MJ, Patte C, Couanet D, et al. Childhood malignant lymphoma of bone. Med Pediatr Oncol 1991;19:22–27.
63. Clayton F, Butler JJ, Ayala AG, et al. Non-Hodgkin's lymphoma in bone. Cancer 1987;60:2494–2501.
64. Spjut HJ, Ayala AG. Skeletal tumors in children and adolescents. Hum Pathol 1983;14:628–642.
65. Braunstein EM. Hodgkin disease of bone: radiographic correlation with the histological classification. Radiology 1980;137:643–646.
66. Linden A, Zankovich R, Theissen P, et al. Malignant lym-

phoma: bone marrow imaging versus biopsy. Radiology 1989;173:335–339.
67. Schicha H, Franke M, Smolorz J, et al. Diagnostic strategies and staging procedures for Hodgkin's lymphoma: bone marrow scintigraphy and magnetic resonance imaging. Recent Results in Cancer Research 1989;771:112–119.
68. Nyman R, Rehn S, Glimelius B, et al. Magnetic resonance imaging in diffuse malignant bone marrow diseases. Acta Radiol 1987;28:199–205.
69. Greco A, Jelliffe AM, Maher EJ, et al. MR imaging of lymphomas: impact on therapy. J Comput Assist Tomogr 1988;12:785–791.
70. Castellino RA. Hodgkin disease: imaging studies and patient management. Radiology 1988;169:269–270.
71. Shawker TH, Dunnick NR, Head GL, et al. Ultrasound evaluation of American Burkitt's lymphoma. J Clin Ultrasound 1979;7:279–283.
72. Haddy TB, Sandlund JT, Magrath IT. Testicular involvement in young patients with non-Hodgkin's lymphoma. Am J Pediatr Hematol/Oncol 1988;10:224–229.
73. Levine C, Vrlenich L. Renal lymphoma in ataxia-telangiectasia: CT contribution. J Comput Assist Tomogr 1989;13:537–539.
74. Patel PJ, Bahakim HM, Kolawole TM. Renal sonography in childhood lymphoma. Urol Int 1990;45:34–37.
75. Zwanger-Mendelsohn S, Chreck EH, Doshi V. Burkitt lymphoma involving the epididymis and spermatic cord: sonographic and CT findings. AJR 1989;153:85–86.
76. Leonard MP, Schlegel PN, Crovatto A, et al. Burkitt's lymphoma of the testis: an unusual scrotal mass in childhood. J Urol 1990;143:104–106.
77. Clayton F, Butler JJ, Ayala AG, et al. Non-Hodgkin's lymphoma in bone. Cancer 1987;60:2494–2501.
78. Rabalais GP, Buchino JJ, Shearer LT. A 12-year-old girl with a rash and pulmonary infiltrations. J Pediatr 1988;112:1008–1013.
79. Yousem SA, Weiss LM, Colby TV. Primary pulmonary Hodgkin's disease: a clinicopathologic study of 15 cases. Cancer 1986;57:1217–1224.
80. Coon WW, Dabich L, Votaw ML. Indications for, and morbidity associated with, operative staging in patients with lymphoma. Am J Surg 1982;143:178–182.
81. Leventhal BG, Donaldson SS. Hodgkin's disease. In: Pizzo PA, Poplack DG, eds. Principles and practice of pediatric oncology. Philadelphia: JB Lippincott, 1989:457–476.
82. Muraji T, Hays DM, Siegel SE. Evaluation of the surgical aspects of staging laparotomy for Hodgkin's disease in children. J Pediatr Surg 1982;17:843–848.
83. Barsky MF, Coates RK, Macdonald DR. Computed tomographic features of primary brain lymphoma. J Can Assoc Radiol 1989;40:80–83.
84. Best JK, Blackledge G, Forbes W St C. Computed tomography of abdomen in staging and clinical management of lymphoma. Br Med J 1978;2:1675–1677.
85. Harnsberger HR, Bragg DG, Osborn AG, et al. Non-Hodgkin's lymphoma of the head and neck: CT evaluation of nodal and extranodal sites. AJR 1987;149:785–791.
86. Radford JA, Cowan RA, Flanagan M, et al. The significance of residual mediastinal abnormality on the chest radiograph following treatment for Hodgkin's disease. J Clin Oncol 1988;6:940–946.
87. Biagini C, Enrici RM, Anselmo AP, et al. The role of restaging laparotomy in Hodgkin's disease. Acta Oncol 1989;28:659–663.
88. Lewis E, Bernardino ME, Salvador PG, et al. Post-therapy CT-detected mass in lymphoma patients: is it viable tissue? J Comput Assist Tomogr 1982;6:792–795.
89. Stolar CJH, Garvin JH, Rustad DG, et al. Residual or recurrent chest mass in pediatric Hodgkin's disease. A surgical problem? Am J Pediatr Hematol/Oncol 1987;9:289–294.
90. Webb WR. MR imaging of treated mediastinal Hodgkin disease. Radiology 1989;170:315–316.
91. Chang PJ, Parker BR, Donaldson SS, et al. Dynamic probabilistic model for determination of optimal timing of surveillance chest radiography in pediatric Hodgkin disease. Radiology 1989;173:71–75.

Differential Diagnosis

Because lymphoma can affect almost any organ or tissue in the body, the differential diagnosis is enormous. Differential diagnosis includes most other benign and malignant tumor masses in children, a range of congenital abnormalities, and a large number of inflammatory disorders. Although far less common than many other disorders, lymphoma should be borne in mind in the differential diagnosis of any perplexing lesion in a child. A thorough knowledge of the pattern of spread of Hodgkin disease and non-Hodgkin lymphoma, and of the biology of these tumors, will help to evaluate the probability of their occurrence in any particular child.

Therapy and Prognosis

TREATMENT OF HODGKIN DISEASE

This tumor is extremely sensitive to radiation therapy or chemotherapy[1] (Table 5–18). Prior to the 1960s treatment was mainly with radiation therapy. To achieve cure, relatively high doses need to be utilized and particularly with moderately extensive disease large areas of the body need to be radiated. The philosophy of radiation therapy is to irradiate all known disease and to prophylactically irradiate the normal lymph node areas immediately adjacent to known areas of disease. Accurate demonstration of the extent of disease by imaging is obviously very important. Commonly used radiation fields include the mantel field above the diaphragm (all neck nodes, axillary, clavicular, mediastinal, and hilar nodes) and an inverted Y field below the diaphragm (all aortic, iliac, and femoral nodes, including the spleen if not resected).

Effective chemotherapy became available in the early 1960s with the development of MOPP (nitrogen mustard vincristine procarbazine and prednisone).[2,3] A number of other drug combinations have since become widely utilized, including ABVD (adriomycin, bleomycin, vinblastine, and dacarbozine). With the development of effective chemotherapy, a philosophy has developed to attempt to reduce the amount of radiation utilized for treatment of Hodgkin disease, especially in children.[1,4] Chemotherapy is now utilized far more frequently, especially for lower-stage diseases, permitting utilization of lower radiation doses and smaller radiation fields[1,5,6] (see Table 5–18). With chemotherapy, imaging is extremely important in monitoring the response of tumor. This is because the number of cycles of chemotherapy to be utilized is frequently dependent on the response. For example, one study recommends utilizing two additional cycles of chemotherapy following complete remission of tumor as identified by imaging[1] (using a minimum of 6 cycles). The trend is to move away from long-term maintenance chemotherapy.[1] Imaging is also particularly important in the detection of relapse. This importance is emphasized when one bears in mind that recovery after relapse can be excellent.

PROGNOSIS OF HODGKIN DISEASE

The overall prognosis with Hodgkin disease is now excellent, in the range of 85 to 90 percent 5-year survival.[1,5,7] The prognosis in children is often better than in adults[1,7] so that a survival of over 90 percent can be expected in most large pediatric series.[1,8] In a large series of patients of all ages with Hodgkin disease reported in 1989,[9] almost all patients went into complete remission, with relapse occurring in about 30 percent. As previously mentioned, recovery after relapse is still excellent. Prognosis, although excellent overall, is still dependent on stage and histology. Prognosis is best for stage I and worst for stage IV disease.[7] With regard to histology, prognosis is best with lymphocyte-predominant histology, decreasing in order with nodular sclerosing, mixed cellularity, and lymphocyte-depleted histology. Fortunately, this latter histology is extremely uncommon in children.[1] Other factors regarding prognosis have been reported. For example, in children (on data collected before 1980), a large mediastinal mass was reported as having a diminished prognosis.[4] Whether this is still true with more modern therapy is not known. Any reports relating prognosis with specific findings must bear in mind that these factors may change as therapy changes. Because prognosis is so very good with Hodgkin disease, therapy protocols are now being directed to reduce the incidence of complications such as radiation therapy to organs, infection, sterility, and second tumors. A second malignancy after childhood Hodgkin disease is a very real problem, being reported in 38 of 979 children[10] (Table 5–19).

TABLE 5–18
Treatment of Hodgkin Disease[1–4]

- Radiation very effective
- Chemotherapy very effective
- Current philosophy is to decrease radiation, especially in children
- Recovery after relapse is excellent
- Combined protocols of chemotherapy and low-dose radiation therapy are common

References

1. Baker L, Parker BR, Donaldson SS, et al. Staging of Hodgkin disease in children: comparison of CT and lymphography with laparotomy. AJR 1990;154:1251–1255.
2. Hoppe RT. The contemporary management of Hodgkin disease. Radiology 1988;169:297–304.
3. Castellino RA. Hodgkin disease: imaging studies and patient management. Radiology 1988;169:269–270.
4. Leventhal BG, Donaldson SS. Hodgkin's disease. In: Pizzo PA, Poplack DG, eds. Principles and practice of pediatric oncology. Philadelphia: JB Lippincott, 1989:457–476.

TREATMENT OF NON-HODGKIN LYMPHOMA[11,12]

Chemotherapy is the main method of treating non-Hodgkin lymphoma, because it is so frequently a diffuse disease.[13] The chemotherapy utilized will vary depending on the histology, with different histologic groups responding differently to various combinations of drugs. Some form of central nervous system prophylaxis is required, especially in patients with lymphoblastic lymphoma. This may be in the form of chemotherapy or radiation therapy. Current protocols attempt to minimize or eliminate radiation therapy, because of the adverse effects on skeletal growth, treatment-related second tumors, and infertility.[13] A 1990 study showed the same survival for stage I and II patients treated with chemotherapy alone as compared to chemotherapy combined with radiation therapy.[13]

For disease in other locations radiation therapy, in general, provides no particular benefit and only increases toxicity. Radiation therapy may, however, be utilized to reduce the size of troublesome symptomatic focal masses, e.g., if there is marked tracheal compres-

TABLE 5–19
Second Malignancy after Childhood Hodgkin Disease (979 Children)[1]

Percentage of children developing a second malignancy	
after 5 yrs	2%
after 10 yrs	5%
after 15 yrs	9%
Nature of second malignancy	
Solid tumor	8 children
Leukemia	17 children
Non-Hodgkin lymphoma	3 children

Reference

1. Makepeace AR, Fermont DC, Bennett MH. Gastrointestinal non-Hodgkin's lymphoma. Clin Radiol 1987;38:609–614.

sion and narrowing or if a lesion is compressing the spinal cord and causing symptoms.

Surgery, apart from biopsy, has a limited role in non-Hodgkin lymphoma with the exception of selected situations in which complete surgical resection is possible. In these cases, surgery improves prognosis. This is particularly possible in some patients with bowel lymphoma—e.g., Burkitt's lymphoma—in whom the bowel disease may be localized at presentation.

PROGNOSIS OF NON-HODGKIN LYMPHOMA

The prognosis with non-Hodgkin lymphoma is summarized in Table 5–20. As can be seen in many patients, an excellent prognosis can occur. There are, however, selected patients in whom the prognosis still remains extremely poor. There are some biochemical factors that have been utilized in attempting to predict prognosis. For example, elevated serum levels of IL-2R or serum LDH are associated with a worse prognosis.[11] Similarly, disease present in the bone marrow and central nervous system carries a worse prognosis. Immunoblastic histology also carries a worse prognosis. Patients who relapse after initial remission have a very poor prognosis (this is the exact opposite of Hodgkin disease) and, therefore, are treated extremely aggressively, including protocols with bone marrow transplantation.[11]

TABLE 5–20
Non-Hodgkin Lymphoma: Prognosis[1–3]

Survival:		
Pre-1960	<20%	
Mid-1970	70%	
1990	Localized lymphoblastic	90%
	Extensive lymphoblastic	60–80%
	Abdominal small cell	60–80%
	If there is marrow or disease	<40%
	Immunoblastic	poor

References
1. Magrath IT. Malignant non-Hodgkin's lymphomas. In: Pizzo PA, Poplack DG, eds. Principles and practice of pediatric oncology. Philadelphia: JB Lippincott, 1989;415–455.
2. Rivera-Luna R, Martinez-Guerra G, Borrego-Roman R. Burkitt's lymphoma. Experience at the Instituto Nacional de Pediatria, Mexico City. Am J Pediatr Hematol/Oncol 1986;8:183–190.
3. Smith SD, Rubin CM, Horvath A, et al. Non-Hodgkin's lymphoma in children. Semin Oncol 1990;17:113–119.

References
1. Hoppe RT. The contemporary management of Hodgkin disease. Radiology 1988;169:297–304.
2. Donaldson SS, Kaplan HS. Complications of treatment of Hodgkin's disease in children. Cancer Treat Rep 1982;66:977–989.
3. Leventhal BG, Donaldson SS. Hodgkin's disease. In: Pizzo PA, Poplack DG, eds. Principles and practice of pediatric oncology. Philadelphia: JB Lippincott, 1989:457–476.
4. Baker L, Parker BR, Donaldson SS, et al. Staging of Hodgkin disease in children: comparison of CT and lymphography with laparotomy. AJR 1990;154:1251–1255.
5. Makepeace AR, Maclennan KA, Hudson GV, et al. Hodgkin's disease in childhood: the British National Lymphoma Investigation Experience (BNLI Report No 27). Clin Radiol 1987;38:7–11.
6. Donaldson SS, Link MP. Combined modality treatment with low-dose radiation and MOPP chemotherapy for children with Hodgkin's disease. J Clin Oncol 1987;5:742–749.
7. Castellino RA. Hodgkin disease: practical concepts for the diagnostic radiologist. Radiology 1986;159:305–310.
8. Castellino RA. Hodgkin disease: imaging studies and patient management. Radiology 1988;169:269–270.
9. Biagini C, Enrici RM, Anselmo AP, et al. The role of restaging laparotomy in Hodgkin's disease. Acta Oncol 1989;28:659–663.
10. Miller ST, Wollner N, Meyers PA. Primary hepatic or hepatosplenic non-Hodgkin's lymphoma in children. Cancer 1983;52:2285–2288.
11. Magrath IT. Malignant non-Hodgkin's lymphomas. In: Pizzo PA, Poplack DG, eds. Principles and practice of pediatric oncology. Philadelphia: JB Lippincott, 1989:415–455.
12. Smith SD, Rubin CM, Horvath A, et al. Non-Hodgkin's lymphoma in children. Semin Oncol 1990;17:113–119.
13. Link MP, Donaldson SS, Berard CW, et al. Results of treatment of childhood localized non-Hodgkin's lymphoma with combination chemotherapy with or without radiotherapy. New Engl J Med 1990;322:1169–1174.

OTHER RETICULOENDOTHELIAL TUMORS

MALIGNANT HISTIOCYTOSIS

Malignant histiocytosis is an aggressive tumor, occurring at a median age of about 2 years.[1,2] The tumor arises from histiocytes[3] and can occur in almost any site in the body.[4]

Clinical findings are widespread lymph node enlargement, together with enlargement of the liver and spleen.[2,4–6] Fever is a common finding. There are frequently skin rashes, disseminated intravascular coagulation, and pancytopenia.[2,4,6] Weight loss and wasting are common.

Imaging findings are predominantly those of enlarged lymph nodes, liver, and spleen (Fig. 5–39). In one study of 23 children,[7] mediastinal adenopathy was identified in 63 percent, interstitial lung disease in 35 percent, pleural effusion in 40 percent, and enlarged retroperitoneal lymph nodes in 43 percent. There are no specific features to suggest the diagnosis.

A B

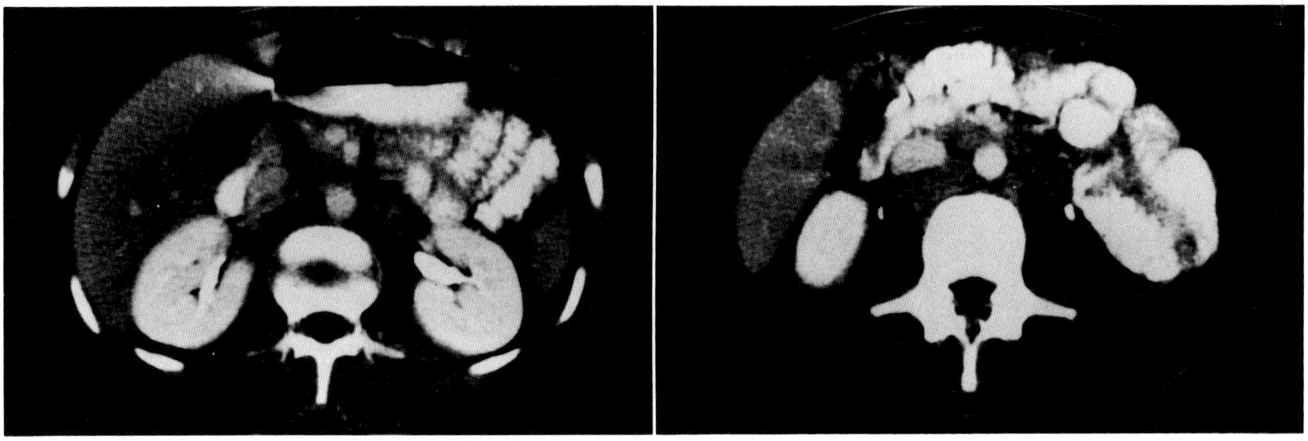

Figure 5–39. **Diagnosis: Malignant histiocytosis.**
***A* and *B*, CT images after oral and intravenous contrast administration. There is extensive lymphadenopathy involving the retrocrural, para-aortic, and some mesenteric lymph nodes (*N*).**

Treatment is predominantly with chemotherapy but prognosis is very poor.[1,2,6]

References

1. Esumi N, Hashida T, Matsumura T. Malignant histiocytosis in childhood. Clinical features and therapeutic results by combination chemotherapy. Am J Pediatr Hematol/Oncol 1986;8:300–307.
2. Hibi S, Esumi N, Todo S, et al. Malignant histiocytosis in childhood: clinical, cytochemical, and immunohistochemical studies of seven cases. Hum Pathol 1988;19:713–719.
3. Kjeldsberg CR, Wilson JF, Berard CW. Non-Hodgkin's lymphoma in children. Hum Pathol 1983;14:612–627.
4. Warnke RA, Kim H, Dorfman RF. Malignant histiocytosis (histiocytic medullary reticulosis). I. Clinicopathologic study of 29 cases. Cancer 1975;35:215–230.
5. Benz-Lemoine E, Brizard A, Huret J-L, et al. Malignant histiocytosis: a specific t(2;5)(p23;q35) translocation? Review of the literature. Blood 1988;72:1045–1047.
6. Dehner LP. Non-Hodgkin's lymphomas and malignant histiocytosis in children. Semin Oncol 1977;4:273–286.
7. Vanel D, Couanet D, Piekarski JD, et al. Radiological findings in 23 pediatric cases of malignant histiocytosis MH. Eur J Radiol 1983;3:60–62.

PLEXIFORM FIBROHISTIOCYTIC TUMOR

Plexiform fibrohistiocytic tumor was first described in 1988.[1] Sixty-five children were reviewed. The mean age was 14 years. Females outnumbered males by 2 to 1. Pathologically, these tumors are slow-growing dermal or subcutaneous masses, rarely greater than 3 cm in size. Microscopically, they consist of histiocytes and fibrous tissue. No imaging findings were described in the report, but I would suspect that nonspecific soft-tissue masses would be identified on ultrasound, CT, or MR. Treatment was by surgery. Thirty-seven percent of the patients recurred. Metastases to regional lymph nodes were identified in 2 patients.

Reference

1. Enzinger FM, Zhang R. Plexiform fibrohistiocytic tumor presenting in children and young adults. An analysis of 65 cases. Am J Surg Pathol 1988;12:818–826.

LEUKEMIA

Leukemia provides an interesting paradox for the pediatric radiologist. This is the most common malignancy in children, yet it is the one for which imaging has the least to contribute. Leukemia causes imaging changes in virtually every organ of the body. Despite this widespread disease, easily detected by imaging, the diagnosis is usually made from examination of peripheral blood and bone marrow biopsy. Imaging is seldom used for the diagnosis of leukemia, has no role to play in determining prognosis, is extremely poor for detection of recurrent disease and is not used routinely for this, and is equally poor and not used for monitoring therapy. Despite all this, an understanding of the disease is important because of its frequency. Radiographic abnormalities may be found incidentally and they need to be recognized. Very recent studies have suggested that MR may have a role in monitoring response to therapy and in early detection of recurrence and this is discussed in detail.

Epidemiology

There are about 4 cases per 100,000 children under the age of 15 years per annum in the United States, which results in about 2,000 new cases per year.[1] The peak age is at about 4 years. There is a definite familial incidence of leukemia, a significant increase following exposure to radiation, an association with many clinical syndromes, including chromosomal abnormalities such as Down syndrome,[2] telangiectasia, Fanconi anemia, and Bloom syndrome. Many environmental factors have also been suggested as contributing to leukemia.

References
1. Poplack DG. Acute lymphoblastic leukemia. In: Pizzo PA, Poplack DG, eds. Principles and practice of pediatric oncology. Philadelphia: JB Lippincott, 1989:323–366.
2. Miller DR. Childhood acute lymphoblastic leukemia: 1. Biological features and their use in predicting outcome of treatment. Am J Pediatr Hematol/Oncol 1988;10:163–173.

Pathology

Over 75 percent of childhood leukemias are acute lymphocytic leukemia (ALL) and this is the type of leukemia that is described in detail in this section. Acute nonlymphocytic leukemia accounts for about 15 percent of pediatric leukemias.[1] It is the most common congenital leukemia and has a worse prognosis than acute lymphocytic leukemia. Chronic leukemias are rare in children, accounting for less than 5 percent. Of these the myelocytic is the most common.

The classification of acute lymphocytic leukemia is complicated. Biologically, acute lymphocytic leukemia is a heterogenous group of disorders that can arise at any point of lymphocyte differentiation. The tumors are classified by many different criteria including the following.

1. Morphology. They are divided by an FAB classification into three types of cells: L1, L2, and L3.
2. Immunology. Eighty percent have a B cell lineage.
3. Cytogenetics. Chromosome abnormalities can be found in leukemic cells in 90 percent of patients.
4. Biochemical characteristics.
5. Cytokinetics, i.e., proliferative activity of these cells.

There is an overlap and no very sharp distinction between acute lymphocytic leukemia and non-Hodgkin lymphoma. The distinction is arbitrarily taken by most workers as the percentage of blast cells in the marrow, tumors with over a certain percentage of blast cells being called acute leukemia.

Eighty percent of the tumors are B cell. The T cell tumors tend to occur in older children, have a higher peripheral white cell count, and have a higher incidence of central nervous system involvement, and more commonly (50 percent) have a mediastinal mass.

Chloroma is a term used to describe focal deposits of leukemic cells seen usually in acute myeloid leukemia.[2] Identification of these deposits may precede the identification of widespread leukemia in the bone marrow. In one study of 8 patients, the mean age was 17 years, much older than in acute lymphocytic leukemia. The chloroma deposits can occur at any site. On CT, they are seen as small nonenhancing nodular masses that can be multiple.[2]

References
1. Fletcher JC, van Eys J, Dorn LD. Ethical considerations in pediatric oncology. In: Pizzo PA, Poplack DG, eds. Principles and practice of pediatric oncology. Philadelphia: JB Lippincott, 1989:309–320.
2. Pomeranz SJ, Hawkins HH, Towbin R. Granulocytic sarcoma (chloroma): CT manifestations. Radiology 1985;155:167–170.

Clinical Presentation

The symptoms of acute leukemia are relatively nonspecific. Two-thirds of the children have fever and hepatosplenomegaly, one-half have enlarged lymph nodes and skin bleeding, one-quarter have bone pain. Signs of anemia, fatigue, and weight loss may also occur.

Imaging Studies

Bone Marrow. MR imaging is increasingly reported as being very sensitive for detection of bone marrow abnormality in children with leukemia. The leukemic cells replace fat in the marrow and cause an increase in T1 relaxation time with resultant decrease in signal intensity on T1 weighted images[1–3] (Fig. 5–40). One study of 11 children with acute lymphocytic leukemia demonstrated increased T1 relaxation time in the spinal marrow in all patients compared to controls.[4] With treatment, the T1 relaxation time returned to normal or close to it. There was reasonable correlation between the measured T1 relaxation time in the spinal marrow and the percentage of blast cells present in the iliac bone marrow biopsy. In another study, T1 relaxation times were measured in the bone marrow in the region of the knee. These workers believed that recurrent tumor could not be reliably differentiated from other causes of prolonged T1 relaxation time.[5] I very much agree with their statements.

Regions of prolonged T1 relaxation time can be seen with necrosis (infarction), localized areas of hemopoiesis, or infection (Fig. 5–41). While there is some enthusiasm for the potential of MR in diagnosis and monitoring of therapy of leukemia by studying the bone marrow, this should be considered experimental at the present time. This is because there are significant problems involved in estimation of the T1 relaxation times; the findings are very nonspecific and can be caused by almost any pathology or even normal increased hemopoiesis. With regard to relapse, it is not known what percentage of marrow needs to be replaced by recurrent tumor before it can be identified on MR imaging. Although MR is more sensitive than other imaging modalities, it may not prove as sensitive as bone marrow biopsy for early detection of relapse. Another problem with MR is that the entire skeleton cannot be surveyed. In addition, relapse not uncommonly occurs at sites other than the bone marrow.

Bone Cortical Abnormality. This is an extremely common finding at presentation in children with leukemia.

A B

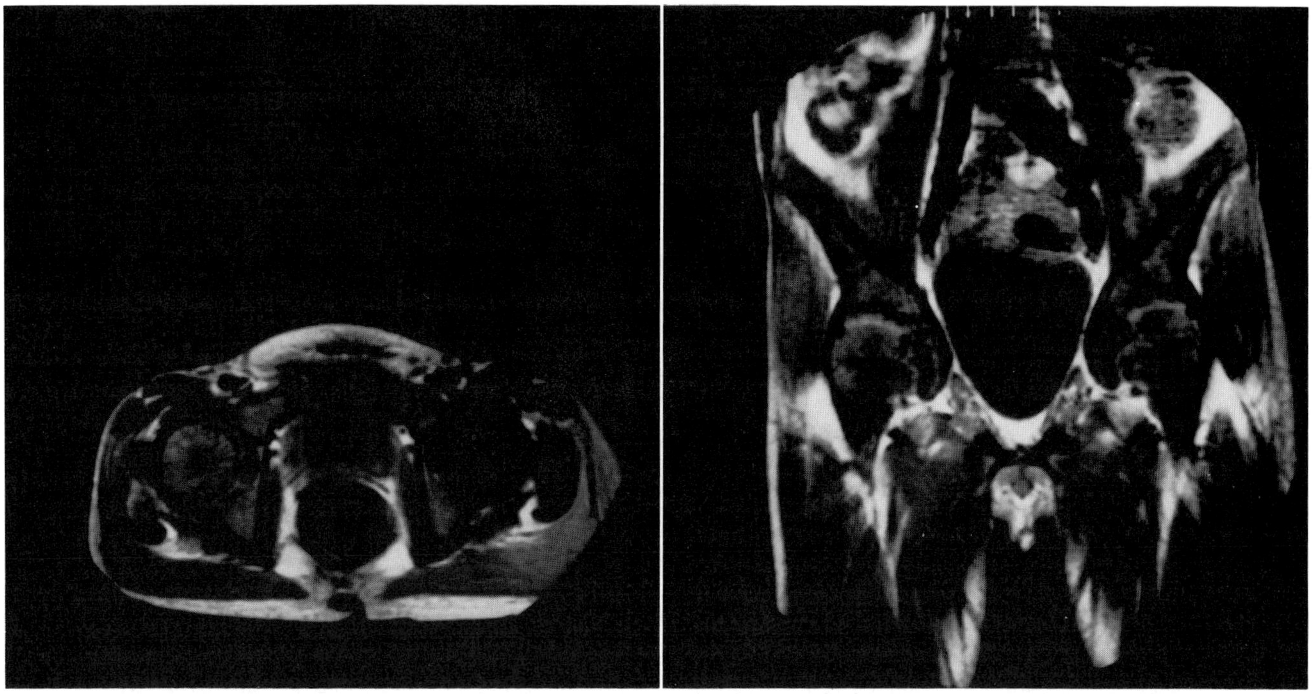

Figure 5–40. **Diagnosis: Leukemia.**
***A* and *B*, Axial and coronal T1 weighted MR images. There is widespread reduction in signal intensity from all of the visualized bone marrow because of diffuse leukemic infiltration.**

In 107 children, at diagnosis, 20 percent had clinical symptoms suggesting bone abnormality and 44 percent had some abnormality on radiograph.[6] The bone abnormalities that are seen include transverse metaphyseal lucent bands, periosteal elevation and thickening, diffuse osteoporosis, focal osteolytic lesions, and pathological fractures.[6–9] A combination of changes is common: in one study, 87 percent of patients had more than one abnormality.[8] The changes in the bone are often symmetrical, usually fairly widespread, and maximal in areas of active bone growth.[8] Demineralization is the most common abnormality seen in the bone, accounting for 60 percent of bone abnormalities in one series[9] and 55 percent in another study of 107 children.[6] Periosteal elevation is usually a single layer involving a long segment of bone.[8] Metaphyseal lucent bands are the next most common abnormality, appearing in about 40 percent of patients with bone change.[9] These are more common in the very young. They are believed to be the result of focal severe osteoporosis.

In a study of 200 children, 7 percent had some bone involvement.[10] The bone changes are not pathognomonic for leukemia. Because the diagnosis is not made from bone imaging, and because the finding of abnormality in the bone does not affect prognosis or therapy, routine bone imaging with isotopes or skeletal survey is not used in leukemia. Children with focal symptoms (usually pain) should have these areas imaged. This is important, because pathological fractures can occur.[10,11]

The osteolytic lesions can be focal or fairly widespread. The most common lytic lesion is seen as a motheaten area of destruction in the diametaphysis. Adjacent areas can grow and coalesce.[8] It is through these areas that pathological fractures occur. Very occasionally sclerotic bone changes will be identified. These patients usually have areas of destruction as well.[8]

The bone changes resolve with therapy. When the patients relapse, the bone abnormalities frequently do not recur.[11]

Central Nervous System. The incidence of central nervous system involvement with leukemia is less than 5 percent at the time of diagnosis. In the early 1970s, up to 80 percent of children developed central nervous system leukemia at some stage. This is now much less common because of prophylactic treatment. Spread of leukemia to the central nervous system occurs either via the blood or by direct involvement from skull bone marrow.[7] Leptomeningeal involvement is the most common. Focal nodules of leukemic infiltration can, however, be identified in the cerebral hemispheres.[12]

At the present time, the overall incidence of central nervous system leukemia is between 2 and 8 percent.[13] On imaging, leptomeningeal leukemia may be difficult to identify. On CT, these lesions frequently will not enhance with intravenous contrast and are, therefore, difficult to see.[14] MR, in the future, may prove better than CT, but this is not yet known. It is anticipated that gadolinium-DTPA will be required to identify disease accurately with MR.

In addition to leukemia itself, several central nervous system complications of prophylactic radiation therapy have been identified. These include cerebral atrophy, leukoencephalopathy, and microangiopathy.[7] Chemotherapy such as methotrexate may also cause abnor-

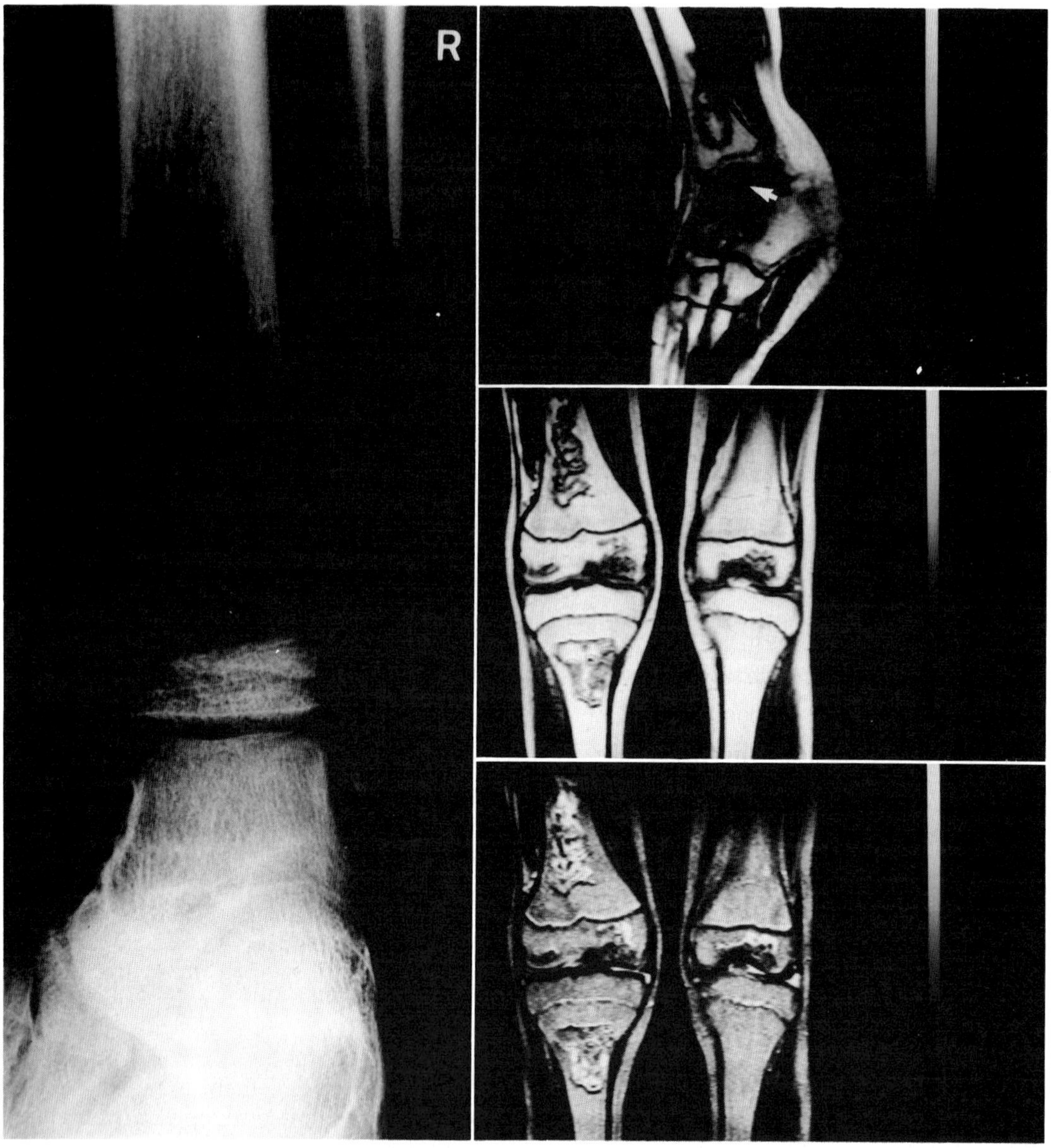

Figure 5-41. **Diagnosis: Complications of leukemia. Marrow infarction.**
***A*, Radiograph of ankle. There is lucency in the medial distal tibia. *B*, MR, T1 weighted image through the ankle. Extensive serpiginous abnormality is seen in the distal tibia consistent with infarction. In addition, there is signal loss in the talus *(white arrow)*, which is unpredicted from plain film findings. *C* and *D*, MR, T1 and T2 weighted images through the knees. Extensive serpiginous abnormality is seen on both sides, consistent with multiple marrow infarct. (From Van Zanten TEG. Nuclear magnetic resonance imaging of bone marrow in childhood leukemia. Clin Radiol 1988;39:77–81.)**

mality. In one study, scattered subcortical calcification on CT were attributed to methotrexate in 10 of 39 patients.[15]

At the present time no routine imaging of CNS is done for diagnosis of leukemic infiltration.

Testis. Occult testicular disease is thought to be present in up to 15 percent of leukemic children at diagnosis.[7] The testis is believed to be a sanctuary site for leukemic cells and late testicular relapse occurs in about 10 percent of patients. This is increasing with prolonged survival and better chemotherapy. Testicular relapse is extremely important, as it may be the initial site of relapse and a site for subsequent seeding of tumor back to the bone marrow. Testicular relapse is more likely in patients in whom the initial white blood cell count was greater than 20,000, the platelet cell count greater than 30,000 per cubic millimeter, and in patients who had enlarged lymph nodes and splenomegaly.[7] The relapse may occur several years after therapy has been stopped. Traditionally, it was believed that ultrasound and other imaging techniques are not adequately sensitive for detection of relapse. There are no large series reported in the last year or two with current high-resolution ultrasound scanners or with current state-of-the-art MR. For many years biopsies were done on patients in remission after therapy had been stopped. About 10 percent of these biopsies were positive.[13] The enthusiasm for performing these biopsies is undergoing reevaluation and is decreasing. One of the reasons is that there is now believed to be a high false negative rate with testicular biopsy.

Ovary. This is a very rare primary site of leukemic relapse. When the ovary is involved, tumor is often found in the uterus and vagina as well. A report of 5 cases and a literature review of 18 additional cases found that ovarian relapse often occurred more than 3 years after initial diagnosis, could involve one or both ovaries, and cause pain as the presenting symptom. Most patients had palpable pelvic masses.[16]

Liver and Spleen. Involvement of the liver and spleen was found in over 60 percent of 755 patients.[17] This incidence approaches 80 percent if there is a mediastinal mass present.[17] Because the identification of disease in the liver and spleen carries no prognostic or therapeutic implications, these organs are not routinely screened. One study utilizing ultrasound[18] reported that leukemia caused diffuse low-level echoes in the liver and spleen that increased in response to therapy.

Chest. An anterior mediastinal mass will be identified in between 5 and 10 percent of leukemic patients at diagnosis.[7] In one large series, a definite mediastinal mass was seen on chest radiograph in 28 of 775 children with acute lymphocytic leukemia.[17] Hilar lymph node enlargement can also be seen.[19] Pulmonary involvement can take the form of diffuse pulmonary infiltrates or a nodular appearance. The appearance may look identical to interstitial pneumonia. The differential diagnosis may be particularly difficult, because patients with pulmonary leukemia may have fever.[13,20] In addition, the pulmonary changes may develop within 24 or 48 hours.[19] The differential diagnosis includes infection, pulmonary edema, pulmonary hemorrhage, pulmonary drug reactions, and transfusion reactions.[19] Although lung involvement is not commonly identified, postmortems of children with leukemia show pulmonary involvement much more often than one would predict from chest radiographs.[21]

Kidney. The kidney is not infrequently involved in acute leukemia. Renal involvement is identified in up to 50 percent of patients at postmortem.[22] The true incidence is not known, because the kidneys are not routinely imaged, again because findings of disease have little impact on therapy or prognosis.

Extensive leukemic infiltration of the kidneys can occur without deterioration of kidney function.[22] Four patterns of abnormality can be identified. There may be unilateral renal enlargement, bilateral renal enlargement, a focal mass in the kidney, or a focal lymph node mass at the hilum of the kidney causing obstruction.[22] Intravenous pyelography will show an increase in renal size and mass effect in some patients. The collecting system may be compressed and distorted. Ultrasound will show decreased echoes in the kidney, increase in renal size, and loss of corticomedullary differentiation. Ultrasound is not as sensitive as CT or MR for detecting change in the kidney. Differential diagnosis includes other causes of diffuse renal enlargement, such as polycystic kidneys and storage disorders, and all other causes of focal renal masses.

Bowel. About 10 percent of children will experience some gastrointestinal abnormality as a result of leukemia.[23] The abnormalities include leukemic infiltration, bowel ulcers and hemorrhage, intussusception, ileus, and typhlitis. These may be caused by the leukemia or chemotoxicity. Decreased immunity will increase the likelihood of infection, abscesses, and typhlitis.

The most troublesome abnormality in the bowel in children with leukemia is typhlitis. This is a necrotizing colitis in the cecum not due to leukemic infiltration. The patients always have a severe neutropenia.[24–26] It can occur in patients with neutropenia caused by other disorders such as aplastic anemia.[25] This disorder involves the cecum and the right colon.[26] There is edema and ulceration followed by secondary infection with a variety of organisms, including clostridia septicum, pseudomonas, and candida.[26,27] In the early 1970s, typhlitis was reported as occurring in terminally ill leukemic children and was found in up to 10 percent of postmortems.[3] With more modern therapy, children are more frequently neutropenic earlier in the disease and typhlitis is being diagnosed more commonly. Imaging is important for diagnosis and management of typhlitis. On plain film radiographs, signs of small bowel obstruction may be seen. Bowel perforation can occur. Gas in the colon may allow identification of thumb printing in the cecum and ascending colon. A mass effect may be seen in the right lower quadrant. Cecal pneumatosis was identified in a quarter of patients and focal distention of the distal ileum in three-quarters.[25] Barium enema will show thick lining of the wall and mucosal folds of the cecum and ascending colon.[25,26] Because of the risks of perforation, barium enema is not the ideal method of investigation. CT is excellent for diagnosis of typhlitis. CT will show cecal wall thickening, thumb printing, and low-density areas caused by hemorrhage and necrosis. An abscess may be identified owing to localized perforation. CT may also be utilized to monitor therapy with findings decreasing with improvement. The treatment of typhlitis is conservative, with surgery being reserved for patients with perforation. Imaging has an important role to play in identification of optimum time for surgery. An occasional complication of typhlitis is marked gastrointestinal hemorrhage, being identified in 3 patients in one study.[28] Angiography in these patients revealed increased vessels, intense mucosal staining and AV shunts. The differential diagnosis of typhlitis includes Henoch Schonlein purpura, hemorrhage with hemolytic uremic syndrome, acute appendicitis, and leukemic infiltration of the bowel. Indolent pneumatosis is usually steroid induced. It is an incidental finding on an abdominal radiograph. It is usually found in children with diminished immunity. It produces no symptoms and resolves spontaneously. Both leukemic cell infiltration or hemorrhage in the bowel tend to be focal and eccentric rather than causing diffuse abnormality as seen with typhlitis. With appendicitis, the degree of thickening of the cecal wall should be much less than is seen with typhlitis.

Eye. This is a rare site of relapse. Leukemia can be seen in the iris or the anterior chamber.

> *Comment.* Leukemia is the most common pediatric malignancy, but the one for which imaging provides the least useful information. Possible significant future roles for imaging will be in detection of relapse in marrow, testis, and central nervous system.

References

1. Moore SG, Gooding CA, Brasch RC, et al. Bone marrow in children with acute lymphocytic leukemia: MR relaxation times. Radiology 1986;160:237–240.
2. Thomsen C, Sorensen PG, Karle H, et al. Prolonged bone marrow T1-relaxation in acute leukaemia. In vivo tissue characterization by magnetic resonance imaging. Mag Reson Imag 1987;5:251–257.
3. Wagner ML, Rosenberg HS, Fernbach DJ, et al. Typhlitis: a complication of leukemia in childhood. AJR 1970; 109:341–350.
4. Jensen KE, Thomsen C, Henriksen O, et al. Changes in T1 relaxation processes in the bone marrow following treatment in children with acute lymphoblastic leukemia. A magnetic resonance imaging study. Pediatr Radiol 1990;20:464–468.
5. Benz-Bohm G, Gross-Fengels W, Bohndorf K, et al. MRI of the knee region in leukemic children. Part II. Follow up: responder, non-responder, relapse. Pediatr Radiol 1990;20:272–276.
6. Rogalsky RJ, Black B, Reed MH. Orthopaedic manifestations of leukemia in children. J Bone Joint Surg 1986;68:494–501.
7. Poplack DG. Acute lymphoblastic leukemia. In: Pizzo PA, Poplack DG, eds. Principles and practice of pediatric oncology. Philadelphia: JB Lippincott, 1989:323–366.
8. Nixon GW, Gwinn JL. The roentgen manifestations of leukemia in infancy. Radiology 1973;107:603–609.
9. Parker BR, Margin S, Castellino RA. Skeletal manifestations of leukemia, Hodgkin disease, and non-Hodgkin lymphoma. Semin Roentgenol 1980;15:302–315.
10. Akber J, Gallagher MT, Mathew L, et al. Destructive skeletal lesions as the primary initial manifestation of acute childhood leukemia. Am J Pediatr Hematol/Oncol 1988;10:258–260.
11. Rosenfield NS, McIntosh S. Prospective analysis of bone changes in treated childhood leukemia. Radiology 1977;123:413–415.
12. Infante AJ, Miller RH, MacRae MA, et al. Intracranial granulocytic sarcoma complicating childhood acute myelomonocytic leukemia. Am J Pediatr Hematol/Oncol 1981;3:173–176.
13. Miller DR. Childhood acute lymphoblastic leukemia: 2. Strategies and innovations for producing more cures. Am J Pediatr Hematol/Oncol 1988;10:174–179.
14. Pedersen H, McConnell J, Harwood-Nash D, et al. Computed tomography in intracranial, supratentorial metastases in children. Neuroradiology 1989;31:19–23.
15. McIntosh S, Fischer DB, Rothman SG, et al. Intracranial calcifications in childhood leukemia. An association with systemic chemotherapy. J Pediatr 1977;91:909–913.
16. Pais RC, Kim TH, Zwiren GT, et al. Ovarian tumors in relapsing acute lymphoblastic leukemia: a review of 23 cases. J Pediatr Surg 1991;26:70–74.
17. Chilcote RR, Coccia P, Sather HN, et al. Mediastinal mass in acute lymphoblastic leukemia. Med Pediatr Oncol 1984;12:9–16.
18. Gore RM, Shkolnik A. Abdominal manifestations of pediatric leukemias: Sonographic assessment. Radiology 1982;143:207–210.
19. Armstrong P, Dyer R, Alford BA, et al. Leukemic pulmonary infiltrates: rapid development mimicking pulmonary edema. AJR 1980;135:373–374.
20. Wells RJ, Weetman RM, Ballantine TVN, et al. Pulmonary leukemia in children presenting as diffuse interstitial pneumonia. J Pediatr 1980;96:262–266.
21. Klatte EC, Yardley J, Smith CB, et al. The pulmonary manifestations and complications of leukemia. AJR 1963;89:598–609.
22. Araki T. Leukemic involvement of the kidney in children: CT features. J Comput Assist Tomogr 1982;6:781–784.
23. Hunter TB, Bjelland JC. Gastrointestinal complications of leukemia and its treatment. AJR 1984;142:513–518.
24. Jaramillo D, Perez-Atayde A, Griscom NT. Apparent association between thymic cysts and prior thoracotomy. Radiology 1989;172:207–209.
25. Frick MP, Maile CW, Crass JR, et al. Computed tomography of neutropenic colitis. AJR 1984;143:763–765.
26. Abramson SJ, Berdon WE, Baker DH. Childhood typhlitis: its increasing association with acute myelogenous leukemia. Radiology 1983;146:61–64.
27. Nixon GW, Gwinn JL. The roentgen manifestations of leukemia in infancy. Radiology 1973;107:603–609.
28. Meyerovitz MF, Fellows KE. Typhlitis: a cause of gastrointestinal hemorrhage in children. AJR 1984;143:833–835.

Differential Diagnosis

Leukemia can present in a wide variety of ways. The differential diagnosis is, therefore, extremely large. Once the diagnosis has been considered it is usually easily made. Many children present with bone or joint pain mimicking juvenile rheumatoid arthritis or diseases causing bone metastases such as neuroblastoma. Other children present with anemia and the differential diagnosis includes all causes of anemia. Similarly all disorders causing hemorrhage and thrombocytopenia are also included in the differential diagnosis.

Therapy and Prognosis

Chemotherapy is the basis of treatment for acute leukemia in children. The chemotherapy regime chosen is very much determined by identifiable prognostic factors, with the most intense therapy utilized in children with poor prognostic factors. Good responders go into remission extremely quickly. If children do relapse, a second remission can be achieved in between 80 and 90 percent. This second remission is most easily achieved in children in whom the relapse was in sanctuary sites (e.g., central nervous system and testicle) rather than in the bone marrow and in patients who are off therapy at the time of relapse.[1]

Children need a minimum of 2 to 3 years of therapy.[1] Radiation therapy has been widely used in recent years as a form of prophylaxis in the central nervous system. This has caused significant reduction in central nervous system disease, but also a significant incidence of side effects. Current therapeutic regimes are aimed at decreasing or avoiding the use of radiation therapy, confining its use to high-risk children.[1] Other regimes attempt a utilization of more intensive chemotherapy, also aimed at reducing or avoiding the requirement for radiation therapy to the central nervous system.

Prognosis in acute lymphocytic leukemia has been related to over 40 different factors.[1] Identification of these prognostic factors is important, because therapy is based on them. Many of these factors are not of great significance. The most important ones are the initial white blood cell count in the peripheral blood, the age of the patient, the rate of initial response, and the FAB characterization of the tumor cells.[2] Factors such as kidney size, bone involvement, liver and spleen involvement are of virtually no prognostic significance.[3] A white blood cell count at diagnosis of over 50,000 per cubic millimeter carries a very poor prognosis.[4] The FAB cell type L3 carries a poor prognosis. Prognosis is worse in children under the age of 2 and over the age of 10 years. Twenty years ago survival in children with acute leukemia was less than 10 percent. This has increased dramatically in recent years, with overall survival now in the range of 65 to 70 percent.[1,2]

Relapse in leukemia is most likely to occur in the marrow, central nervous system, or testicle. Most relapses occur within 24 months after therapy has been stopped.[5]

References

1. Bleyer WA. Remaining problems in the staging and treatment of childhood lymphoblastic leukemia. Am J Pediatr Hematol/Oncol 1989;11:371–379.
2. Miller DR. Childhood acute lymphoblastic leukemia: 1. Biological features and their use in predicting outcome of treatment. Am J Pediatr Hematol/Oncol 1988;10:163–173.
3. Neglia JP, Day DL, Swanson TV, et al. Kidney size at diagnosis of childhood acute lymphocytic leukemia: lack of prognostic significance for outcome. Am J Pediatr Hematol/Oncol 1988;10:296–300.
4. Poplack DG. Acute lymphoblastic leukemia. In: Pizzo PA, Poplack DG, eds. Principles and practice of pediatric oncology. Philadelphia: JB Lippincott, 1989:323–366.
5. Miller DR. Childhood acute lymphoblastic leukemia: 2. Strategies and innovations for producing more cures. Am J Pediatr Hematol/Oncol 1988;10:174–179.

PROBLEMS WITH LEUKEMIA

From a clincal viewpoint, major problems still exist with regard to a standardized staging system and the marked inconsistency between various reports with regard to many of the identified prognostic factors.[1] There is no method available for detection of small foci of residual tumor or very early recurrence.[1] Cranial radiotherapy has resulted in significantly improved survival, but at a price of significant complications.[2] The optimum time for duration of therapy for children with leukemia is still not known.[2] From an imaging point of view, leukemia may be identified as an incidental, unexpected finding when imaging is performed because of unexplained clinical symptoms. Apart from this, the vast majority of leukemic children are imaged usually only for the identification and management of complications of leukemia and not to aid in the management of the disease process itself (see Fig. 5–41). One study done to determine the role of imaging in follow-up of patients in remission covered 29 children.[3] Extensive imaging including CT, ultrasound, gallium scanning, and skeletal survey identified virtually no abnormality. The only two children in whom disease was found had a testicular tumor, which was diagnosed by biopsy and not imaging.[3]

What are the future roles of imaging in leukemia? I remain somewhat skeptical with regard to the ability of MR to be used as a method for screening for relapse. Certainly in the central nervous system, MR can provide outstanding information with regard to secondary effects from radiation therapy. Perhaps it can be used to titrate a dose of prophylactic therapy rather than to detect disease only after such therapy has been completed.

References

1. Bleyer WA. Remaining problems in the staging and treatment of childhood lymphoblastic leukemia. Am J Pediatr Hematol/Oncol 1989;11:371–379.
2. Miller DR. Childhood acute lymphoblastic leukemia: 1. Biological features and their use in predicting outcome of treatment. Am J Pediatr Hematol/Oncol 1988;10:163–173.
3. Parker BR, Margin S, Castellino RA. Skeletal manifestations of leukemia, Hodgkin disease, and non-Hodgkin lymphoma. Semin Roentgenol 1980;15:302–315.

CHAPTER 6
ENDOCRINE TUMORS

NEUROBLASTOMA

Epidemiology

Neuroblastoma occurs with an incidence of approximately 9 cases per million children under the age of 15 years per annum.[1] This translates into approximately 500 new cases presenting each year in the United States,[2,3] which is about 8 percent of all pediatric cancer.[1]

Neuroblastoma is a cancer of the very young, with the mean age at the time of presentation variously reported as 20 months,[4] 2 years,[3] and 2½ years.[5] Seventy-five percent of cases occur under the age of 5 years.[2] Unlike Wilms tumor, neuroblastoma can be present at birth. The percentage of cases presenting in the first year of life ranges from 15 percent,[1] 25 percent,[6,7] up to 33 percent.[2] Certain subgroups of neuroblastoma patients are particulalry common in the first year of life. This includes patients with a cervical location of the primary tumor[8] and patients with stage IV-S neuroblastoma. These latter patients are almost invariably under the age of 1 year, with several series reporting that 100 percent of patients are less than 1 year old.[7,9–11] Of all tumors presenting in the neonatal period (the first month of life), neuroblastoma is the most common, accounting for 50 percent of such malignancies.[12]

Although there are isolated reports of the association of neuroblastoma with, for example, the fetal hydantoin syndrome,[13] Beckwith syndrome,[14] and clusters of tumor within families,[15] there is no consistent link with any teratogen or genetic disease.[3]

> *Comment:* Unlike Wilms tumor, no high-risk groups for the development of neuroblastoma have been identified and there is no routine imaging screening recommended.

References

1. Brodeur GM, Seeger RC, Barrett A, et al. International criteria for diagnosis, staging, and response to treatment in patients with neuroblastoma. J Clin Oncol 1988;6:1874–1881.
2. Davis S, Rogers MAM, Pendergrass TW. The incidence and epidemiologic characteristics of neuroblastoma in the United States. Am J Epidemiol 1987;126:1063–1074.
3. Kushner DH, Cheung N-KV. Neuroblastoma. Pediatr Ann 1988;17:269–283.
4. Martin-Simmerman P, Cohen MD, Siddiqui A, et al. Calcification and uptake of Tc-99m diphosphonates in neuroblastomas: concise communication. J Nucl Med 1984;25:656–660.
5. Dehner LP. Pediatric surgical pathology, 2nd ed. Baltimore: Williams & Wilkins, 1987:562–574.
6. Cassady JR. A hypothesis to explain the enigmatic natural history of neuroblastoma. Med Pediatr Oncol 1984;12:64–67.
7. Grosfeld JL, Baehner RL. Neuroblastoma: an analysis of 160 cases. World J Surg 1980;4:29–38.
8. Cushing BA, Slovis TL, Philippart AI, et al. A rational approach to cervical neuroblastoma. Cancer 1982;50:785–787.
9. Evans AE, Chatten J, D'Angio GJ, et al. A review of 17 IV-S neuroblastoma patients at the Children's Hospital of Philadelphia. Cancer 1980;45:833–839.
10. Evans AE, Baum E, Chard R. Do infants with stage IV-S neuroblastoma need treatment? Arch Dis Child 1981;56:271–274.
11. Franken EA, Smith WL, Cohen MD, et al. Hepatic imaging in stage IV-S neuroblastoma. Pediatr Radiol 1986;16:107–109.
12. Forman HP, Leonidas JC, Berdon WE, et al. Congenital neuroblastoma. Evaluation with multimodality imaging. Radiology 1990;175:365–369.
13. Allen RW, Ogdon B, Bentley FL, et al. Fetal hydantoin syndrome, neuroblastoma, and hemorrhagic disease in a neonate. JAMA 1980;244:1464–1465.
14. Emery LG, Shields M, Shah NR, et al. Neuroblastoma associated with Beckwith-Wiedemann syndrome. Cancer 1983;52:176–179.
15. Hayes FA, Smith EI. Neuroblastoma. In: Pizzo PA, Poplack DG, eds. Principles and practice of pediatric oncology. Philadelphia: JB Lippincott, 1989:607–622.

Pathology

Neuroblastoma arises from neural crest tissue[1,2] and, therefore, can be found at any site along the sympathetic nervous system chain or in the adrenal medulla.[3] It has very rarely been reported in the pancreas.[4] Neuroblastoma is unique among all human cancer in that it has an unusual ability to regress spontaneously with complete resolution of tumor or to mature without therapy into a benign ganglioneuroma.[5] Spontaneous regression is particularly common in the very young, and this may allow many cases of neuroblastoma to escape clinical detection completely.[6] This supposition is supported by the finding of neuroblastoma cells on histologic section of the adrenal medulla in a high percentage of early aborted fetuses. Following almost complete resection of a neuroblastoma, microscopic residual tumor can also resolve spontaneously without the need for further treatment.[7,8]

The distribution of the anatomic site of the primary tumor is described in Table 6–1. As can be seen, approximately 40 percent of the tumors arise from the adrenal gland. Different series report slight modifications of this distribution. Note that in up to 10 percent of patients, the location of the primary tumor may not be determined. I anticipate that with the improved imaging ability of a new generation of CT and ultrasound machines and with increased use of magnetic resonance imaging the number of primary tumors that go undetected will decrease.

> *Comment:* Many children with neuroblastoma will present with signs and symptoms of disseminated disease. If the primary tumor is not detected clinically, the radiologist will be called upon to locate this primary tumor, and knowledge of the distribution and location of primary tumors is important. Spontaneous regression will result in a small number of primary tumors that are never found by imaging. Failure to locate a primary tumor should not exclude a diagnosis of neuroblastoma.

Neuroblastomas are usually solid tumors of varying size. They are often very large in the abdomen and pelvis and smaller in the chest and neck. The large tumors often show areas of hemorrhage and necrosis on cut sections. These are identified on imaging with particular characteristics, depending on the modality utilized. There are a few reports of truly cystic neuroblastomas,[9–11] but these are extremely rare. These patients all tend to be less than 3 months old, with the diagnosis having been made antenatally in 2 patients.[10] The cystic areas are well defined and may be true cysts or may represent areas of very old resolving hemorrhage. The cysts may be single or multiple and may vary in size up to 5 cm in diameter. There may be no large areas of microscopic tumor, with neuroblastoma being identified only histologically in the walls of the cystic area.

TABLE 6–1
Anatomic Site of Primary Neuroblastoma

Site	Percentage of Cases
Adrenal gland	40
Other abdominal sites	25
Posterior mediastinum	15
Neck	5
Pelvis	5
Unknown	10

> *Comment:* Hemorrhage and necrosis are common in large tumors and cause a heterogeneous appearance on imaging.

Neuroblastoma may remain localized or demonstrate extensive local spread. Stage I lesions are well encapsulated, round, or ovoid, with no local invasion. Sympathetic chain tumors lie in the paravertebral sulcus[12] and may show permeative spread along neurovascular bundles.[12] This growth may extend through the intervertebral foramina, causing extradural compression of the spinal cord.[6] These "dumbbell" lesions can occur at any level in the spinal cord.[13] Adrenal primary tumors spread in the perirenal space along the vessels. It has been demonstrated that the anterior renal fascia extends across the midline, as does the perirenal space behind it.[14] The tumor grows in the perirenal space to encase and displace the aorta and inferior vena cava and then spreads along major branches of the aorta through the peritoneal folds and ligaments in which these vessels lie, e.g., into the gastrohepatic ligament.[14] The tumor may also spread along the renal vessels, invading the hilum of the kidney.[15] Invasion of the inferior vena cava rarely occurs.

> *Comment:* The permeative spreading of neuroblastoma accounts for the extensive encasement of the aorta and inferior vena cava, and the extension of this tumor into the spinal canal, which is not seen with many other tumors, for example, Wilms tumor.

At the time of initial diagnosis, metastatic spread is present in up to 70 percent of patients with neuroblastoma. Two distinct patterns of spread can be identified, depending on the age of the patient. In the very young, up to 1 year of age, metastases are predominantly to liver, bone marrow, and skin, with some spread to lymph nodes. Over the age of 1 year, metastatic spread is predominantly to bone cortex, lymph nodes, liver, and bone marrow. Stage IV-S neuroblastoma occurs almost exclusively under the age of 1 year; the location of metastasis in these patients is seen in Table 6–2. In a literature review of 126 patients with stage IV-S neuroblastoma, 4 percent were found to be over the age of 1 year at the time of presentation.

Bone cortical metastases may be single, but are frequently multiple. They may be symmetrical. They are particularly common in the skull and are seen in any bone except for the hands, feet, and clavicles. In the skull, the metastases often have a large soft-tissue component, which may project outward as a clinically de-

TABLE 6-2
Location of Metastases in Patients with Stage IV-S Neuroblastoma[1,2]

Location	Percentage of Cases
Liver	83–94
Skin	18–26
Bone marrow	33–50

References
1. Franken EA, Smith WL, Cohen MD, et al. Hepatic imaging in stage IV-S neuroblastoma. Pediatr Radiol 1986;16:107–109.
2. Evans AE, Baum E, Chard R. Do infants with stage IV-S neuroblastoma need treatment? Arch Dis Child 1981;56:271–274.

tectable lump or inward as a space-occupying lesion displacing the dura. Primary dural metastases are also common. These lie on the outer surface of the dura, causing invagination of the dura. They rarely penetrate through the dura. They may invade or erode the adjacent bone and may penetrate all the way through it.[6,16,17] These metastases may invade and erode the margins of the sutures, creating a false impression of suture widening and raised intracranial pressure. Metastases to the sphenoid bone may extend into the orbit, causing proptosis. Primary orbital soft-tissue metastases also occur. Bone marrow metastases are present in between 40 and 60 percent of patients at the time of initial presentation.[18,19] These may occur as single or multiple focal deposits of tumor, or in severe cases there may be extensive infiltration of tumor throughout the bone marrow space.

In older patients, liver metastases tend to be well defined and single or multiple. In the very young, they are commonly seen as diffuse infiltrating tumor, replacing the entire liver. Metastases may even occur to ectopic liver tissue.[20] Lymph node metastases are common at any age. The involved lymph nodes may become extremely large.

Other sites of metastases are rare, but recognition and knowlege of them is important. Neuroblastoma can occasionally be found in the pancreas and spleen. Focal testicular metastases have been identified[21]; these were identified without diffuse metastatic spread in other locations. Kidney, ovary, thymus, brain, eyes, and heart are other described locations for metastases.[22,23] Lung metastases tend to be found in patients with widespread disseminated disease and in these patients are not an infrequent incidental finding at postmortem, although they may not have been diagnosed before death.[24] They may be identified in up to 22 percent of such postmortems.[25] Lung involvement with neuroblastoma may be the result of direct invasion of the lung, infiltration of the pulmonary lymphatics, or diffuse hematogenous spread.[24] Primary brain parenchymal metastases from neuroblastoma have been described in three cases.[16] In most cases, this is believed to be caused by local invasion of the spinal canal, with penetration through the meninges and subsequent CSF spread.[16] Note that raised intracranial pressure in patients with neuroblastoma can occur. It may be caused by parenchymal metastases, space occupation by large dural metastases, or obstruction of venous sinuses by compression of dural metastases.[16,17]

> *Comment:* Location of metastases is age dependent, and imaging studies seeking these lesions need to take into account the age of the patient. Bone marrow and bone cortical metastases are independent events. While spread can occur from marrow to cortex, or from cortex to marrow, this is frequently not the case. Separate imaging techniques must, therefore, be utilized to seek marrow metastases and cortical metastases.

Unlike Wilms tumor, which is bilateral in a significant number of cases, neuroblastoma almost always has a single primary lesion. There are isolated case reports of simultaneous primary lesions in the adrenal and posterior mediastinal or in both adrenal glands.[26]

There are three different staging systems about which the radiologist must be aware. These are the Evans (Table 6–3), Pediatric Oncology Group (Table 6–4), and International Staging System (Table 6–5). The Evans System has been in widespread use for almost 20 years. It is the classification system used by the Children's Cancer Study Group, and it has also been used in many other studies of neuroblastoma. Changes in the

TABLE 6-3
Evans Staging System for Neuroblastoma

Stage	Description
I	Tumor is confined to organ of origin (totally excised)
II	Tumor extends beyond organ of origin, but does not cross the midline; regional lymph nodes may be involved
III	Tumor extends beyond midline to encroach on tissues on opposite side
IV	Distant metastases (skeletal, other organs, soft tissues, distant lymph nodes)
IV-S	Localized primary tumor not crossing midline with remote disease confined to liver, subcutaneous tissues, and bone marrow, but without evidence of bone cortex involvement

Notes:
1. IV-S tumor definition does not have an age limit, although almost all cases turn out to be <1 year old.
2. Midline extension is not to be diagnosed on the basis of a pedunculated tumor overhanging the midline. There must be direct tumor infiltration across the midline.

TABLE 6–4
Pediatric Oncology Group Staging System for Neuroblastoma[1,2]

Stage	Description
A	Complete resection of localized primary tumor
B	Incomplete resection of primary tumor. Nodes and liver negative
C	Complete or incomplete resection of primary tumor; nodes positive, liver negative
D	Disseminated metastatic tumor

References
1. Bousvaros A, Kirks DR, Grossman H. Imaging of neuroblastoma: an overview. Pediatr Radiol 1986;16:89–106.
2. Hayes FA, Smith EI. Neuroblastoma. In: Pizzo PA, Poplack DG, eds. Principles and practice of pediatric oncology. Philadelphia: JB Lippincott, 1989:607–622.

TABLE 6–5
International Staging System for Neuroblastoma[1]

Stage	Description
1	Localized tumor confined to the area of origin; complete gross excision with or without microscopic residual disease; identifiable ipsilateral and contralateral lymph nodes negative microscopically
2A	Unilateral tumor with incomplete gross excision; identifiable ipsilateral and contralateral lymph nodes negative microscopically
2B	Unilateral tumor with complete or incomplete gross excision; with positive ipsilateral regional lymph nodes; identifiable contralateral lymph nodes negative microscopically
3	Tumor infiltrating across the midline with or without regional lymph node involvement; or, unilateral tumor with contralateral regional lymph node involvement; or, midline tumor with bilateral regional lymph node involvement
4	Dissemination of tumor to distant lymph nodes, bone, bone marrow, liver, or other organs (except as defined in stage 4S)
4S	Localized primary tumor as defined for stage 1 or 2 with dissemination limited to liver, skin, or bone marrow

Reference
1. Brodeur GM, Seeger RC, Barrett A, et al. International criteria for diagnosis, staging, and response to treatment in patients with neuroblastoma. J Clin Oncol 1988;6:1874–1881.

knowledge of the biological behavior and therapy of neuroblastoma have resulted in several valid criticisms of this staging mechanism. First, it takes no account of the resectability of the tumor and second, patients may be placed at stage II or III regardless of the presence or absence of tumor in regional lymph nodes.[6,27] Recent studies have indicated that prognosis is dependent upon the tumor resection and that it is also dependent upon the presence or absence of lymph node tumor in stage II disease.[28] The Pediatric Oncology Group Staging System (Table 6–4) takes account of these factors. In order to permit a comparison of children in different countries, an International Staging System for neuroblastoma has recently been described and it is believed that this system will get widespread acceptance[19] (Table 6–5). Tables 6–6 and 6–7 illustrate the distribution of patients among the various stages at the time of presentation. Up to 60 percent of patients will have disseminated disease at the time of presentation.

TABLE 6–6
Stage of Patients with Neuroblastoma (All Ages)[1–3]

Stage	Percentage of Patients
I	3–13
II	11–20
III	8–16
IV	43–60
IV-S	9–10

References
1. Grosfeld JL, Baehner RL. Neuroblastoma: an analysis of 160 cases. World J Surg 1980;4:29–38.
2. Bousvaros A, Kirks DR, Grossman H. Imaging of neuroblastoma: an overview. Pediatr Radiol 1986; 16:89–106.
3. Foglia RP, Fonkalsrud EW, Feig SA, et al. Accuracy of diagnostic imaging as determined by delayed operative intervention for advanced neuroblastoma. J Pediatr Surg 1989;24:708–711.

TABLE 6–7
Stage of Neonatal (<1 Month Old) Neuroblastoma[1]

Stage	Number	Percentage
I	1	6
II	3	17
III	0	0
IV	3	17
IV-S	10	60

Reference
1. Isaacs H Jr. Congenital and neonatal malignant tumors. A 28-year experience at Children's Hospital of Los Angeles. Am J Pediatr Hematol/Oncol 1987;9:121–129.

> *Comment:* The radiologist must be aware of the new International Staging System for Neuroblastoma.
>
> Up to 60 percent of patients have metastatic disease at presentation. Extensive use of imaging to seek metastatic disease is, therefore, very appropriate.
>
> Primary neck tumors are much more commonly stage I or II.[29]

Evaluation of catecholamine concentration in the urine provides a good tumor marker in patients with neuroblastoma. Catecholamines (VMA, HVA) are produced by between 85 and 95 percent of neuroblastomas.[3,30–32] The urine concentration of catecholamine falls in response to therapy.[6]

> *Comment:* Measurement of urinary catecholamine excretion is helpful in diagnosis and monitoring of therapy in patients with neuroblastoma.

Histologic subclassification of neuroblastoma has recently become important.[31,33] For many years neuroblastomas were categorized as either pure neuroblastoma or ganglioneuroblastoma, with some belief that the latter tumors did better. This designation has, however, been criticized as it is arbitrary and subject to marked sampling areas.[31] as most neuroblastomas have a very variable histologic appearance through the tumor. The Shimada classification[33] has the advantage of relying on few subjective observations. Tumors are classified as stroma rich or stroma poor, depending on the content of background stroma and an MKI index (mitotic karyorrhexis) is calculated. This index is the number of cells per 5,000 showing mitosis or nuclear fragmentation. In addition, tumors are classified as undifferentiated or differentiated.[33] The combination of these findings together with the patient's age is very helpful in prognosis and this is discussed in some detail later.

Pathology techniques continue to improve. A study published in 1991 reported use of immune staining of marrow aspirates using labeled antibody to neuroblastoma cells. Examination of marrow aspirates in 197 patients was performed. Using routine stains, 46 percent of patients showed tumor in the bone marrow. Using the new immune stains, 67 percent of patients were positive for tumor.[34] Of particular significance was the fact that in patients with stage II or III, the demonstration of these "occult" marrow metastases using immune stains indicated a significantly worse prognosis.

References

1. Carlsen NLT, Nielsen OH, Hertz H. Neuroblastoma. Acta Paediatr Scand 1981;70:61–66.
2. Triche TJ, Askin RB. Neuroblastoma and the differential diagnosis of small-, round-, blue-cell tumors. Hum Pathol 1983;14:569–578.
3. Grosfeld JL, Baehner RL. Neuroblastoma: an analysis of 160 cases. World J Surg 1980;4:29–38.
4. Chapman P, Carter RL, Clifford P. The diagnosis and surgical management of olfactory neuroblastoma: the role of craniofacial resection. J Laryngol Otol 1981;95:785–799.
5. Evans AE, D'Angio GJ, Propert K, et al. Prognostic factors in neuroblastoma. Cancer 1987;59:1853–1859.
6. Kushner DH, Cheung N-KV. Neuroblastoma. Pediatr Ann 1988;17:269–283.
7. Hayes FA, Smith EI. Neuroblastoma. In: Pizzo PA, Poplack DG, eds. Principles and practice of pediatric oncology. Philadelphia: JB Lippincott, 1989:607–622.
8. Cassady JR. A hypothesis to explain the enigmatic natural history of neuroblastoma. Med Pediatr Oncol 1984;12:64–67.
9. Garick DJ, Kodroff MB, Marrow HG, et al. Thoracic neuroblastoma presenting as a cystic hygroma. Arch Dis Childh 1988;63:1270–1271.
10. Atkinson GO, Zaatari GS, Lorenzo RI. Cystic neuroblastoma in infants: radiographic and pathologic features. AJR 1986;146:113–117.
11. Hendry GMA. Cystic neuroblastoma of the adrenal gland—a potential source of error in ultrasound diagnosis. Pediatr Radiol 1982;12:204–206.
12. Adam A, Hochholzer L. Ganglioneuroblastoma of the posterior mediastinum: a clinicopathologic review of 80 cases. Cancer 1981;47:373–381.
13. Punt J, Pritchard J, Pincott JR, et al. Neuroblastoma: a review of 21 cases presenting with spinal cord compression. Cancer 1980;45:3095–3101.
14. Oliphant M, Berne AS. Mechanism of direct spread of abdominal neuroblastoma: CT demonstration and clinical implications. Gastrointest Radiol 1987;12:59–66.
15. Oliphant M, Berne AS. Aggressive neuroblastoma simulating Wilms tumor. Radiology 1988;167:878.
16. Dresler S, Harvey DG, Levisohn PM. Retroperitoneal neuroblastoma widely metastatic to the central nervous system. Ann Neurol 1979;5:196–198.
17. Latchaw RE, L'Heureaux PRL, Young G, et al. Neuroblastoma presenting as central nervous system disease. AJNR 1982;3:623–630.
18. Belasco J. Occult neuroblastoma: difficulties of diagnosis. Am J Dis Child 1979;133:858–859.
19. Brodeur GM, Seeger RC, Barrett A, et al. International criteria for diagnosis, staging, and response to treatment in patients with neuroblastoma. J Clin Oncol 1988;6:1874–1881.
20. Tsuchida Y, Yokomori K, Saito S, et al. Stage IV-S neuroblastoma involving the liver and ectopic liver. Cancer 1984;53:1609–1611.
21. Casola G, Scheible W, Leopold GR. Neuroblastoma metastatic to the testis: ultrasonographic screening as an aid to clinical staging. Radiology 1984;151:475–476.
22. Filiatrault D, Hoyoux C, Benoit P, et al. Renal metastases from neuroblastoma. Pediatr Radiol 1987;17:137–138.
23. Gallet BL, Egelhoff JC. Unusual CNS and orbital metastases of neuroblastoma. Pediatr Radiol 1989;19:287–289.
24. Stigall R, Smith WL, Franken EA, et al. Intrapulmonic metastatic neuroblastoma. Ann Radiol 1979;22:223–227.
25. Towbin R, Gruppo RA. Pulmonary metastases in neuroblastoma. AJR 1982;138:75–78.
26. Kramer SA, Bradford WD, Anderson EE. Bilateral adrenal neuroblastoma. Cancer 1980;45:2208–2212.
27. Hayes FA, Green A, Hustu HO, et al. Surgicopathologic staging of neuroblastoma: prognostic significance of regional lymph node metastases. J Pediatr 1983;102:59–62.
28. Ninane J, Pritchard J, Jones PHM, et al. Stage II neuroblastoma. Adverse prognostic significance of lymph node involvement. Arch Dis Child 1982;57:438–442.
29. Cushing BA, Slovis TL, Philippart AI, et al. A rational ap-

proach to cervical neuroblastoma. Cancer 1982;50:785–787.
30. Friedland GW, Crowe JE. Neuroblastoma and other adrenal neoplasms. In: Parker BR, Castellino RA, eds. Pediatric oncologic radiology. CV Mosby, 1977:267–271.
31. Dehner LP. Classic neuroblastoma: histopathologic grading as a prognostic indicator. The Shimada System and its progenitors. Am J Pediatr Hematol/Oncol 1988;10:143–154.
32. Finklestein JZ. Neuroblastoma: it is time for a new approach. Am J Pediatr Hematol/Oncol 1988;10:155–160.
33. Shimada H, Chatten J, Newton WA, et al. Histopathologic prognostic factors in neuroblastic tumors: definition of subtypes of ganglioneuroblastoma and an age-linked classification of neuroblastomas. JNCI 1984;73:405–416.
34. Moss TJ, Reynolds CP, Sather HN, et al. Prognostic value of immunocytologic detection of bone marrow metastases in neuroblastoma. N Engl J Med 1991;342:219–226.

Clinical Presentation

Clinical signs and symptoms are summarized in Table 6–8. There are a number of points regarding the clinical findings that need to be discussed.

1. Unlike Wilms tumor, patients with neuroblastoma are often quite sick at the time of presentation, with systemic symptoms being present in over two-thirds of patients. This is because of the widespread metastatic disease present in so many patients.
2. The clinical features are caused by local effects, effects of metastatic disease, or a variety of other effects, including hormone production by the tumor.
3. There is often delay in making the diagnosis with a significant period of time from the initial onset of symptoms until neuroblastoma is diagnosed.[1]
4. Opsomyoclonus consists of acute cerebellar ataxia with jerky muscle movements and abnormal jerky eye movements.[2] About 50 percent of patients with this clinical syndrome have neuroblastoma. Of all patients with neuroblastoma, about 2 percent have opsomyoclonus.[2] Of interest are the facts that the primary tumor is more frequently in the chest,[3] these patients often have a better prognosis than other patients with neuroblastoma,[3] and the symptoms may persist even after removal of the primary tumor.[4]
5. Hypertension is relatively uncommon, occurring in less than 10 percent of patients.[3]
6. In neonates with stage IV-S neuroblastoma, the liver may be massively enlarged. This enlargement can cause severe symptoms of respiratory embarrassment. Compression of the inferior vena cava may obstruct blood flow from the kidneys and result in renal failure.
7. Refractory diarrhea is a presenting sign in less than 10 percent of patients. This diarrhea is caused by the secretion of vasoactive intestinal polypeptide (VIP) from the tumor.[5,6]

References

1. Wilson LMK, Draper GJ. Neuroblastoma, its natural history and prognosis: a study of 487 cases. Br Med J 1974;3:301–307.
2. Altman AJ, Baehner RL. Favorable prognosis for survival in children with coincident opso-myoclonus and neuroblastoma. Cancer 1976;37:846–852.
3. Bousvaros A, Kirks DR, Grossman H. Imaging of neuroblastoma: an overview. Pediatr Radiol 1986;16:89–106.
4. Kushner DH, Cheung N-KV. Neuroblastoma. Pediatr Ann 1988;17:269–283.
5. Grosfeld JL, Baehner RL. Neuroblastoma: an analysis of 160 cases. World J Surg 1980;4:29–38.
6. Tiedemann K, Pritchard J, Long R, et al. Intractable diarrhoea in a patient with vasoactive intestinal peptide-secreting neuroblastoma. Eur J Pediatr 1981;137:217–219.

Imaging Studies

IMAGING BY MODALITY

Chest Radiograph. A posterior mediastinal neuroblastoma may be an incidental finding on a chest radiograph performed for other reasons (Fig. 6–1). A chest radiograph should be obtained in all patients with suspected or known neuroblastoma in any location. Primary thoracic neuroblastomas can be located in the apex of the thorax or in the posterior mediastinum (Fig. 6–2). The tumors are usually of moderate size but can occasionally be very large. They appear as homogenous soft-tissue densities with no cavitation. Calcification is only recognized in about 15 percent of patients. Most of the tumors have a vertical elongated shape with tapered edges rather than the formation of a sulcus adjoining the superior and inferior aspects of the tumor with the mediastinal shadows (Fig. 6–2). The margin of the tumor appears smooth or lobulated.

Malignancy is strongly suspected by the identification of separation of the ribs, invasion of the ribs or ad-

Figure 6–1. Diagnosis: Neuroblastoma. Incidental finding in a newborn.
Chest radiograph. There is a right superior/posterior mediastinal mass, which was an incidental finding on chest radiograph. At surgery this was a neuroblastoma. *Arrow* = tumor.

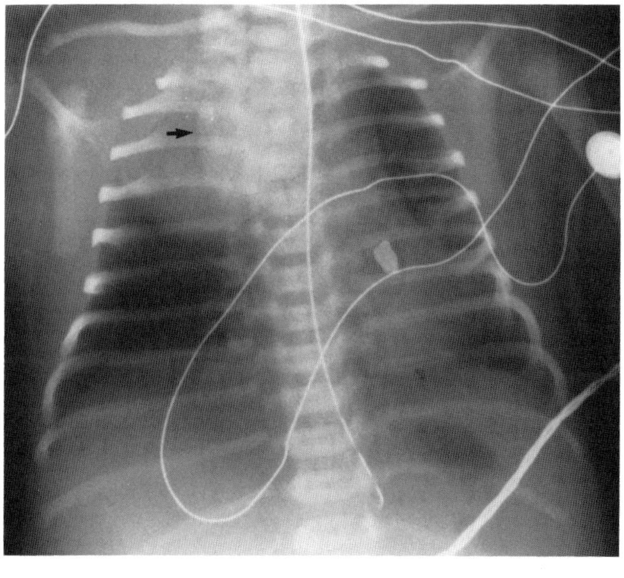

TABLE 6-8
Clinical Signs and Symptoms of Neuroblastoma

Local effects
- Neck tumors[1]—incidental mass, dysphagia, cough, wheeze, dyspnea
- Mediastinal tumors—incidental chest radiograph abnormality, dyspnea, wheeze, Horners syndrome[2] and heterochromia (each iris is a different color)[3,4]
- Chylothorax from lymphatic obstruction[5]
- Abdominal tumor—Nil, pain, incidental mass, hypertension (from compression of renal vessels)[6]
- Pelvic—altered bowel or bladder habit, pain
- Spinal invasion—acute or chronic neurologic dysfunction (bowel, bladder paralysis)

Effects of metastatic disease
- Skull—scalp mass, pain, proptosis[7]
- Liver—abdominal mass (especially in babies)[8,9]
- Systemic effects—ill, fatigue, weight loss, poor appetite, anemia, bruising

Other effects
- Opsomyoclonus[10]
- Refractory diarrhea[11]
- Flushing and sweating[12]

References

1. Smith MCF, Smith RJH, Bailey CM. Primary cervical neuroblastoma in infants. J Laryngol Otol 1985;99:209–214.
2. Beckerman BL, Seaver R. Congenital Horner's syndrome and thoracic neuroblastoma. J Pediatr Ophthalmol 1978;15:24–25.
3. Cushing BA, Slovis TL, Philippart AI, et al. A rational approach to cervical neuroblastoma. Cancer 1982;50:785–787.
4. Kushner DH, Cheung N-KV. Neuroblastoma. Pediatr Ann 1988;17:269–283.
5. Easa D, Balaraman V, Ash K, et al. Congenital chylothorax and mediastinal neuroblastoma. J Pediatr Surg 1991;26:96–98.
6. Bousvaros A, Kirks DR, Grossman H. Imaging of neuroblastoma: an overview. Pediatr Radiol 1986;16:89–106.
7. Aghadiuno PU, Thomas SM, Ogan O, et al. Olfactory neuroblastoma. A case report in an African child. J Laryngol Otol 1983;97:261–265.
8. Isaacs H Jr. Congenital and neonatal malignant tumors. A 28-year experience at Children's Hospital of Los Angeles. Am J Pediatr Hematol/Oncol 1987;9:121–129.
9. Forman HP, Leonidas JC, Berdon WE, et al. Congenital neuroblastoma. Evaluation with multimodality imaging. Radiology 1990;175:365–369.
10. Altman AJ, Baehner RL. Favorable prognosis for survival in children with coincident opso-myoclonus and neuroblastoma. Cancer 1976;37:846–852.
11. Tiedemann K, Pritchard J, Long R, et al. Intractable diarrhoea in a patient with vasoactive intestinal peptide-secreting neuroblastoma. Eur J Pediatr 1981;137:217–219.
12. Friedland GW, Crowe JE. Neuroblastoma and other adrenal neoplasms. In: Parker BR, Castellino RA, eds. Pediatric oncologic radiology. CV Mosby, 1977: 267–271.

jacent vertebra, or widening of the intervertebral foramina. Invasion of the pleura is suspected by the identification of a pleural effusion.[1] Pulmonary involvement with neuroblastoma[2,3] is often an incidental finding at postmortem, with the chest radiograph taken before death appearing normal. When the chest radiograph is abnormal, the pattern is varied and nonspecific. There may be a diffuse interstitial abnormality, an appearance resembling pulmonary edema, diffuse or focal, small or large unilateral or bilateral nodules.[2,3] It must be emphasized that findings of pulmonary disease in neuroblastoma are exceedingly uncommon. Widening of the paravertebral stripe in the lower thorax may be an indication of lymph node spread from an abdominal primary tumor, into the para-aortic lymph nodes and through the diaphragm hiatus. Bone metastasis to spine or ribs may be identified on the chest radiograph.

Abdominal Radiograph. This should be obtained in all patients with neuroblastoma. This radiograph may be entirely normal. A mass lesion may be suspected by displacement of bowel or by loss of the outline of the psoas muscle. Tumor calcification may be detected in up to

A B C

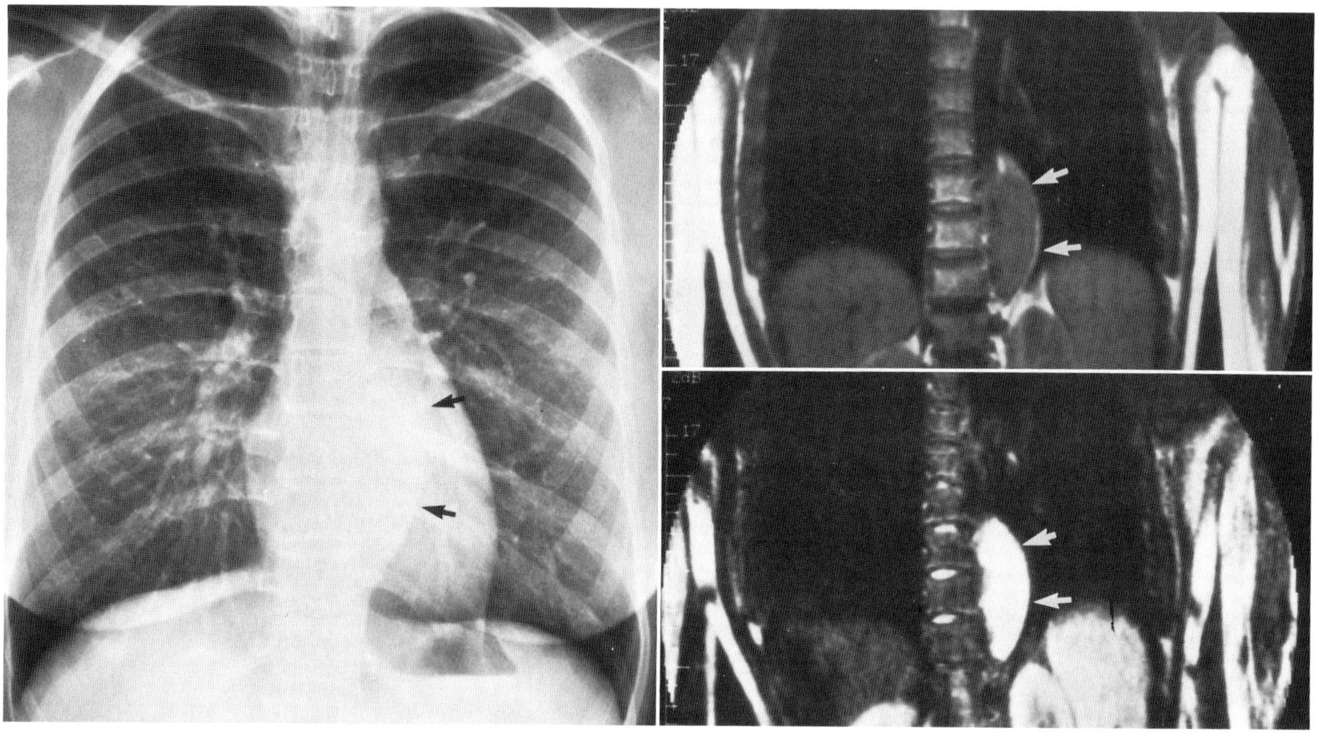

Figure 6–2. Diagnosis: Thoracic neuroblastoma.
A, **Chest radiograph. A posterior mediastinal paraspinal mass is identified *(arrows)*. *B* and *C*, MR, T1, and T2 weighted coronal images. The tumor is well identified *(arrows)*. Note the tapered superior and inferior margins. The lesion is of similar intensity to liver on T1 and very bright on T2 weighted image.**

two-thirds of patients.[4] Metastatic disease to bones may be identified. Direct invasion of the spinal canal is suspected by the presence of vertebral abnormality.

Intravenous Urogram. Until about 10 years ago this investigation was widely used to evaluate neuroblastoma. There should be no place for its current use. Unfortunately, the use of intravenous pyelography is still recommended in some imaging protocols. Intravenous pyelography will miss over one-third of abdominal tumors.[5] It cannot define the size of the tumor or its local or distant spread in the abdomen.[5] Intravenous pyelography provides no information that is not readily available from other imaging modalities.

Angiography. Angiography was once a part of the routine evaluation of abdominal tumors. Over the past 10 years it has seldom been used. Two recent reports suggest specific indications for which an angiogram might be helpful. In planning radical excision of a tumor, either on presentation or following chemotherapy or radiation therapy, it might be helpful for the surgeon to know if the kidney has been invaded and requires resection with the tumor mass. Angiographic signs of renal invasion are tumor vessels arising from the renal capsular, perforating, or intrarenal arteries.[6] To predict the resectability of tumor around the aorta, a lateral angiogram has been used. Calculations of the distance between the spine and the aorta, between the superior mesenteric artery and the aorta, and the angle between the superior mesenteric artery and the aorta have been found to be helpful in predicting resectability of the tumor.[7] While these angiographic findings may be helpful to some surgeons, my own view is that modern CT, ultrasound, and MR should provide at least the equivalent information, if not more. I do not believe that angiography has any place in the evaluation of patients with neuroblastoma.

Plain Film Radiographs of the Bones. These may show evidence of metastatic spread or local invasion. Long bone metastases from neuroblastoma have a variety of appearances.[8–10] The lesions classically are found at the ends of long bones, are sometimes symmetrical, and have poorly marginated lytic zones with irregular mottling (Fig. 6–3). They may, however, occur at any location in the bones (Fig. 6–4), may have areas of sclerosis (Fig. 6–5), may have more well-defined areas of lysis, can fracture (Fig. 6–6), and can be associated with significant adjacent soft-tissue mass lesions. In the skull, the lesions again appear as irregular areas of lysis, with localized areas of sclerosis and thickening as well.[10] In more long-standing cases, there may be a hair-on-end appearance.[8] The sutures appear widened because of erosion of the suture margins by tumor or to actual widening from raised intracranial pressure. In the spine, plain film findings of direct spinal spread of tumor may be seen in up to 75 percent of patients.[11,12] A paraspinal mass may be identified. The interpedicular distance may appear widened and the pedicle might be destroyed. The intervertebral foramina are enlarged. In long-standing cases, scalloping of the posterior vertebral body and widening of the spinal canal can be iden-

A B C

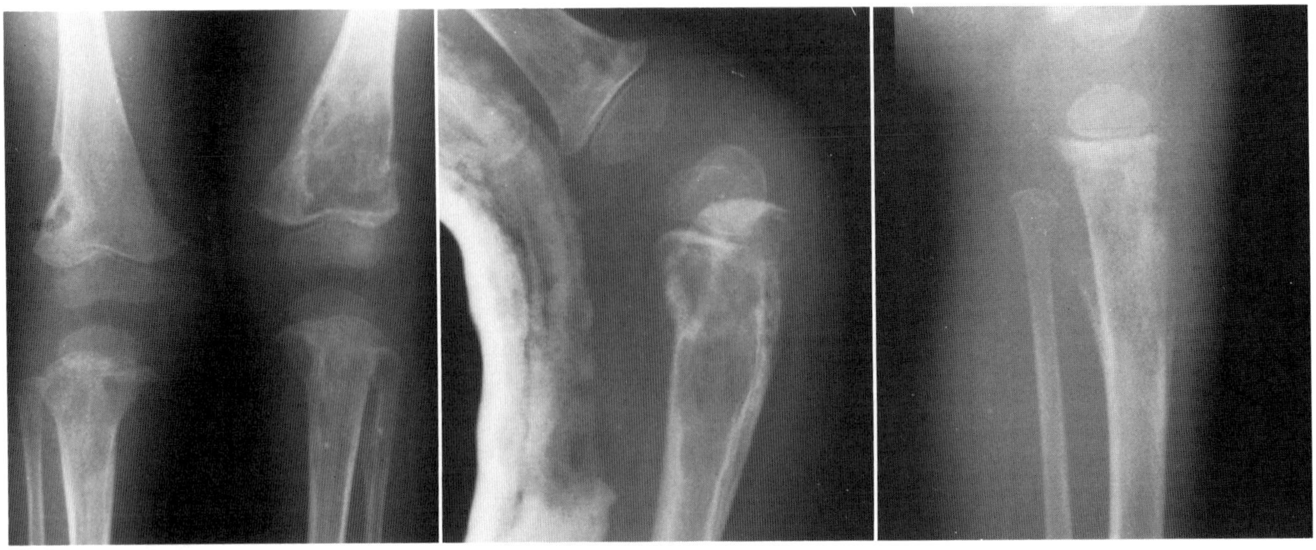

Figure 6-3. **Diagnosis: Neuroblastoma. Typical appearance of bone metastases. *A* through *C*, Plain film radiographs of leg bones. There are widespread lesions in the distal femurs and proximal tibias. The lesions are somewhat symmetrical in appearance. The lesions show predominantly destructive changes with periosteal reaction.**

tified.[8,11,12] Routine screening of the entire skeleton with radiographs is not recommended, because of the superior sensitivity of bone isotope scanning. Bone lesions are, however, commonly seen on chest and abdominal radiographs obtained in patients with neuroblastoma.

Figure 6-4. **Diagnosis: Neuroblastoma. Bone metastases. Plain film radiograph of pelvis and proximal femur. Lytic lesions are seen in both proximal femurs *(arrows)* and also distributed throughout both iliac wings. This is a fairly typical appearance.**

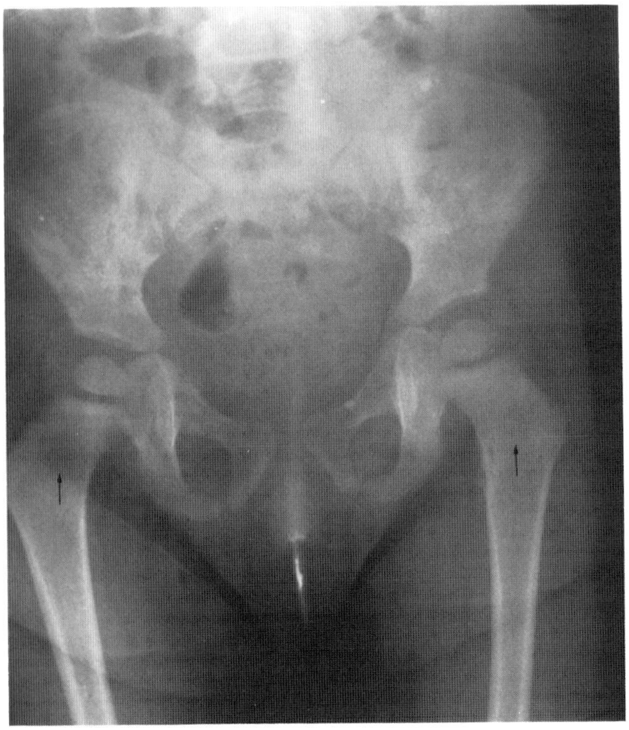

Radiographs should be obtained of any bone in which there are clinical symptoms (e.g., pain) or in which there is abnormality demonstrated by bone isotope scan.

Ultrasound. This is widely utilized as the initial screening modality in patients in whom an abdominal mass has been detected clinically. For this reason patients with neuroblastoma will frequently have ultrasound studies (Fig. 6–7). The ultrasound appearance of neuroblastoma must, therefore, be known. When CT and MR are available, ultrasound often has only a minor role to play in the management of patients with neuroblastoma. Ultrasound identifies a mass lesion, which typically is very echogenic. Some workers believe that the degree of heterogeneity helps differentiate neuroblastoma from Wilms tumor, purely on the ultrasound appearance,[13] but this differentiation should not be relied on. Areas of hemorrhage and necrosis appear as low-intensity regions. Well-defined oval or round foci of increased echoes in part of the tumor mass have been described as relatively specific features for neuroblastoma, correlating with pathologic nodules surrounded by collagen in 4 of 10 patients[14] (Fig. 6–8).

My own belief is that there is a wide range of appearances of neuroblastoma and other abdominal tumors, and that ultrasound cannot and should not be used to make a specific diagnosis. The diagnosis can be suspected from ultrasound and confirmed more accurately by other means. The typical adrenal neuroblastoma will appear as a mass lesion in the region of the adrenal gland above the kidney, causing displacement of the kidney. The size will vary considerably. The soft-tissue components of the tumor will be of moderate echogenicity. Areas of hemorrhage may appear as low or high echogenicity, with areas of necrosis being of relatively low echogenicity. Areas' of calcification will cause strong echoes, usually with shadowing. Ultra-

A B

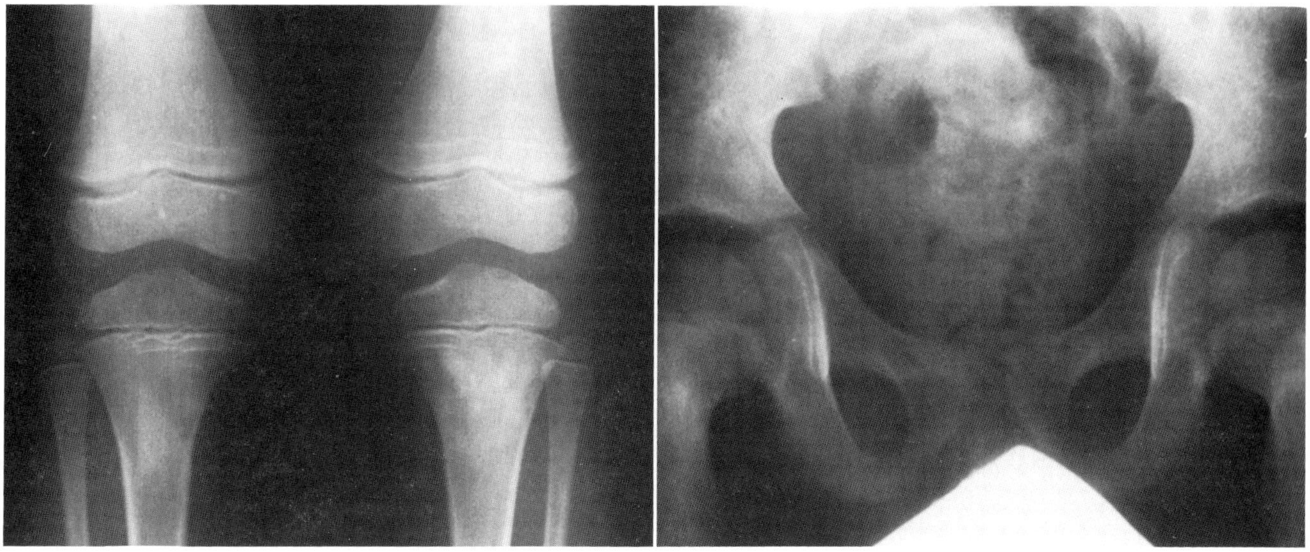

Figure 6–5. **Diagnosis: Neuroblastoma. Blastic (sclerotic) bone metastases.**
***A* and *B*, Plain film radiographs of pelvis, proximal femur, and knees. Symmetrical, moderately defined blastic lesions are seen in the proximal tibias, proximal femurs, and in the roofs of both hip joints.**

sound is probably not as sensitive as CT for detection of calcium. As with other modalities, ultrasound cannot specifically identify the origin of the tumor mass from the adrenal gland or from the sympathetic chain. Origin from the adrenal gland can be inferred with a large suprarenal tumor.

Rare cases of cystic neuroblastoma have been described. These occur in the abdomen, chest, or neck.[15–18] The cysts are usually well defined and echo free. They may be single or multiple and vary in size up to several centimeters in diameter. Adjacent abnormal soft tissue may be identified or may be absent on ultrasound (seen only on histology). The importance of these lesions is that they may be mistaken for other pathology. One case with a cystic neck neuroblastoma was initially mistakenly diagnosed as a cystic hygroma.[17]

Metastatic disease may be identified with ultrasound (Fig. 6–9). Lymph node metastases are identified as en-

Figure 6–6. **Diagnosis: Neuroblastoma. Pathological bone fractures.**
***A* and *B*, Plain film radiographs. Two different patients show lytic lesions and pathologic fractures in the proximal humerus and distal femur, respectively.**

A B

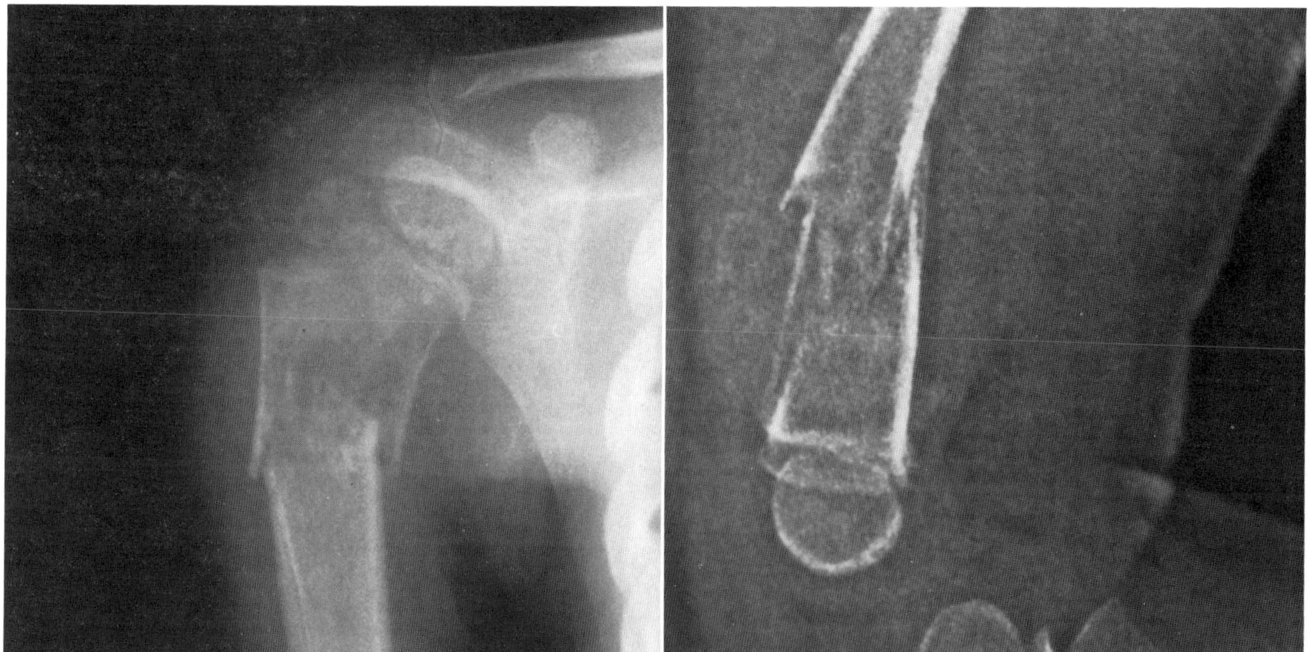

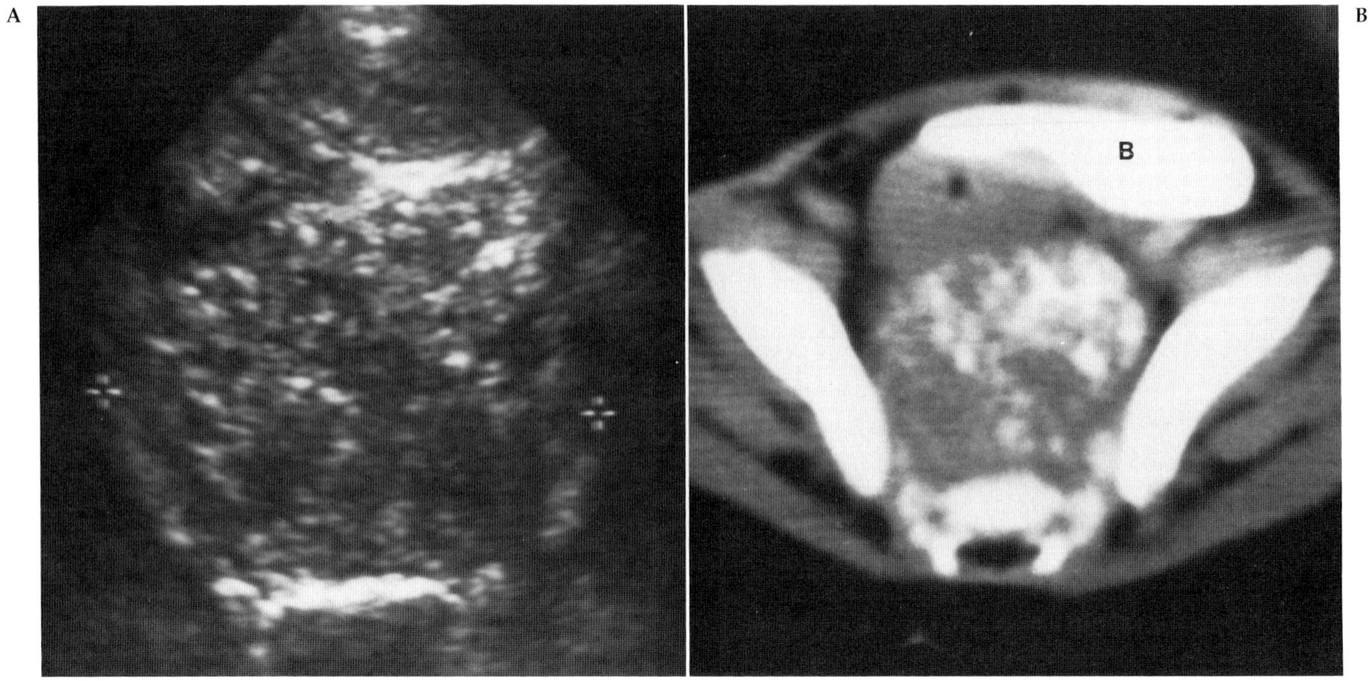

Figure 6-7. Diagnosis: Pelvic neuroblastoma.
A, Ultrasound. There is a large mass lesion of mixed moderate and high echogenicity. Very strong echoes with shadowing are evidence of calcium within the tumor. The margins of the lesion are not well seen. ***B***, CT. A large heavily calcified pelvic mass is seen. *B* = bladder. The margins of the mass are better defined than with ultrasound. All pelvic tumors will lie in the midline. According to the Evans classification, they are stage II if there are metastases to unilateral abdominal lymph nodes and stage III if there are metastases to bilateral abdominal lymph nodes.

larged lymph nodes with either increased or decreased echoes. Visualization of some lymph nodes may be obscured by overlying bowel gas. Metastatic disease of organs is seen as nonspecific focal lesions of either increased or decreased echogenicity compared to the

Figure 6-8. Diagnosis: Neuroblastoma.
Ultrasound. There is a large mass in the abdomen. Within the lesion is a region of increased echogenicity *(solid arrows)* that correlates pathologically with a region of tumor cells surrounded by collagen. *Open arrow* = aorta. (From Amundsen GM. Neuroblastoma: a specific sonographic tissue pattern. AJR 1987;148:943–945.)

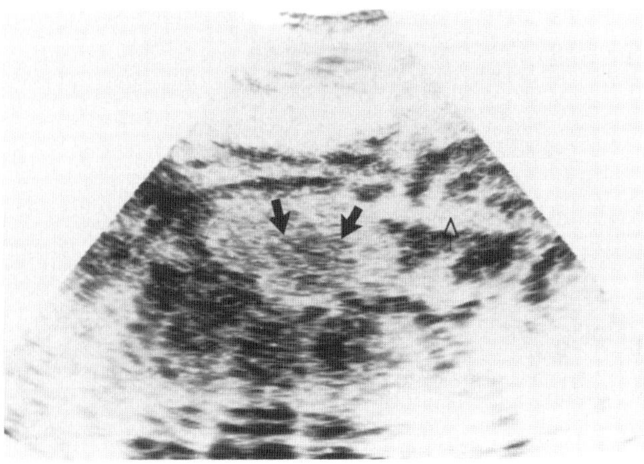

tissue of the metastatic organ.[5,19,20] In the liver of patients with stage IV-S neuroblastoma, focal abnormality is frequently not identified. The liver is markedly enlarged and there may be a diffuse increase in the echoes within the liver.[15] Ultrasound probably has little role to play in the routine evaluation of metastatic spread of neuroblastoma, because other more sensitive modalities are available. It has no role to play in the skeletal system.

CT. This is an extremely important modality for imaging of neuroblastoma, except for the skeletal system. It should be used for evaluation and staging of the primary tumor, detection of lymph node and liver metastases, and for the evaluation of skull metastases. CT will identify virtually all of the primary tumors that can be identified on any imaging modality. The tumor, regardless of site, is seen as a soft-tissue lesion usually with fairly well-defined margins (Fig. 6–10). Calcification will be identified on CT in up to 90 percent of patients[5,21–23] (Fig. 6–11). On noncontrast scans, the tumors may appear homogeneous or of mixed soft-tissue intensity.[24] They are more frequently nonhomogeneous.[5] Following injection of intravenous contrast, the inhomogeneity becomes more apparent with viable areas of tumor enhancing and enhancement not occurring in areas of hemorrhage or necrosis[5,24] (Fig. 6–11).

There are no diagnostic features by which the diagnosis of neuroblastoma can absolutely be made. The ap-

A

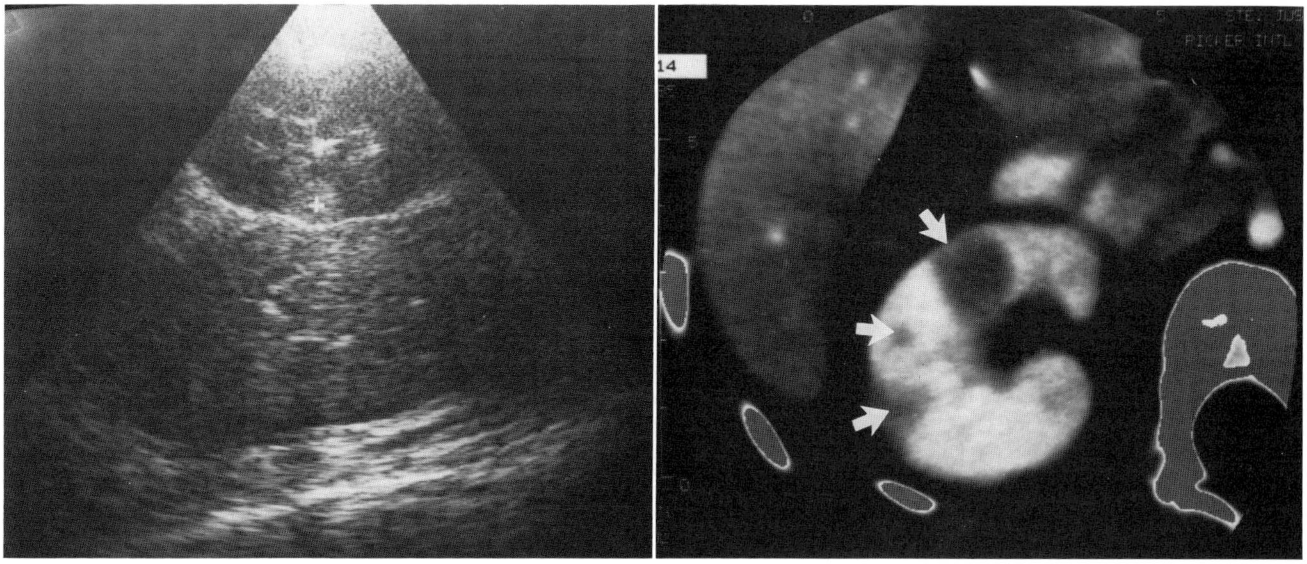

B

Figure 6–9. **Diagnosis: Renal metastases from neuroblastoma. The patient had a left adrenal neuroblastoma. The metastases were identified in the right kidney 10 months later.**
A, **Longitudinal view of right kidney. A 1 cm capsular hypoechogenic metastasis is seen in the anterior part of the kidney (+).** ***B,*** **CT after bolus injection of contrast. Three hypointense metastatic lesions are identified** ***(arrows).*** **The anterior lesion corresponds to the ultrasound. (From Filiatrault D. Renal metastases from neuroblastoma. Pediatr Radiol 1987;17:137–138.)**

pearance of calcium in a tumor mass in the neck, posterior mediastinum, retroperitoneum, or pelvis very strongly suggests the diagnosis of neuroblastoma. Origin from the adrenal gland cannot be detected, but can be inferred by the location of the tumor above the kidney with displacement of the kidney. The kidney is usually displaced inferiorly, but may on occasion be displaced laterally or even anteriorly by an adrenal neuroblastoma (Fig. 6–12). Occasionally, there may be difficulty differentiating a retroperitoneal right upper quadrant tumor from a tumor in the posterior aspect of the right lobe of the liver. Obliteration of the perinephric fat between the right kidney and the psoas muscle is excellent evidence of a retroperitoneal rather than a hepatic mass[23] (Fig. 6–12). Anterior displacement of the inferior vena cava, renal vessels, duodenum, or adjacent colon strongly suggests a retroperitoneal tumor.[23]

CT is very good for demonstrating local spread of tumor. Tumor spread medially behind the anterior renal fascia, with displacement and encasement of the great vessels, is well identified[26] (Fig. 6–13). The relationship of this spread to the midline is important for categorization of the patient as stage III. CT is better than ultrasound in this regard. Renal invasion by neuroblastoma

Figure 6–10. **Diagnosis: Left adrenal neuroblastoma.**
CT. Fairly typical appearance of a neuroblastoma (*N*). The tumor lies anterosuperior to the left kidney. There are moderately well-defined margins.

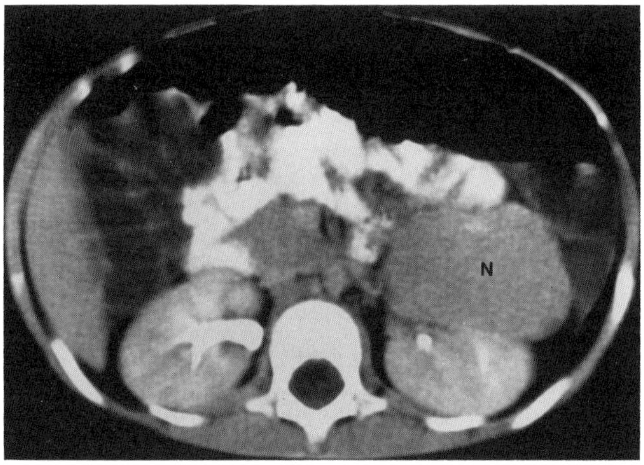

Figure 6–11. **Diagnosis: Neuroblastoma. Typical appearance.**
CT. There is a gigantic right-sided neuroblastoma with central calcification surrounding a central area of necrosis, which is not enhanced following intravenous contrast injection.

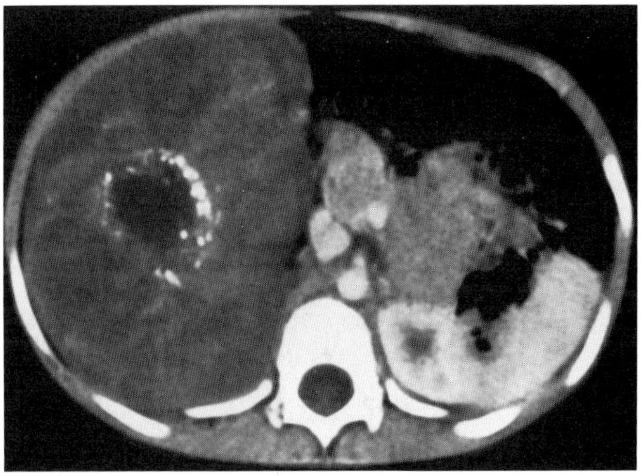

A B

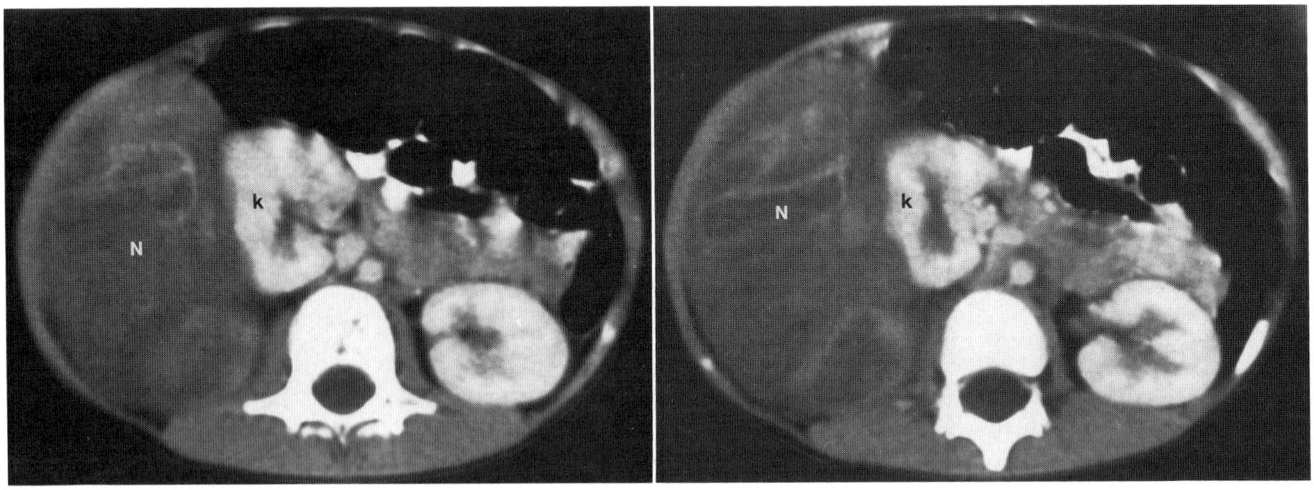

Figure 6-12. **Diagnosis: Right adrenal neuroblastoma with unusual displacement of the right kidney. *A* and *B*, CT images. There is a very large right adrenal neuroblastoma (*N*). The right kidney (*K*) is displaced medially and anteriorly. This is an unusual finding.**

is being increasingly recognized[26-28] (Figs. 6–14 and 6–15). The invasion often occurs from the hilum of the kidney into the deeper kidney tissue. Occasionally, the tumor may appear to be completely intrarenal and is believed by some to actually arise within the kidney substance.[27,28] These tumors cannot be differentiated preoperatively from a Wilms tumor purely on the CT appearance of the primary mass. Lymph node spread is suspected by the detection of the enlargement of lymph nodes. There are no absolute measurements available to differentiate normal from enlarged lymph nodes. It is known that tumor may be present in small lymph nodes, and enlargement of lymph nodes can be the result of reactive inflammation and not tumor.

Liver metastases on CT scan have a varied appearance. They may appear as focal low-intensity areas.[9] In stage IV-S neuroblastoma, where there is diffuse infiltration of the liver with tumor, the CT shows hepatomegaly. Attenuation will frequently be decreased and irregular, but focal lesions cannot be appreciated. Renal metastases can also be seen on CT (see Fig. 6–9). Lung metastases can be diffuse or focal (Fig. 6–16). The extension of sympathetic chain neuroblastoma into the spinal canal may be suspected by CT, but CT alone is not as accurate for its detection as CT myelography, performed after the subarachnoid injection of nonionic contrast.[5]

Demonstration of the relationship of the tumor mass to the great vessels of the abdomen is important, and for this reason CT scan should be performed dynamically following bolus injection of intravenous contrast material to ensure maximum opacification of the blood vessels. Inability to find a large vein in small neonates, and the variable time taken for vessel opacification, means that excellent vessel opacification will not be achieved in every patient. In patients with skull or orbital bone metastases demonstrated clinically or by other imaging modalities, CT (or MR) should be performed as well. These bone lesions frequently have a large soft-tissue component, and estimation of this, prior to treatment, is helpful, as subsequent scans can be used to monitor therapy (Fig. 6–17). Other bone lesions also may have soft-tissue extension (Fig. 6.18) CT is excellent for evaluation of the primary tumor and metastatic spread to all sites. Certain specific questions are still, however, better answered by utilizing other imaging modalities. This is discussed further later.

Magnetic Resonance. This holds great promise and will probably have an important role to play in evaluation of neuroblastoma.[15,29-32] The advantages of MR are its ability to image in multiple planes, improved soft-tissue contrast resolution, and excellent visualization of blood vessels, which is important for surgical planning (Fig. 6–19). MR is proving very accurate in identification of the primary tumor mass, and is at least as good as other imaging modalities.[29,32,33] The internal structure of the tumor may appear homogeneous on some pulse sequences and varied on others.

Figure 6-13. **Diagnosis: Neuroblastoma. Local spread.**
***A* through *F*, Series of 6 contiguous CT images obtained after bolus injection of IV contrast. They show a very large neuroblastoma arising from the right adrenal gland. The tumor is clearly crossing the midline and is, therefore, stage III. Much of the tumor lying to the left of the spine probably lies in lymph nodes. Note that the primary tumor cannot be differentiated from contiguous involved large lymph nodes. As the tumor has grown and infiltrated in the perirenal space, it has completely encased the aorta, displaced, encased, and separated the superior mesenteric artery and vein, and elevated the pancreas, pushing it forward. The tumor has also invaded the upper pole of the right kidney. *Black A* = aorta. *White A* = superior mesenteric artery. *V* = superio mesenteric vein. *P* = pancreas. *K* = kidney.**

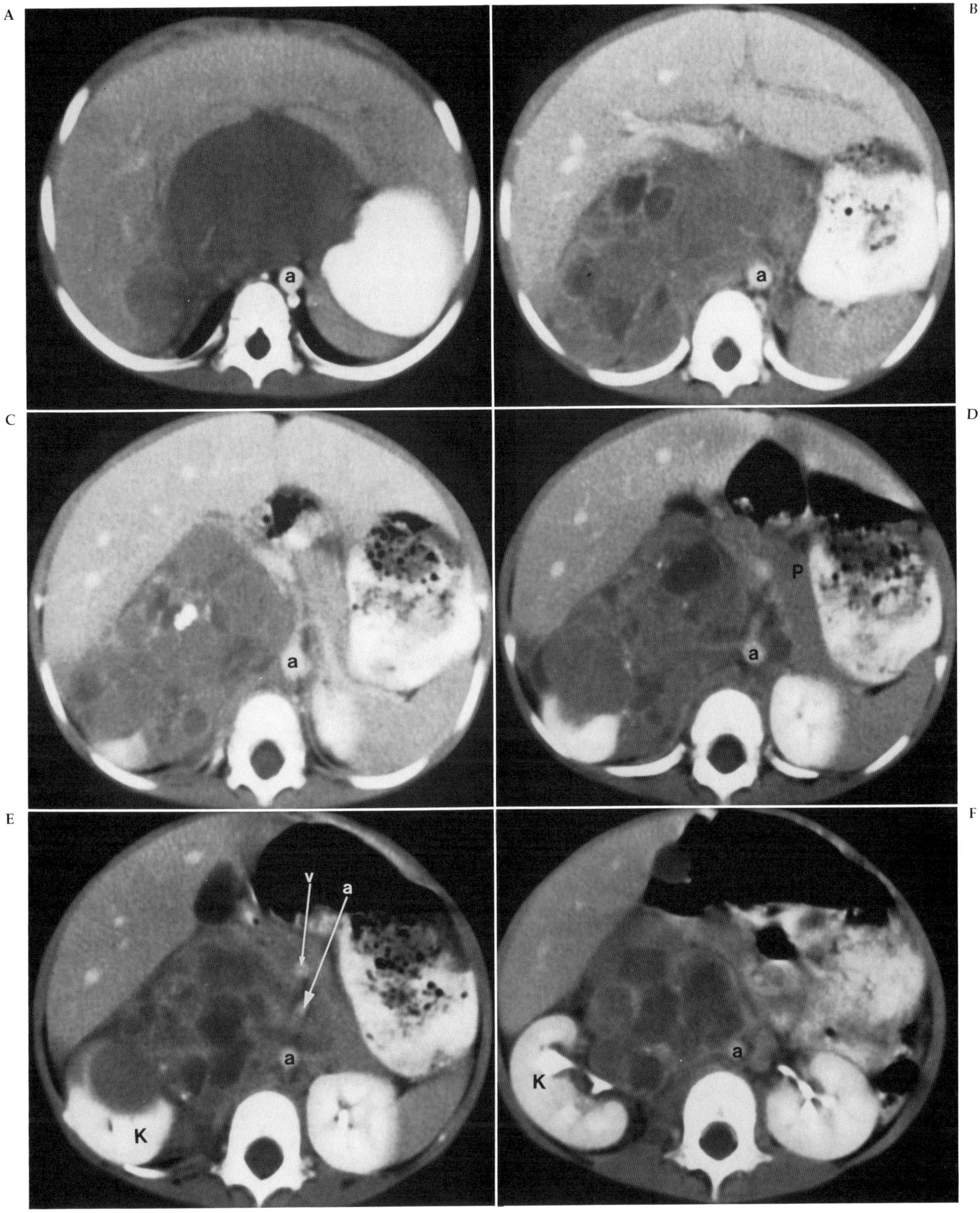
A
a
B
a
C
a
D
P
a
E
v
a
a
K
F
a
K

A B

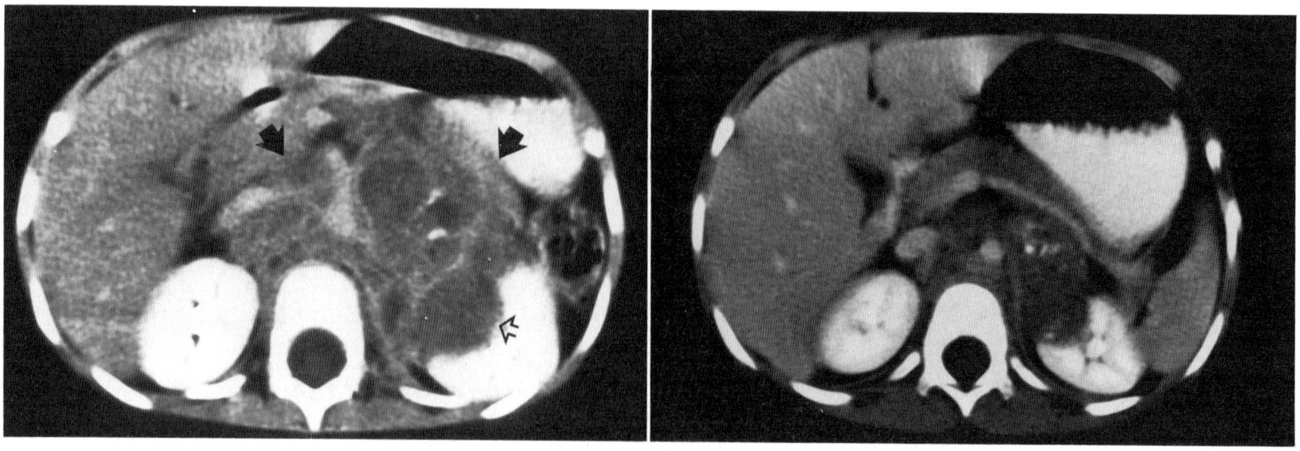

Figure 6-14. **Diagnosis: Neuroblastoma with renal invasion. Also marked decrease on chemotherapy. *A,* CT scan. There is gigantic left-sided neuroblastoma *(arrows).* The lesion is invading the hilum of the left kidney *(open arrow). B,* Same patient after chemotherapy. There is marked reduction in the size of the tumor. Again note the invasion of the hilum of the left kidney.**

In general, the tumor has characteristics of prolongation of T1 and T2 relaxation time with bright signal on T2 weighted images and lower signal on T1 weighted images (Figs. 6–2, 6–19, and 6–20). As the kidney normally has fairly long T1 and T2 relaxation times, it may occasionally be difficult to separate the tumor from the kidney. Areas of calcification, unless very large, will not be identified on the MR images. Areas of hemorrhage and necrosis will have varying appearance on different pulse sequences (Fig. 6–20). Hemorrhage may appear very bright on T1 pulse sequences. Changes in intensity of signal may be seen with therapy,[29] but the exact significance is not known. As with CT, MR can identify spread to lymph nodes and liver. At the present time there are no reports to suggest that MR is superior to CT in detecting tumor in very small lymph nodes or in the differentiation of inflamed from pathologic lymph nodes. In the liver, focal metastases are seen as areas of signal intensity lower than normal liver on T1 and higher than normal liver on T2 weighted pulse sequences. In stage IV-S neuroblastoma, MR is superior to CT and utlrasound[34] (Fig. 6–21). Like these other modalities, MR shows hepatomegaly. T2 weighted MR pulse sequences show a widespread nodular increase in signal intensity involving almost the entire liver. MR is outstanding for the identification of tumor spread into the extradural space[32] and it should replace CT myelography for this.

Of particular help is the ability of MR to image in the

Figure 6-15. **Diagnosis: Neuroblastoma with false appearance of renal invasion.**
CT. There is a small left adrenal neuroblastoma (*N*). There is a poorly defined interface *(arrow)* between the neuroblastoma and the left kidney (*K*). At surgery no tumor invasion of the kidney was identified. The appearance is thought to be caused by partial volume effect at the superior aspect of the left kidney.

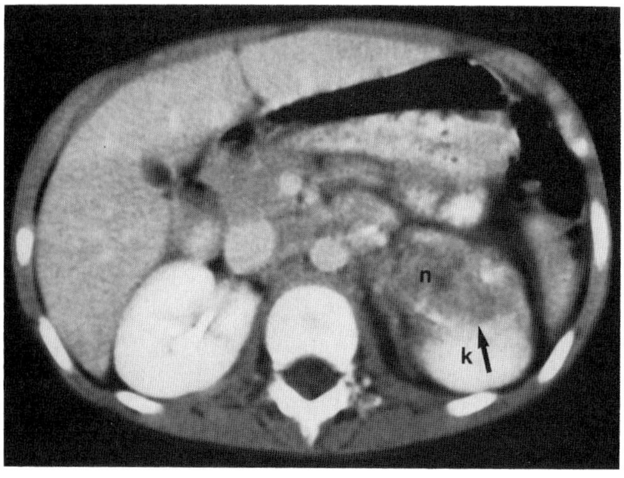

Figure 6-16. **Diagnosis: Neuroblastoma. Lung metastases at the time of initial presentation.**
CT. At least two nodular metastatic lesions *(arrows)* are seen in the right lower lobe. These both resolved with chemotherapy. This appearance is very unusual in that lung metastases from neuroblastoma are usually a terminal event and are usually diffuse and infiltrating.

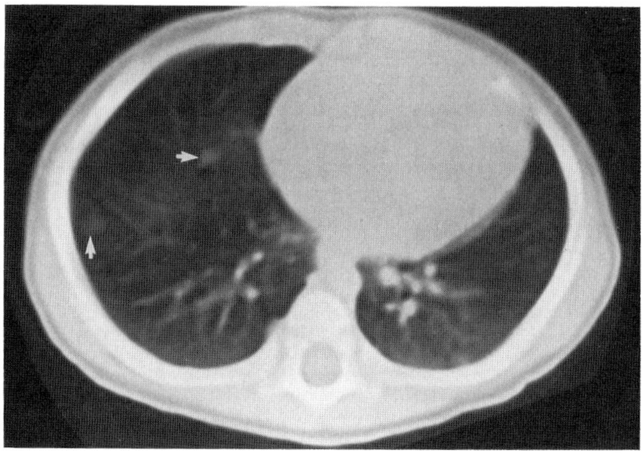

A B C

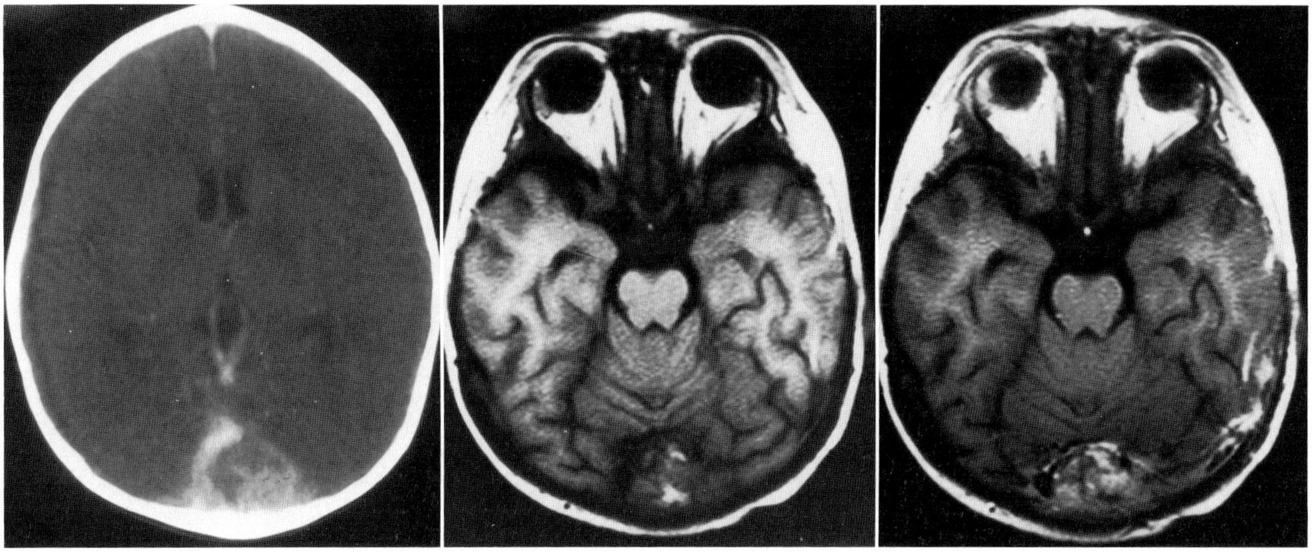

Figure 6–17. **Diagnosis: Neuroblastoma. Skull metastasis with large extradural soft-tissue components. *A*, CT. There is a large posterior metastatic lesion. *B* and *C*, T1 weighted axial MR images without and with gadolinium-DTPA. The lesion is well identified. There is moderate enhancement with gadolinium-DTPA.**

coronal plane (Fig. 6–22). The dumbell-shaped tumor with the isthmus passing through the intervertebral foramen is well identified, together with the total extent of the extradural component of the tumor. MR is proving better than CT for the demonstration of the relationship of tumor to the great vessels in the abdomen,[29] with excellent visualization of vessels being achieved without the need for administration of contrast agent (Fig. 6–23). MR is very sensitive for detection of bone marrow metastases (Fig. 6–24), but the appearance of marrow abnormality is very nonspecific (Fig. 6–25). Imaging in multiple planes may be required for optimal vessel visualization. The coronal plane is particularly helpful. MR imaging techniques in general should involve the utilization of a minimum of two pulse sequences and a minimum of two imaging planes. As with CT, MR is excellent for identification of the extent of soft-tissue tumor present with skull, extradural, and orbital metastases (Fig. 6–26). With other bone metastasis MR identifies soft-tissue abnormality very well (Fig. 6–27).

Figure 6–18. **Diagnosis: Neuroblastoma. Rib metastasis with a large soft-tissue component.**
CT image through the thorax. There is a metastatic lesion to a left anterior rib. A large soft-tissue component *(arrow)* projects into the thoracic cavity.

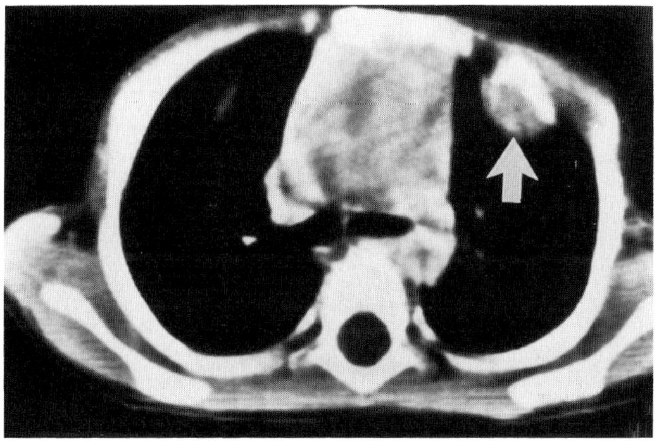

Radionuclide Isotopes. These are extremely valuable in evaluation of patients with neuroblastoma. Technetium 99m MDP bone scan should be utilized to evaluate the skeleton in every patient with known or suspected neuroblastoma (Fig. 6–28). This technique has consistently been shown to be more sensitive than skeletal radiography (skeletal survey).[5,35] The primary tumor frequently takes up the radioisotope, with such uptake being identified in between 66 and 74 percent of patients[21,23] (Fig. 6–28). Uptake may occasionally be helpful in identifying the location of a previously obscured primary neuroblastoma. It would also be helpful (in the absence of bone lesions) in differentiation of neuroblastoma from Wilms tumor in those few cases in which this distinction is not clear on CT (for example, in those patients with neuroblastoma that has invaded the kidney). The uptake of isotope by the primary tumor is proportional to the size of the tumor but is independent of the stage of the tumor, the extent of production of catecholamines by the tumor,[23] and the amount of calcium seen within the tumor.[21,23] Calcification within neuroblastoma has previously been demonstrated not to be the result of dystrophic deposition of calcium in areas of necrosis; it is seen in areas of viable tumor.[23] It has been suggested that the degree of uptake of a bone-seeking isotope in the primary tumor is proportional to the activity of calcium metabolism occurring within the primary tumor mass.[23]

Although the primary tumor mass will frequently take up the technetium 99m MDP, the main role of this

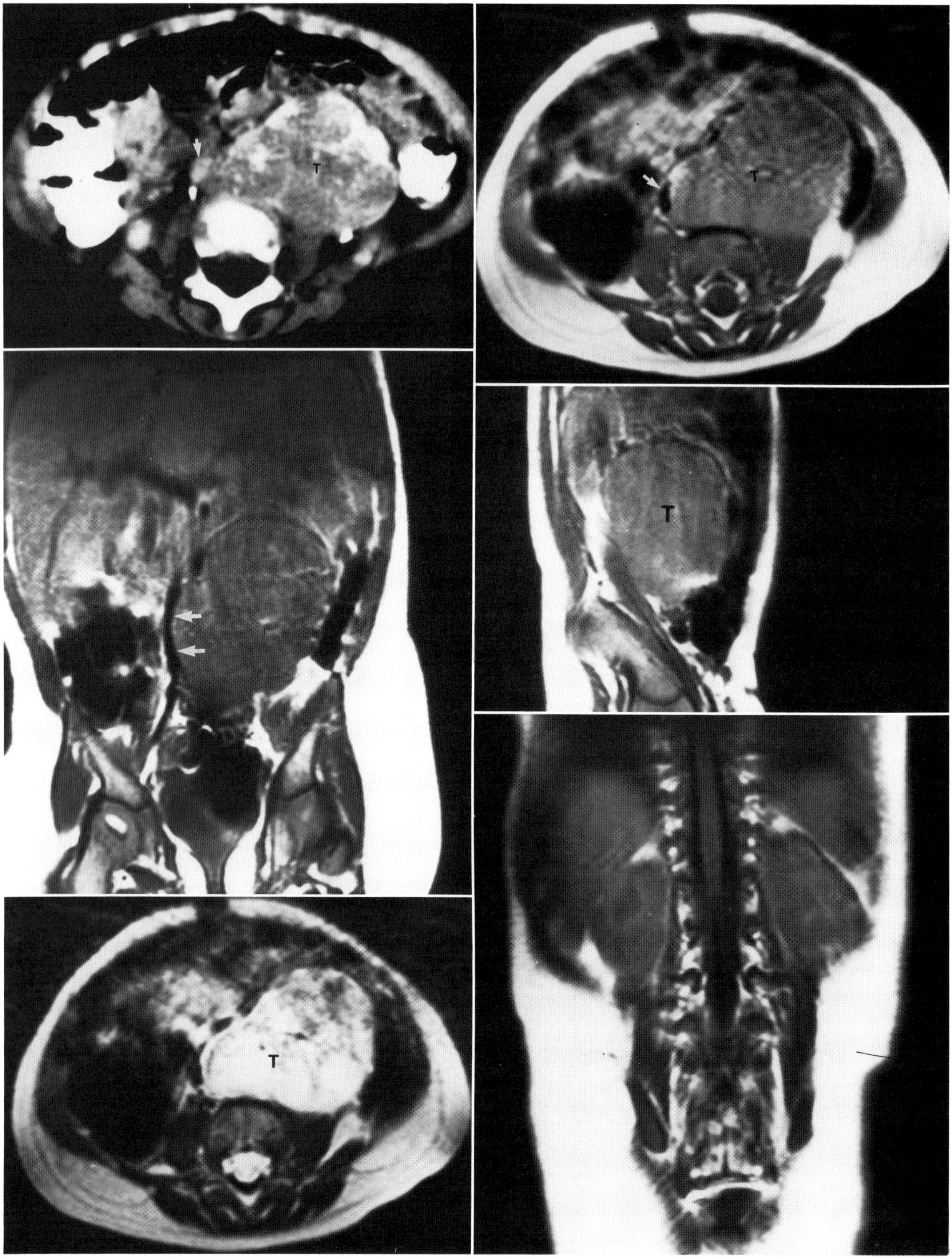
T

Figure 6–19. Diagnosis: Neuroblastoma. Comparison of MR and CT, and MR characteristics. There is a left-sided sympathetic chain tumor (*T*).
A, CT. A large tumor is well defined. It is heavily calcified. It is difficult to differentiate the aorta *(arrow)* from tumor. ***B*** through ***D***, MR, T1 weighted images. The tumor margins are well defined. Calcium is of low signal intensity and much less well defined than on the CT images. The aorta *(arrows)* is, however, much better defined. It is displaced by the tumor but not invaded or occluded. Note that the tumor is of intermediate signal intensity. **E**, MR, T2 weighted image. Axial plane corresponding to image ***A***. The tumor is now of very bright signal intensity. Some of the very low signal intensity areas represent the calcification. ***F***, Coronal image through the spinal canal. The cord is well identified. No tumor is seen in the spinal canal.

A

B

C

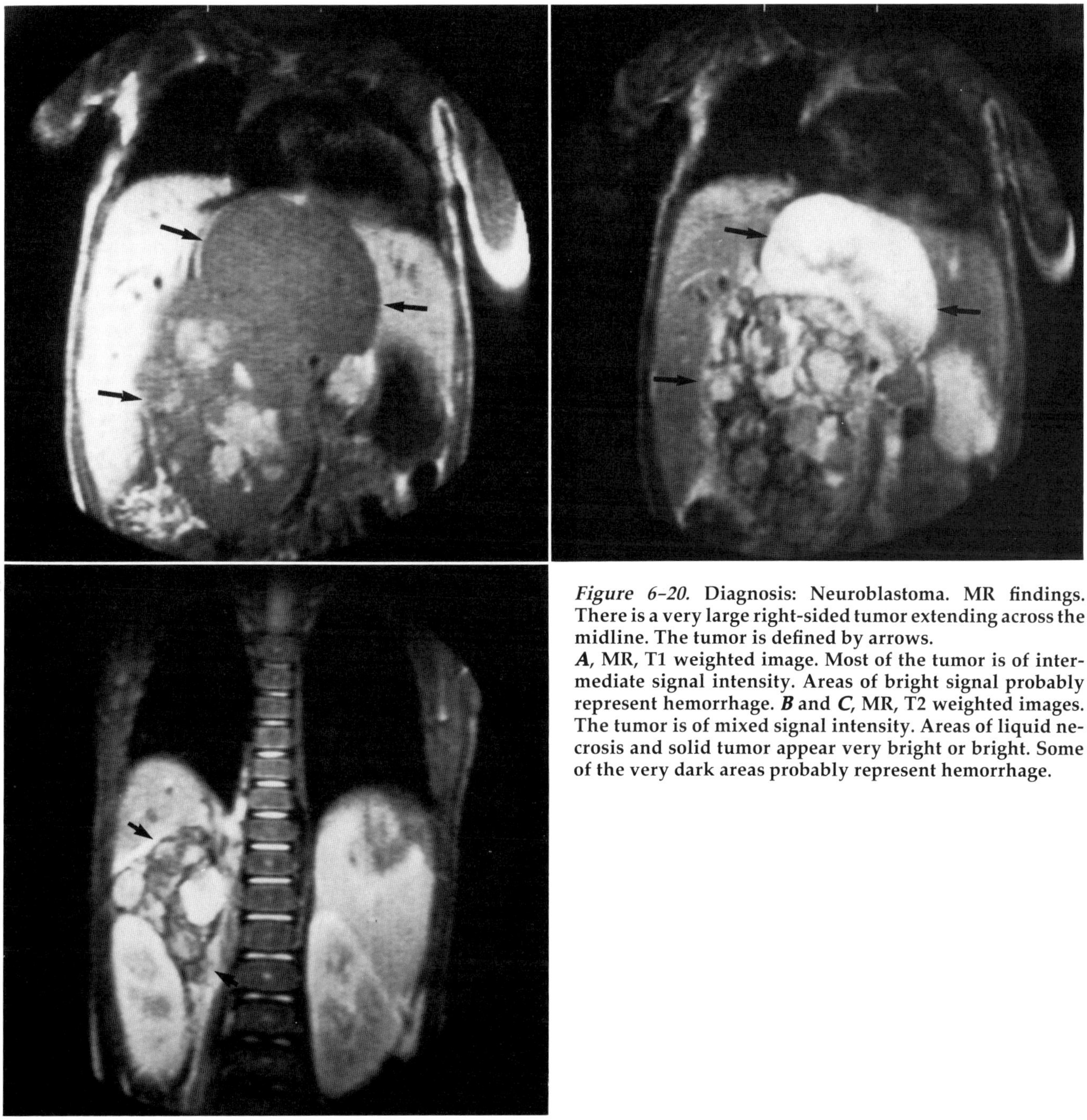

Figure 6–20. Diagnosis: Neuroblastoma. MR findings. There is a very large right-sided tumor extending across the midline. The tumor is defined by arrows.
A, MR, T1 weighted image. Most of the tumor is of intermediate signal intensity. Areas of bright signal probably represent hemorrhage. ***B*** and ***C***, MR, T2 weighted images. The tumor is of mixed signal intensity. Areas of liquid necrosis and solid tumor appear very bright or bright. Some of the very dark areas probably represent hemorrhage.

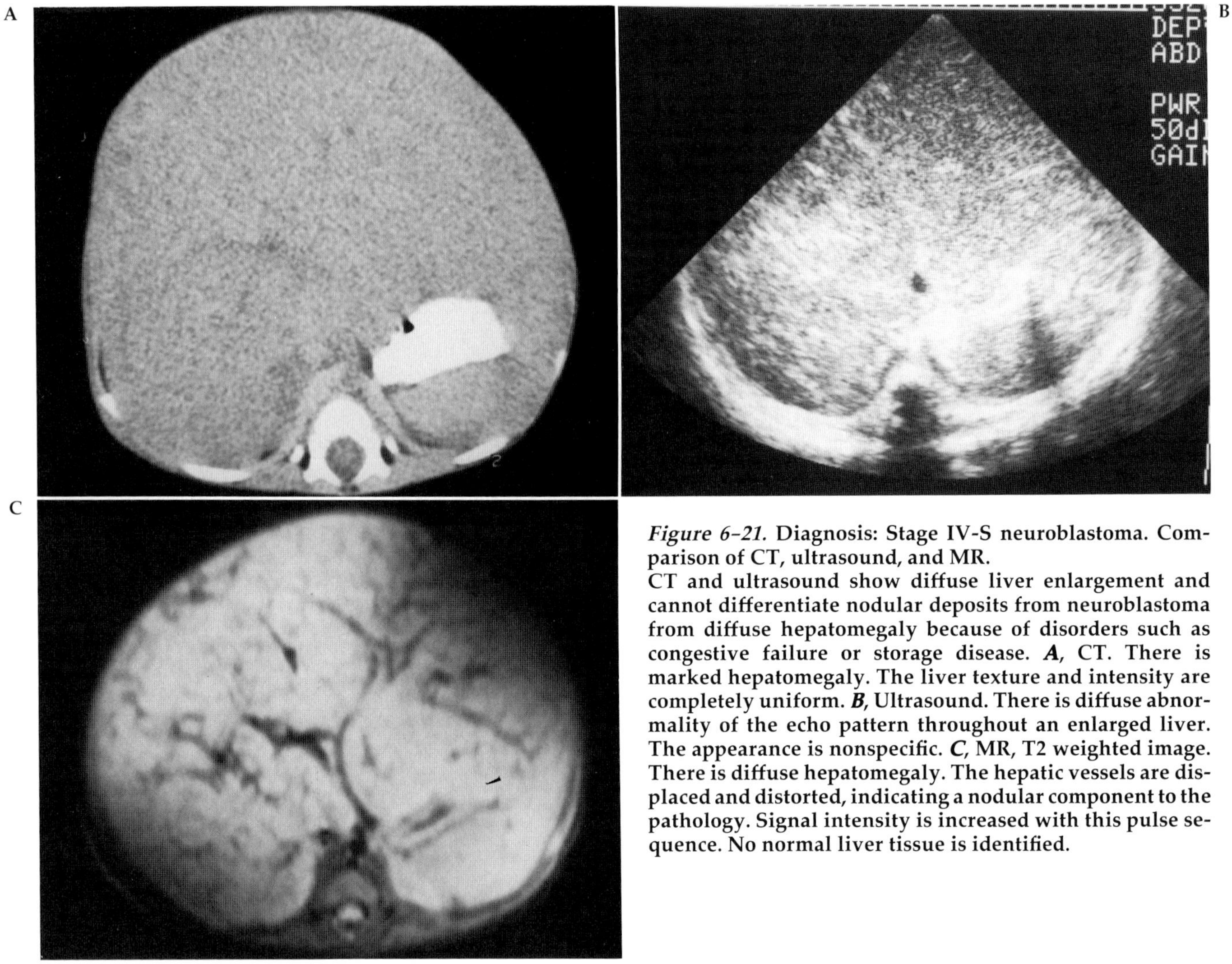

Figure 6-21. **Diagnosis: Stage IV-S neuroblastoma. Comparison of CT, ultrasound, and MR.**
CT and ultrasound show diffuse liver enlargement and cannot differentiate nodular deposits from neuroblastoma from diffuse hepatomegaly because of disorders such as congestive failure or storage disease. *A,* CT. There is marked hepatomegaly. The liver texture and intensity are completely uniform. *B,* Ultrasound. There is diffuse abnormality of the echo pattern throughout an enlarged liver. The appearance is nonspecific. *C,* MR, T2 weighted image. There is diffuse hepatomegaly. The hepatic vessels are displaced and distorted, indicating a nodular component to the pathology. Signal intensity is increased with this pulse sequence. No normal liver tissue is identified.

test is in the detection of bone metastasis either on initial presentation or on follow-up. The advantage of MDP is its extreme sensitivity.[35,36] One disadvantage is that uptake is not specific, occurring with many disorders, including infection, trauma, and other tumors. Another disadvantage is that the amount of metastatic tumor cannot be quantified and that while uptake, in general, will decrease with response to therapy there is no good correlation between the change in the degree of uptake with response. Improvement (decrease) in the MDP uptake may lag behind response for a long, variable time. Increasing uptake or new areas of uptake probably do indicate new tumor, however. The relative lack of specificity is often not a clincial problem, as the presence of tumor can usually be inferred if there are multiple areas of increased uptake. With a single area, or only two or three areas, of increased isotope uptake, plain film radiographs may in many cases confirm the presence of tumor. A normal radiograph excludes a fracture but not tumor. Until recently, in cases with single hot lesions on bone scan and a normal radiograph, biopsy was usually required to confirm the diagnosis. As is discussed later MIBG scan may prove extremely helpful in these cases.

Technetium-labeled sulfur colloid scanning has been utilized to seek liver metastases.[5,37] These lesions are seen as focal or diffuse patchy areas of decreased uptake. Because false negative results are common[37] and because of the availability of CT and MR, sulfur colloid scanning of the liver is no longer performed for the evaluation of patients with neuroblastoma. This agent is, however, also taken up by normal red marrow, and it has proven extremely sensitive for the detection of marrow metastases from neuroblastoma.[38] In this study, four patients had an abnormal sulfur colloid scan, indicating marrow metastasis, confirmed by marrow biopsy, with normal MDP bone scan and normal plain film radiographs of the area. Unfortunately, this study has not been widely acknowledged, and few if any centers routinely use sulfur colloid bone marrow scanning in the evaluation of patients with neuroblastoma. This test should be more widely used, at least in an experimental mode. One disadvantage of the test is that normal yellow marrow does not take up the isotope and this may be confused with areas of metastasis. Provided

A B C D

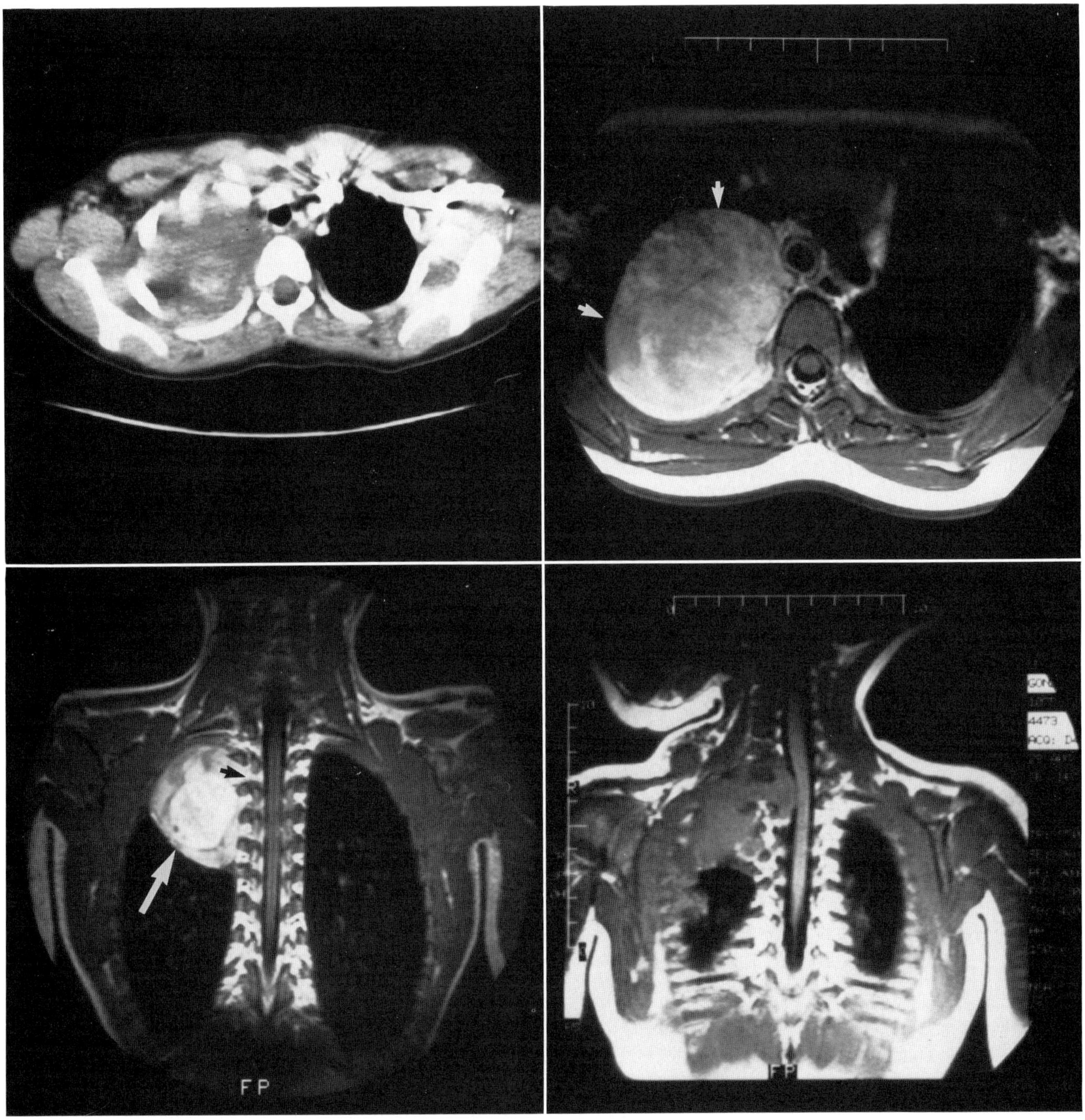

Figure 6–22. **Diagnosis: Apical thoracic neuroblastomas in two patients.**
Case 1: Tumor extension into the intervertebral foramina but not into the extradural space. *A*, CT. A large calcified tumor is seen in the apex of the right side of the chest. The margins of the tumor are not well defined. *B*, Transverse MR. The tumor is extremely well defined *(arrows)*, with sharp margins. Posteriorly, there is a clear interface between tumor and chest wall. *C*, Coronal MR. The large tumor *(large arrow)* is again clearly identified. There is extension into the intervertebral foramen *(little arrow)*
Case 2: Extension into the extradural space. *D*, Coronal MR T1 weighted image. The tumor shows extension into the subarachnoid space with displacement of the spinal cord.

that one has a knowledge of the normal distribution of red and yellow marrow, this should not be a problem. In addition, most neuroblastomas occur in the very young child, an age during which most of the skeleton still contains red marrow. At birth, the spine, pelvis, and long bones contain red marrow. There is a slow replacement of red marrow with yellow marrow, starting peripherally and moving toward the hips and shoulders so that by about the age of 10 or 12, an adult pattern of marrow has been achieved, with red marrow confined

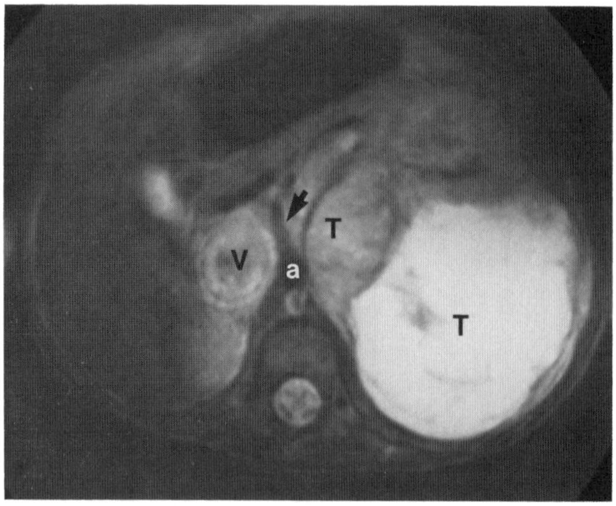

Figure 6-23. Diagnosis: Neuroblastoma.
Vessel visualization. There is a large left-sided adrenal tumor (*T*). Tumor is seen invading the vena cava (*V*). The aorta (*A*) and celiac artery *(arrow)* are well identified without the need for intravenous contrast.

to the spine, pelvis, proximal humeri, and proximal femurs.

During the past 10 years, there have been several reports utilizing iodine-labeled metaiodobenzylguanidine (MIBG) to evaluate patients with neuroblastoma.[39–47] This agent resembles norepinephrine and is an analog of guanethidine. It is metabolized by the neuroblastoma and, therefore, taken up by the tumor. The dose is 0.5 mCi per 1.73 m^2. Scans are obtained at 48 and 72 hours.[43] The great advantage of this agent is that it is extremely specific. While it is also taken up by carcinoid tumors, pheochromocytomas, and thyroid tumors, these tumors are exceedingly rare in the very young so that uptake in a young infant is virtually diagnostic of a neuroblastoma. The agent may be taken up by either the primary tumor[44] (Fig. 6–29) or metastasis in any site (Fig. 6–30). Iodine 131 has been most used, but when available iodine 123 is advantageous both with regard to image quality and patient dose.[41,45,46] Disadvantages of iodine 123 are a greatly increased cost and a shorter half life, which means the material must be used on the

Figure 6-24. Diagnosis: Neuroblastoma. Bone marrow metastases.
***A* through *C*, MR, T1 weighted images. Several low-intensity areas seen in the right iliac bone. These are caused by metastatic tumor replacing normal fatty marrow. *D*, MR, T2 weighted image. The marrow metastasis *(arrow)* appears of very bright signal.**

A B C D

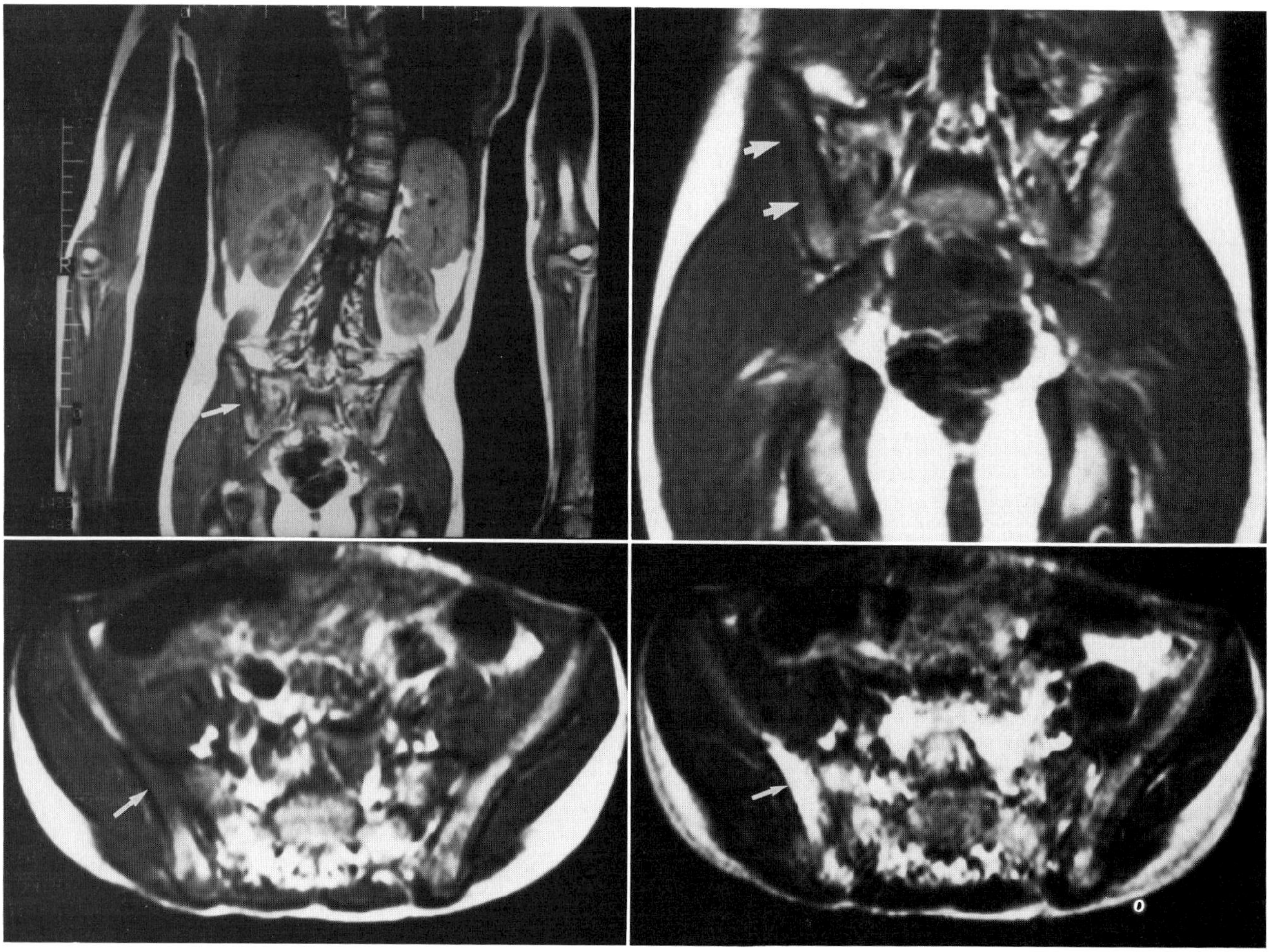

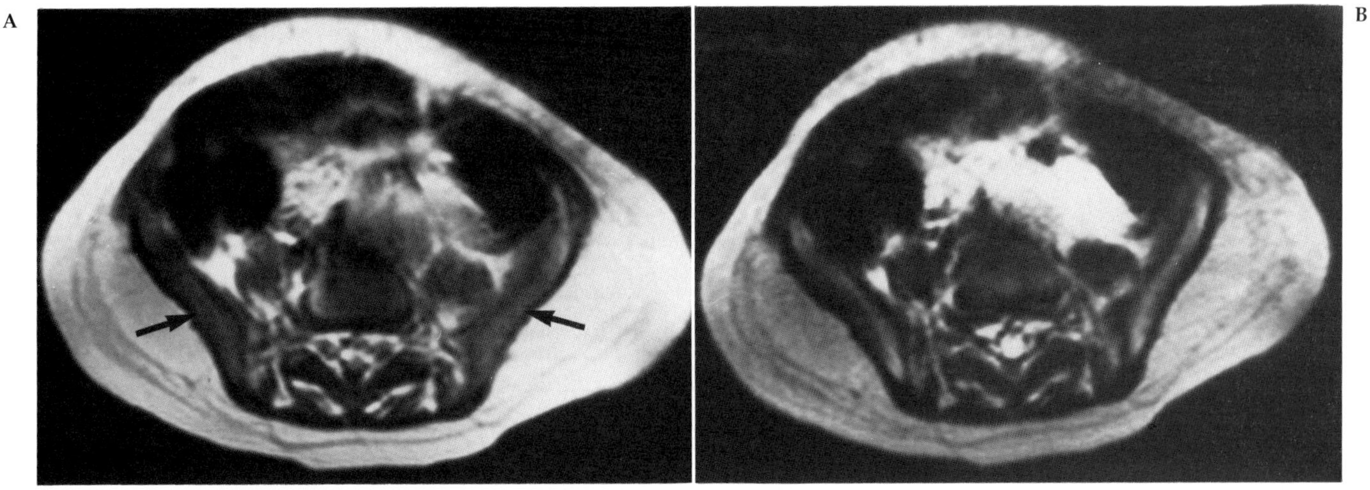

Figure 6-25. **Diagnosis: Neuroblastoma. False positive marrow abnormality.**
***A*, MR, axial T1 weighted image. Diminished signal is seen in the bone marrow of both iliac crests. *B*, MR, T2 weighted image. There is slight increase in signal intensity from the marrow in both iliac crests. MIBG scan was negative. Iliac crest marrow biopsies were negative. The cause of the low signal in the bone marrow was prossibly increased hemopoietic marrow due to anemia.**

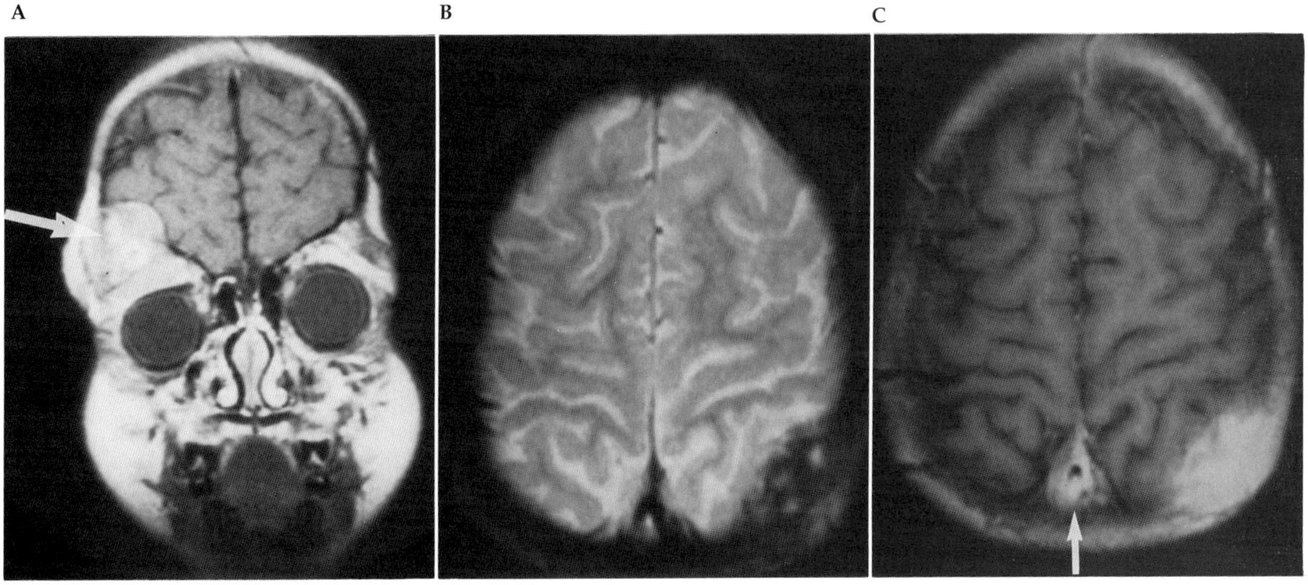

Figure 6-26. **Diagnosis: Neuroblastoma. Skull and orbital metastases.**
***A*, Coronal MR, T1 weighted image after gadolinium-DTPA administration. There is a large enhancing metastatic lesion in the roof of the right orbit *(arrow)*. *B* and *C*, Axial T1 weighted images before and after gadolinium-DTPA administration. A left posterior metastatic lesion is seen. There is a large extradural component extending into the cranium. A second lesion is seen encasing the superior sagittal sinus just above the torcular *(arrow)*.**

day that it is produced. Disadvantages of MIBG imaging are that lesions may occasionally be missed, with absence of uptake in the primary tumor or metastases identified by other modalities. In addition, there is normal uptake in the salivary glands, liver, and heart,[46] and since 90 percent of the agent is excreted by the kidneys they too may appear hot. It may also be that mature ganglioneuroma cells as well as neuroblastoma cells can take up MIBG, so that mature ganglioneuroma cannot be differentiated from neuroblastoma in a residual mass following chemotherapy. A final, and major, disadvantage of MIBG scanning is that uptake in the bone is nonspecific and cortical metastasis cannot be differentiated from marrow metastasis. This is especially important in neuroblastoma, as cortical metastases are far more sinister than bone marrow metastases.

Suggested uses of iodine-labeled MIBG scanning are in the diagnosis of neuroblastoma, staging neuroblastoma, differential diagnosis, monitoring therapy, and treating the patient. There have been several reports of labeling of MIBG with very high doses of radioactive iodine, and patients treated in this manner have shown some remission, but no cure, in up to 35 percent of cases.[47] At this stage, MIBG scanning does have a rou-

A B

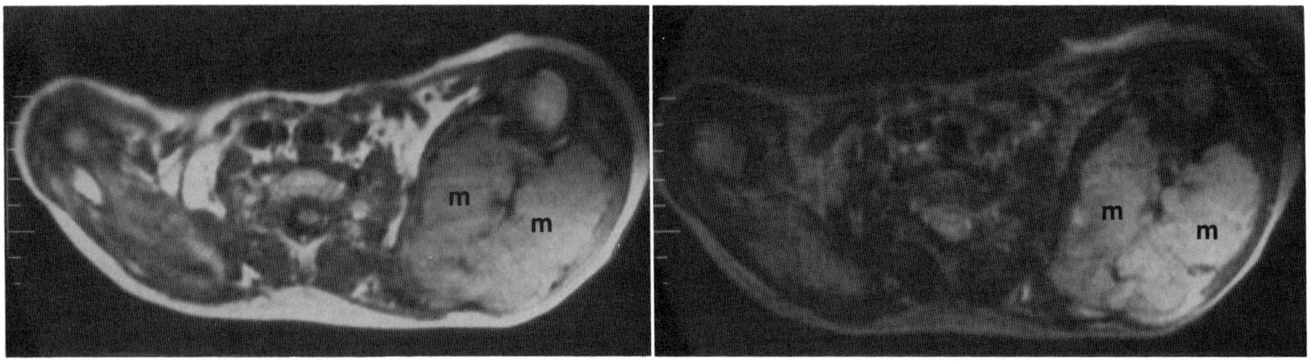

Figure 6–27. **Diagnosis: Neuroblastoma. Metastatic spread to the left scapula with a large soft-tissue component.**
A **and** ***B*****, T1 and T2 weighted MR images. The metastasis (*****M*****) is extremely well identified. It is very large. The signal intensity increases with T2 weighting.**

tine role to play in imaging of patients with neuroblastoma. A recent study of 37 patients reported uptake of MIBG in over 90 percent of primary tumors and a sensitivity of about 70 percent for detection of metastases or local relapse.[46] In another study,[48] MIBG uptake occurred in 11 of 12 primary tumors. It may be used as a study complementary to MDP scanning for evaluation of the skeleton in the initial screening of the patient. It should always be used for further evaluation of a patient with a single hot spot on MDP bone scan with a normal radiograph. Uptake of MIBG in this region confirms the presence of neuroblastoma and avoids the necessity for biopsy. There is probably little role for MIBG imaging in the early evaluation of response to therapy, as CT or MR can more accurately define reduction in volume of soft-tissue tumor masses. In the patient, believed to be in remission by clinical evaluation, VMA determinations, and other imaging, MIBG should always be performed, as the presence of any uptake will indicate the persistence of viable tumor. It is not known whether absence of uptake completely confirms remission. I suspect that it does not, as it would be unrealistic to expect MIBG scanning to detect microscopic residual foci of tumor, for example, in the primary tumor bed.

COMPARISON OF DIFFERENT IMAGING MODALITIES

Unfortunately, there are no definitive studies published recently regarding the relative value of the different imaging modalities for answering different questions in the evaluation of neuroblastoma. All of the different modalities have not been compared. Many of the publications utilize techniques that are no longer state of the art; many of the studies utilize small numbers of patients without controls, without good baseline standards, and without being prospectively planned. The following discussion is based on the data available from studies that have been performed, combined with impressions from personal experience (Fig. 6–31).

Primary Tumor Imaging. CT is the imaging modality of choice; MR provides complementary information (Fig. 6–32). Early reports in 1978 indicated a preference for CT and ultrasound over the traditional evaluation of abdominal radiograph and intravenous urogram.[49] While ultrasound is excellent in many patients, it has the disadvantages of not allowing viewing of the retroperitoneum completely in all patients because of overlying bowel gas, the inability to monitor tumor shrinkage as accurately as CT, and a poorer detection rate for liver metastatic spread. There are no studies comparing ultrasound and CT for vessel visualization, but I believe that ultrasound, particularly with color Doppler, will prove excellent (Fig. 6–33). Prior to surgical resection, if vessels have not been well opacified on CT, and if MR is not available or has not been performed, color Doppler ultrasound is suggested. This should be performed in addition to and not instead of CT. In one study comparing CT and ultrasound in the evaluation of neonatal neuroblastoma,[15] CT was better than ultrasound for identification of the primary tumor, which was missed in one case by ultrasound. In addition, liver disease was more readily identified with CT. In another study,[22] CT was determined to be better than ultrasound or intravenous pyelography in the detection and delineation of the primary tumor mass.

CT may not identify tumor found at surgery. In patients who had CT, MR, or both (and in whom delayed surgery was performed in stage III or IV patients treated initially with chemotherapy),[50] discordance was identified in 10 of 26 patients. There were five reports of false positive studies for imaging, and in the other cases more extensive tumor was found at surgery than was suggested by imaging. Unfortunately, in this paper surgery was taken as the standard and there is no way of knowing if surgery in fact missed tumor. In a 1983 Children's Cancer Study Group Report,[51] 22 patients with stage IV tumor in clinical and radiologic complete remission had surgery performed approximately 6 months after initial diagnosis. In 12 of these 22 patients, some residual tumor was identified at surgery. While it is impossible for imaging to detect microscopic residual tumor, I suspect that the results with more modern imaging techniques would now be much better than in the report of patients imaged prior to 1983. The question as to whether or not a complete remission can be diagnosed

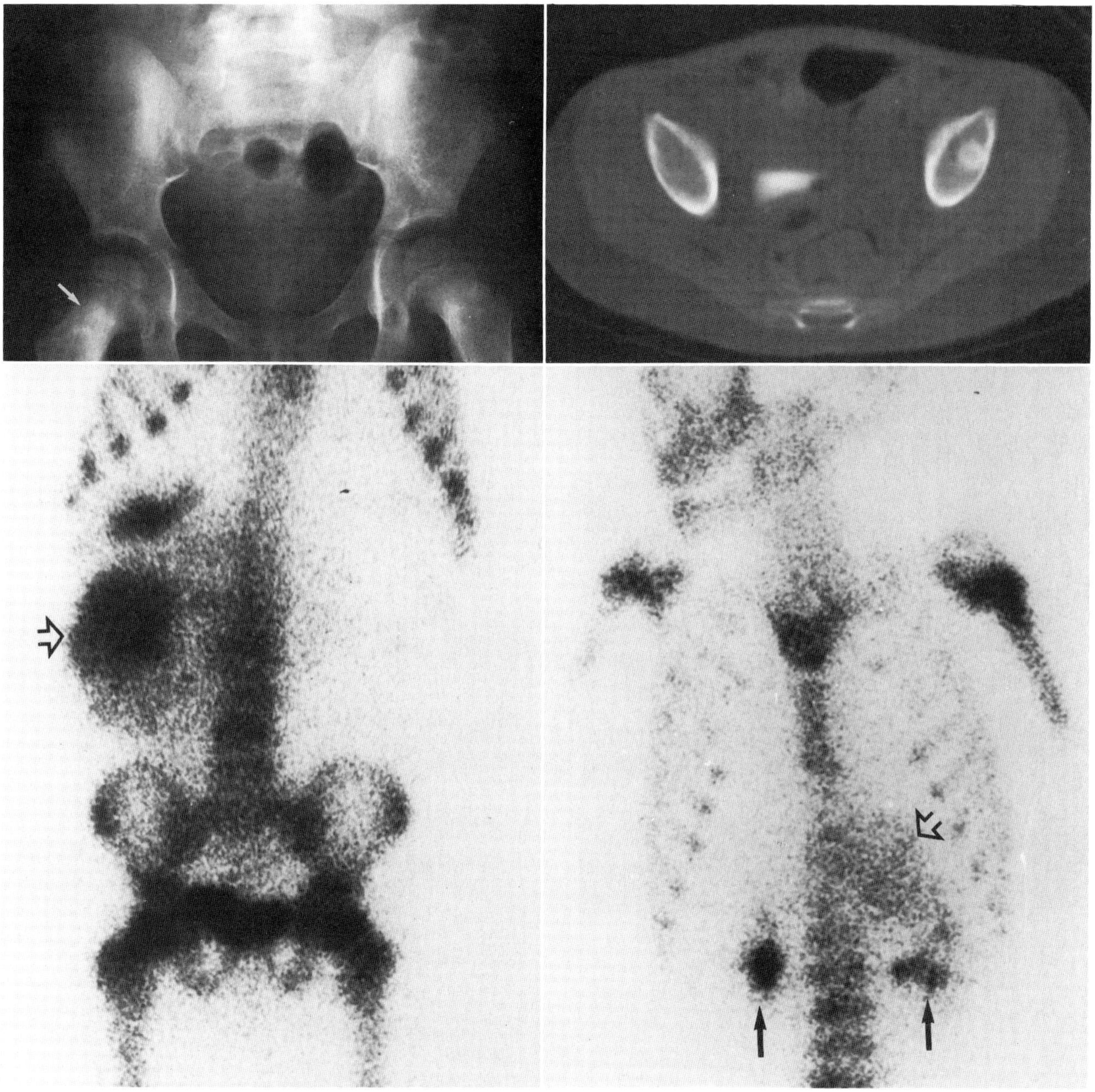

Figure 6–28. **Diagnosis: Neuroblastoma. MDP technetium 99m detection of metastases and uptake in primary tumor.**
A, **Radiograph of pelvis. A sclerotic lesion *(arrow)* is seen in the proximal right femur. There is suspicion of sclerotic abnormality on the left side in the iliac bone just above the hip joint. *B,* CT. This shows a sclerotic lesion in the left iliac bone. *C* and *D,* Posterior and anterior bone scan images. The increased uptake in the left iliac bone and both proximal femurs consistent with metastatic disease. Note also intense uptake by the primary tumor mass *(open arrow).* Uptake by both kidneys *(arrows)* is a normal finding.**

without surgery is an important one. I believe that in the presence of a negative CT, MR, and MIBG imaging, it would be extremely unlikely for surgery to identify significant residual tumor.

Bone Metastases. Two studies comparing skeletal survey and bone scan, MIBG and MDP bone scan, are summarized in Tables 6–9 and 6–10. As can be seen, bone scan is superior to skeletal survey. MDP bone scan and MIBG scan are complementary.

Liver Metastases. CT is the recommended modality for detection of liver metastases, although I think that MR may prove more sensitive than CT in the future. No

A

B

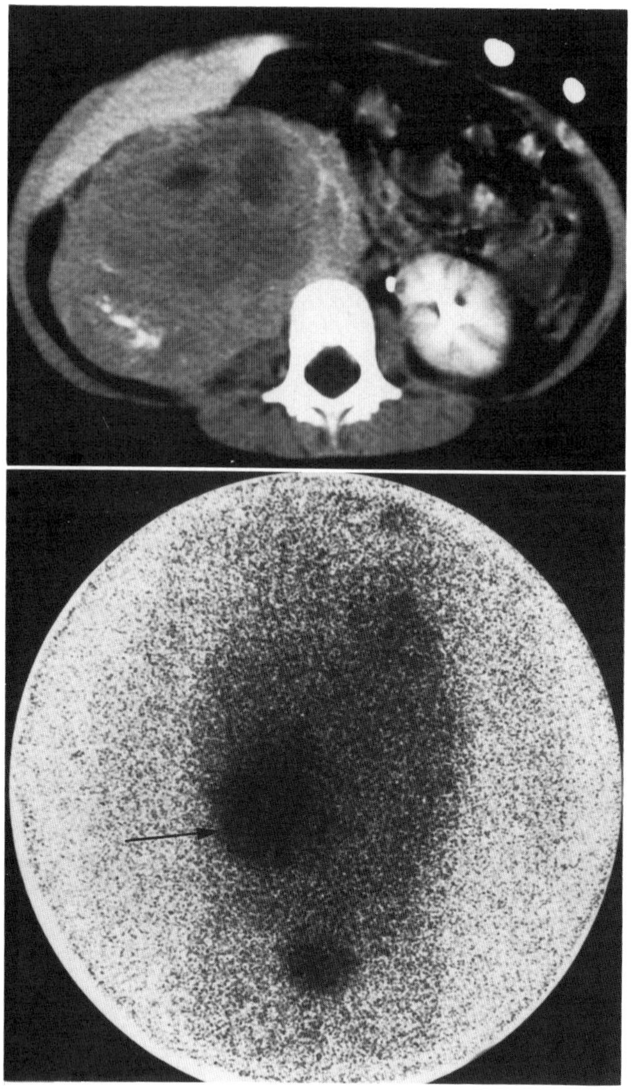

Figure 6–29. **Diagnosis: Neuroblastoma. MIBG uptake by primary tumor.**
***A*, CT. There is a large right-sided calcified neuroblastoma.**
***B*, Anterior view of MIBG scan. There is intense uptake of the isotope by the primary tumor mass *(arrow)*.**

studies comparing these two modalities have been performed.

Extradural Extension of Tumor. No comparative studies have been reported, but when these are done, I believe that MR will prove to be the modality of choice.

Bone Marrow Metastases. At the present time, little imaging is routinely done to evaluate the bone marrow for metastatic tumor. There are two very good modalities for this. Sulfur colloid bone scan, as discussed previously, will show bone marrow metastatic disease not identified on plain film radiographs or on MDP bone scan. MR imaging[29] is exquisitely sensitive for the detection of bone marrow disease. The appearance is nonspecific and it is difficult to screen the entire skeleton. However, if MR is routinely utilized for the evaluation of the primary tumor, and for the evaluation of the spine for extradural spread, large segments of the bony

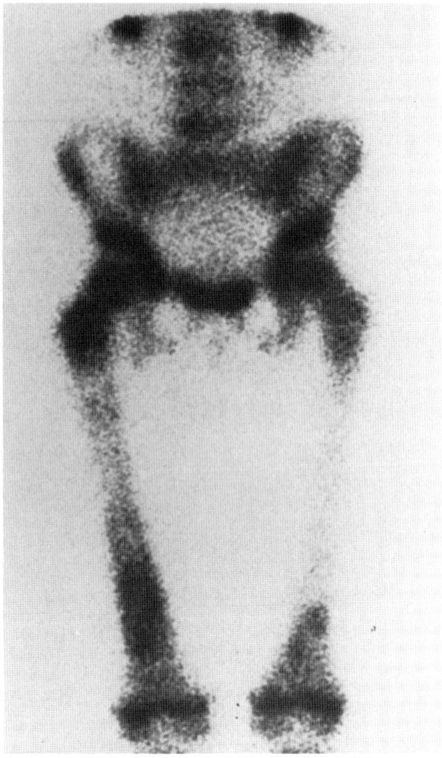

Figure 6–30. **Diagnosis: Neuroblastoma. Metastases identified with Iodine MIBG isotope scanning.**
Uptake of isotope in multiple bone metastases is identified.

skeleton, including the pelvis, proximal femurs, and a large amount of the spine, will be available for evaluation. Positive information from these scans can be used to guide marrow biopsy. At the present time, most protocols utilize a bone marrow biopsy and a bone marrow aspirate obtained from each iliac crest as the definitive means for identification of bone marrow tumor. The dangers of errors of this approach are obvious, because bone marrow spread is frequently not diffuse but patchy and metastatic tumor can easily be missed.

RECOMMENDED USE OF IMAGING MODALITIES FOR INITIAL EVALUATION AND FOLLOW-UP IN PATIENTS WITH SUSPECTED OR KNOWN NEUROBLASTOMA

Hunt the Primary Tumor. There are a number of situations in which a child will be strongly suspected or even known to have a neuroblastoma but in whom the site of the primary tumor is not known. These situations need to be elaborated.

1. In children presenting with opsomyoclonus, it is known that up to 50 percent will have neuroblastoma. The primary tumor is frequently in the chest[52] and is very often small.
2. Children with neuroblastoma may present with signs and symptoms caused by metastases. Bone marrow biopsy and urine catecholamine evaluation may be positive, indicating the presence of a neuroblastoma, and

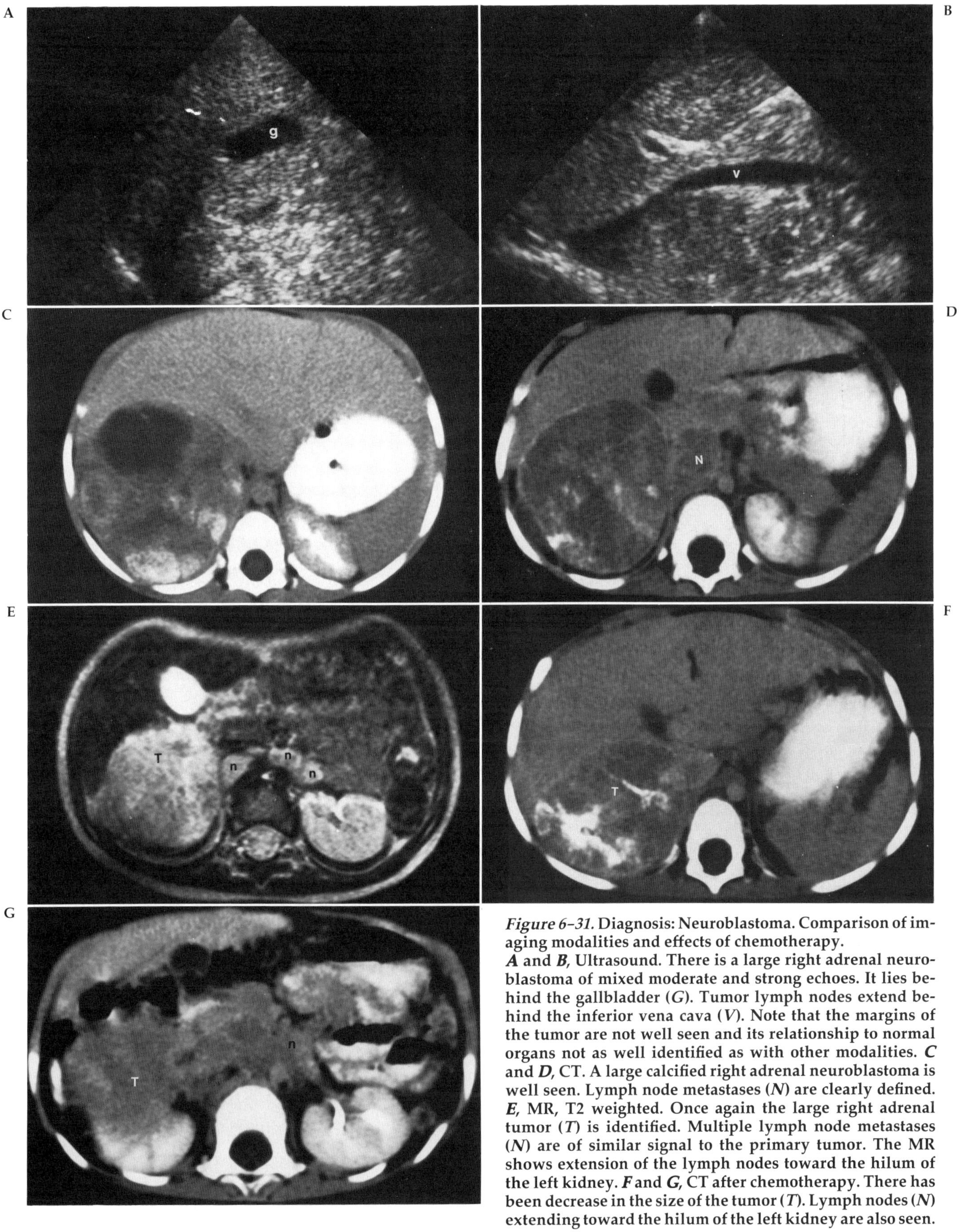

Figure 6–31. Diagnosis: Neuroblastoma. Comparison of imaging modalities and effects of chemotherapy.
A and ***B***, Ultrasound. There is a large right adrenal neuroblastoma of mixed moderate and strong echoes. It lies behind the gallbladder (*G*). Tumor lymph nodes extend behind the inferior vena cava (*V*). Note that the margins of the tumor are not well seen and its relationship to normal organs not as well identified as with other modalities. ***C*** and ***D***, CT. A large calcified right adrenal neuroblastoma is well seen. Lymph node metastases (*N*) are clearly defined. ***E***, MR, T2 weighted. Once again the large right adrenal tumor (*T*) is identified. Multiple lymph node metastases (*N*) are of similar signal to the primary tumor. The MR shows extension of the lymph nodes toward the hilum of the left kidney. ***F*** and ***G***, CT after chemotherapy. There has been decrease in the size of the tumor (*T*). Lymph nodes (*N*) extending toward the hilum of the left kidney are also seen.

imaging is then required to identify the location of the primary tumor.

3. In Japan, routine screening of 170,000 6-month-old children by doing spot urine tests for catecholamines identified 32 positive tests. Primary tumors were found in only 15 of these patients. If routine screening is introduced in the United States as advocated,[53] imaging will be required to identify primary tumors in patients with positive urine screening tests.

My approach to this problem would be initially to perform a chest radiograph and plain film radiograph of the abdomen. Particularly in the chest, this may well identify the primary tumor. If these studies are negative, one is faced with a choice of three modalities: CT, MDP, or MIBG scanning. I have no strong preference for the order in which these tests are performed. Any could be the first test to identify the tumor. If negative, one would need to proceed with all three tests to maximize opportunity of identification of tumor. In addition, MR, particularly coronal imaging, could be utilized effectively. Both of the radioisotope tests are sensitive, but will still probably miss between 10 and 20 percent of the primary tumors. CT will probably miss fewer tumors than this, but there is extensive radiation, as the patient may have to be scanned from the base of the skull down through the entire pelvis. A possible cause of error with CT is that in a few patients with abdominal tumors, the

Figure 6–32. **Diagnosis: Left adrenal neuroblastoma. Comparison of different modalities.**
A, **Ultrasound. There is a large mass that has predominantly moderate and strong echoes. The margins of the lesion, its total extent, and its relationship to other structures is not as well identified with ultrasound as it is with other modalities. *B,* CT. Large tumor mass lies anterior to the left kidney (*K*). The lesion crosses the midline and is, therefore, stage III. The aorta (*A*) is moderately well seen but other major vessels are not well visualized. Low-intensity areas in the lesion could be caused by hemorrhage or necrosis. *C,* MR spin density image obtained slightly superior to the CT image. A large tumor mass is well identified. On this image, necrosis is of intermediate intensity whereas hemorrhage is bright. The aorta, inferior vena cava, and superior mesenteric vessels appear dark because of flow voids and are seen much better than on a CT image. *D,* Coronal T1 weighted image. This clearly differentiates hemorrhage, which appears very bright, from the rest of the tumor. *H* = hemorrhage.**

A B

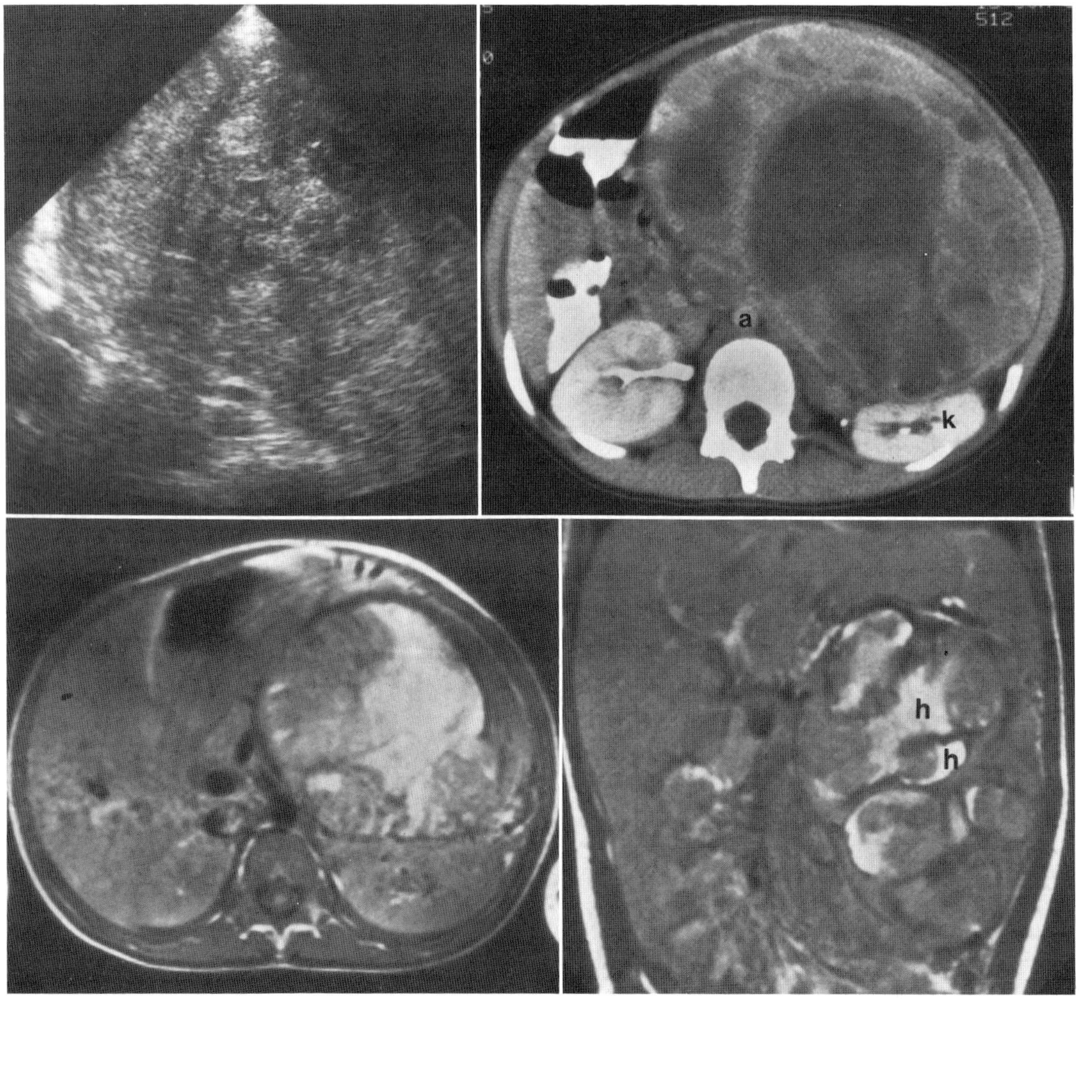

C D

TABLE 6–9
Comparison of Skeletal Survey and Bone Scan

Both Abnormal*	Skeletal Survey Abnormal	Tc99m MDP Bone Scan Abnormal	Total
26[1]	2	17	45
31[2]	5	10	46

*The bone scan showed more lesions than the skeletal survey in over 80 percent of these cases.

References

1. Baker M, Siddiqui AR, Provisor A, et al. Radiographic and scintigraphic skeletal imaging in patients with neuroblastoma. J Nucl Med 1983;21:467–469.
2. Heisel MA, Miller JH, Reid BS, et al. Radionuclide bone scan in neuroblastoma. Pediatrics 1983;71:206–209.

TABLE 6–10
Comparison of MIBG and MDP for Detection of Bone Metastases[1]

Both Negative	Both Positive	Only MIBG Positive	Only MDP Positive	Total
11	5	2	5	23

Reference

1. Heyman S, Evans AE, D'Angio GJ. I-131 metaiodobenzylguanidine: diagnostic use in neuroblastoma patients in relapse. Med Pediatr Oncol 1988;16:337–340.

only identifiable abnormality may be a small focus of calcification, which may even be confused with opacified bowel loops.[54] MR might prove sensitive, but although it has been shown to be excellent at demonstrating large neuroblastomas, there are no reports comparing it with other modalities for the identification of small lesions 1 to 2 cm in size. In the abdomen, these small lesions may be confused with bowel loops. MR's role should probably still be considered experimental. I do not utilize ultrasound for screening for primary tumors. Most of the thorax and significant areas of the abdomen will be obscured by bowel gas. If the ultrasound is positive, I would proceed to CT anyway. If the ultrasound is negative, CT will be required.

Further Evaluation of a Known Primary Tumor Mass (Fig. 6–34). CT and MR are the imaging modalities of choice. Ideally, I would perform both studies. There is insufficient experience with MR to recommend completely replacing CT with MR. MR, however, has already been demonstrated to be excellent for identification of primary tumor and to be better than CT for evaluation of the major blood vessels in relation to the tumor and for the evaluation of extradural spread. I suspect too that in time it will prove more sensitive for the detection of liver metastases. MR image quality is not as consistently good as CT and in some patients is greatly degraded by motion. For these reasons I think both modalities are justified. Both have the advantage, compared to other modalities, of permitting the evaluation of tumor volume. This is most easily achieved with CT, where slice thickness and table shift are accurately known.

Tumor volumes are easily calculated by tracing the cross-sectional area of each image, multiplying the various areas by the slice thickness, and adding each together. Current national protocols use a product of the greatest two diameters of a tumor to evaluate its size.[39] This should no longer be done, as it can in no way compare with the accuracy of tumor volume estimation by CT, which is widely available throughout many countries. Evaluation of tumor resectability is best achieved with a combination of CT and MR, with utilization of color Doppler ultrasound in selected patients, as previously discussed. Current aggressive surgical techniques attempt resection of as much tumor as possible without sacrifice of vital vessels or organs. The above combination of imaging modalities should evaluate the margins of the tumor well, detect invasion of local organs such as kidney, detect the relationship of the tumor to the aorta, inferior vena cava, and major branches of these vessels (Fig. 6–35), and detect the presence and extent of extradural spread of tumor.[27]

One controversial issue is whether or not to perform myelography if MR is not available. This is routinely performed in some centers if there is a neuroblastoma not arising from the adrenal gland (i.e., a paraspinal neuroblastoma). My own view is that this is not necessary and that many patients can be spared the unpleasant myelogram. Most patients with significant extradural spread have some neurological symptoms at the time of presentation.[12] In one series, 19 of 20 patients had symptoms.[11] In another series, 18 of 21 patients had evidence of plain film spine abnormality.[12] As extradural spread is identified only in about 10 percent of patients,[9] and as most of these patients with significant spread have neurological abnormalities on plain film spine radiographs, I believe that CT myelography should be performed only in patients with either plain film radiographic or clinical abnormality. Approximately 90 percent of patients will thus be spared the myelogram. A small amount of invasion through the intervertebral foramen will be detected at surgery, and in the absence of clinical symptoms the preoperative detection of this tumor spread does not alter therapy.

Screening for Bone Cortical and Marrow Metastases. Tc99m MDP and I-123 MIBG scans should be done on initial presentation in all patients. If both studies are negative, no further imaging of bone is required. Prior to MIBG scanning, there were isolated reports of bones with extensive destruction being falsely negative on MDP scan. The combination of MDP and MIBG should, I think, detect all patients with skeletal metastases so that routine skeletal survey should no longer be per-

A B

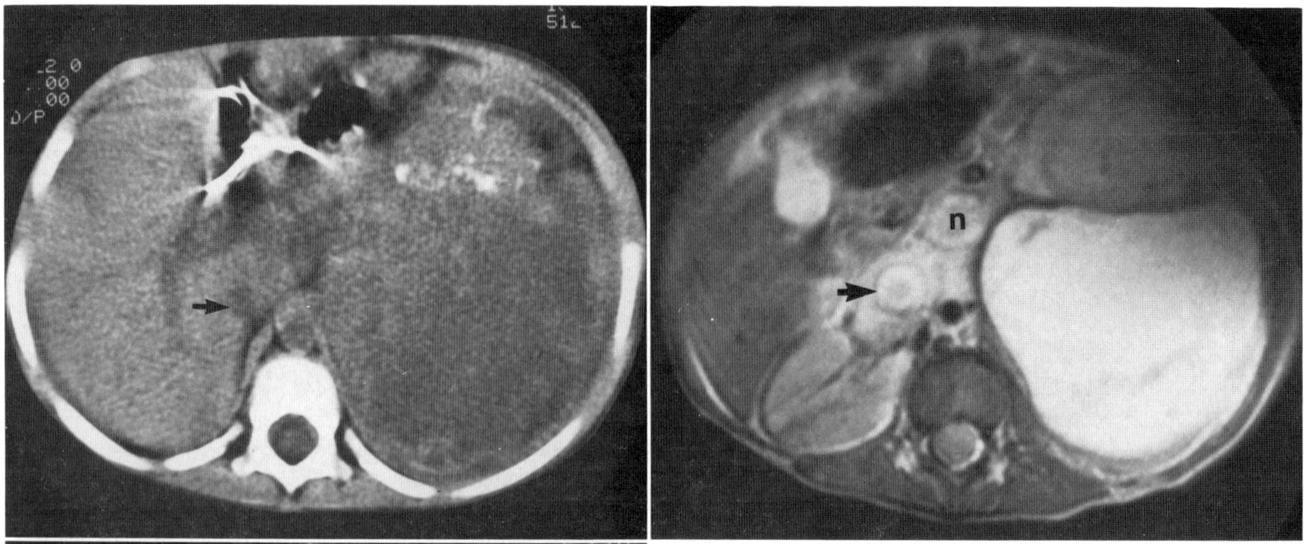

C

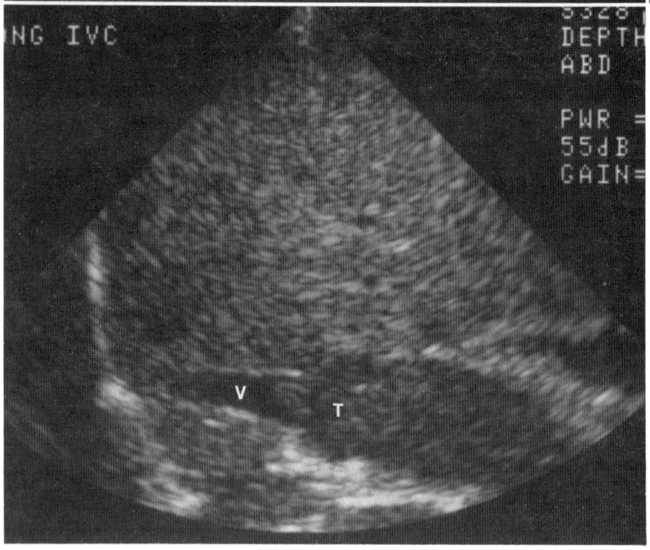

Figure 6–33. Diagnosis: Neuroblastoma with invasion of the inferior vena cava.
A, CT. There is a large calcified left adrenal neuroblastoma. Low intensity is seen in the region of the inferior vena cava *(arrow)*, but tumor cannot be differentiated from a nonopacified vessel. ***B***, MR. The large left neuroblastoma is again identified. Tumor is seen in the inferior vena cava *(arrow)*. The appearance is, however, not greatly dissimilar from that seen in the more anteriorly placed lymph node (*N*). ***C***, Longitudinal ultrasound. Tumor (*T*) is clearly identified in the inferior vena cava. *V* = normal vena cava superior to the tumor.

A

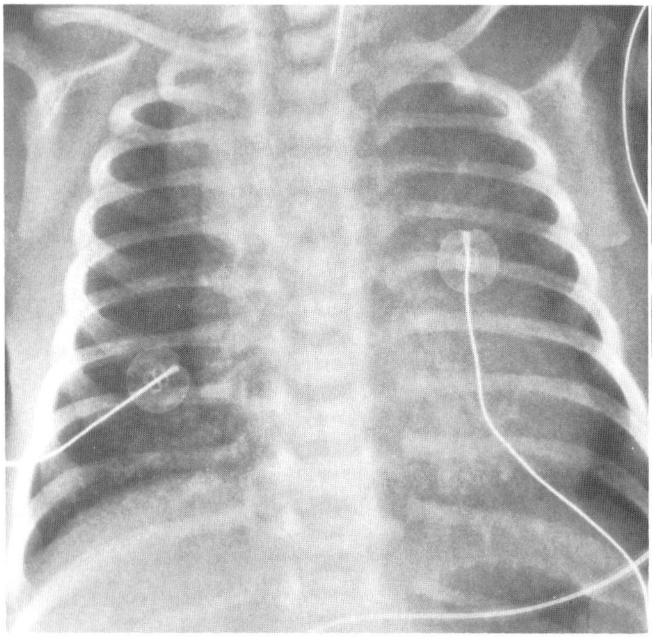

B

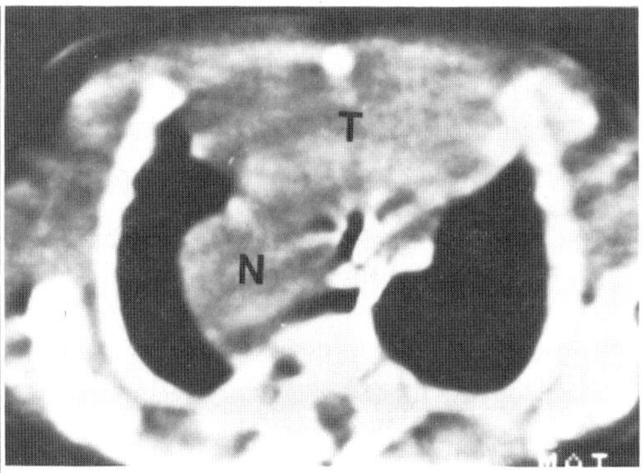

Figure 6–34. Diagnosis: Neuroblastoma with severe tracheal compression.
A, Chest radiograph. The trachea is intubated and pushed slightly to the left. There is an anterior mediastinal mass, but on this image, thymus cannot be differentiated from neuroblastoma. The displacement of the trachea is abnormal. ***B***, CT. There is a large anterior thymus (*T*) and a posterior neuroblastoma (*N*) that extends into the mid mediastinum and compresses the trachea, significantly narrowing the airway.

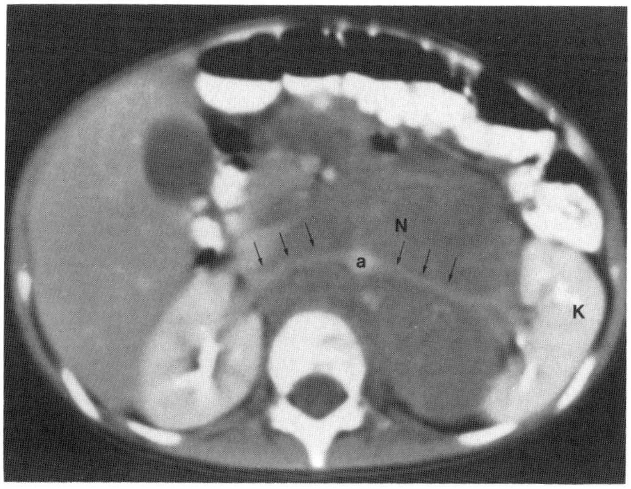

Figure 6–35. **Diagnosis: Neuroblastoma, nonresectable. Giant neuroblastoma (*N*) is displacing the left kidney (*K*). The aorta (*A*) is completely encased by tumor. Both renal arteries *(arrows)* are also completely encased so that the tumor cannot be resected without sacrificing the aorta and both kidneys.**

formed even in those patients in whom both these studies are negative. As previously discussed, the bone marrow has not been imaged in any of the national protocols. I suggest that bone marrow scan be performed in all patients and that areas of imaged bone marrow, on MR, be carefully evaluated for abnormality.

Metastases to Local Lymph Nodes and Liver. Metastases to local lymph nodes and liver on initial presentation are imaged by CT and MR.

Skull Metastases. If skull metastases are identified clinically or on isotope scanning, head and orbit CT should be performed.

Follow-up Studies. There is much less data available with neuroblastoma than with Wilms tumor regarding the nature of the timing and location of relapse and tumor spread. What is known is that patients with stage I or stage II tumor with negative lymph nodes very rarely relapse. If these patients are monitored clinically and with urine determination of catecholamine excretion, it could be argued that limited, if any, imaging follow-up studies should be performed. It is extremely important that the degree of intensity of imaging follow-up be related to the likelihood of significant yield, so that if these patients are imaged, the amount of imaging done should definitely be less than in patients who are stage III or IV. One study suggests that 80 percent of recurrences will occur within 18 months of initial diagnosis.[55] However, it is known that neuroblastomas can relapse unexpectedly for many years and, therefore, it is difficult to define the optimum time for stopping imaging surveillance. The site of recurrence in one study of 52 patients is indicated in Table 6–11, which shows the pattern, in general terms, of the distribution of tumor on initial presentation (Fig. 6–36). Based on available reports the following is suggested:

1. For stage I and stage II tumors with no lymph node disease, either no imaging or a baseline CT and bone scan performed approximately 3 months after initial surgery. MIBG might be performed in addition to or instead of the bone scan, particularly if the primary tumor is known to have taken up this agent before resection.
2. Regular CT scans (every 3 to 6 months) should be done to evaluate the response to therapy in patients with residual nonresected primary tumor. These scans could be repeated more frequently at times of change of therapy (e.g., altered chemotherapy, presurgery, pre-bone marrow transplantation). The scans could be done less frequently when a state of stable residual tumor is reached or when no detectable tumor is left. They should be stopped a few months after therapy is terminated. If a patient has been in a state of remission for a significant period of time (e.g., 2 years), it may be appropriate to stop imaging and continue surveillance with clinical evaluation and urine catecholamine determination.
3. Skull metastases can be evaluated with CT. Liver metastases can similarly be evaluated with CT at the same time the primary tumor is being evaluated. The bones can be evaluated with either MDP or, if available, MIBG. If the patient has been shown on presentation to have bone metastases on MDP, which have not been demonstrated with MIBG, the MDP should be utilized for follow-up. On the other hand, if the patient is known to have previously had bone metastases that have taken up MIBG, this may be the modality of choice, as it is probably more sensitive than MDP for evaluation of response to treatment. It is known that MDP scan can remain positive even after tumor resolution. The duration of surveillance should probably follow the same guidelines as the surveillance of the primary tumor mass.
4. Any patient developing a single hot lesion on MDP scan should have plain radiograph and MIBG scan to help evaluate whether this lesion is a true metastasis or not.
5. Additional imaging should be performed any time there is a change in the clinical status of the patient or a significant alteration in the urine catecholamine secretion.

There are no absolute recommendations for specific studies, anatomical areas, or timing of follow-up. Selec-

TABLE 6–11
Neuroblastoma: Site of Tumor Recurrence or Development of New Tumor in 51 Patients[1]

Site	No. of Patients
At primary site	13
Bone marrow	11
Bone cortex	12
Liver	3
Lymph nodes	9
Brain	3

Reference

1. Stark DD, Brasch RC, Moss AA, et al. Recurrent neuroblastoma. The role of CT and alternative imaging tests. Radiology 1983;148:107.

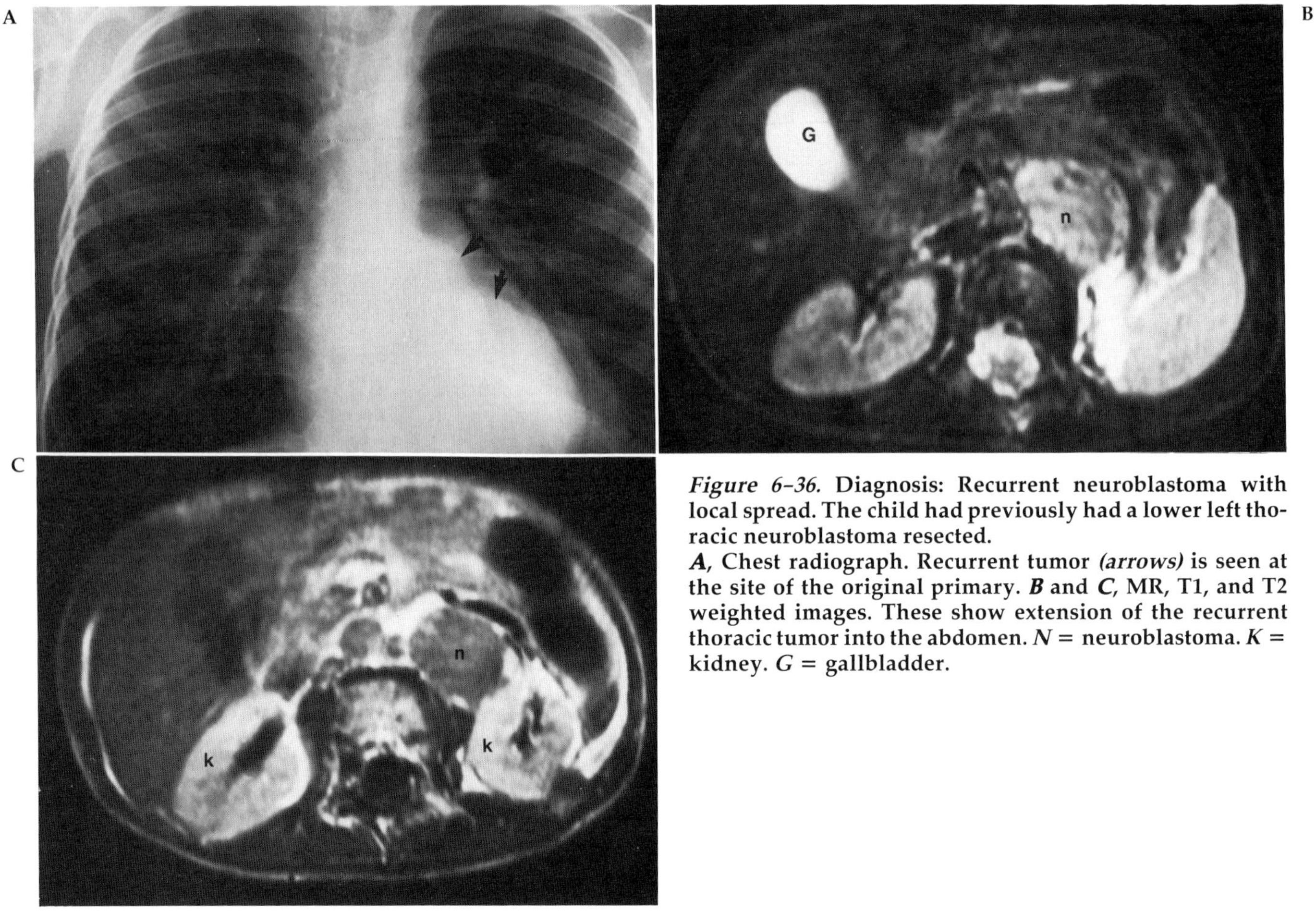

Figure 6-36. **Diagnosis: Recurrent neuroblastoma with local spread. The child had previously had a lower left thoracic neuroblastoma resected.**
***A*, Chest radiograph. Recurrent tumor *(arrows)* is seen at the site of the original primary. *B* and *C*, MR, T1, and T2 weighted images. These show extension of the recurrent thoracic tumor into the abdomen. *N* = neuroblastoma. *K* = kidney. *G* = gallbladder.**

tion and timing of modalities should be based on the patient's tumor stage and the clinical situation, with maximum intensity of imaging effort at those times in which there is a significant clinical change or an alteration in therapy is contemplated.

References

1. Reed JC, Hallet KK, Feigin DS. Neural tumors of the thorax: subject review from the AFIP. Radiology 1978;126:9–17.
2. Stigall R, Smith WL, Franken EA, et al. Intrapulmonic metastatic neuroblastoma. Ann Radiol 1979;22:223–227.
3. Towbin R, Gruppo RA. Pulmonary metastases in neuroblastoma. AJR 1982;138:75–78.
4. Friedland GW, Crowe JE. Neuroblastoma and other adrenal neoplasms. In: Parker BR, Castellino RA, eds. Pediatric oncologic radiology. CV Mosby, 1977:267–271.
5. Bousvaros A, Kirks DR, Grossman H. Imaging of neuroblastoma: an overview. Pediatr Radiol 1986;16:89–106.
6. Hata Y, Uchino J, Sasaki F, et al. Kidney-preserving radical tumor resection in advanced neuroblastoma. J Pediatr Surg 1989;24:382–385.
7. Saeki M, Hagane K, Nakano M. Radiologic evaluation of surgical resectability in abdominal neuroblastoma. J Pediatr Surg 1989;24:378–381.
8. Latchaw RE, L'Heureux PRL, Young G, et al. Neuroblastoma presenting as central nervous system disease. AJNR 1982;3:623–630.
9. Armstrong EA, Harwood-Nash DCF, Ritz CR, et al. CT of neuroblastomas and ganglioneuromas in children. AJNR 1982;3:401–406.
10. Chirathivat S, Post MJD. CT demonstration of dural metastases in neuroblastoma. J Comput Assist Tomogr 1980;4:316–319.
11. Holgersen LO, Santulli, TV, Schullinger JN, et al. Neuroblastoma with intraspinal (dumbbell) extension. J Pediatr Surg 1983;18:406–411.
12. Punt J, Pritchard J, Pincott JR, et al. Neuroblastoma: a review of 21 cases presenting with spinal cord compresson. Cancer 1980;45:3095–3101.
13. Hartman DS, Sanders RC. Wilms' tumor versus neuroblastoma: usefulness of ultrasound in differentiation. J Ultrasound Med 1982;1:117–122.
14. Amundson GM, Trevenen CL, Mueller DL, et al. Neuroblastoma: a specific sonographic tissue pattern. AJR 1987;148:943–945.
15. Forman HP, Leonidas JC, Berdon WE, et al. Congenital neuroblastoma. Evaluation with multimodality imaging. Radiology 1990;175:365–369.
16. Hendry GMA. Cystic neuroblastoma of the adrenal gland—a potential source of error in ultrasound diagnosis. Pediatr Radiol 1982;12:204–206.
17. Garick DJ, Kodroff MB, Marrow HG, et al. Thoracic neuroblastoma presenting as a cystic hygroma. Arch Dis Childh 1988;63:1270–1271.
18. Atkinson GO, Zaatari GS, Lorenzo RI. Cystic neuroblas-

toma in infants: radiographic and pathologic features. AJR 1986;146:113–117.
19. Casola G, Scheible W, Leopold GR. Neuroblastoma metastatic to the testis: ultrasonographic screening as an aid to clinical staging. Radiology 1984;151:475–476.
20. Filiatrault D, Hoyoux C, Benoit P, et al. Renal metastases from neuroblastoma. Pediatr Radiol 1987;17:137–138.
21. Podrasky AE, Stark DD, Hattner RS, et al. Radionuclide bone scanning in neuroblastoma: skeletal metastases and primary tumor localization of 99mTc-MDP. AJR 1983;141:469–472.
22. Stark DD, Moss AA, Brasch RC, et al. Neuroblastoma: diagnostic imaging and staging. Radiology 1983;148:101–105.
23. Martin-Simmerman P, Cohen MD, Siddiqui A, et al. Calcification and uptake of Tc-99m diphosphonates in neuroblastomas: concise communication. J Nucl Med 1984;25:656–660.
24. Peretz GS, Lam AH. Distinguishing neuroblastoma from Wilms tumor by computed tomography. J Comput Assist Tomogr 1985;9:889–893.
25. Engel IA, Auh YH, Rubenstein WA, et al. Large posterior abdominal masses: computed tomographic localization. Radiology 1983;149:203–209.
26. Oliphant M, Berne AS. Aggressive neuroblastoma simulating Wilms tumor. Radiology 1988;167:878.
27. Rosenfield NS, Leonidas JC, Barwick KW. Aggressive neuroblastoma simulating Wilms tumor. Radiology 1988;166:165–167.
28. Shende A, Wind ES, Lanzkowsky P. Intrarenal neuroblastoma mimicking Wilms' tumor. New York St J Med 1979;79:93.
29. Cohen MD, Weetman R, Provisor A, et al. Magnetic resonance imaging of neuroblastoma with a 0.15-T magnet. AJR 1984;143:1241–1248.
30. Belasco J. Occult neuroblastoma: difficulties of diagnosis. Am J Dis Child 1979;133:858–859.
31. Casselman JW, Smet MH, Van Damme B, et al. Primary cervical neuroblastoma: CT and MR findings. J Comput Assist Tomogr 1988;12:684–686.
32. Oliphant M, Berne AS. Mechanism of direct spread of abdominal neuroblastoma: CT demonstration and clinical implications. Gastrointest Radiol 1987;12:59–66.
33. Cohen MD, Klatte EC, Smith JA, et al. Nuclear magnetic resonance evaluation of fifty children with cancer. Ann Radiol 1985;28:339–343.
34. Harris TM, Cohen MD. Abdominal magnetic resonance imaging. Pediatr Radiol 1989;20:10–19.
35. Gilday DL, Ash JM, Reilly BJ. Radionuclide skeletal survey for pediatric neoplasms. Radiology 1977;123:399–406.
36. Heisel MA, Miller JH, Reid BS, et al. Radionuclide bone scan in neuroblastoma. Pediatrics 1983;71:206–209.
37. Franken EA, Smith WL, Cohen MD, et al. Hepatic imaging in stage IV-S neuroblastoma. Pediatr Radiol 1986;16:107–109.
38. Siddiqui AR, Oseas RS, Wellman HN, et al. Evaluation of bone-marrow scanning with technetium-99m sulfur colloid in pediatric oncology. J Nucl Med 1979;20:379–386.
39. Brodeur GM, Seeger RC, Barrett A, et al. International criteria for diagnosis, staging, and response to treatment in patients with neuroblastoma. J Clin Oncol 1988;6:1874–1881.
40. Gerrard M, Eden OB, Merrick MV. Imaging and treatment of disseminated neuroblastoma with ^{131}I-metaiodobenzylguanidine. Br J Radiol 1987;60:393–395.
41. Hoefnogel CA, Voute PA, deKraker J, et al. Radionuclide diagnosis and therapy of neural crest tumors using iodine 133 metaiodobenzylguanidine. J Nucl Med 1987;28:308–314.
42. Shulken B, Shen SW, Sisson JC, et al. Iodine 131-MIBG scintigraphy of the extremities in metastatic pheochromocytoma and neuroblastoma. J Nucl Med 1987;28:315–318.
43. Heyman S, Evans AE, D'Angio GJ. I-131 metaiodobenzylguanidine: diagnostic use in neuroblastoma patients in relapse. Med Pediatr Oncol 1988;16:337–340.
44. Hattner RS, Huberty JP, Engelstad BL, et al. Localization of M-iodo(^{131}I)benzylguanidine in neuroblastoma. AJR 1984;143:373–374.
45. Velchik MG, Alavi A, Kressel HY, et al. Localization of pheochromocytoma: MIGB, CT, and MRI correlation. J Nucl Med 1989;30:328–336.
46. Feine U, Muller-Schauenburg W, Treuner J, et al. Metaiodobenzylguanidine (MIBG) labeled with ^{123}I/^{131}I in neuroblastoma diagnosis and follow-up treatment with a review of the diagnostic results of the international workshop of pediatric oncology held in Rome, September 1986. Med Pediatr Oncol 1987;15:181–187.
47. Moyes JSC, Babich JW, Carter R, et al. Quantitive study of radio-iodinated MIBG uptake in children with neuroblastoma: correlation with tumor histology. J Nucl Med 1989;30:474–479.
48. Jacobs A, Delree M, Desprechins B, et al. Consolidating the role of I-MIBG-scintigraphy in childhood neuroblastoma: five years of clinical experience. Pediatr Radiol 1990;20:157–159.
49. Berger PE, Kuhn JP, Munschauer RW. Computed tomography and ultrasound in the diagnosis and management of neuroblastoma. Radiology 1978;128:663–667.
50. Foglia RP, Fonkalsrud EW, Feig SA, et al. Accuracy of diagnostic imaging as determined by delayed operative intervention for advanced neuroblastoma. J Pediatr Surg 1989;24:708–711.
51. Sitarz A, Finklestein J, Grosfeld J, et al. An evaluation of the role of surgery in disseminated neuroblastoma: a report from the Children's Cancer Study Group. J Pediatr Surg 1983;18:147–151.
52. Ziegelbaum MM, Kay R, Rothner AD, et al. The association of neuroblastoma with myoclonic encephalopathy of infants: the use of magnetic resonance as an imaging modality. J Urol 1988;139:81–82.
53. Woods WG, Tuchman M. Neuroblastoma: the case for screening infants in North America. Pediatrics 1987;79:869–873.
54. Donaldson JS, Gilsanz V, Miller JH. CT scanning in patients with opsomyoclonus: importance of nonenhanced scan. AJR 1986;146:781–783.
55. Stark DD, Brasch RC, Moss AA, et al. Recurrent neuroblastoma. The role of CT and alternative imaging tests. Radiology 1983;148:107.

Differential Diagnosis

The differential diagnosis of neuroblastoma varies depending on the anatomic location of the primary tumor. Disorders that should be considered in the differential diagnosis are listed in Table 6–12. In most cases, it should be relatively easy to make the diagnosis of neuroblastoma prior to biopsy. The diagnosis is made from

TABLE 6–12
Differential Diagnosis of Neuroblastoma

Neck primary
- Infected lymph nodes
- Lymphoma
- Cystic hygroma

Posterior mediastinum
- Other neurogenic tumors
- Extramedullary hemopoesis
- Abscess

Adrenal
- Wilms tumor
- Teratoma
- Rhabdomyosarcoma
- Abscess
- Pancreatic tumor
- Lymphoma
- Other adrenal tumors

Nonadrenal, abdomen, and pelvis
- Teratoma
- Rhabdomyosarcoma
- Abscess
- Lymphoma

the location of the primary tumor, knowledge of the age of the patient, the pattern of metastatic spread if present, with strong reinforcement by the identification of uptake of MDP of MIBG in the primary tumor and the results of catecholamine concentration in the urine. A few specific points in differential diagnosis are discussed further.

In a few cases, particularly in which there is renal invasion, it may be difficult on imaging studies of the primary tumor mass to differentiate Wilms tumor from neuroblastoma. MIBG, MDP, and catecholamine results will resolve the difficulty in most cases.

It may sometimes be difficult to differentiate adrenal hemorrhage in the newborn from congenital neuroblastoma. It has been said that decrease in size of the lesion with time on sequential ultrasound images favors adrenal hemorrhage. This is not true, as a spontaneously resolving neuroblastoma will show the same pattern. Again uptake of isotopes and catecholamine excretion should be utilized to make the determination, rather than ultrasound or CT imaging of the primary tumor. Because of its ability to categorize the presence of blood, MR might be helpful, although there are no published cases demonstrating this hypothesis.

Therapy and Prognosis

Prognosis of neuroblastoma is poor and has not altered significantly in the last 30 to 40 years. The overall cure has remained at approximately 35 percent.[1,2]

Any evaluation of the therapy of neuroblastoma must take into account the well-documented ability of the tumor to spontaneously regress without any interventional therapy.[3,4]

The survival of neuroblastoma by stage from several reported references is summarized in Table 6–13. As can be seen, stage I disease has an excellent prognosis whereas stage IV has a uniformly dismal prognosis. Survival by age is given in Table 6–14. There is a very definite more favorable prognosis in patients under the age of 1 year. There are a number of clearly defined prognostic factors that give a markedly improved survival with neuroblastoma. These are summarized in Table 6–15 and include the patient's age, a nonabdominal site of the primary tumor, a tumor of stage I, II, or IV-S, and the results of several laboratory evaluations.

Elevated serum ferritin and elevated serum neuron specific enolase are nonspecific indicators of a worse prognosis. Of great significance is the recent determination of worsening prognosis, regardless of stage, if the patient is demonstrated to have increased replication (>10) of a segment of DNA that has been designated the n myc oncogene. About 30 percent of all patients with neuroblastoma will have increased amplification of this n myc oncogene. The correlation between the number of replications of this oncogene and prognosis is not absolute, but it does appear to be independent of patient stage so that even patients with a favorable stage, and even a favorable age, have a much worse prognosis if they are demonstrated to have multiple copies of this oncogene. Increased replications

TABLE 6–13
Neuroblastoma Survival by Stage

Stage	Survival (percentage)					
Ref. no.	(1)	(2)	(3)	(4)	(5)	(6)
I	100	100	95–100	94	100	96
II	82	74	85–90	79	93	89
III	42	35	50–60	50	81	50
IV	30	10	10–15	—	23	—
IV-S	—	75	60–65	—	90	—

References

1. Evans AE, D'Angio GJ, Propert K, et al. Prognostic factors in neuroblastoma. Cancer 1987;59:1853–1859.
2. Grosfeld JL, Baehner RL. Neuroblastoma: an analysis of 160 cases. World J Surg 1980;4:29–38.
3. Copeland DR, van Eys J. Childhood cancer survivors: living beyond cure. Am J Pediatr Hematol/Oncol 1987;91:56–57.
4. Finklestein JZ. Neuroblastoma: it is time for a new approach. Am J Pediatr Hematol/Oncol 1988;10:155–160.
5. Rosen EM, Cassady R, Frantz CN, et al. Neuroblastoma: the Joint Center for Radiation Therapy/Dana-Farber Cancer Institue/Children's Hospital experience. J Clin Oncol 1984;2:719–732.
6. Evans AR, Brand W, deLorimier A, et al. Results in children with local and regional neuroblastoma managed with and without vincristine, cyclophosphamide, and imidazolecarboxamide. Am J Clin Oncol 1984;6:3–8.

TABLE 6-14
Neuroblastoma Survival by Age[1]

Age	Percentage
<1 yr	74
−2 yrs	43
−3 yrs	18
>3 yrs	14
Overall	36

Reference

1. Grosfeld JL, Baehner RL. Neuroblastoma: an analysis of 160 cases. World J Surg 1980;4:29–38.

TABLE 6-15
Factors Giving Improved Survival in Neuroblastoma[1-4]

Age < 1 year
Nonabdominal site of primary
Stage I, II, or IV-S
Few copies (<10) of n myc oncogene
Serum neuron specific enolase < 100 ng per ml
Serum ferritin < 150 ng per ml
Favorable Shimada histology

References

1. Evans AE, D'Angio GJ, Propert K, et al. Prognostic factors in neuroblastoma. Cancer 1987;59:1853–1859.
2. Grosfeld JL, Baehner RL. Neuroblastoma: an analysis of 160 cases. World J Surg 1980;4:29–38.
3. Tesoro JD, Nessi R. Late metastasis from neuroblastoma mimicking Ewing's sarcoma. Pediatr Radiol 1980;10:107–109.
4. D'Angio GJ. Neuroblastoma overview—1986. Med Pediatr Oncol 1987;15:159–162.

of the n myc oncogene were found in 19 of 33 patients with stage IV neuroblastoma. These patients had a worse prognosis than those in whom the n myc oncogene was not increased.[5] The implications of this for the radiologist are quite significant. Future therapeutic protocols may well be altered to reflect the results of the determination of these laboratory tests, and follow-up imaging protocols will need to be altered accordingly. In addition, these tests can identify patients, even with favorable stage, at high risk for relapse. These patients should obviously be followed much more intensively with imaging than low-risk patients.

A final characterization that is proving extremely useful in terms of prediction of outcome is the Shimada classification. This is quite complicated. Patients are designated into a favorable or poor prognosis group depending on criteria that have been described in the pathology section of this chapter and that are summarized in Table 6–16. In a very large number of patients, this classification has proved valuable: 87 percent of good-prognosis patients have survived, whereas only 7 percent of the poor-prognosis group have survived. Future therapeutic decisions will be affected by the Shimada grading, and radiologists will need to alter imaging protocols accordingly. Therefore, although complicated, knowledge of this system is essential.

> *Comment:* Powerful predictors of prognosis can be identified for neuroblastoma.

Stage IV-S tumor is an unusual tumor with a high rate of spontaneous regression and a high survival rate despite the presence of disseminated metastasis (except to bone). There is debate as to the optimum treatment for these patients. The primary tumor, if identified, should be resected.[6] Even without further treatment most patients will survive and the risks of relapse need to be balanced against the side effects of chemotherapy. Reported overall survival ranges between 60 and 90 percent for patients with stage IV-S neuroblastoma.[7-9] Deaths tend to be most common in infants under the age of 6 weeks.[2,7,10] In a literature review of 126 cases of stage IV-S neuroblastoma, there were 32 deaths. Eight of these deaths were attributed to therapy. Of the 126 patients 102 had received either chemotherapy, radiation therapy, or both. This study found no difference in mortality between treated and untreated groups of patients.[11] Most of these deaths appear to be related to mechanical problems caused by massive hepatomegaly. The very large liver causes respiratory embarrassment and also renal failure. These patients are also at risk for sepsis. In another report of 137 cases, the increased mortality under the age of 6 weeks was confirmed. The absence of skin lesions in this group was associated with a much worse outcome. The presence or absence of marrow metastases did not influence the outcome.[8]

Surgery has an important role to play in the management of children with neuroblastoma. In stage I patients and in those stage II patients with no lymph node disease, surgery alone can be completely curative. With re-

TABLE 6-16
Shimada "Histology"—Poor-Prognosis Groups[1]

Patients are assigned a poor prognosis if they have any of the following:

- Stroma rich + nodular tumor
- Stroma poor + over 5 years old
- Stroma poor, aged 1½ to 5 years with either MKI > 100 or undifferentiated tumor
- Stroma poor, aged < 1½ years, with MKI > 200

Reference

1. Shimada H, Chatten J, Newton WA, et al. Histopathologic prognostic factors in neuroblastic tumors: definition of subtypes of ganglioneuroblastoma and an age-linked classification of neuroblastomas. JNCI 1984;73:405–416.

gard to the effect of surgery on the outcome of stage IV patients, there is confusing information. In one study, it was demonstrated that of those stage IV patients who did survive, all had complete resection of the primary tumor at some stage.[12] In another study, in 1983, reviewing 191 stage IV patients from the CCSG, it was found that initial complete resection or delayed radical surgery resulted in no improvement in prognosis.[13] The philosophy of surgical intervention in neuroblastoma seems to be to remove as much tumor as possible without sacrificing the abdominal aorta or inferior vena cava, major branches of these vessels (with the exception of the inferior mesenteric artery), or major organs.[7] In patients with stage I, II, or III disease, an attempt is made to resect as much tumor as possible at time of presentation. In patients with stage IV disease, the patient is first treated with chemotherapy, and radical surgery is attempted only if there has been clinical and radiographic evidence of remission of metastatic disease.

Many patients with stage III and IV disease will show significant shrinkage in the size of the primary tumor with chemotherapy (see Fig. 6–14). Tumor increase can also be seen (Fig. 6–37). In up to 60 percent of cases, chemotherapy may result in clinical resolution of the primary tumor.[14] Because of this favorable response, if initial surgery is not able to resect the tumor, it is advocated that second delayed surgery be performed. Two, three, or four attempts at surgical resection may be performed after chemotherapy.[15] This delayed surgery can render patients with stage III and IV disease free of local tumor[15,16] and can improve survival. In one study in stage III patients, complete resection of tumor either initially or after chemotherapy resulted in survival in 20 of 26 patients compared to survival in 9 of 32 patients when resection was impossible.[16] The major serious complication of aggressive surgery is laceration of large vessels, which occurred in 5 of 46 cases in one series.[17] Postoperative intussusception, involving only the small bowel, has a significantly increased incidence in patients with neuroblastoma, occurring in 4 of 28 patients in one series.[18] This intussusception presents with abdominal pain and obstruction within the first 10 days following surgery.[18]

Comment: Radical surgery is important for survival in neuroblastoma. This requires accurate definition of the local spread of tumor and its relationship to adjacent major structures and organs. Modern imaging technology should be able to provide this information accurately and patients should be aggressively imaged prior to any surgical intervention. It is equally important that the radiologist take time to review all of the imaging directly with the surgeon who will be performing the operation. Unfortunately, much information available in the images is frequently not conveyed to the surgeon.

A wide variety of chemotherapeutic agents have been utilized in neuroblastoma.[19] They are not utilized for patients with stage I or II disease but are used in all patients with stage III and IV disease.[20] Chemotherapy will, in most cases, result in reduction of the extent of primary and metastatic tumor,[14,20] and aggressive therapeutic regimens have resulted in improved length of survival in patients with stage IV disease, although the final outcome has not improved in the past few decades. More recent approaches have been to use large doses of chemotherapy with total body irradiation followed by bone marrow transplantation. These studies are ongoing and it is not yet known whether this approach will result in an improved survival for stage IV patients. Radioactive I^{131} MIBG has been used to treat a few patients; long-term outcome is not known.[20]

Radiation therapy cannot cure neuroblastoma.[21] It is not used in patients with stage I disease or those with stage II disease and negative lymph nodes.[22] There is some debate with regard to its use in patients with stage II disease and affected lymph nodes. In patients with stage III and IV disease, radiation therapy helps in reducing the size of the primary tumor. It will also, in most patients, produce symptomatic relief from metastatic

Figure 6–37. **Diagnosis: Tumor growth on chemotherapy.**
***A*, CT. There is a moderately large tumor lying anterior to the left kidney. *B*, One year later the tumor is now markedly enlarged. The left kidney is invaded.**

A

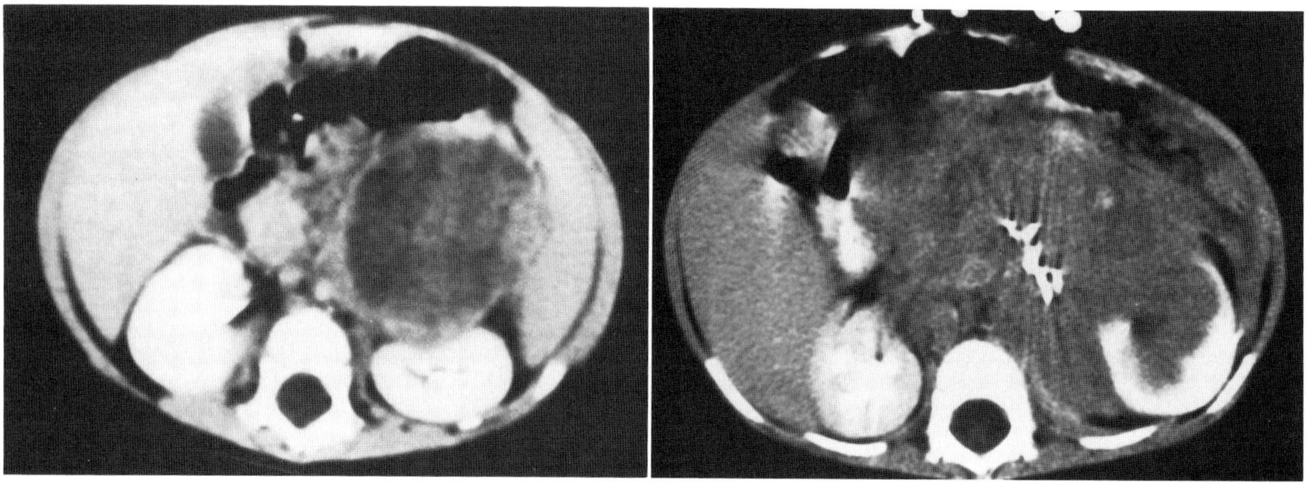

B

TABLE 6–17
Definitions of Response to Treatment[1]

Response	Primary	Metastases	Markers
Complete response	No tumor	No tumor (chest, abdomen, liver, bone, bone marrow, nodes)	HVA/VMA normal
Very good partial response	Reduction >90% but <100%	No tumor (as above except bone); no new bone lesions, all preexisting lesions improved	HVA/VMA decreased
Partial response	Reduction 50–90%	No new lesions; 50–90% reduction in measurable sites; 0 to 1 bone marrow samples with tumor; bone lesions same as very good partial response	HVA/VMA decreased 50 to 90%
Mixed response	No new lesions; >50% reduction of any measurable lesion (primary or metastases) with <50% reduction in any other; <25% increase in any existing lesion.*		
No response	No new lesions; <50% reduction but <25% increase in any existing lesion*		
Partial disease relapse	Any new lesion; increase of any measurable lesion by >25%; previous negative marrow positive for tumor		

*Quantitative assessment does not apply to marrow disease.

Note: Evaluations of primary and metastatic disease as outlined in Table 6–3.

Reference

1. Brodeur GM, Seeger RC, Barrett A, et al. International criteria for diagnosis, staging, and response to treatment in patients with neuroblastoma. J Clin Oncol 1988;6:1874–1881.

disease but will not cure the metastases.[7] Low-dose total body radiation is used prior to bone marrow transplantation.

In order to achieve uniformity between different centers, the International Staging System for Neuroblastoma has recommended a standardized definition of varying responses to therapy. This information is provided in Table 6–17.

References

1. Carlsen NLT, Nielsen OH, Hertz H. Neuroblastoma. Acta Paediatr Scand 1981;70:61–66.
2. Grosfeld JL, Baehner RL. Neuroblastoma: an analysis of 160 cases. World J Surg 1980;4:29–38.
3. Evans AE, D'Angio GJ, Propert K, et al. Prognostic factors in neurblastoma. Cancer 1987;59:1853–1859.
4. Hayes FA, Smith EI. Neuroblastoma. In: Pizzo PA, Poplack DG, eds. Principles and practice of pediatric oncology. Philadelphia: JB Lippincott, 1989:607–622.
5. Tsuda H, Shimosato Y, Upton MP, et al. Retrospective study on amplification of N-myc and c-myc genes in pediatric solid tumors and its association with prognosis and tumor differentiation. Laboratory Investigation 1988;59:321–329.
6. Evans AE, Baum E, Chard R. Do infants with stage IV-S neuroblastoma need treatment? Arch Dis Child 1981;56:271–274.
7. Evans AE. Staging and treatment of neuroblastoma. Cancer 1980;45:1799–1802.
8. Stephenson SR, Cook BA, Mease AD, et al. The prognostic significance of age and pattern of metastases in stage IV-S neuroblastoma. Cancer 1986;58:372–375.
9. Garick DJ, Kodroff MB, Marrow HG, et al. Thoracic neuroblastoma presenting as a cystic hygroma. Arch Dis Childn 1988;63:1270–1271.
10. Evans AE, Chatten J, D'Angio GJ, et al. A review of 17 IV-S neuroblastoma patients at the Children's Hospital of Philadelphia. Cancer 1980;45:833–839.
11. McWilliams NB. IV-S neuroblastoma: treatment controversy revisited. Med Pediatr Oncol 1986;14:41–44.
12. Hata Y, Naito H, Sasaki F, et al. Fifteen years' experience of neuroblastoma: a prognostic evaluation according to the Evans and UICC staging systems. J Pediatr Surg 1990;25:326–329.
13. Sitarz A, Finklestein J, Grosfeld J, et al. An evaluation of the role of surgery in disseminated neuroblastoma: a report from the Children's Cancer Study Group. J Pediatr Surg 1983;18:147–151.
14. Ikeda K, Nakagawara A, Yano H, et al. Improved survival rates in children over 1 year of age with stage III or IV neuroblastoma following an intensive chemotherapeutic regimen. J Pediatr Surg 1989;24:189–193.
15. Foglia RP, Fonkalsrud EW, Feig SA, et al. Accuracy of diagnostic imaging as determined by delayed operative intervention for advanced neuroblastoma. J Pediatr Surg 1989;24:708–711.
16. Haase GM, Wong KY, deLorimier AA, et al. Improvement in survival after excision of primary tumor in stage III neuroblastoma. J Pediatr Surg 1989;24:194–200.
17. Azizkhan RG, Shaw A, Chandler JG. Surgical complications of neuroblastoma resection. Surgery 1985;97:514–517.
18. Cohen MD, Baker M, Grosfeld JL, et al. Post-operative intussusception in children with neuroblastoma. Br J Radiol 1982;55:197–200.
19. Finklestein JZ, Klemperer MR, Evans A, et al. Multiagent chemotherapy for children with metastatic neuroblastoma: a report from Childrens Cancer Study Group. Med Pediatr Oncol 1979;6:179–188.
20. Mastrangelo D. Editorial: the treatment of neuroblastoma with ^{131}I-MIBG. Med Pediatr Oncol 1987;15:157–158.
21. Kushner DH, Cheung N-KV. Neuroblastoma. Pediatr Ann 1988;17:269–283.
22. Bousvaros A, Kirks DR, Grossman H. Imaging of neuroblastoma: an overview. Pediatr Radiol 1986;16:89–106.

ADENOCYSTIC CARCINOMA OF THE LACRIMAL GLAND

Adenocystic carcinoma of the lacrimal gland is very rare. It presents as a firm soft-tissue mass in the upper outer corner of the orbital margins. Apart from the location of the tumor there are no specific features to suggest the correct diagnosis. Ultrasound shows a solid well-defined mass[1] of soft tissue and CT similarly shows a nonspecific well-defined mass[1] (Fig. 6–38).

These tumors require wide surgical excision and tend to recur.

Reference

1. Dagher G, Anderson RL, Ossoinig KC, et al. Adenoid cystic carcinoma of the lacrimal gland in a child. Arch Ophthalmol 1980;98:1098–1100.

ADRENAL CARCINOMA

Epidemiology

Adrenal carcinomas are very rare tumors in childhood.[1] In a large literature review, only 200 cases could be identified.[2] Over 75 percent of the patients are under the age of 5 years,[2,3] with the most common age being in the range of 3 to 5 years. They are more common in females than in males.[4,5] There is an increased incidence in association with clinical syndromes such as hemihypertrophy and Beckwith syndrome.[2,3]

Pathology

Over 75 percent of adrenal carcinomas in children are functional, producing hormones.[3] Two-thirds of these functioning tumors produce androgenic steroids, causing precocious puberty in males and virilization in females.[6] Most of the remaining functioning tumors produce cortisol.[2–4] Adrenal carcinomas will very rarely produce aldosterone or feminizing hormones.[2,3]

These tumors tend to be locally aggressive with invasion. Metastases, when they occur, are to the lung, liver, lymph nodes, and bone.[2,3,6] There may be direct venous spread into the inferior vena cava.[6] When present, the tumor in the inferior vena cava is extremely friable and there is a high risk of tumor embolization.[6]

Microscopically, it may be difficult to differentiate benign adenomas from malignant carcinomas, as the adenomas often have pleomorphic cells and also demonstrate local invasion.[2,3]

A

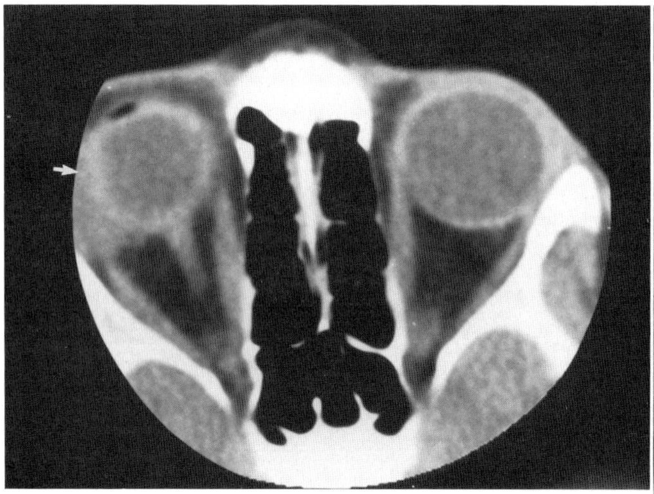

B

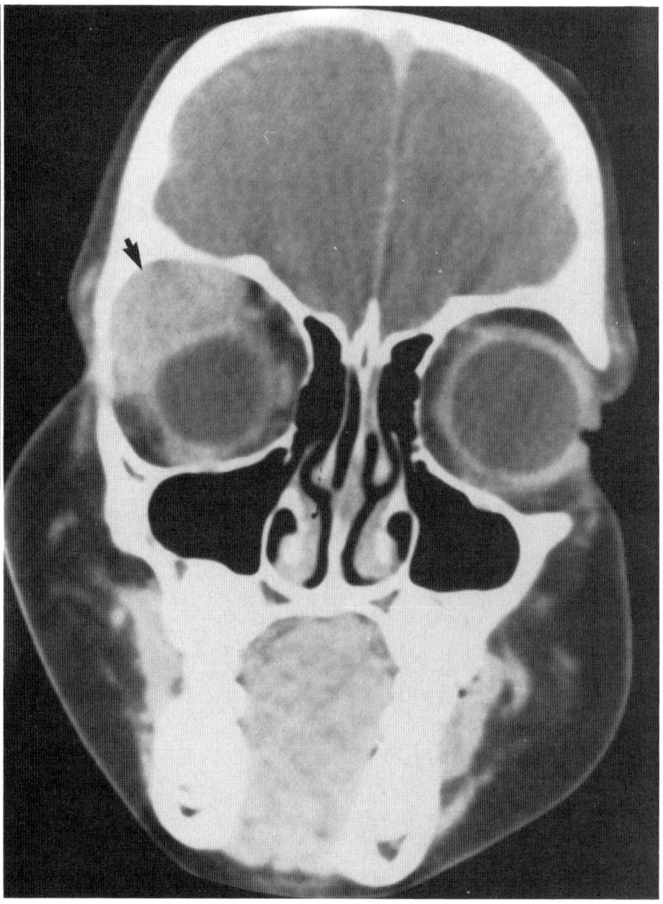

Figure 6–38. **Diagnosis: Lacrimal gland carcinoma (adenocystic carcinoma).**
A **and** ***B*****, CT. There is a large soft-tissue mass lesion in the upper outer quadrant of the right orbit** ***(arrows).*** **It is causing some compression of the eyeball.**

Clinical Presentation

The clinical signs and symptoms are usually those caused by increased hormone production rather than the presence of an abdominal mass or metastatic disease.

Imaging

Traditionally, intravenous pyelography was used to determine the presence of an adrenal mass by renal displacement. This was positive in about 60 percent of patients.[3,4] Ultrasound, CT, and MR can now relatively easily identify adrenal carcinomas and metastases (Fig. 6–39). The tumors are large at the time of diagnosis, with a mean diameter in 14 children of 8 cm and a range of 2½ to 20 cm[5] (Fig. 6–40). Hemorrhage and necrosis are not uncommon,[6] causing inhomogeneity on the imaging studies. On ultrasound, a stellate-shaped echogenic star caused by radiating echogenic scars has been described.[3,6] MR findings in 2 patients reveal tumors with signal intensity on T1 weighted images similar to that of liver. Vena caval extension can be identified with ultrasound or MR. In 3 patients, the caval tumor extended all the way into the right atrium.[6]

Differential Diagnosis

The differential diagnosis includes other adrenal tumors (Fig. 6–41). The stellate scar pattern on the ultrasound and the clinical findings resulting from hormone production are usually adequate to strongly suspect the correct diagnosis. Neuroblastoma is distinguished by calcification, extensive lymph node metastases, the more common presence of distant metastases at the time of diagnosis, and elevation of urine catecholamine levels. Other retroperitoneal tumors are differentiated by the absence of hormone production. The clinical differential diagnoses include idiopathic precocious puberty, congenital adrenal hyperplasia, and hormone production from hepatic or ovarian tumors.

Therapy and Prognosis

Surgical resection is the main form of therapy.[3] The tumors are not responsive to radiation therapy. Chemotherapy is usually reserved for patients with metastases or persistent elevation of hormonal levels after resection of the primary tumor.[3] The prognosis has traditionally been poor,[6] but has recently been said to be improving.[2] Prognosis is better in the very young and also better if

A B C

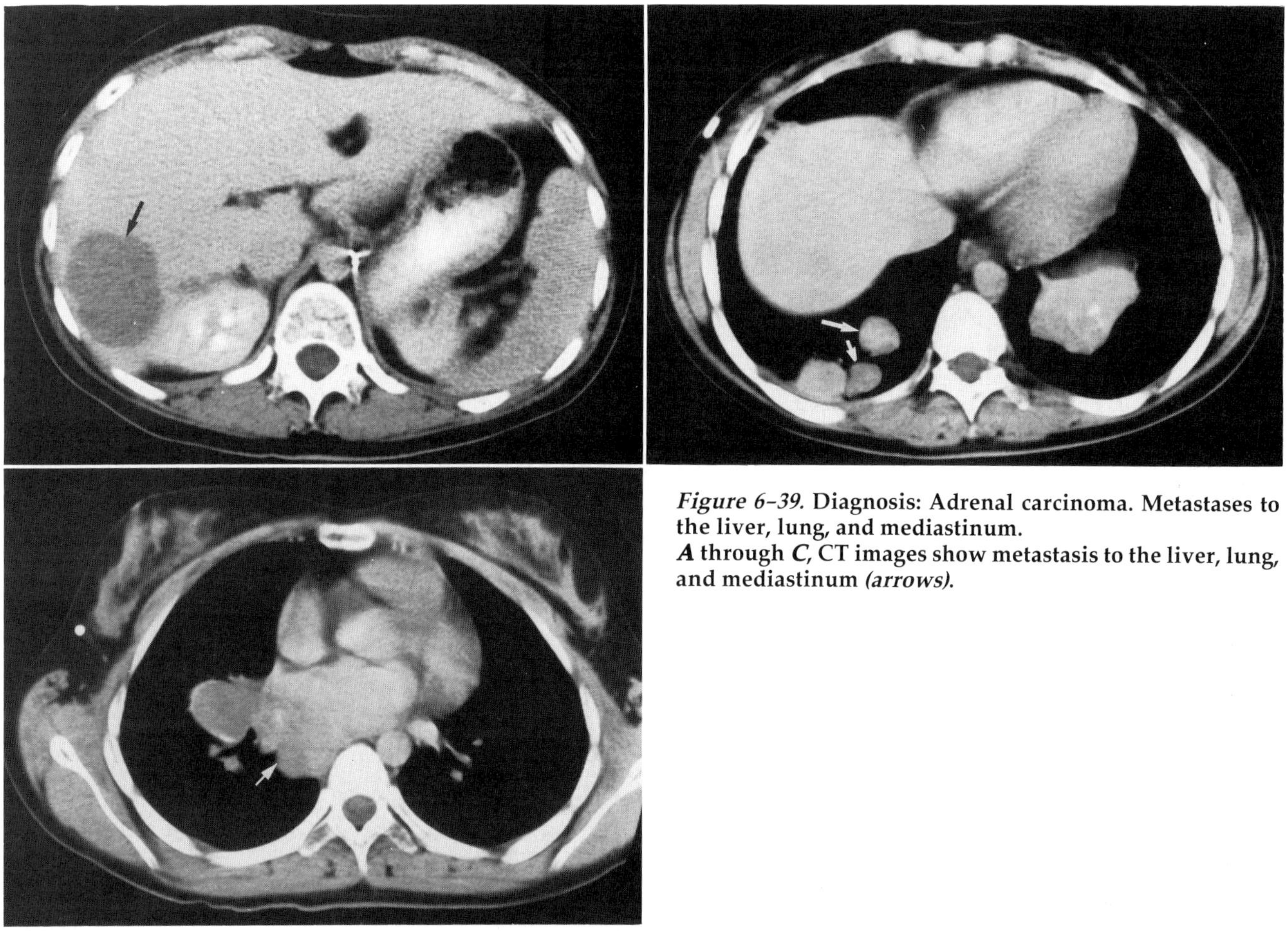

Figure 6–39. **Diagnosis: Adrenal carcinoma. Metastases to the liver, lung, and mediastinum.**
A **through** ***C*****, CT images show metastasis to the liver, lung, and mediastinum** ***(arrows).***

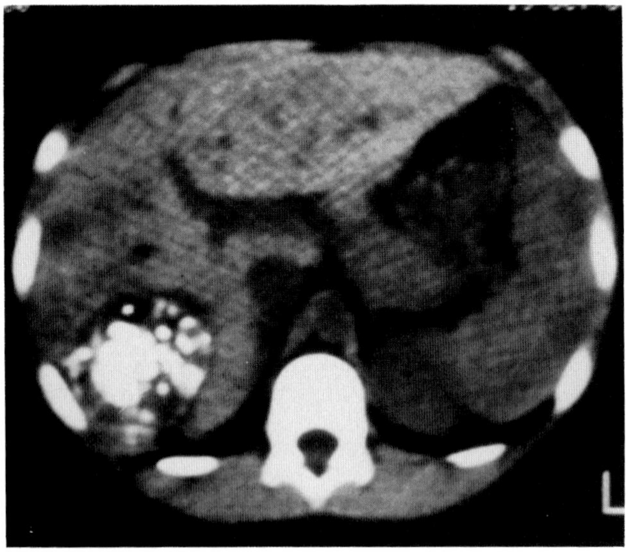

Figure 6-40. **Diagnosis: Adrenocortical carcinoma. There is a large, heavily calcified right adrenal tumor mass. On imaging, this cannot be differentiated from neuroblastoma. (From Morales L. Adrenocortical tumors in childhood. A report of four cases. J Pediatr Surg 1989;24:276–281.)**

the tumors are functioning.[3] If recurrence occurs, it usually does so within 1 to 2 years of tumor resection.[2]

References

1. Crock PA, Clark ACL. Combination chemotherapy for adrenal carcinoma: response in a 5½-year-old male. Med Pediatr Oncol 1989;17:62–65.
2. Lee PDK, Winter RJ, Green OC. Virilizing adrenocortical tumors in childhood: eight cases and a review of the literature. Pediatrics 1985;76:437–444.
3. Morales L, Rottermann RM, Julia V. Adrenocortical tumors in childhood: a report of four cases. J Pediatr Surg 1989;24:276–281.
4. Stewart DR, Jones PHM, Jolleys A. Carcinoma of the adrenal gland in children. J Pediatr Surg 1974;9:59–67.
5. Prando A, Wallace S, Marins JLC, et al. Sonographic findings of adrenal cortical carcinomas in children. Pediatr Radiol 1990;20:163–165.
6. Godine LB, Berdon WE, Brasch RC, et al. Adrenocortical carcinoma with extension into inferior vena cava and right atrium: report of 3 cases in children. Pediatr Radiol 1990;20:166–168.
7. Dehner LP. Non-Hodgkin's lymphomas and malignant histiocytosis in children. Semin Oncol 1977;4:273–286.

OVARIAN TUMORS[1–4]

Malignant tumors of the ovary are very uncommon in children. The most common age of presentation is around puberty.

Pathologically these tumors are classified as follows:

Germ cell, 70%
Epithelial, 15%
Stroma, 10%
Miscellaneous, 5%

The germ cell tumors are discussed in detail in Chapter 9 in the section dealing with germ cell tumors.

At this stage it should be noted that for most of the ovarian tumors imaging usually cannot differentiate between the various tumor types, nor can it differentiate accurately between benign and malignant tumors (Fig. 6–42). Malignancy is suggested by local invasion, ascites, lymphadenopathy, and by the presence of distant metastases, but malignancy can be present in the absence of any of these findings.

Clinical symptoms of ovarian tumors are also nonspecific. Patients may present with abdominal pain, an abdominal mass, or secondary effects from hormone production.

Figure 6-41. **Diagnosis: Virilizing benign adrenal adenoma.**
***A*, Abdominal radiograph. Faint speckled calcification is visualized in the region of the right adrenal gland. This cannot be differentiated from other tumors such as neuroblastoma. *B*, CT. There is a 1-inch-diameter adrenal adenoma (*A*) with peripheral calcification.**

A

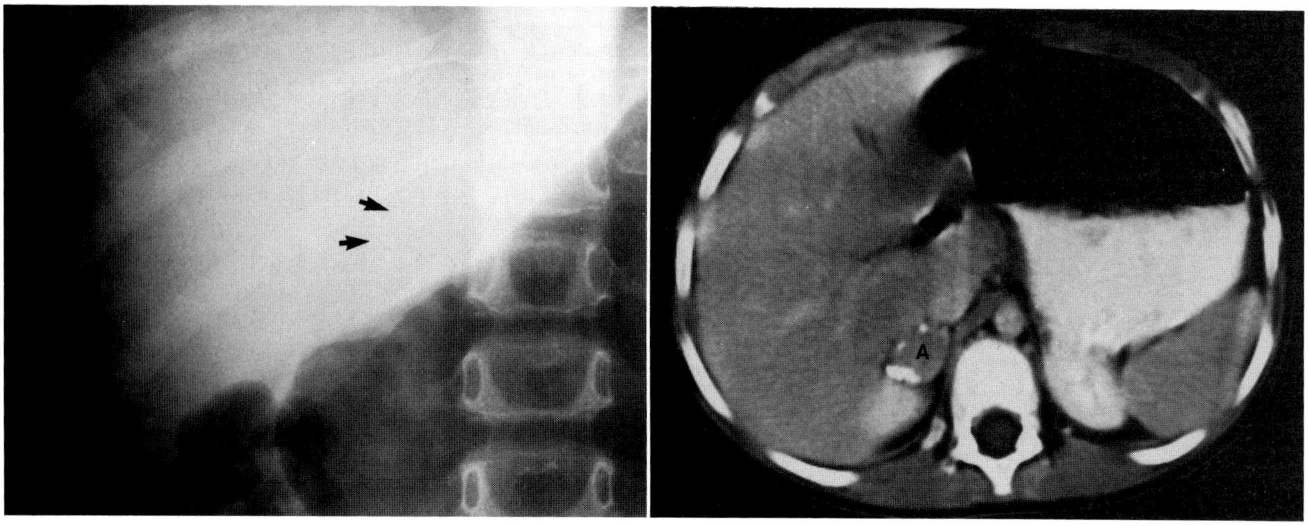

B

A

B

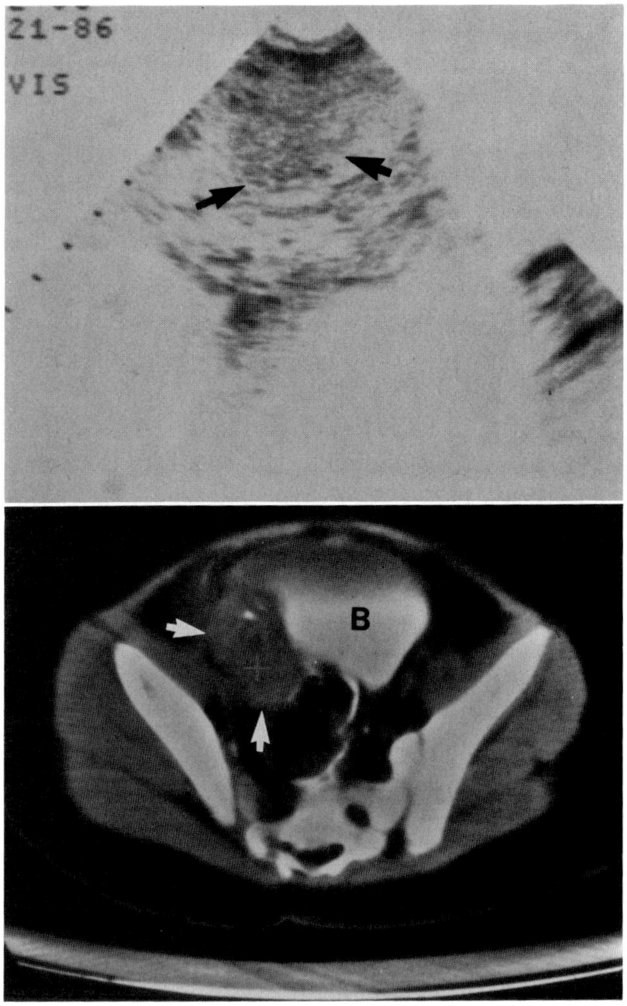

Figure 6–42. **Diagnosis: Ovarian hemangioma. *A,* Ultrasound. A nonspecific pelvic mass is identified *(arrows). B,* CT. The mass lesion arises in the region of the right ovary *(arrows).* It is indenting the bladder (*B*). A small area of calcium is seen within it. The appearance is nonspecific.**

EPITHELIAL TUMORS

These are usually cystadenomas or cystadenocarcinomas. These tend to be large tumors with a predominantly cystic component (Fig. 6–43).

STROMAL TUMORS

Stromal tumors include granulosa cell tumors (Fig. 6–44), arrhenoblastoma, and gynandroblastoma. The granulosa cell tumors produce estrogen and cause precocious puberty. Ten percent are bilateral. They are usually not malignant. The arrhenoblastomas are extremely rare. They usually cause virilization and occasionally precocious puberty.

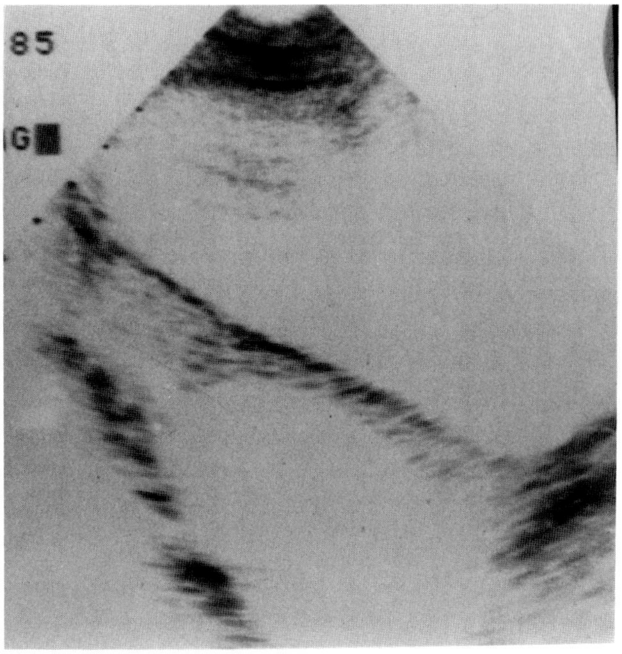

Figure 6–43. **Diagnosis: Ovarian cyst adenocarcinoma. Ultrasound. There is a gigantic abdominal tumor that is predominantly cystic. Multiple tumor septa are identified separating the cystic spaces.**

GONADOBLASTOMA

Gonadoblastomas are mixed germ cell and stromal tumors. They occur only in dysgenetic gonads associated with chromosome abnormalities. They usually present around puberty. One-third are bilateral.[1] They can produce estrogens.[4] They are usually fairly benign but can be mixed with choriocarcinoma. Treatment is resection.[4]

References

1. Sty JR, Wells RG. Other abdominal and pelvic masses in children. Semin Roentgenol 1988;23:216–231.
2. Togashi K, Nishimura K, Itoh K, et al. Ovarian cystic teratomas: MR imaging. Radiology 1987;162:669–673.
3. Dagher G, Anderson RL, Ossoinig KC, et al. Adenoid cystic carcinoma of the lacrimal gland in a child. Arch Ophthalmol 1980;98:1098–1100.
4. Chernausek SD, Leslie ND, Bloch CA, et al. Endocrine disorders in children. Surg Clin N Am 1985;65:1527–1537.

PHEOCHROMOCYTOMA[1–4]

Pheochromocytoma are rare tumors in children. There is an increased incidence in association with disorders such as von Recklinghausen's disease, MEN syndrome,

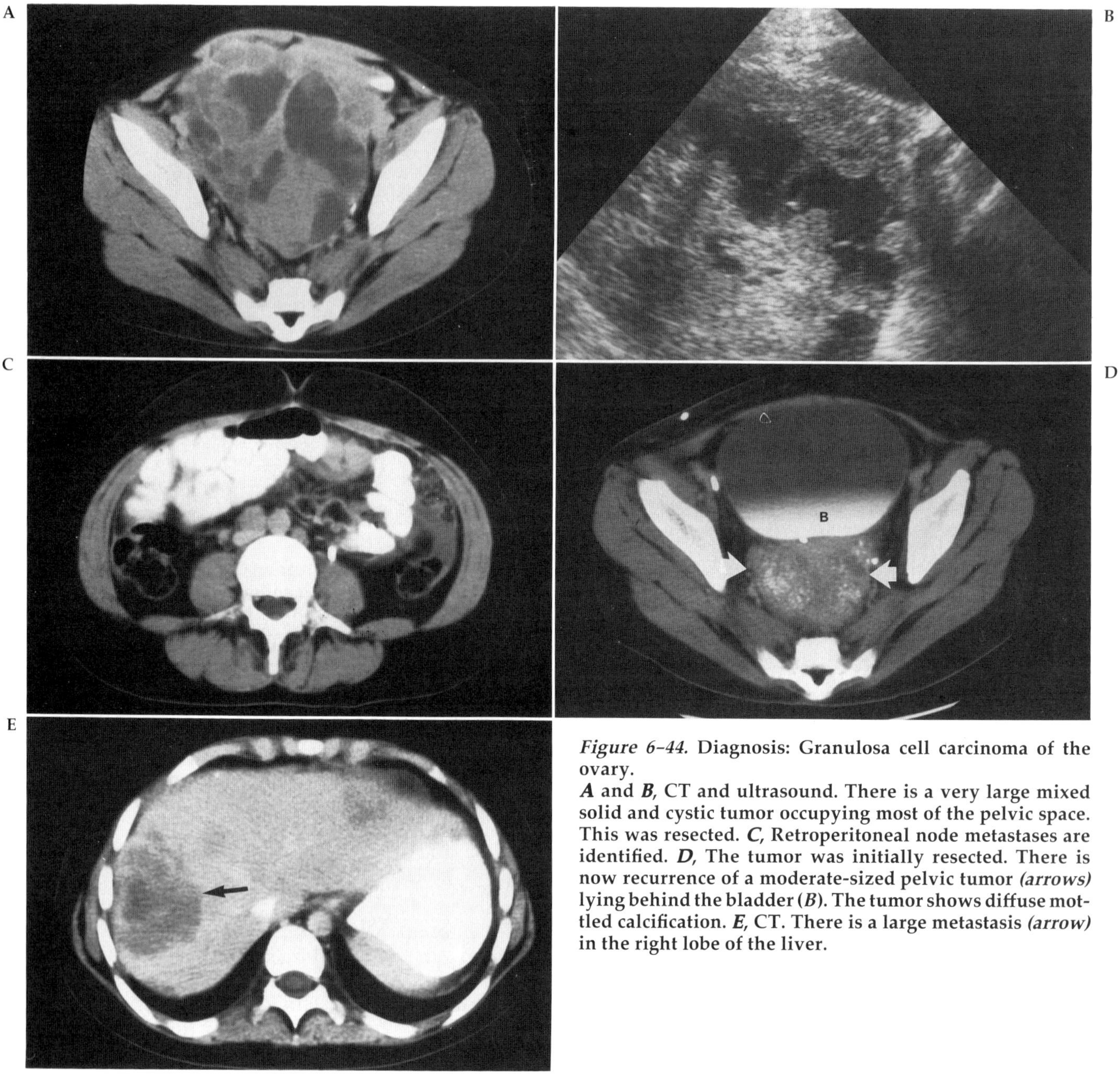

Figure 6–44. **Diagnosis: Granulosa cell carcinoma of the ovary.**
A **and** ***B,*** **CT and ultrasound. There is a very large mixed solid and cystic tumor occupying most of the pelvic space. This was resected.** ***C,*** **Retroperitoneal node metastases are identified.** ***D,*** **The tumor was initially resected. There is now recurrence of a moderate-sized pelvic tumor** ***(arrows)*** **lying behind the bladder (*B*). The tumor shows diffuse mottled calcification.** ***E,*** **CT. There is a large metastasis** ***(arrow)*** **in the right lobe of the liver.**

von Hippel-Lindau disease, and Sturge Weber syndrome. Twenty-five to 30 percent are bilateral.[1]

In children, less than 10 percent of the tumors are malignant. They are more commonly nonadrenal in location than in adults. The most common sites are around the aorta or adjacent to the bladder.[1] It should be noted that the term paraganglioma is sometimes used to refer to a nonadrenal pheochromocytoma.

These tumors are usually fairly easily identified on imaging, often being over 4 to 6 cm in size at the time of diagnosis. They can be seen with CT, MR, or ultrasound (Fig. 6–45) and are frequently positive on MIBG scanning.[4] MIBG is useful as an initial screening test in patients with suspected pheochromocytoma, with the tumor presence being confirmed and better defined with subsequent CT or MR.[4] On CT, they appear as nonspecific fairly uniform soft-tissue masses. On MR, the tumors show features consistent with long T1 and very long T2 relaxation times. They are of lower intensity than liver on T1 weighted images and characteristically extremely bright on T2 weighted images, which in some cases may cause them to be mistaken for a cyst. Imaging cannot differentiate benign from malignant tumors by the appearance of the primary tumor.

The clinical presentation is usually raised blood pressure, with headache being common.[4] The diagnosis is usually strongly suspected because of positive biochemical tests before imaging is commenced.

A B

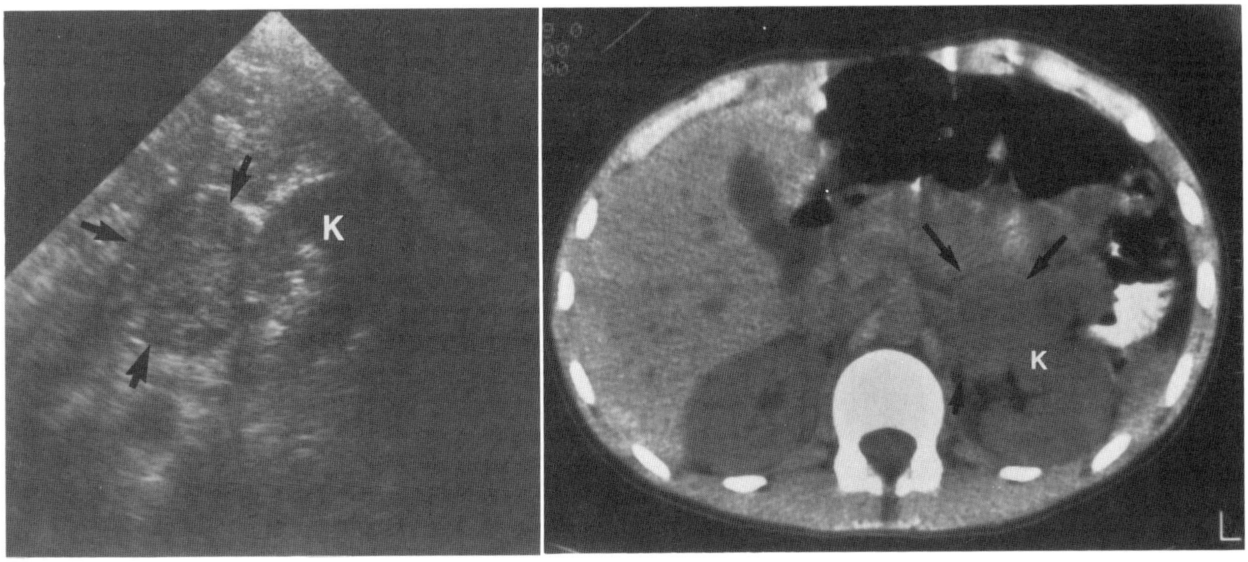

Figure 6-45. Diagnosis: Pheochromocytoma.
A, Ultrasound. There is a large echogenic mass lesion *(arrows)* lying anterior to the right kidney. The appearance is relatively nonspecific. ***B***, CT. This again identifies a homogenous soft-tissue mass lesion *(arrows)* lying anterior to the right kidney. *K* = kidney.

References
1. Dehner LP. Pediatric surgical pathology, 2nd ed. Baltimore: Williams & Wilkins, 1987:560–562.
2. Levine E, de Vries P, Wetzel LH. MR imaging of inferior vena caval recurrence of extraadrenal pheochromocytoma. J Comput Assist Tomogr 1987;11:717–718.
3. Schmedtje JF, Sax S, Pool JL, et al. Localization of ectopic pheochromocytomas by magnetic resonance imaging. AM J Med 1987;83:770–775.
4. Velchik MG, Alavi A, Kressel HY, et al. Localization of pheochromocytoma: MIGB, CT, and MRI correlation. J Nucl Med 1989;30:328–336.

TESTICULAR TUMORS[1–12]

Tumors of the testis are not uncommon in children. They are classified as follows.[2,3,12]

Primary malignant tumors of the testis
- Germ cell tumors, 70%
- Stromal tumors, 20%
- Gonadoblastoma, 5%
- Carcinoid

Paratesticular tumors
- Rhabdomyosarcoma

Metastatic tumors
- Leukemia
- Lymphoma
- Neuroblastoma
- Wilms tumor

Most testicular tumors present as a slow-growing testicular mass.[6] They are often painless. Hydrocele may be present in up to 25 percent of patients.[4,6]

The imaging appearance of the various testicular tumors is not widely described, because many of these tumors are resected before local imaging is performed. With the advent of high-resolution small-part ultrasound transducers, and also the excellent visualization of the testes with MR imaging, it is anticipated that imaging will be performed more frequently in the future as an initial part of the management of a patient with a scrotal or testicular mass.

GERM CELL TUMORS

Germ cell tumors are described in detail in the section on germ cell tumors in Chapter 9.

METASTATIC TUMORS

Metastatic tumors are described in the sections dealing with each of the specific primary tumors.

STROMAL TUMORS

Stromal tumors include Leydig cell tumors, Sertoli cell tumors, and granulosa cell tumors. These germinal cell tumors produce estrogens or androgens. Clinical symptoms include enlargement of the genitals, gynecomastia, local testicular mass, and virilization.[10]

The Leydig cell tumors produce androgens.[10,12,13] They cause precocious puberty. The peak age is about 4 years. They are invariably benign and do not metastasize. Treatment is local surgical excision.[12]

The Sertoli cell tumors have a peak incidence of 18 months of age, with most children being less than 6 months.[12] They present as a testicular mass, with or without signs of precocious puberty. The masses are usually small at the time of diagnosis. The tumors are usually benign but can occasionally metastasize, with metastatic spread being identified in 1 of 22 patients in one series.[12] Treatment is surgical excision.

GONADOBLASTOMA

Gonadoblastoma is described in detail in the section on ovarian tumors.

References

1. Casola G, Scheible W, Leopold GR. Neuroblastoma metastatic to the testis: ultrasonographic screening as an aid to clinical staging. Radiology 1984;151:475–476.
2. Flamant F, Nihoul-Fekete C, Patte C. Optimal treatment of clinical stage I yolk sac tumor of the testis in children. J Pediatr Surg 1986;21:108–111.
3. Kaplan GW, Cromie WC, Kelalis PP, et al. Prepubertal yolk sac testicular tumors—report of the testucular tumor registry. J Urol 1988;140:1109–1112.
4. Exelby PR. Testis cancer in children. Semin Oncol 1979;6:116–121.
5. Barth RA, Teele RL, Colodny A, et al. Asymptomatic scrotal masses in children. Radiology 1984;152:65–68.
6. Exelby PR. Testicular cancer in children. Cancer 1980;45:1803–1809.
7. Fernandes ET, Etcubanas E, Bar BN, et al. Two decades of experience with testicular tumors in children at St Jude Children's Research Hospital. J Pediatr Surg 1989;24:677–682.
8. Husband JE, Hawkes DJ, Peckham MJ. CT estimations of mean attenuation values and volume in testicular tumors: a comparison with surgical and histologic findings. Radiology 1982;144:553–558.
9. Livingstone RR, Sarembock LA. Testicular tumours in children. S African Med J 1986;70:168–169.
10. Chernausek SD, Leslie ND, Bloch CA, et al. Endocrine disorders in children. Surg Clin N Am 1985;65:1527–1537.
11. Perry C, Servadio C. Seminoma in childhood. J Urol 1980;124:932–933.
12. Brosman SA. Testicular tumors in prepubertal children. Urology 1979;13:581–588.
13. Dehner LP. Pediatric surgical pathology, 2nd ed. Baltimore: Williams & Wilkins, 1987:712–736.

THYROID TUMORS[1]

Thyroid tumors are very rare in children. Only about 10 percent are malignant. A history of prior radiation therapy to the neck region is extremely common. The mortality for all of these tumors is less than 20 percent.

Thyroid tumors are classified as papillary, follicular, or medullary.

PAPILLARY TUMORS

Papillary tumors are the most common thyroid tumors in children, with a mean age at presentation of 12 to 14 years. Half are multifocal. Ninety percent have spread to local lymph nodes, and the clinical presentation is often that of lymphadenopathy that has been present for a long time. Twenty to 50 percent have lung metastases at the time of diagnosis.

FOLLICULAR TUMORS

Follicular tumors represent less than 10 percent of thyroid cancer in children. These are well-defined tumors that may be single or multiple.

MEDULLARY TUMORS

Medullary tumors represent only 2 to 3 percent of thyroid malignancy in children. Most of them are part of the MEN-II syndrome. Local metastases to lymph nodes are common.

Reference

1. Dehner LP. Pediatric surgical pathology, 2nd ed. Baltimore: Williams & Wilkins, 1987:524–540.

CHAPTER 7
MUSCULOSKELETAL TUMORS

BONE AND SOFT-TISSUE TUMORS

Malignant tumors of the bones and soft tissues are rare in children, occurring with much less frequency than in adults. Although most of these tumors are more common in adults, a few occur more commonly in children (e.g., osteogenic sarcoma). A special fascination of musculoskeletal malignant tumors is the intellectual challenge they offer the radiologist. Bone tumors have always been of particular interest to radiologists because of the possibility of differentiating the various tumors from each other, and from benign lesions, on the plain film radiograph. The advent of newer imaging technologies such as computerized tomography (CT) and magnetic resonance (MR) imaging has provided new information with regard to bone lesions and has for the first time permitted a clear imaging definition of primary soft-tissue tumors.

Careful analysis of the plain film radiograph may lead in many cases to a confident definitive diagnosis. In other patients, a combination of information from various imaging modalities leads to a specific diagnosis, while in yet other patients, the results of imaging provide only a lengthy differential diagnosis. Musculoskeletal tumor investigation requires a close collaborative effort with integration of the imaging findings, clinical information, and the pathologic histology of the tumor. In some tumors, the histologic diagnosis is easy, whereas in other patients, it is extremely difficult, with the pathologist relying on radiologic information to help with his or her differential diagnosis.

Malignant lesions of bone and soft tissue are most easily classified by reference to their cell of origin (Table 7–1). In some tumors, the precise cell of origin of the malignancy is not known and considerable controversy rages. This is true, for example, of Ewing sarcoma, the origin of which, some pathologists believe, is a primitive mesenchymal cell, while others provide evidence for a neural origin.

Of the primary bone malignant tumors, osteogenic sarcoma and Ewing sarcoma are by far the most common. Table 7–2 identifies the incidence of the various primary bone tumors in children. Osteogenic sarcoma and Ewing sarcoma together account for over 80 percent of these lesions. All the other primary bone tumors in children, and almost all the primary soft-tissue malignancies (with the exception of rhabdomyosarcoma),

TABLE 7–1
Classification of Malignant Tumors of Musculoskeletal System by Their Tissue of Origin

Origin	Tumor
Bone	Osteosarcoma
Cartilage	Chondrosarcoma
Fibrous tissue	Fibrosarcoma, malignant fibrous histiocytosis
Vascular tissue	Hemangiopericytoma
Fat	Liposarcoma, lipoblastomatosis
Unknown	Ewing
Neural	Neurofibrosarcoma
Muscle	Rhabdomyosarcoma

TABLE 7–2
Distribution of Primary Malignant Bone Tumors in Children[1]

Tumor	Percentage
Osteogenic sarcoma	56
Ewing	31
Primary lymphoma	4
Chondrosarcoma	4
Fibrosarcoma	3
Other	2

Reference
1. Spjut HJ, Ayala AG. Skeletal tumors in children and adolescents. Hum Pathol 1983;14:628–642.

are extremely rare. Table 7–3 lists the large number of rare tumors that can be found in the musculoskeletal system in children. Rhabdomyosarcoma is discussed in Chapter 9, which deals with tumors that can be found in multiple organs and tissues.

Imaging is important at every stage in the evaluation of a child with a musculoskeletal tumor. Imaging plays a role in identifying the original lesion, providing a differential diagnosis, staging the tumor, and monitoring therapy.

Staging of primary musculoskeletal tumors is not as developed as, for example, with Wilms tumor or neuroblastoma. Although a generalized staging system for malignant bone tumors has been suggested (Table 7–4), this type of classification has not received widespread acceptance. The major requirement in staging of the musculoskeletal tumors is determining the presence or absence of metastatic disease.

Conventional radiography, isotope scanning, CT, MR, and ultrasound have all been used in the evaluation of musculoskeletal tumors.

Conventional Radiography

The plain film radiograph is still the best modality for the initial evaluation of a bone tumor.[1,2] It provides the best information with regard to the aggressiveness and rate of growth of the lesion. In addition, the pattern of bone destruction, the appearance of the periosteal reaction, and the pattern of matrix mineralization if present still provide probably the best differential diagnosis for a primary bone tumor. Plain film radiographs should be obtained at initial presentation of any primary bone tumor, for the evaluation of new local symptoms or pain in any distant bone site, for the further evaluation of any "hot spot" identified on bone MDP isotope scan, and sequentially for the monitoring of the response of any bone tumor to chemotherapy or radiation therapy. Plain film radiographs of bone have no role to play in the routine screening of the entire skeleton for metastatic deposits from primary bone tumors. The plain film radiograph should be carefully evaluated, with particular attention being paid to the margin of the lesion, the periosteal reaction, and the matrix mineralization (Table 7–5). In addition, much useful information with regard to the differential diagnosis between benign and malignant bone tumors can be obtained by careful evaluation of the location of the lesion both along the length of the shaft of the bone and with attention to the transverse location from the marrow to the bone surface. A guide to the usefulness of this evaluation is given in Table 7–6.

TABLE 7–3
List of Uncommon Musculoskeletal Malignant Tumors in Children

Adamantinoma
Alveolar soft-part sarcoma
Chondrosarcoma
Clear-cell sarcoma
Epithelioid sarcoma
Fibrosarcoma
Hemangiopericytoma
Juvenile angiofibroma
Liposarcoma and lipoblastomatosis
Malignant fibrous histiocytoma
Melanotic neuroectodermal tumor
Mesenchymoma
Primitive neuroectodermal tumor
Synovial cell sarcoma

TABLE 7–4
Staging of Malignant Bone Tumors[1]

Stage	Description
I	Low grade and no metastases
II	High grade and no metastases
	Intramedullary
	Extramedullary
III	Metastatic disease is present

Reference

1. Link MP, Eilber F. Osteosarcoma. In: Pizzo PA, Poplack DG, eds. Principles and practice of pediatric oncology. Philadelphia: JB Lippincott, 1989:689–711.

TABLE 7–5
Plain Film Radiograph Analysis of Bone Tumors

Margin of lesion—indicator of biologic activity. In increasing order of activity, the margin may be:
- Sharp (geographic)
  - Sclerotic—enchondroma, chondromyxoid fibroma, osteoblastoma, cyst, cortical defect
  - Nonsclerotic—giant cell tumor, aneurysmal bone cyst
- Slightly ill defined
  - Low-grade malignancy
  - Infection
- Permeative
  - Malignancy
- Moth eaten
  - Malignancy
  - Hyperemia—infection
  - Hyperparathyroidism

Periosteal reaction—nonspecific indicator of biologic activity of a lesion

Matrix mineralization
- Fairly homogeneous—suggests osteoid matrix
- Punctate, stippled, granular—suggests cartilage matrix

TABLE 7–6
Differential Diagnosis of Benign and Malignant Bone Tumors: Usefulness of Location

	Epiphysis	Metaphysis	Diaphysis
Exophytic	—	Osteochondroma Osteogenic sarcoma Parosteal aneurysmal bone cyst	Osteochondroma Parosteal osteogenic sarcoma Parosteal aneurysmal bone cyst
Cortex	—	Fibrous cortical defect Osteoid osteoma Periosteal osteogenic sarcoma	Fibrous cortical defect Osteoid osteoma
Eccentric	Chondroblastoma Infection Eosinophilic granuloma Giant cell tumor	Osteogenic sarcoma Giant cell tumor Chondromyxoid fibroma	Chondromyxoid fibroma
Central		Enchondroma Bone cysts	Malignant histiocytosis Ewing sarcoma Fibrous dysplasia Bone cysts

Note: Exceptions occur to all of the above. The table should be used as a useful guideline only.

Bone Isotope Scan

The bone isotope scan (with technetium 99m) has a limited role in the evaluation of the primary bone tumor. In a symptomatic child, it is extremely unlikely that the plain film radiograph in the location of the primary bone tumor will be abnormal. For determining the extent of local spread of a primary bone tumor, CT and MR are more accurate than MDP bone isotope scan. Similarly, the scan is of limited value in following the response of the primary bone tumor to chemotherapy or radiation therapy, as the response seen on the bone scan will frequently lag a long time behind the histopathologic response.

The major role for bone isotope scanning is in the detection of metastatic disease, and for this the isotope scan is the imaging modality of choice. A large number of nonmalignant lesions can also cause focal increased activity on the radionuclide bone scan (Table 7–7), and the specificity of the bone scan is greatly improved by further analysis of plain film radiographs obtained of regions of "hot spots" on isotope images. Very rarely, metastatic disease may be missed, for example, in areas of extensive destruction, if the area of abnormality is obscured by previously administered barium or by a bladder that is full with urine containing the radioisotope.

In addition, for routine screening for metastatic disease the MDP bone scan should also be performed in all patients with focal bone pain, not at the location of the primary tumor, in whom the plain film radiograph is negative.

TABLE 7–7
Nonmalignant Causes of Increased Activity in Radionuclide Bone Scans[1]

Normal structures
- Base of skull
- Costochondral junctions
- External occipital protuberance
- Paranasal sinuses
- Inferior tip of scapulae
- Spinous processes of vertebrae
- Sternum
- Sternoclavicular joints
- Sternomanubrial joint
- Sacroiliac joints
- Unfused epiphyses

Benign soft-tissue abnormalities
- Calcific tendinitis
- Cellulitis
- Injection site of scan agent
- Myositis ossificans
- Operative site

Benign osseous abnormalities
- Benign cartilage tumors
- Bone infarct
- Fibrous dysplasia
- Healing fractures
- Inflammatory arthritis
- Metabolic bone disease
- Osteoarthritis
- Osteoid osteoma
- Osteomyelitis
- Surgical or biopsy site

Reference
1. Gold RI, Seeger LL, Bassett LW, et al. An integrated approach to the evaluation of metastatic bone disease. Radiol Clin N Am 1990;28:471–483.

Computed Tomography

CT should be performed for evaluation of all primary bone tumors, as it provides much greater information with regard to periosteal reaction, cortical destruction, and matrix mineralization than does MR.[3] It is much less useful for primary soft-tissue tumors. In occasional patients, e.g., those with fatty tumors, CT scan will provide some tissue specificity. There is debate with regard to the relative accuracy of CT and MR for identification of extent of marrow spread of a primary bone tumor. Unfortunately, many of the comparative studies claiming superiority for MR have utilized CT scanning techniques that are suboptimal. For example, CT is improved by the utilization of thin sections and also by the utilization of pixel histograms of the bone marrow rather than direct subjective evaluation of marrow intensity. In practice it probably matters little if CT gives a small error (of less than a centimeter) compared to MR, as most surgical approaches to primary bone tumor resection strive to leave a clear tumor-free margin of at least 6 to 7 cm. As discussed below, MR should be performed in addition to CT for evaluation of all patients with primary bone tumors.

CT is the modality of choice for screening for lung metastases.

Magnetic Resonance

MR is the imaging modality of choice for the evaluation of primary soft-tissue malignant tumors. Many workers, and I would agree, believe that MR alone is adequate and that an additional CT scan may provide equal but very rarely additional information over that provided by the MR scan. The only potential advantage of CT is an identification of calcium in a soft-tissue lesion, but if this is to be important in the differential diagnosis, it is usually identified quite readily on the plain film radiograph. With regard to primary bone tumors, MR is complementary to CT, providing better definition of the margins of the lesion.[2,3] In one study of 40 soft-tissue sarcomas reported in 1988, MR was superior to CT. In 23 percent of patients, it showed tumor in muscle groups that was not identified by CT. Demonstration of this additional tumor influenced surgery.[4] As with CT, MR cannot differentiate histology in most of the soft-tissue tumors,[5] although it probably provides slightly more tissue specificity than does CT. MR can identify fat; a low signal on T1 and T2 pulse sequences probably suggests the presence of fibrous tissue; and a serpiginous low-intensity signal on T1 and T2 weighted images suggests the presence of a vascular tumor such as hemangioma.

For bone metastases neither MR nor CT should be routinely used. While MR is sensitive for detection of marrow abnormality, it does not provide a global picture of the entire skeleton. Either CT, MR, or both of these modalities could be used for further evaluation of potential metastatic lesions identified on bone scan or plain film radiograph.

Ultrasound

Ultrasound is extremely poor for identification of primary bone tumors. With regard to soft-tissue tumors or the soft-tissue component of bone tumors, ultrasound is reasonably good, but does not compare favorably with either CT or MR.[6] Ultrasound, therefore, has little role to play in the evaluation of musculoskeletal tumors in children.

Comment. Plain film radiographs, MR, and CT are the best modalities for evaluating primary bone tumors.

References
1. Stoker DJ. Management of bone tumours—the radiologist's role. Clin Radiol 1989;40:233–239.
2. Dalinka MK, Zlatkin MB, Chao P, et al. The use of magnetic resonance imaging in the evaluation of bone and soft-tissue tumors. Radiol Clin N Am 1990;28:461–470.
3. Tehranzadeh J, Mnaymneh W, Ghavam C, et al. Comparison of CT and MR imaging in musculoskeletal neoplasms. J Comput Assist Tomogr 1989;13:466–472.
4. Demas BE, Heelan RT, Lane J, et al. Soft-tissue sarcomas of the extremities: comparison of MR and CT in determining the extent of disease. AJR 1988;150:615–620.
5. Sundaram M, McGuire MH, Herbold DR. Magnetic resonance imaging of soft tissue masses: an evaluation of fifty-three histologically proven tumors. Mag Reson Imag 1988;6:237–248.
6. Glasier CM, Seibert JJ, Williamson SL, et al. High resolution ultrasound characterization of soft tissue masses in children. Pediatr Radiol 1987;17:233–237.

CONVENTIONAL OSTEOSARCOMA

Osteosarcoma is defined as any malignant bone tumor that contains osteoid.[1] The histologic appearance of osteosarcomas is extremely varied, but all of these tumors are linked together by the common finding of the presence of osteoid.

The classification of osteosarcoma is important and confusing. The importance of recognizing various well-defined subgroups of osteosarcoma is that some of these subtypes have a very different prognosis and, therefore, require different therapy. In addition, while the radiologist is comfortable with recognition of a typical classic osteogenic sarcoma, failure to appreciate the existence of the wide variety of different subtypes will inevitably result in incorrect diagnoses, with many of these lesions being missed. Delayed diagnosis will have a harmful effect on the child.

The confusion with regard to the classification of osteosarcoma is that the various classification systems that have been suggested are not based on a single parameter such as histology, but instead blend together a mixture of parameters, including histology, location, behavior, and predisposing factors. While there is no absolute universal agreement, the classification outlined in Table 7–8 includes most of the well-recognized subgroups of osteosarcoma and provides a workable reference. The manner in which the anatomic location and histologic grade blend together to provide the classification is summarized in Table 7–9. Each of the types of osteosarcoma is discussed here. For many of the different subtypes certain features, such as age at presentation, therapy, or prognosis, may be identical to those found with the classic, conventional osteosarcoma. This tumor is described in great detail. The various subtypes are described briefly, with emphasis on the features that distinguish these tumors from conventional osteosarcoma.

Comment: Osteosarcoma is not a single tumor but exists in several well-recognized forms.

Epidemiology

The incidence of newly diagnosed cases of osteosarcoma in children is approximately 4.8 per million children per year.[2] Osteosarcoma accounts for approximately 60 percent of malignant bone tumors in children[3] and causes about 50 percent of all deaths from bone tumors in children.[4] The median age for diagnosis is 18 years,[5] with 80 percent of all cases of osteosarcoma occurring under the age of 30 years,[6] 70 percent of cases occurring under the age of 20 years, and 10 percent of cases occurring under the age of 10 years.[7,8] Fifty percent of osteosarcomas occur between the age of 10 and 19 years.[4] This peak in the incidence of osteosarcoma comes during the adolescent growth spurt, which is believed to be an etiologic factor.[3] The peak in females occurs at a slightly younger age than males, corresponding to their earlier growth spurt.[3] In addition, osteosarcoma is found most commonly at sites of maximal bone growth, at the proximal humerus and around the knee joint. The overall incidence is higher in males than in females.[2]

Unlike Wilms tumor, in which there are very clearly defined correlations with genetic and congenital syndromes, this association does not exist strongly with osteosarcoma. A wide variety of etiologic factors have been described in association with osteosarcoma (Table 7–10), but it must be emphasized that the vast majority of tumors occur without any association with any of these etiologic factors. The most important of these factors is radiation therapy, with up to 3 percent of all osteosarcomas occurring following radiation. The time lag between the radiation and the development of the osteosarcoma can be as little as 4 years.[9] With regard to hereditary bilateral retinoblastoma and osteosarcoma, it was previously believed that radiation therapy was the etiologic factor for the associated osteosarcoma. More

TABLE 7–8
Classification of Osteosarcoma[1–3]

- Conventional
  - Osteoblastic
  - Chondroblastic
  - Fibroblastic
- Telangiectatic
- Parosteal
- Periosteal
- High-grade surface
- Intracortical
- Small cell
- Intraosseous well differentiated (central low grade)
- Extraosseous

Note: This classification is not ideal, as it is based on a mixture of histology, location, and behavior, but the various types are well recognized in the literature.

References

1. Carrasco CH, Charnsangavej C, Raymond AK, et al. Osteosarcoma: angiographic assessment of response to preoperative chemotherapy. Radiology 1989;170:839–842.
2. Lindell MM, Shirkhoda A, Raymond AK, et al. Parosteal osteosarcoma: radiologic-pathologic correlation with emphasis on CT. AJR 1987;148:323–328.
3. Unni KK, Dahlin DC. Osteosarcoma: pathology and classification. Semin Roentgenol 1989;24:143–152.

TABLE 7–9
Correlation of Anatomic Location and Grade with Tumor "Type"[1,2]

Anatomic Location	Grade	Tumor Type
Medullary	Low	Intraosseous well differentiated
	High	Conventional (osteoblastic, chondroblastic, fibroblastic)
		Telangiectatic
		Small cell
Cortical		Intracortical
Surface	Low	Parosteal
	Intermediate	Periosteal
	High	High-grade surface

References

1. Carrasco CH, Charnsangavej C, Raymond AK, et al. Osteosarcoma: angiographic assessment of response to preoperative chemotherapy. Radiology 1989;170:839–842.
2. Lindell MM, Shirkhoda A, Raymond AK, et al. Parosteal osteosarcoma: radiologic-pathologic correlation with emphasis on CT. AJR 1987;148:323–328.

TABLE 7–10
Etiologic Factors Associated with Osteosarcoma

Radiation therapy[1–8]
Bilateral retinoblastoma[9]
Osteogenesis imperfecta[9,10]
Rothmund Thomson syndrome[11]
Cyclophosphamide[12,13]
Fibrous dysplasia[14]
Benign cartilage bone tumors[2]
Association with HLA-A11 phenotype[15]
Hodgkin disease[16]

References
1. Stark P, Smith DC, Watkins GE, et al. Primary intrathoracic extraosseous osteogenic sarcoma: report of three cases. Radiology 1990;174:725–726.
2. Unni KK, Dahlin DC. Osteosarcoma: pathology and classification. Semin Roentgenol 1989;24:143–152.
3. Lorigan JG, Libshitz HI, Peuchot M. Radiation-induced sarcoma of bone: CT findings in 19 cases. AJR 1989;153:791–794.
4. Link MP, Eilber F. Osteosarcoma. In: Pizzo PA, Poplack DG, eds. Principles and practice of pediatric oncology. Philadelphia: JB Lippincott, 1989:689–711.
5. Arthur RJ, Brunelle F. Computerised tomography in the evaluation of expansile lesions arising from the skull vault in childhood—a report of 5 cases. Pediatr Radiol 1988;18:294–301.
6. Katzman H, Waugh T, Berdon W. Skeletal changes following irradiation of childhood tumors. J Bone Joint Surg 1969;51-A:825–842.
7. Dewar JM, Courtney JT, Byrne MJ, et al. Esophageal cancer in a young woman after treatment for osteosarcoma. Med Pediatr Oncol 1988;16:287–289.
8. Lee Y-Y, Van Tassel P, Nauert C, et al. Craniofacial osteosarcomas: plain film, CT, and MR findings in 46 cases. AJR 1988;150:1397–1402.
9. Dehner LP. Pediatric surgical pathology, 2nd ed. Baltimore: Williams & Wilkins, 1987:972–984.
10. Schajowicz F, McGuire MH, Araujo ES, et al. Osteosarcomas arising on the surfaces of long bones. J Bone Joint Surg 1988;70-A:555–564.
11. Baro PR, Bastart FM, Bartrina JR, et al. Case report 529. Skeletal Radiol 1989;18:136–139.
12. McClay EF. Epidemiology of bone and soft tissue sarcomas. Semin Oncol 1989;16:264–272.
13. Gohakar D, Borges A, Shetty P. Osteogenic sarcoma developing after successful therapy of acute lymphocytic leukemia. Am J Pediatr Hematol Oncol 1986;8:259–260.
14. Taconis WK. Osteosarcoma in fibrous dysplasia. Skeletal Radiol 1988;17:163–170.
15. Shimizu T, Chigira M, Nagase M, et al. HLA phenotypes in patients who have osteosarcoma. J Bone Joint Surg 1990;72:68–73.
16. Niebrugge D, Monzon C, Perry MC, et al. Osteogenic sarcoma following Hodgkin's disease. Cancer 1981;48:416–418.

recent work suggests that osteosarcoma can occur even without the use of radiation therapy.[3] Of particular interest is a recent paper[10] describing the association of an HLA-A11 phenotype in 50 percent of 20 patients with osteosarcoma, with a prevalence of only 16 percent in control patients.

> *Comment:* Most osteosarcomas occur spontaneously without identification of predisposing factors.

References
1. Dahlin DC, Unni KK. Osteosarcoma of bone and its important recognizable varieties. Am J Surg Pathol 1977;1:61–72.
2. Tebbi CK, Gaeta J. Osteosarcoma. Pediatr Ann 1988;17:285–299.
3. Link MP, Eilber F. Osteosarcoma. In: Pizzo PA, Poplack DG, eds. Principles and practice of pediatric oncology. Philadelphia: JB Lippincott, 1989:689–711.
4. Dehner LP. Pediatric surgical pathology, 2nd ed. Baltimore: Williams & Wilkins, 1987:972–984.
5. Bentzen SM, Poulsen HS, Kaae S, et al. Prognostic factors in osteosarcomas. A regression analysis. Cancer 1988;62:194–202.
6. Edeiken-Monroe B, Edeiken J, Jacobson HG. Osteosarcoma. Semin Roentgenol 1989;24:153–173.
7. Gillespy T, Manfrini M, Ruggieri P, et al. Staging of intraosseous extent of osteosarcoma: correlation of preoperative CT and MR imaging with pathologic macroslides. Radiology 1988;167:765–767.
8. Taylor WF, Ivins JC, Pritchard DJ, et al. Trends and variability in survival among patients with osteosarcoma: a 7-year update. Mayo Clin Proc 1985;60:91–104.
9. Arthur RJ, Brunelle F. Computerised tomography in the evaluation of expansile lesions arising from the skull vault in childhood—a report of 5 cases. Pediatr Radiol 1988;18:294–301.
10. Shimizu T, Chigira M, Nagase M, et al. HLA phenotypes in patients who have osteosarcoma. J Bone Joint Surg 1990;72:68–72.

Pathology

The *anatomic location* of a conventional osteosarcoma is important. It occurs in only a few characteristic sites, and location of a lesion in alternate sites makes the diagnosis of osteosarcoma less likely. Osteosarcoma is a tumor of the long bones. In one study of 125 patients, 95 percent were identified in the long bones of the arm and leg.[1] Within these bones the distal femur and proximal tibia are the most favored sites. Between 55 and 70 percent of all conventional osteosarcomas occur in the region of the knee joint.[1–3] This has been a consistent finding in many large series of patients. In a Children's Cancer Study Group study of 135 patients, 8 percent of the osteosarcomas occurred in unusual sites, including the ribs, pelvis, spine, calcaneus, and skull.[4] Osteosarcoma of the hands and feet is extremely rare.[5] Up to 5 percent of lesions may be found in the jaw.[6] Within the long bones the epicenter of the tumor is in the metaphysis in almost all cases.[5] It can occasionally be in the diaphysis and even more uncommonly in the epiphysis. One recent study reported 1 patient with an osteosarcoma arising within the epiphysis and reviewed 8 other patients described in the literature.[7] Recognition of the occurrence of osteosarcoma in the epiphysis is important in the differential diagnosis of primary epiphyseal bone lesions. Other rare sites for osteosarcoma include the nasal bone[8] and the meninges.[9]

> *Comment:* Osteosarcoma occurs in areas of rapid bone growth. Seventy percent are found in the metaphyses around the knee joint. It does, however, occur in unusual sites and knowledge of this is important if the correct diagnosis is to be made.

Macroscopically, the osteosarcomas arise eccentrically in the metaphyses of the long bones. They very quickly penetrate the cortex elevating the periosteum and spread into the soft tissue. They also spread quickly into the bone marrow. Extensive spread in the bone marrow may be identified with contiguous spread in the shaft of the marrow space being much greater than the longitudinal extent of cortical or soft-tissue tumor abnormality. Areas of hemorrhage and necrosis are commonly identified in the tumor. The soft-tissue component of the tumor is frequently quite large. In one series, 80 percent of the tumors were greater than 6 cm in diameter at the time of diagnosis.[10]

> *Comment:* Absence of extensive marrow abnormality, and of any soft-tissue component to a bone tumor, makes diagnosis of osteosarcoma very unlikely (except for uncommon purely blastic osteosarcomas).

Skip lesions are defined as areas of osteogenic sarcoma, distinctly separate from the primary tumor, but occurring in the same bone or in an immediately adjacent bone.[11,12] They are believed to be due to spread of tumor within a bone through marrow sinusoids and to adjacent bone through venous channels.[13] The issue of skip lesions is contentious and hotly debated, with some authorities claiming that they are extremely rare[5] and others reporting them in up to 25 percent of patients.[2] In one large series, skip metastases were identified in only 0.7 percent of 282 patients.[14] In another study, CT identified no skip lesions in 48 cases.[15] Resolution of this conflict is of much more than passing academic interest, as therapy is greatly influenced by their presence or absence.

Pathologically, skip metastases were found in 10 of 40 specimens.[11] The skip metastases may be proximal or distal to the primary tumor.[14] They are not multifocal tumors, but represent areas of local metastatic spread. There are many reasons for the widely differing reported occurrence of skip metastases. The most likely explanation is that in many patients, neither the pathologist nor the radiologist comprehensively evaluates the entire bone and the entire adjacent bones. For example, the pathologist may only sample selected sites or the pathology specimen may not include the entire bone.

With regard to imaging, lesions will be missed if the entire bone is not included in the imaging protocol. Of particular importance, these lesions will frequently not be diagnosed if the radiologist is unaware of their existence and does not specifically look for them. In the past, skip lesions were more frequently diagnosed by the pathologist. In one 1975 study of 40 patients, 10 children had skip lesions, of which only 2 were diagnosed by imaging.[16] I believe that modern-day imaging, particularly MR, should permit the preoperative identification of almost all macroscopic skip metastases. In one patient, MR identified a skip lesion confirmed on pathology, but missed on radiograph, CT, and bone scan.[12] No other publications to support this hypothesis are available.

> *Comment:* The radiologist must be aware of the entity of skip metastases and must carefully evaluate the entire bone to detect them.

Multifocal osteosarcoma (osteosarcomatosis) is a term that has caused confusion in the literature and that I believe should no longer be utilized. As originally described it referred to those patients in whom there were multiple bone lesions in the absence of lung metastases, but the term has more recently been expanded to include patients with multiple bone lesions and lung metastases.[17] The term multifocal osteosarcoma was originally introduced in the belief that this was an unusual variant of osteosarcoma with multiple primary tumors in the bone. A careful recent review[17] of 15 patients under the age of 18 years identified a dominant lesion in all patients and concluded that the other bone lesions were metastases (Table 7–11). In another study,[18] a dominant lesion was identified in 8 of 9 patients. The dominant lesion is almost always in the distal femur.[5,18] The pattern of metastatic spread in the bones is somewhat unusual in that up to 90 percent of the metastases are well defined and sclerotic[5] and that the bones are symmetrically involved in up to 80 percent of patients.[17] Most recent reports state that patients with these symmetrical bone metastases may have lung metastases as well.[17–19] Early work suggested that the dominant lesion was more anaplastic than usual,[5] but a recent large series indicates that the dominant lesion is identical to a typical conventional osteosarcoma.[17] If radiologists are still to utilize the term multifocal osteosarcoma, they should use it purely as a descriptive term for those patients in whom there are bilateral, often symmetrical, multiple blastic bone metastases. The overall incidence of metastases with this appearance ranges from 0.3 percent[5] to 4.2 percent.[17]

Metastases from osteosarcoma can present in almost any region of the body. It is assumed that over 80 per-

TABLE 7-11
Osteosarcomatosis*[1]

Bones	
Dominant lesion present	100%
No. of involved sites of metastasis	8.1 ± 8.6
Symmetry	80%
Lung metastases	73% (on chest radiographs)

*15 patients under 18 years of age.

Reference
1. Hopper KD, Moser RP, Haseman DB, et al. Osteosarcomatosis. Radiology 1990;175:233–239.

cent of patients have micrometastases at the time of diagnosis.[20] By far the most common site is the lung and the next most common is bone. All other sites of metastases are uncommon (Table 7–12). Several points are of interest to the radiologist. Many lung metastases are calcified, and it is important not to mistake a pulmonary metastasis for a benign calcified lesion such as histoplasmosis. Since lung metastases are frequently bilateral, the identification of one metastasis should evoke an intense search for additional lesions. The presence of calcium within many of the metastases accounts for the uptake of technetium 99m MDP by many of these lesions. Two important points regarding metastases from osteosarcoma have emerged in recent years. Both of these impact on the radiologist. The first point is that bone metastases, which were previously thought to be extremely uncommon in the absence of lung metastasis, have now been recognized to occur not infrequently in the absence of lung metastasis. Second, current improved therapy and increased survival for patients with osteogenic sarcoma is causing a change in the pattern of recognized metastasis,[17,21] with nonpulmonary metastasis being recognized far more often than previously. For example, bone metastases have now been reported in up to 36 percent of patients.[17]

> *Comment:* Changing patterns of metastasis from osteosarcoma are occurring in response to more prolonged survival from more effective chemotherapy. Imaging of these nonpulmonary sites must become more intensive.

Microscopically, conventional osteosarcomas show three predominant cell types: osteoblastic, fibroblastic, and chondroblastic. All three types are usually present and their distribution is quite varied even in one tumor. The tumors are classified according to the dominant type (Table 7–13). Prognosis is not dependent on the type. The importance of this subdivision is that the presence of any osteoid within the tumor, no matter how little, classifies the tumor as an osteogenic sarcoma.[5] Even if the tumor is almost entirely cartilage, it will not be called a chondrosarcoma, but an osteosarcoma, if osteoid is present.

TABLE 7-12
Sites and Patterns of Metastasis in Osteosarcoma

- Lung
  - Most common
    - Present in up to 40% of cases on initial diagnosis[1]
    - Present in up to 80% of cases within 2 years
  - First site in 90% of cases[2]
  - 20–50% bilateral on initial presentation[3,4]
  - 90% have lung metastases at death[2]
- Bone
  - 15–50% of cases[2,5]
- Uncommon sites
  - Myocardium[6]
  - Brain[2,5]
  - Mediastinal nodes[7]
  - Inferior vena cava[8]
  - Kidney[9]
  - Liver[10]
  - Pericardium[2]
  - Adrenal[2]
  - Nodes[2,11]

References
1. Dehner LP. Pediatric surgical pathology, 2nd ed. Baltimore: Williams & Wilkins, 1987:972–984.
2. Link MP, Eilber F. Osteosarcoma. In: Pizzo PA, Poplack DG, eds. Principles and practice of pediatric oncology. Philadelphia: JB Lippincott, 1989:689–711.
3. Tebbi CK, Gaeta J. Osteosarcoma. Pediatr Ann 1988;17:285–299.
4. Han M-T, Telander RL, Pairolero PC, et al. Aggressive thoracotomy for pulmonary metastatic osteogenic sarcoma in children and young adolescents. J Pediatr Surg 1981;16:928–933.
5. Danziger J, Wallace S, Handel SF, et al. Metastatic osteogenic sarcoma to the brain. Cancer 1979;43:707–710.
6. Watts FB, Zingas AP, Das L, et al. Computed tomographic diagnosis of an intracardiac metastasis from osteosarcoma. CT 1983;7:271–272.
7. van Zanten TEG, Golding RP, Taets ven Amerongen AHM. Osteosarcoma with calcific mediastinal lymphadenopathy. Pediatr Radiol 1987;17:258–259.
8. deSantos LA, Bernardino ME, Murray JA. Computed tomography in the evaluation of osteosarcoma: experience with 25 cases. AJR 1979;132:535–540.
9. Lockhart SK, Coan JD, Jaffe N, Osteosarcoma metastatic to the kidney. Clin Imag 1989;13:154–156.
10. Shapiro RS, Mendelson DS, Norton KI, et al. Case report: calcified liver metastases from osteosarcoma. CT: J Comput Tomogr 1988;12:196–198.
11. English R, Dicks-Mireaux C, Malone M, et al. Osteosarcoma—presumed lymph node metastases in two cases. Skeletal Radiol 1989;18:289–293.

The initial response of osteosarcoma to chemotherapy is necrosis rather than fibrosis.[5] There is a decrease in size of the soft-tissue component of the tumor, an in-

TABLE 7-13
Pathologic Subtypes of Conventional Osteosarcoma*[1,2]

Predominant Tissue Type	Name	Percentage of All Conventional Osteosarcomas
Cartilage	Chondroblastic osteosarcoma	25
Fibrous tissue	Fibroblastic osteosarcoma	25
Osteoid	Osteoblastic osteosarcoma	50

*Note: All three types contain some osteoid.

References
1. Link MP, Eilber F. Osteosarcoma. In: Pizzo PA, Poplack DG, eds. Principles and practice of pediatric oncology. Philadelphia: JB Lippincott, 1989:689–711.
2. Unni KK, Dahlin DC. Osteosarcoma: pathology and classification. Semin Roentgenol 1989;24:143–152.

TABLE 7-14
Criteria of Histologic Response of Osteosarcoma to Preamputation Chemotherapy[1]

Grade of Histologic Response	Criteria
I	No effect identified
II	5–95% of viable tumor cells remaining
III	Scattered foci of viable tumor cells; less than 5% of tumor cells remaining
IV	No viable tumor cells in extensive sampling

Reference
1. Rosen G, Caparros B, Huvos AG, et al. Preoperative chemotherapy for osteogenic sarcoma: selection of postoperative adjuvant chemotherapy based on the response of the primary tumor to preoperative chemotherapy. Cancer 1982;49:1221–1230.

crease in matrix mineralization, and finally restructuring of destroyed bone. The response to initial chemotherapy, as evaluated by the pathologist, is extremely important in defining patient's subsequent chemotherapy.[22] This response is graded into four types, representing from no response to 100 percent necrosis of the tumor. This classification of response is summarized in Table 7–14.

References
1. Price CHG, Shuber K, Salzer-Kuntschik M, et al. Osteosarcoma in children. A study of 125 cases. J Bone Joint Surg 1975;57-B:341–345.
2. Dehner LP. Pediatric surgical pathology, 2nd ed. Baltimore: Williams & Wilkins, 1987:972–984.
3. Edeiken J, Raymond AK, Ayala AG, et al. Small-cell osteosarcoma. Skeletal Radiol 1987;16:621–628.
4. Heller RM, Dominguez R, Ertel IJ, et al. A review of the unusual appearance or atypical location of osteogenic sarcoma in childhood. RadioGraphics 1984;4:507–515.
5. Dahlin DC, Unni KK. Osteosarcoma of bone and its important recognizable varieties. Am J Surg Pathol 1977;1:61–72.
6. Finkelstein JB. Osteosarcoma of the jaw bones. Radiol Clin N Am 1970;8:425–436.
7. Palatiel H, Wilkinson RH, Kozakewich HPW. Case report 507. Skeletal Radiol 1988;17:527–530.
8. Sigh J, Gluckman JL, Kaufman RA, et al. Osteosarcoma of the nasal bone in a child. Head Neck Surg 1982;4:246–250.
9. Wang A-M, Fitzgerald TJ, Lichtman AH, et al. Neuroradiologic features of primary falx osteosarcoma. AJNR 1986;7:729–732.
10. Taylor WF, Ivins JC, Pritchard DJ, et al. Trends and variability in survival among patients with osteosarcoma: a 7-year update. Mayo Clin Proc 1985;60:91–104.
11. Enneking WF, Kagan A. The implications of "skip" metastases in osteosarcoma. Clin Orthop Rel Res 1975;111:33–41.
12. Wetzel LH, Schweiger GD, Levine E. MR imaging of transarticular skip metastases from distal femoral osteosarcoma. J Comput Assist Tomogr 1990;14:315–317.
13. Wuisman P, Enneking WF. Prognosis for patients who have osteosarcoma with skip metastasis. J Bone Joint Surg 1990;72:60–67.
14. Malawer MM, Dunham WK. Skip metastases in osteosarcoma: recent experience. J Surg Oncol 1983;22:236–245.
15. Coffre C, Vanel D, Contesso G, et al. Problems and pitfalls in the use of computed tomography for the local evaluation of long bone osteosarcoma: report on 30 cases. Skeletal Radiol 1985;13:147–153.
16. Enneking WF, Kagan A. "Skip" metastases in osteosarcoma. Cancer 1975;36:2192–2205.
17. Hopper KD, Moser RP, Haseman DB, et al. Osteosarcomatosis. Radiology 1990;175:233–239.
18. Parham DM, Pratt CB, Parvey LS, et al. Childhood multifocal osteosarcoma. Clinicopathologic and radiologic correlates. Cancer 1985;55:2653–2658.
19. Edeiken-Monroe B, Edeiken J, Jacobson HG. Osteosarcoma. Semin Roentgenol 1989;24:153–173.
20. Hudson M, Jaffe MR, Jaffe N, et al. Pediatric osteosarcoma: therapeutic strategies, results, and prognostic factors derived from a 10-year experience. J Clin Oncol 1990;18:1988–1997.
21. Tebbi CK, Gaeta J. Osteosarcoma. Pediatr Ann 1988;17:285–299.
22. Rosen G, Caparros B, Huvos AG, et al. Preoperative chemotherapy for osteogenic sarcoma: selection of postoperative adjuvant chemotherapy based on the response of the primary tumor to preoperative chemotherapy. Cancer 1982;49:1221–1230.

Clinical Presentation

The clinical findings in patients with osteosarcoma are few. The patients are usually well and do not present with widespread signs of systemic disease. The most common clinical presentation is the presence of focal pain at the site of the primary tumor together with the presence of a mass in some patients.[1,2] The pain is usually increased with patient activity[2] and in some patients an episode of trauma initially draws attention to the underlying tumor.[2] The median duration from the onset of symptoms until the time of diagnosis is about 3 months,[2,3] but in some patients, unfortunately, diagnosis is often delayed for over 6 months.[1] The reason for this is that mild trauma from athletic participation is frequent in teenagers and the pain from an osteogenic sarcoma often needs to be present for some length of time before the patient seeks medical assistance.

Alkaline phosphotates concentration in the serum is elevated in up to 40 percent of patients with osteosarcoma,[1] but this is a relatively nonspecific finding. No other serum markers for this tumor exist.

References

1. Link MP, Eilber F. Osteosarcoma. In: Pizzo PA, Poplack DG, eds. Principles and practice of pediatric oncology. Philadelphia: JB Lippincott, 1989:689–711.
2. Tebbi CK, Gaeta J. Osteosarcoma. Pediatr Ann 1988;17:285–299.
3. Taylor WF, Ivins JC, Pritchard DJ, et al. Trends and variability in survival among patients with osteosarcoma: a 7-year update. Mayo Clin Proc 1985;60:91–104.

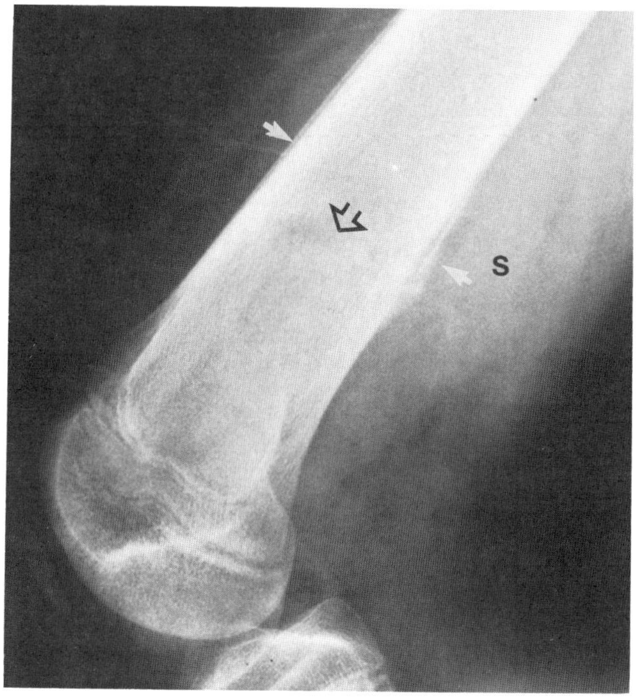

Figure 7-1. Diagnosis: Osteosarcoma. Classic plain film findings.
There is a tumor of the distal femur. There is a well-defined periosteal reaction *(arrows)*. A large soft-tissue (*S*) component of the tumor is seen posteriorly. There is poorly defined destruction *(open arrow)*. The periosteal reaction shows the formation of the Codman triangle.

Imaging Studies

The objectives of imaging are to identify a lesion, define its local extent as accurately as possible, identify metastases, and monitor response to therapy. The various modalities used in the evaluation of osteosarcoma are first described in detail, following which they are integrated to answer specific clinical questions.

DESCRIPTION BY MODALITY

Plain Film Radiograph. A plain film radiograph of the primary lesion is extremely important and should be performed in all patients. The classic conventional osteosarcoma will be seen as a destructive lesion with some sclerosis involving the metaphysis of one of the long bones, especially around the knee joint (Fig. 7–1). The destruction will have permeative, poorly defined margins (Fig. 7–2). The cortex will be broken and a periosteal reaction will be present (Fig. 7–1). A soft-tissue mass may be identifiable even on the plain film radiograph (Fig. 7–1). Unfortunately, not all patients have this classic appearance; there is a wide range.[1] Occasionally, even when symptoms are present, the plain film radiograph may appear fairly normal, with only subtle erosion or a subtle periosteal reaction (Fig. 7–3). Unfortunately, at this stage the lesion is sometimes missed and only diagnosed retrospectively following further progression. While most lesions show a mixture of destruction with either matrix mineralization or reactive new bone formation (Fig. 7–4), both extremes of

Figure 7-2. Diagnosis: Osteosarcoma. Typical findings.
Plain film radiograph. Distal femur. The tumor has a moderate-sized soft-tissue component that shows heavy periosteal and tumor matrix calcification. There is permeative bone destruction with very poorly defined margins *(arrows)*.

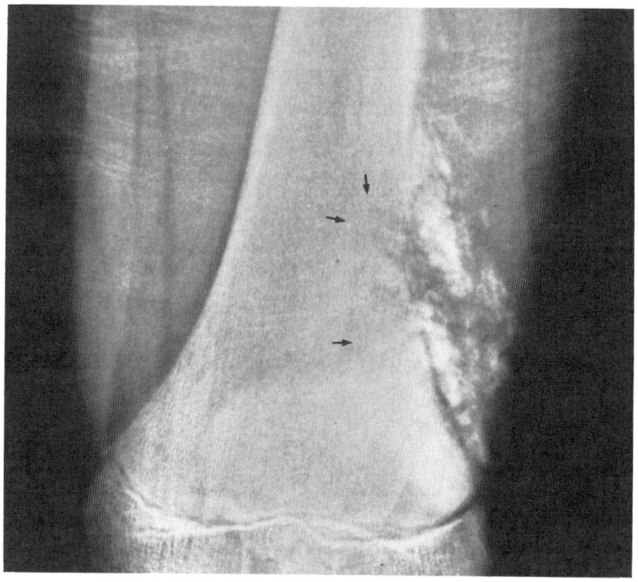

A

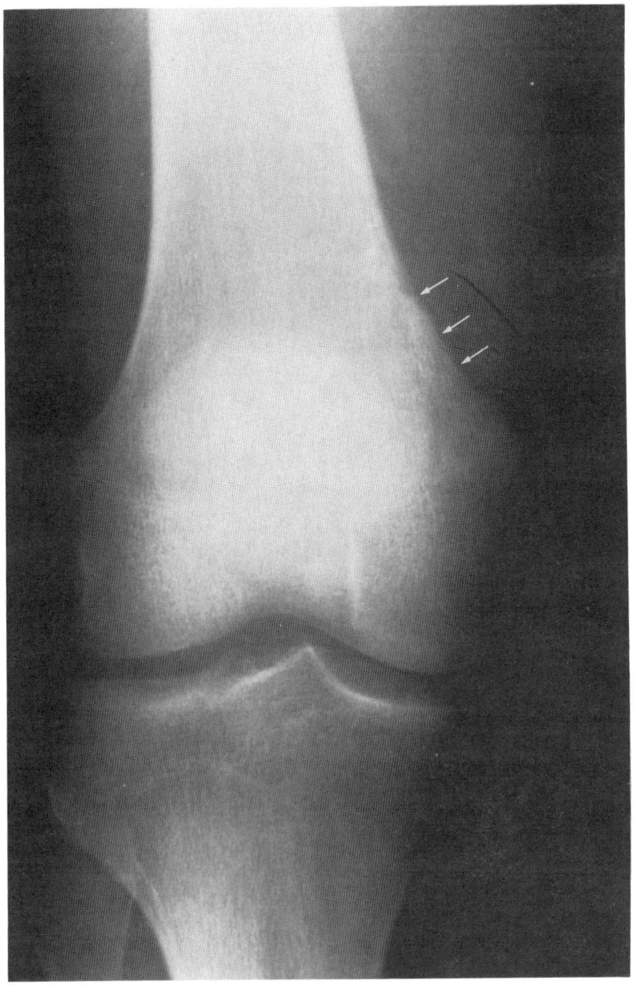

B

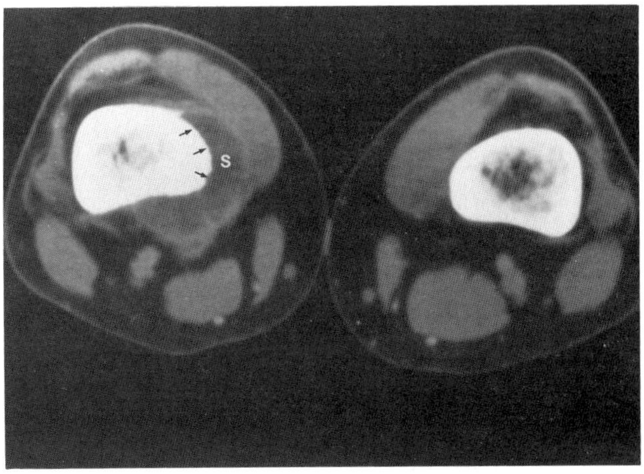

Figure 7–3. **Diagnosis: Osteosarcoma. Subtle plain film radiographic findings.**
A, **Plain film radiograph. There is subtle but definite cortical destruction of the medial aspect of the distal femur *(arrows).* This could easily be missed. *B,* CT. This shows definite cortical destruction with significant irregularity of the cortical margin *(arrows).* A moderate soft-tissue tumor mass (*S*) is also identified.**

this spectrum exist. Approximately 15 percent of lesions may appear purely lytic, with or without a periosteal reaction.[2] The rare lesions arising in the epiphysis are almost always predominantly lytic in nature. The importance of recognition of this pattern is that these purely lytic lesions may show little destruction, may have little periosteal reaction, and, therefore, may easily be misdiagnosed as a more benign lesion. In one large series of 50 patients,[3] 70 percent showed a mixed pattern of lysis and blastic response, 16 percent were lytic, and 14 percent were blastic. The very blastic lesions may also be misdiagnosed as a more benign lesion. They too are often well defined without significant periosteal reaction or soft-tissue extensions. (CT and MR of these lesions may also show a relative lack of involvement of the bone marrow beyond the blastic margins identified on the plain film radiograph.)

Most osteosarcomas will lie in the metaphysis, but up to 18 percent may be seen in the diaphysis (Figs. 7–5 and 7–6). It is important, therefore, not to exclude the diagnosis of osteosarcoma merely because a malignant looking bone lesion lies in the diaphysis. At one time it was believed that invasion from the metaphysis into the epiphysis was relatively uncommon. New imaging modalities, however, demonstrate that this occurs not infrequently and in one series was identified in up to 36 percent of patients.[3] Most osteosarcomas will demonstrate some degree of periosteal reaction. This is very varied in appearance. For example, in one series, it had a sunburst appearance (Fig. 7–7) in 44 percent of patients, was irregular and thick (22 percent) (Fig. 7–6), laminated (20 percent), and demonstrated a Codman triangle in 60 percent[3] (see Fig. 7–1). The pattern of periosteal reaction should not be relied upon to make the diagnosis of osteosarcoma. Cortical destruction is present in almost all cases; it will be seen on the plain film radiograph in many patients but may require further imaging for its identification. A soft-tissue component of the tumor is present in almost all cases and it too may require CT or MR to be identified: On the plain film radiograph it is most likely to be seen only when large or if matrix mineralization is present. Matrix mineralization is classically fairly homogeneous or clumped (Fig. 7–6). Although not stressed in the literature, my own view is that it is sometimes extremely difficult to differentiate calcium deposition in the tumor matrix (matrix mineralization) from reactive sclerosis of normal bone, a fragmented periosteal reaction, or both. Fracture may occur through the tumor (Fig. 7–8).

The general appearance, on plain films, of osteosar-

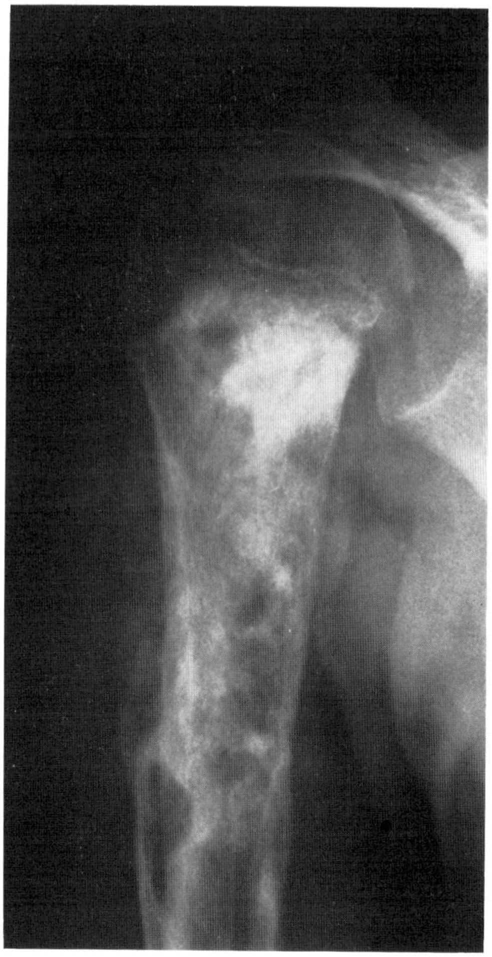

Figure 7–4. **Diagnosis: Osteosarcoma with mixed lytic and blastic reactions.**
Plain film radiograph. There is a large tumor of the proximal right humerus. The tumor shows typical appearance of mixed areas of lysis together with blastic areas of new bone formation.

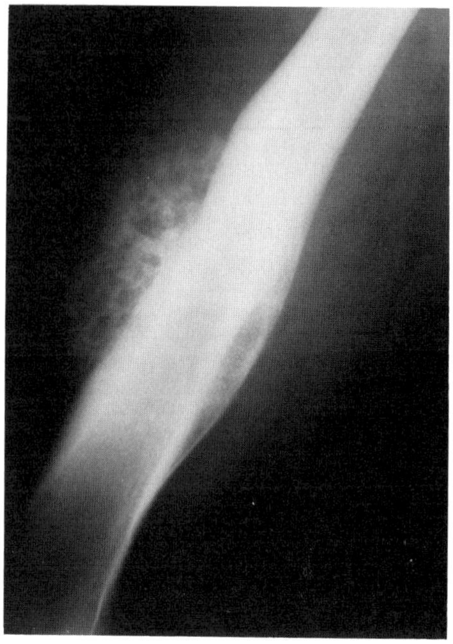

Figure 7–5. **Diagnosis: Osteosarcoma. Diaphyseal location. Plain film radiograph. There is lesion of the mid shaft of the femur. There is some reactive sclerosis of the cortex with an extensive mottled periosteal reaction.**

Figure 7–6. **Diagnosis: Osteosarcoma of mid shaft of femur. Plain film radiograph. The location of the tumor in the mid shaft of the bone is uncommon. There is extensive blastic reaction, with the bone appearing fairly sclerotic. An irregular thick periosteal reaction is seen *(large arrow).* Homogenous clumps of soft-tissue matrix mineralization are present *(small arrows).***

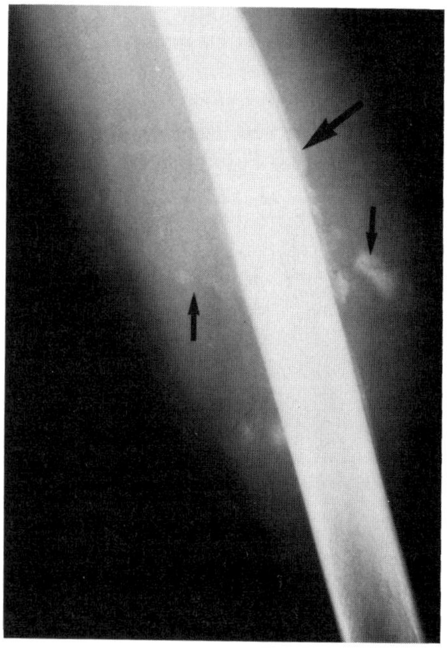

coma outside of the long bones follows the same principles as in the long bones. Again the appearance is varied, with a mixed invasive lytic and blastic response being the most common (Fig. 7–9). As with the long bones, cortical destruction and soft-tissue extension of the tumor are usually also present (Fig. 7–9). The variations seen in the long bones are also described: For example, in one patient with a primary tumor of the calcaneus, the plain film showed a diffusely blastic abnormality.[4]

> *Comment:* The typical osteosarcoma is easy to diagnose. Knowledge of the wide spectrum of appearance on the plain film will help reduce misdiagnoses of the slightly atypical lesions. This is important, as variations are not uncommon. High-quality images are needed if early lesions are not to be missed.

MDP Technetium 99m Radioisotope Scan. MDP technetium 99m radioisotope scan is valuable in the overall

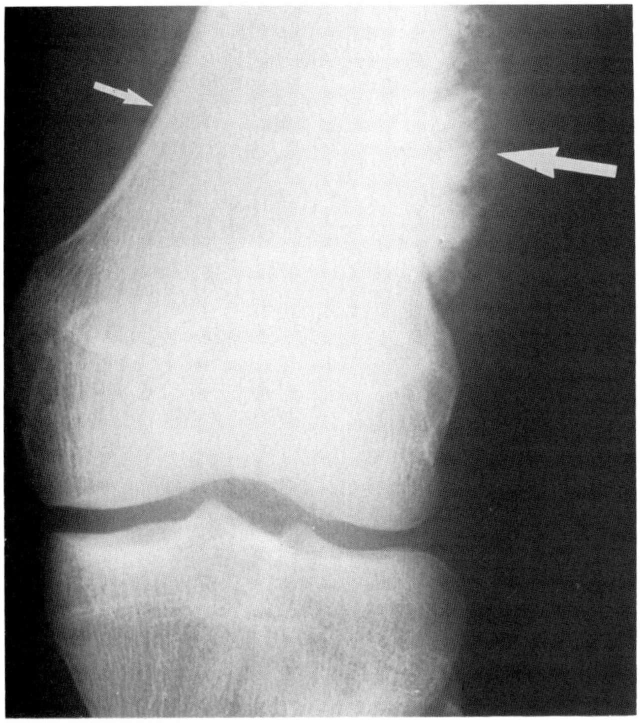

Figure 7-7. **Diagnosis: Osteosarcoma. Periosteal reaction. Plain film radiograph. There is a tumor of the distal femur. The periosteal reaction is linear *(small arrow)* on the medial aspect of the bone and shows a sunburst appearance laterally *(large arrow).***

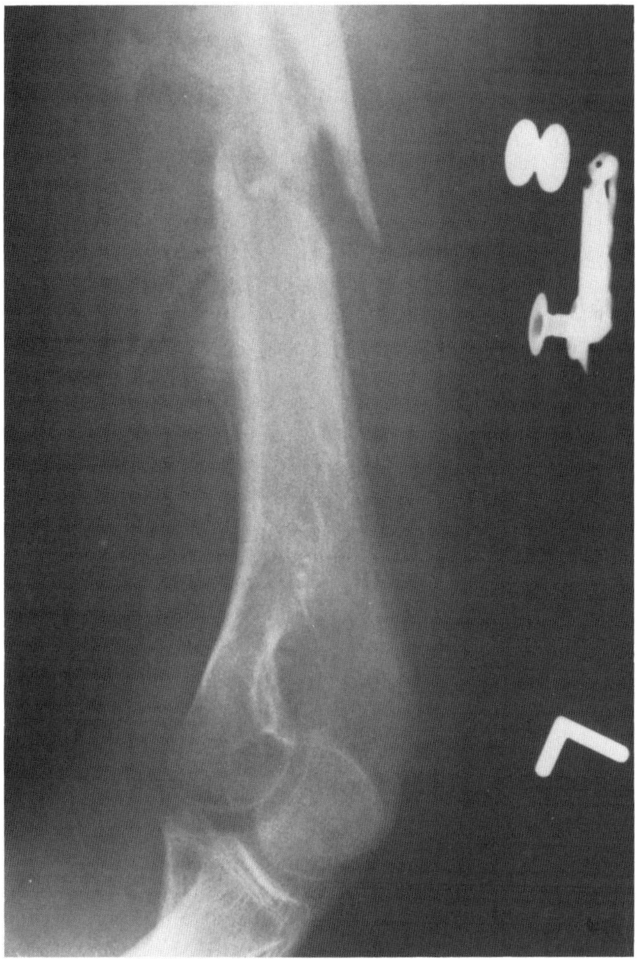

Figure 7-8. **Diagnosis: Osteosarcoma. Pathologic fracture. Plain film radiograph. There is a destructive lesion in the mid shaft of the left humerus with periosteal reaction and a large soft-tissue component. A fracture has occurred through the lesion.**

evaluation of patients with osteosarcoma. Virtually 100 percent of the primary lesions will demonstrate uptake of this radioisotope. The uptake is slightly less in purely lytic lesions than in other types. There is intense uptake of the MDP by the bone component of the lesion,[5] with frequent uptake in the soft-tissue component of the tumor as well.[5] MDP is extremely sensitive for detection of the primary tumor. It is, however, nonspecific. Although intensity of uptake is frequently higher in malignant tumors than in benign bone tumors,[5] this difference is inadequate to make reliable differentiation in an individual patient. The uptake of MDP in the primary tumor does not correlate with pathology for evaluation of the local extent of the tumor. This is because an extended pattern of uptake is frequently seen.[5] This is caused either by hyperemia from the tumor or minor trauma from an abnormal gait owing to pain from the tumor.[3] The extended pattern of uptake may be seen in the same bone as the osteosarcoma, across a joint, or in an adjacent limb. This pattern is seen in up to 80 percent of patients. In one series of 40 patients, all showed uptake of MDP by the primary tumor and 19 showed an augmented uptake as well.[3] Fortunately, both CT and MR are excellent modalities for evaluation of local extent of tumor, so that one need not attempt to utilize MDP bone scan for this.

The main role of MDP scanning is to screen the rest of the skeleton for metastases both on initial presentation and on follow-up.[6] It is the modality of choice for this. In addition, metastases in other sites will frequently be identified on MDP radioisotope scanning. This is because many of these metastases actively metabolize calcium and therefore take up the bone-seeking agent (Fig. 7–10). In the lung, MDP scanning has no role to play in routine screening for metastases. This is because CT scan is far more sensitive and the MDP scan will only detect relatively large lesions. However, if a single lesion is detected on CT scan, the presence of uptake of MDP would be extremely strong evidence for the presence of a metastasis rather than an incidental benign lung lesion. Uptake in lung metastases has been reported in 20 to 39 percent of cases with metastases.[7,9] Metastases in unusual sites are not infrequently first discovered as incidental findings on MDP bone scan study. This is because, if asymptomatic, these other unusual sites may not routinely be screened with other imaging modalities. A routine MDP scan has little role in the evaluation of response of primary tumor to chemotherapy.[5,8] Experimentally, positive emitted tomography

A B

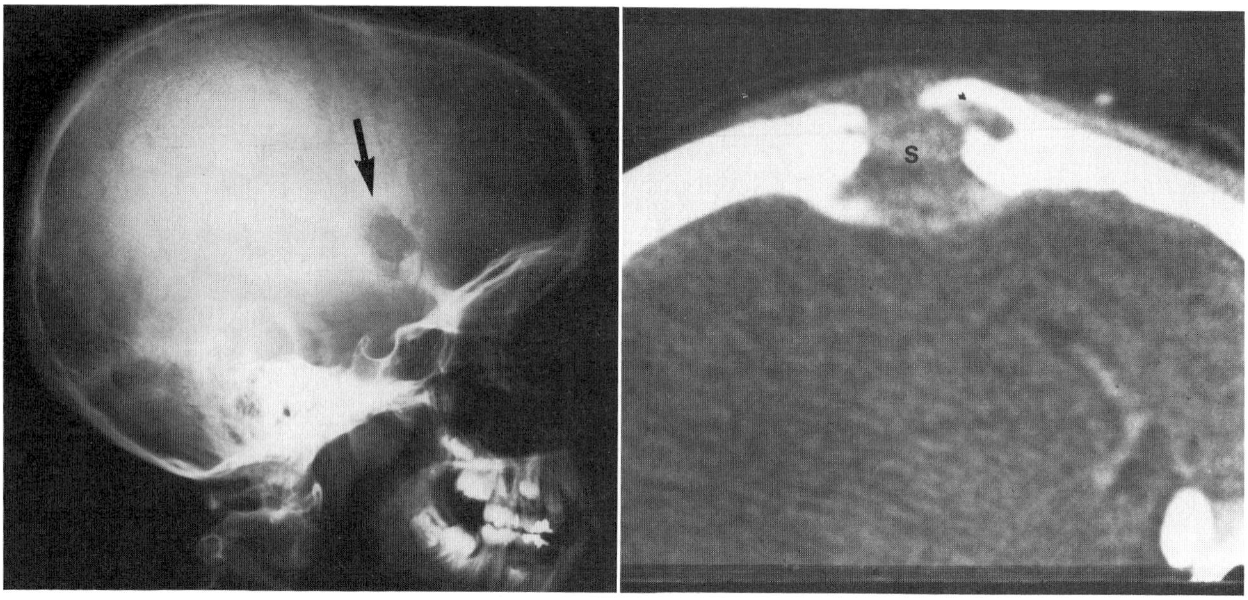

Figure 7–9. **Diagnosis: Osteosarcoma of skull.**
***A*, Lateral view of skull. There is a lytic lesion *(arrow)* in the parietotemporal region. It has a scalloped, irregular, slightly sclerotic border. *B*, CT. After intravenous contrast injection, there is localized destruction of both inner and outer table of the skull with an enhancing soft-tissue (*S*) mass. (From Kornreich L. Osteogenic sarcoma of the calvarium in children: CT manifestations. Neuroradiology 1988;30:439–441.)**

(PET) studies of glucose metabolism have shown some correlation of utilization rates with histologic grading of tumor.[9] As yet this has no clinical application.

CT. CT scan is routinely used for evaluation of osteosarcoma. As early as 1979, in a study of 25 patients, it was demonstrated that CT was better than plain film radiograph for demonstration of the soft-tissue extent and of the marrow spread of the primary osteosarcoma.[10] Accurate definition of tumor has become particularly important in recent years with new trends in surgery involving limb salvage and transbone rather than transarticular amputation. There is debate regarding the relative merits of CT and MR (Figs. 7–11, 7–12, and 7–13). Many reports since 1979 confirm the excellence of CT for demonstrating the local extent of osteosarcoma. MR may, however, be even better. For example, in one study, MR was found to be superior to CT for demonstration of the soft-tissue mass, less effective for demonstration of cortical destruction and calcification, and equivalent for demonstration of marrow spread.[11] In a study of 55 cases in 1983, CT was better than plain film radiograph for demonstration of soft-tissue tumor,[3] and it showed the relationship of the tumor to the great vessels adequately in 29 of 35 patients. In another study of 17 patients, CT was found to provide all information necessary for performance of limb salvage surgery.[12]

From a technical point of view, CT scanning should be performed using high-resolution contiguous slices. The entire affected bone must be scanned without any interslice gaps. Thin slices are helpful particularly close to the joint, when it is desirable to demonstratea penetration of tumor into the joint. Administration of a bolus of intravenous contrast will improve visualization of the soft-tissue component of the tumor and potentially will improve visualization of adjacent important blood vessels. There are no reported prospective studies looking at the advantages of intravenous contrast and comparing them to either noncontrasted CT scans or to MR.

The CT appearance of primary osteogenic sarcoma reflects the varied patterns that have been described in detail for the plain film (Fig. 7–14). On CT, a nutrient vessel may mimic the appearance of a skip lesion.[13] Comparison with the other side will avoid this pitfall. CT is more sensitive than the plain film for demonstration of periosteal reaction, matrix mineralization, soft-tissue tumor, and bone marrow spread. The global picture provided by the plain film radiograph and the pattern of permeative destruction together with the changing interface between normal and abnormal bone is, however, still best appreciated on the plain film radiograph and this is important in differential diagnosis.[13] CT is equally effective in evaluation of osteosarcoma in unusual sites. For example, in two patients with skull osteosarcoma, CT was able to demonstrate full thickness bone abnormality with soft-tissue masses both internally and externally, and an intact dura[14] (Fig. 7–9).

CT is without doubt the modality of choice for detection of lung metastases. There is universal agreement with this statement. From a technique viewpoint, contiguous 1 cm slices should be obtained throughout both lung fields. There is no requirement to give intravenous contrast and, in fact, this may be unhelpful as it may obscure subtle calcification in some of the metastatic le-

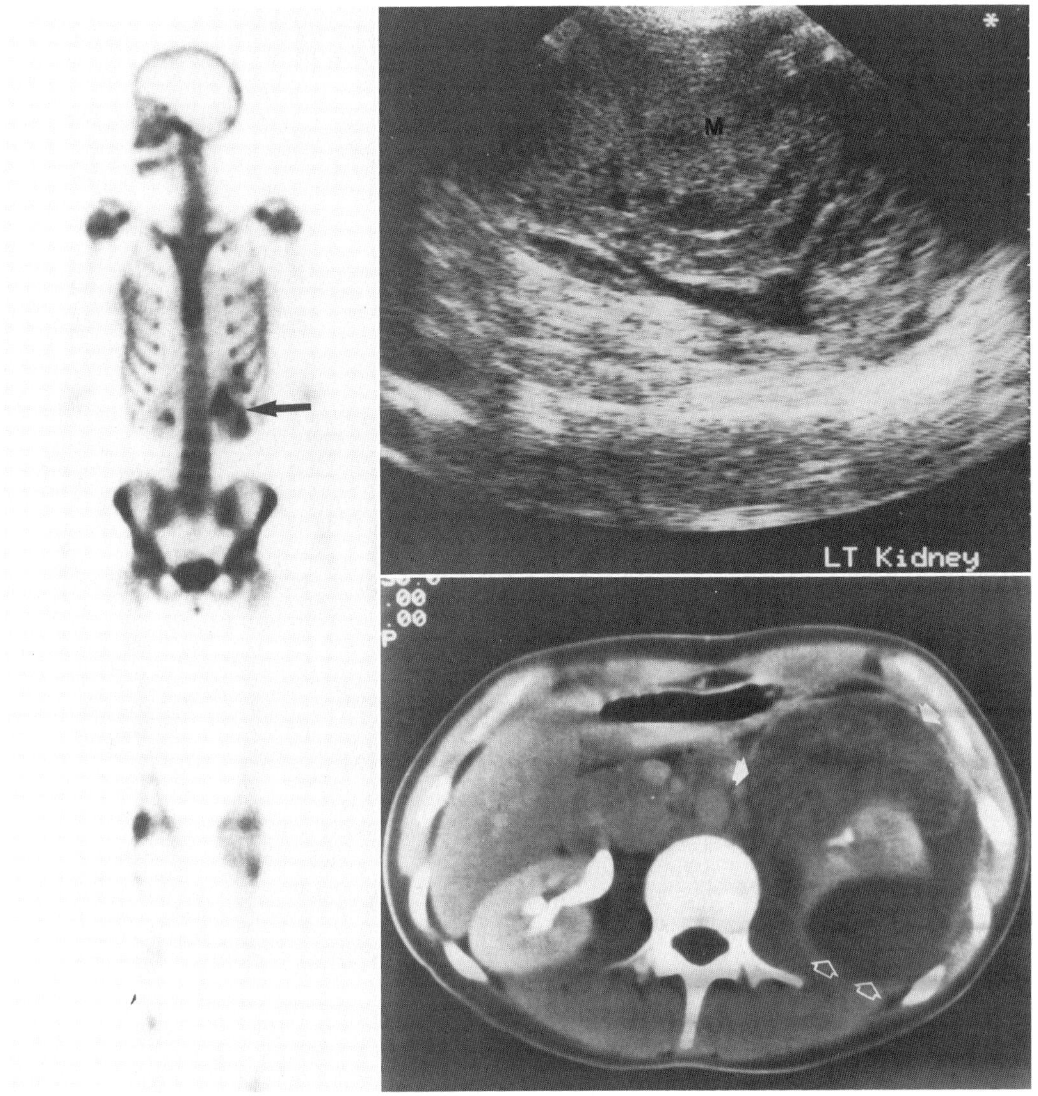

Figure 7–10. **Diagnosis: Osteosarcoma. Kidney metastasis. The lesion was identified as an incidental finding on a bone scan.**
***A,* Anterior view of technetium 99m MDP bone scan showing areas of increased uptake in the upper and lower pole of the left kidney *(arrow)*. *B,* Sagittal sonogram of the left kidney demonstrates a large noncalcified mass (*M*) occupying most of the mid and anterior aspects. No normal renal parenchyma could be identified. *C,* Enhanced CT scan after intravenous contrast. There is a large renal mass, which is fairly solid anteriorly *(closed arrows)* and partially cystic posterolaterally *(open arrows)*. (From Lockhart S. Osteosarcoma metastatic to the kidney. Clin Imag 1989;13:154–156.)**

sions. No studies have been reported comparing chest CT with and without contrast. The lung lesions appear as well-defined focal soft-tissue densities with the number of metastases detected ranging from one to a large number. Fifty percent of the lesions will be subpleural.[7] When a large number of lesions are present, they may vary considerably in size. Lesions as small as a couple of millimeters in diameter may be detected. Calcification is often present in the larger lesions. Because metastases from osteosarcoma are often treated aggressively with surgery, accurate definition of these lesions by CT is important. There is some evidence that prognosis is better if the lesions are resected while still small, again emphasizing the importance of early diagnosis with CT.

MR. On MR imaging normal bone cortex produces virtually no signal while the appearance of the bone marrow depends on the amount of fat present within it. Yellow bone marrow has a very bright signal on both T1 and T2 weighted pulse sequences. The signal of red bone marrow is slightly less on the T1 weighted pulse sequences. Interpretation of marrow spread of osteogenic sarcoma requires a knowledge of the normal conversion of red to yellow bone marrow. At birth, red hemopoietic bone marrow extends all the way to the ankles and wrists. There is a gradual conversion, starting peripherally and moving centrally, of red to fatty

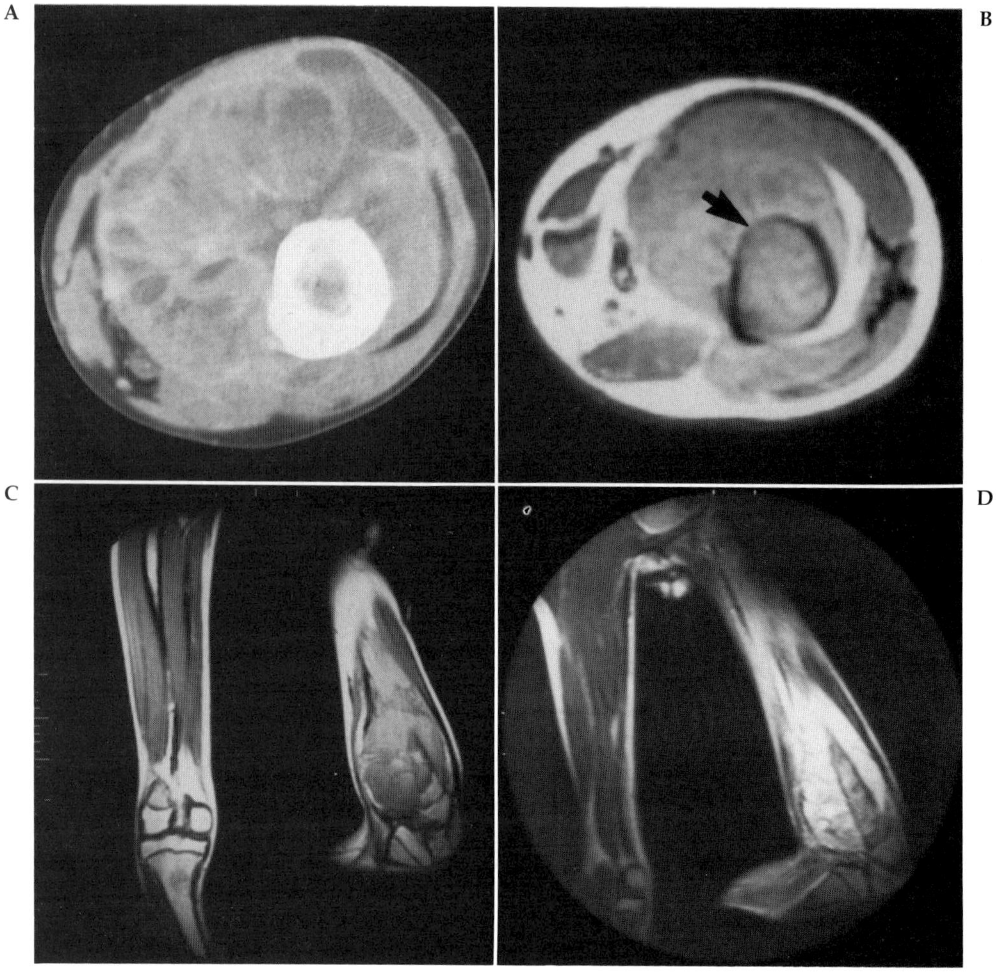

Figure 7-11. **Diagnosis: Osteosarcoma. CT and MR findings. Tumor of distal femur. *A*, CT. The tumor has a very large soft-tissue component. The cortical margin is irregular. Increased density is seen in the marrow space from tumor infiltration. *B*, MR, T1 weighted image. This is obtained at a higher level than *A*. There is a large soft-tissue component to the tumor. Cortical abnormality is not as clearly seen as with CT but there is a definite increase in signal in the cortex, particularly anteriorly *(arrow)*. *C* and *D*, T1 weighted and T2 weighted coronal images through different segments of the tumor. These again demonstrate a very large soft-tissue tumor that is of muscle signal intensity on the T1 weighted image and very bright on the T2 weighted image.**

yellow marrow, so that by the mid teenage years the adult pattern is reached in which the red marrow is confined to the axial skeleton and the proximal humeri and femurs. The pattern of conversion from the periphery centrally involves one bone and then the adjacent bone. Within any particular bone, conversion starts in the diaphysis and spread toward both metaphyses. Normal red marrow should not be mistaken for tumor on T1 weighted images. It can be differentiated by comparison with the opposite side and with knowledge of the normal conversion patterns described here (Fig. 7–15).

Cortical destruction by tumor is seen as a loss of the normal sharply defined cortex with some increase in signal seen within it. Current MR is far more sensitive for detection of cortical abnormality than it was several years ago. While there are no prospective studies comparing high-resolution thin-slice CT with high-resolution thin-slice MR, I think that CT with bone window settings will prove more sensitive than MR for the detection of very subtle cortical destruction. The same also applies for identification of periosteal reaction. Originally it was felt that MR could not detect abnormality of the periosteum, but more recent work clearly indicates that this is not true. MR can detect large areas of new bone formation or matrix mineralization, but it is not as sensitive as CT for detection of small areas of matrix calcification.[15] In one study of 27 patients,[16] MR and CT were compared to findings at pathology and surgery. MR, it was concluded, was better than CT for identification of bone marrow and muscle compartment tumor, equivalent to CT for identification of the joint and cortical tumor, and also for identification of the relationship of tumor to the neurovascular bundles. In another study, MR was found to be better for identification of soft-tissue tumor, equivalent to CT for identification of intraosseous spread, and worse than CT for detec-

A

B, C

D, E

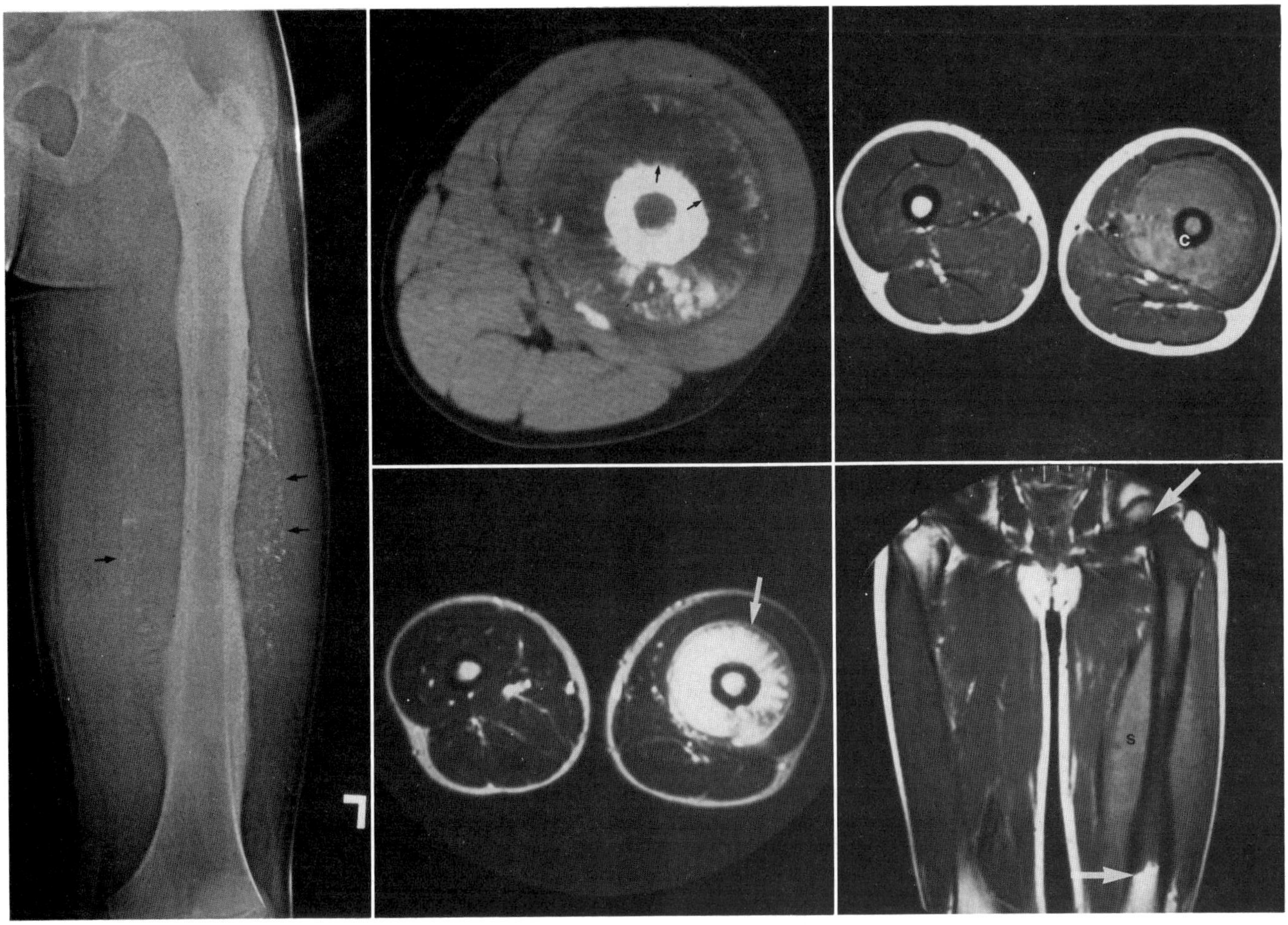

Figure 7-12. Diagnosis: Osteosarcoma. Comparison of CT and MR.
A, Plain film radiograph. This shows a large lesion arising in the diaphysis of the left femur and extending into both metaphyseal regions. Histologically, this was a chondroblastic osteosarcoma. The elevated peripheral margin of the periosteum is defined by arrows. ***B,*** CT image through the mid part of the lesion. The central marrow abnormality is less easy to appreciate than on the MR images (***C*** and ***D***). The marginal irregularity of the cortex *(small arrows)* is well seen. Extensive moderately heavily calcified tumor has elevated the periosteum so that the tumor has a well-defined peripheral margin. ***C,*** MR, T1 weighted image. Marrow abnormality is much easier to appreciate on this MR image. The entire marrow is of very low signal compared to the bright signal of the opposite side. The cortex (*C*) is seen as a low-intensity area surrounding the bone marrow. The subtle cortical irregularity seen on the CT image cannot be easily appreciated. The soft-tissue component of the tumor is well defined. Calcification is seen as low-intensity areas within the tumor. This is not as well seen as with the CT scan. ***D,*** MR, T2 weighted image. The bone marrow has increased in signal intensity and now appears similar to normal marrow. The soft-tissue tumor is now extremely bright and contrast between it and normal muscles is much greater than was seen with CT or the T1 weighted MR image. A rim of edema *(arrow)* surrounding the tumor is more easily appreciated with this image than with the T1 weighted MR image or with the CT. ***E,*** MR coronal T1 weighted image. This image depicts nicely the superior inferior extent of the soft-tissue (*S*) component of the tumor. It shows the marrow extent of the tumor much more clearly than the axial MR images. It shows much greater superior and inferior extent of tumor than was appreciated on other CT slices. The superior and inferior boundaries between normal and abnormal marrow are indicated by *arrows.* Note that proximally the tumor extends almost to the growth plate. MR is particularly good for identification of the soft-tissue and marrow extent of tumor. CT defines cortical irregularity and soft-tissue calcification better than MR.

A

B

C

D

E

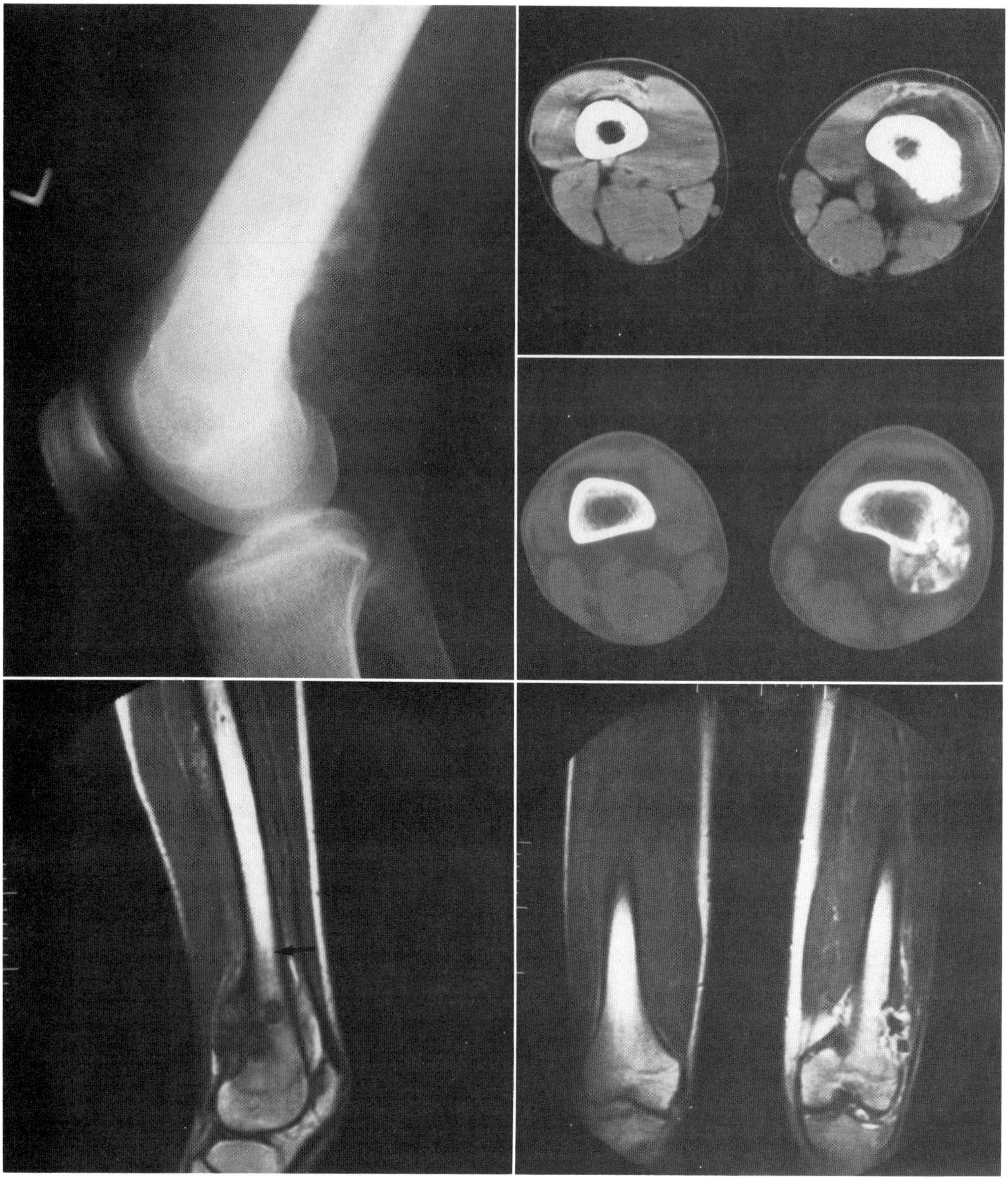

Figure 7-13. Diagnosis: Osteosarcoma of distal femur. Comparison of MR and CT findings. ***A***, Plain film radiograph. There is a classic osteosarcoma of the distal femur with some sclerosis of the shaft and an adjacent soft-tissue mass showing periosteal and matrix mineralization. ***B*** and ***C***, CT images. These show the irregularity of the cortical margin and heavily calcified soft-tissue component of the tumor. Note that on the inferior image (***C***) there is a large posterolateral component to the tumor, but the trabecular pattern in the inferior aspect of the marrow space is not greatly dissimilar from the opposite side. Therefore, one cannot appreciate the presence of tumor in the marrow cavity at this level. ***D*** and ***E***, MR, sagittal T1 and coronal T2 weighted images. The soft-tissue component of the lesion is of low intensity on the T1 weighted image. There are some areas of increased signal on T2 but large areas remain dark because of the extensive calcification identified on the CT images. The superior extent of the tumor is well seen *(arrow).* Inferiorly, figure ***D*** shows extensive low-signal intensity through the growth plate involving almost all of the epiphysis. This involvement of marrow, almost to the joint surface, is greater than could be appreciated from CT images.

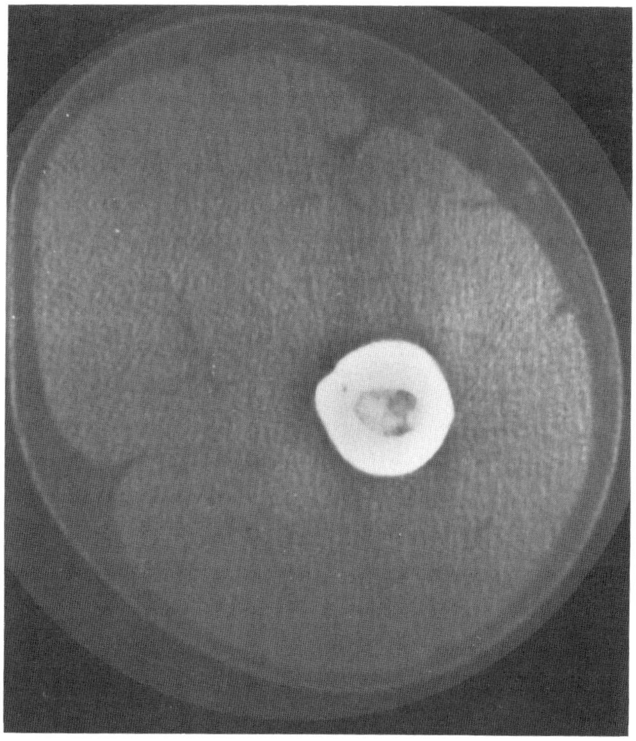

Figure 7-14. **Diagnosis: Osteosarcoma. CT appearance of blastic tumor.**
CT image shows extensive tumor calcification of the bone marrow component of the lesion.

Figure 7-15. **Diagnosis: Normal bone marrow. Changes of conversion of hemopoietic to fatty marrow.**
MR axial spin density image. Signal intensity is greater in the diaphysis than in either end of the femur. This is because conversion is occurring from hemopoietic (red) to fatty (yellow) marrow. The patchy nature of the signal is caused by incomplete conversion. It is extremely important not to mistake this appearance for metastatic lesions from osteosarcoma. The bilateral symmetry is very helpful in this regard.

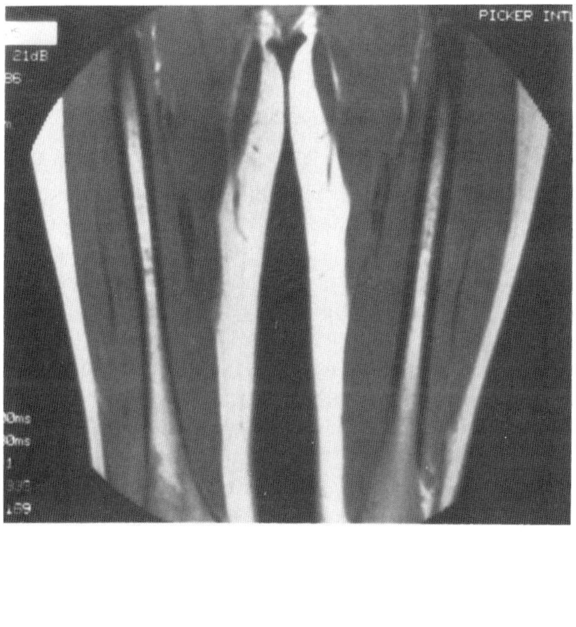

tion of tumor calcification, cortical destruction, and periosteal reaction.[17] There will not be agreement between the different reported studies comparing CT and MR, because the techniques utilized for each of the modalities always vary. A fair reflection of current thinking, however, is that MR is superior to CT for identifying the soft-tissue component of the tumor, at least as good as if not better than CT for delineation of bone marrow spread and joint involvement, worse than CT for calcification identification, and worse than or equivalent to CT for identification of cortical and periosteal abnormality (see Figs. 7–11, 7–12, and 7–13).

Signal intensity of abnormal tissue in osteogenic sarcoma is variable (see Figs. 7–11, 7–12, and 7–13). Cortical abnormality is seen as an increase in signal on either T1 or T2 weighted pulse sequences (Fig. 7–16). Periosteal elevation and thickening is seen as a very low signal intensity circumferential band separate from and elevated from the cortex. The thickness of this reaction and its homogeneity will correspond to some extent to that seen on the plain film radiograph. Bone marrow abnormality is best appreciated on T1 weighted images and is seen as a reduction in signal intensity compared to normal bone marrow. On T2 weighted images, the tumor in the bone marrow has a high signal intensity but normal marrow also has a high signal because of fat. Tumor is, therefore, not well appreciated in the bone marrow on T2 weighted images. In contrast to this, T2 weighted images are best for identification of soft-tissue tumor. On these pulse sequences, the tumor appears of bright signal intensity, much greater than normal muscle. On T1 weighted pulse sequences, the tumor is frequently of similar intensity, slightly greater or slightly less than normal muscle, and it is not as clearly visualized. STIR pulse sequences, in which normal bone marrow signal is suppressed, are particularly helpful for identification of marrow tumor. With these pulse sequences normal marrow is dark and tumor by contrast is bright.

As mentioned, the soft-tissue component of the tumor is usually of high signal on T2 weighted pulse sequences and similar signal to muscle on T1 weighted sequences. There is, however, some variation from this in almost all patients as the tumors are heterogeneous and not homogeneous. Areas of osteoid, for example, will produce a signal lower than muscle on both T1 and T2 weighted pulse sequences.[18] Similarly, areas of fibrosis will be of low signal on both pulse sequences. Hemorrhage will vary in signal intensity on T1 and T2 weighted pulse sequences depending on its age, and areas of necrosis, particularly if liquefied, will be extremely bright on T2 weighted pulse sequences. Various histologic subtypes of osteosarcoma cannot be differentiated by MR,[19] and it is not possible to differentiate osteosarcoma from other malignant or benign bone lesions purely on the signal characteristics.

One area of some contention regards the presence or absence of edema and the ability of MR to differentiate tumor from edema. Edema, like tumor, will be of relatively low signal intensity on T1 pulse sequences with

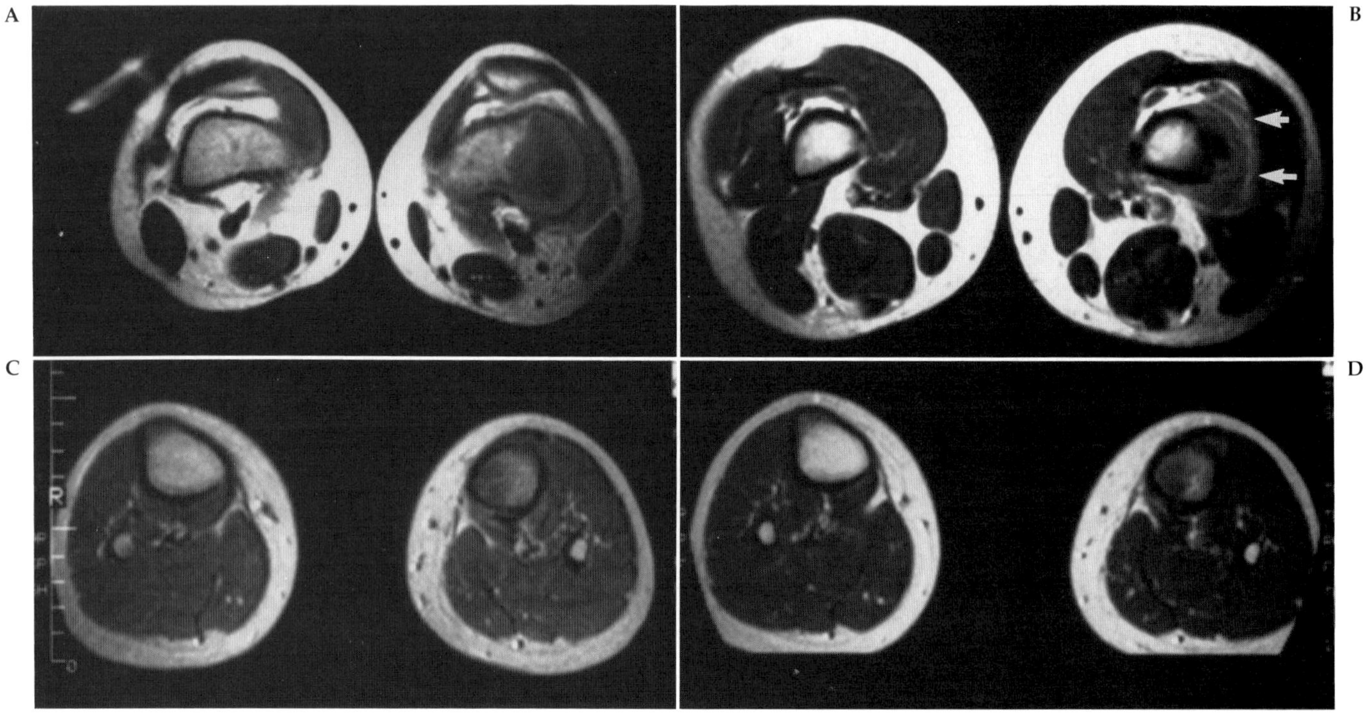

Figure 7–16. **Diagnosis: Osteosarcoma. Gadolinium-DTPA enhancement (2 cases). *A* and *B*, MR, T1 weighted images, before and after gadolinium-DTPA administration. There is mild patchy increase in signal intensity *(arrows)* following administration of gadolinium-DTPA. *C* and *D*, MR, T1 weighted images, before and after gadolinium-DTPA administration. The tumor does not enhance.**

increasing signal intensity seen with T2 weighting. In one study, it was concluded that edema around the soft-tissue component of the tumor is seen as strandy fingerlike areas of increased signal on T2 weighted images extending between the muscles especially along the normal fascial plane. The primary soft-tissue tumor by contrast was more homogeneous and better defined. In the bone marrow, several studies have demonstrated excellent correlation between tumor extent as predicted by MR and comparison with pathology. Most reports seem to indicate that edema is not a major factor in the bone marrow and that the abnormality identified on MR represents tumor. A single case, recently reported,[19] had what was believed to be extensive marrow edema, although this was not confirmed histologically. Until this problem is resolved the cautious surgeon will leave a wide margin of normal tissue adjacent to all identifiable abnormalities on the MR images, not attempting to base surgical decisions on MR differentiation of tumor and edema.

From a technical point of view MR images must cover the entire affected limb in order to detect skip lesions. Images should be obtained with a minimum of T1 and T2 weighted pulse sequences and also STIR pulse sequences. At least two imaging planes should be utilized. Although the images obtained in the coronal and sagittal planes are very attractive, the axial plane has the advantage of excluding partial volume effects caused by curvature of the long bones and, in addition, provides the most easily interpretable comparison with the opposite normal side. Another advantage of the axial plane is that it facilitates research comparisons with CT. My own preference is to perform the bulk of the imaging in the axial plane with additional images obtained in the coronal plane as time permits. The choice of imaging coil provides a conflict. Circular coils will best permit comparison with the opposite side and also most readily permit evaluation of the entire bone. Surface coils will provide better resolution. Again my preference is to utilize a circular coil for initial screening and then to supplement this with surface coil imaging and thin slices to resolve specific problems, e.g., better delineation of the relationship of the tumor to a joint surface (Fig. 7–16). Gadolinium-DTPA has not been widely used. In one recent study giving gadolinium-DTPA and performing rapid sequence, serial, gradient echo images, it was found that the slope of increase in signal intensity was slightly more in malignant than in benign bone tumors. There was, however, still significant overlap and this technique could not be utilized as a clear indicator of malignancy. Gadolinium-DTPA was also helpful in differentiating necrosis and edema from tumor. Necrosis and edema showed less rapid increase in signal intensity than did soft-tissue tumor. While the soft-tissue component of the tumor did increase with gadolinium-DTPA, the contrast difference between the tumor and normal muscle was still less than could be obtained with noncontrast enhanced T2 weighted images. The contrast between the tumor and normal marrow following gadolinium-DTPA administration was less than that seen with T1 weighted images without gadolinium-DTPA administration.

When available, MR should be performed in all patients with osteosarcoma as it provides unique information that impacts significantly on patient management. It is the best modality for identifying the soft-tissue component of the tumor and its relationship to adjacent muscles and the neurovascular bundle. It is probably the best modality for identifying tumor spread within the bone marrow, skip lesions, epiphyseal extension of the tumor, and invasion of the tumor into the joint space. Compared to CT, MR has less artifact from any surgical implants.

Angiography. Angiography was once utilized fairly extensively for the evaluation of osteosarcoma. On angiograms, 90 percent of osteosarcomas appear very vascular,[3,20] 75 percent of tumors demonstrate a marked capillary blush, and in 35 percent of cases significant arterial venous shunts can be seen.[3] Angiography has now been superseded by CT (which shows the neurovascular bundle reasonably well) and to a greater extent by MR. Angiography cannot identify joint involvement with tumor, cannot show accurately the soft-tissue component of the tumor, and cannot differentiate tumor blood vessels from reactive hyperemia.[3] In one center, angiography following intra-arterial chemotherapy is still utilized as a means of evaluating tumor response to chemotherapy.

Most of the above descriptions of the appearance of osteosarcoma with the various different imaging modalities refer to the long bones. The comments are applicable to tumors occurring in the pelvis as well (Fig. 7–17). In the craniofacial area, however, the osteosarcomas have a somewhat different appearance (Fig. 7–18). While uncommon overall, when they do occur in the head, they are particularly common in the upper or lower jaw. In the maxilla, they tend to be found on the alveolar ridge and in the mandible in the body (Fig. 7–19). A fairly characteristic very early sign of osteosarcoma in the mandible is widening of the periodontal membrane (Fig. 7–19). The radiographic findings in 32 patients with craniofacial osteosarcoma are summarized in Table 7–15.

IMAGING EVALUATION OF RESPONSE TO THERAPY

The demands of imaging must change with and reflect alterations in therapy. Prior to the 1970s most nonmetastatic osteosarcomas were treated by amputation through the next most proximal joint. Imaging was required to raise the suspicion of the diagnosis of osteosarcoma to a level at which biopsy was performed. Imaging was also utilized to detect metastasis. Because the primary tumor was resected with the amputation, no further imaging of the primary tumor was required (or possible).

The modern therapeutic approach for osteosarcoma is to treat almost all patients with initial chemotherapy. The reasons for this are first to evaluate the sensitivity of tumor to specific chemotherapeutic agents. (This information is utilized for planning continued chemotherapy following surgery.) Second, tumor shrinkage, which can be achieved in the majority of patients, facilitates local resection of the primary tumor with limb salvage.

For these reasons it has become imperative to develop imaging techniques sensitive enough to detect early response or failure to respond to chemotherapy. See Table 7–14 for the pathologic classification of response. All of the imaging modalities can be utilized to evaluate tumor response, but some are much better than others, either because they are more sensitive, more specific, or detect response earlier after commencement of chemotherapy. In general terms, any reduction in the size of the soft-tissue component of the tumor is an indication of a favorable response to chemotherapy. Conversely, an increase in size of tumor is usually an indication of poor response, although occasionally it might be caused by a large hemorrhage. Only MR can identify hemorrhage with accuracy.[21] It is important to note that the size of the soft-tissue component of tumor may not decrease significantly even with a good response.[21] This may be due to the fact that the

TABLE 7–15
Craniofacial Osteosarcoma: 32 Cases[1]

No. Cases	Site	Soft-Tissue Mass	Lytic/ Blastic	Periosteal Reaction	Soft-Tissue Matrix Ca^{++}	Chondroblastic Histology
11	Maxilla (8/11 in body)	All	6/2	0	6	80%
13	Mandible (all in alveolar ridge)	All	4/6	3	8	80%
8	Skull	All	All lytic	0	4	0%

Reference

1. Lee Y-Y, Van Tassel P, Nauert C, et al. Craniofacial osteosarcomas: plain film, CT, and MR findings in 46 cases. AJR 1988;150:1397–1402.

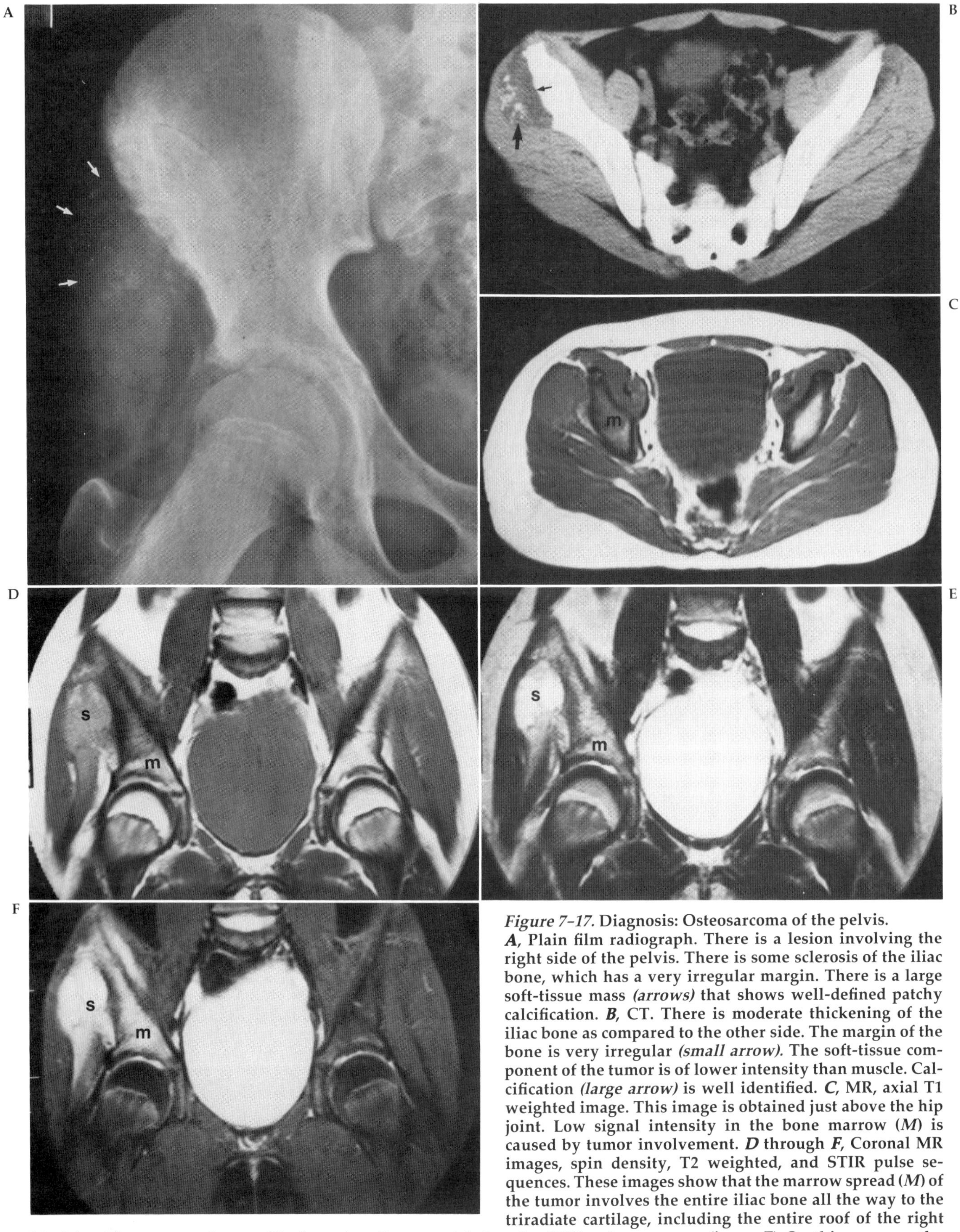

Figure 7–17. Diagnosis: Osteosarcoma of the pelvis. ***A,*** Plain film radiograph. There is a lesion involving the right side of the pelvis. There is some sclerosis of the iliac bone, which has a very irregular margin. There is a large soft-tissue mass *(arrows)* that shows well-defined patchy calcification. ***B,*** CT. There is moderate thickening of the iliac bone as compared to the other side. The margin of the bone is very irregular *(small arrow).* The soft-tissue component of the tumor is of lower intensity than muscle. Calcification *(large arrow)* is well identified. ***C,*** MR, axial T1 weighted image. This image is obtained just above the hip joint. Low signal intensity in the bone marrow (*M*) is caused by tumor involvement. ***D*** through ***F,*** Coronal MR images, spin density, T2 weighted, and STIR pulse sequences. These images show that the marrow spread (*M*) of the tumor involves the entire iliac bone all the way to the triradiate cartilage, including the entire roof of the right hip joint. The marrow abnormality is most easily appreciated on the STIR pulse sequence *(image F).* On this sequence the abnormal marrow appears of bright signal. Note that normal marrow on the opposite side is of very low signal. The large soft-tissue component (*S*) of the tumor is seen on all three pulse sequences. Maximum contrast between it and normal muscle is seen on the STIR and T2 weighted sequences. Calcification is not appreciated. This tumor was a chondroblastic osteosarcoma. MR showed marrow extent far better than CT or plain film. Plain film and CT showed the tumor calcification. This was important in that the calcification is the only clue that this tumor is an osteosarcoma rather than a Ewing sarcoma.

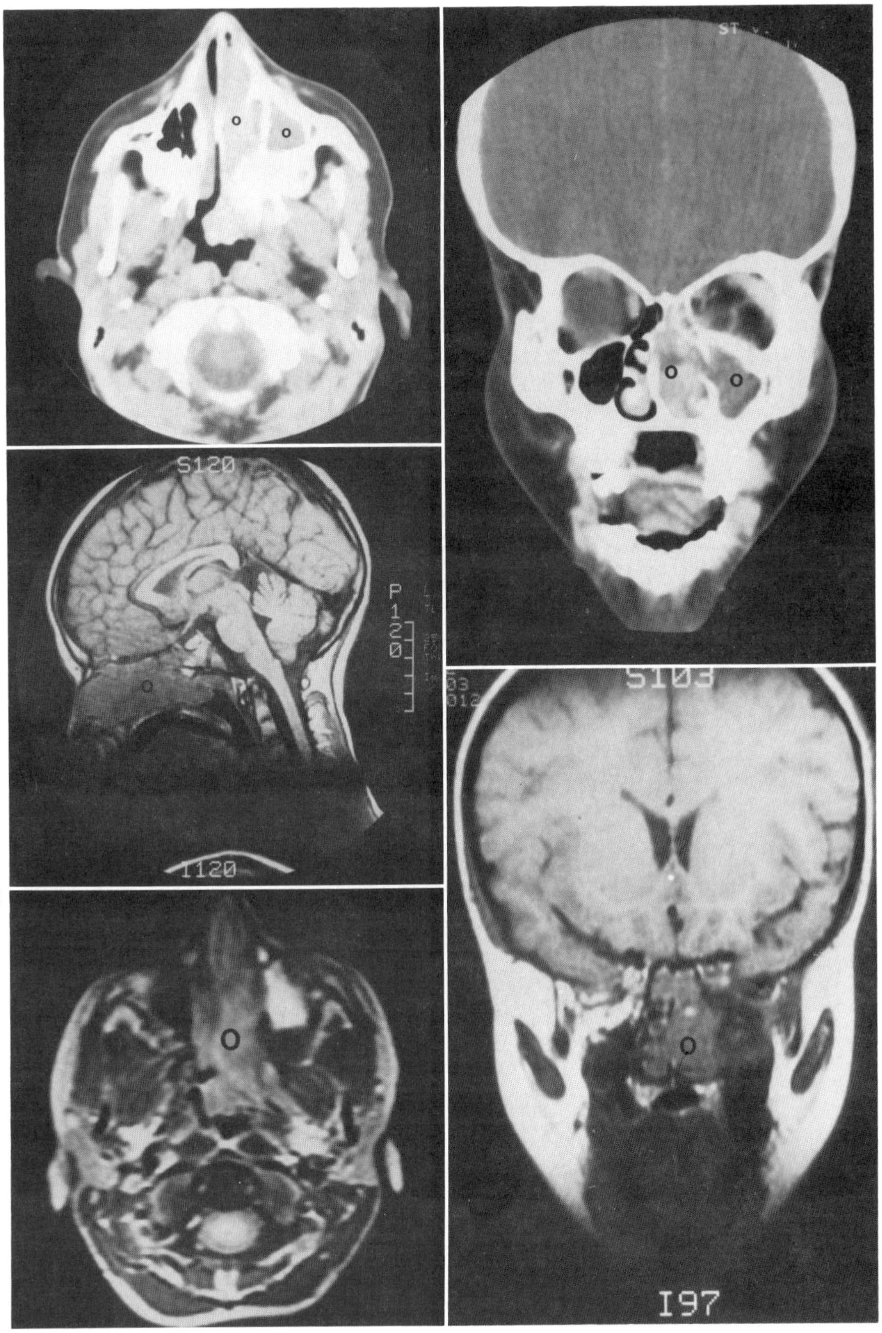

Figure 7–18. **Diagnosis: Osteosarcoma of the skull.**
***A* and *B*, CT axial and coronal images. Extensive osteosarcoma (*O*) is seen involving the left side of the nose and the left maxillary sinus. The nasal septum is displaced to the right. The medial wall of the maxillary sinus is completely destroyed. *C* through *E*, MR sagittal, coronal, and axial images. The soft-tissue component of the osteosarcoma (*O*) is fairly well seen. The bone destruction is not as clearly identified as on the CT image. This child had previously been treated for bilateral retinoblastomas.**

response is predominantly tumor necrosis rather than fibrosis. At this stage it should be noted that there is one variant of osteosarcoma in which it is extremely difficult to evaluate any response to chemotherapy by any imaging modality. This is the purely blastic form of conventional osteosarcoma. In these tumors, almost the entire tumor mass consists of the heavily mineralized blastic tumor, with little if any soft-tissue component and little if any extension in the bone marrow space. As bone healing is normally indicated by increase in density and as these tumors have little soft-tissue component, there are no criteria by which to evaluate their response. The changes seen, with the various imaging modalities, of all the other types of conventional osteosarcoma are discussed in more detail here.

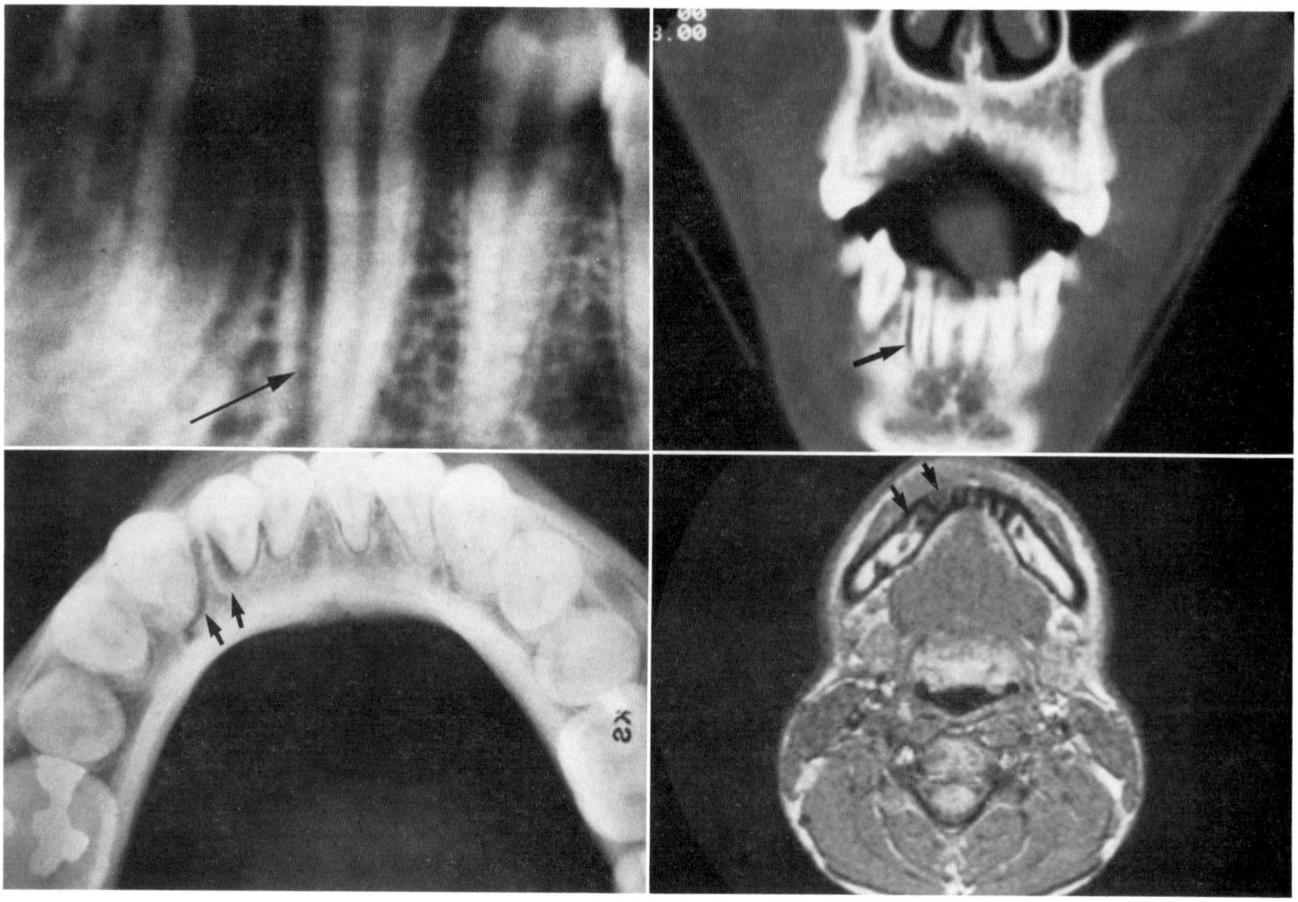

Figure 7–19. **Diagnosis: Osteosarcoma of the mandible.**
***A*, Plain film radiograph. This shows thickening of the periodontal membrane *(arrow)*. *B* and *C*, CT images. These confirm the thickening of the periodontal membrane *(arrows)*. *D*, MR, T1 weighted image. This shows extensive signal loss in the bone marrow *(arrows)*, indicating much more extensive disease than could be appreciated from the other images.**

Plain Film Radiograph. On plain film radiographs soft-tissue mass may be seen to decrease in size. The periosteal reaction becomes more solid and there is bridging of regions of cortical destruction. The periosteum becomes incorporated into the adjacent cortex and the pattern of permeative destruction decreases. The bony portion of the tumor becomes more sclerotic.[8,21,22] Unfortunately, all of the above changes occur late and the plain film radiograph is not nearly as sensitive as other modalities for detection of earlier response to therapy.

Angiography. On angiography, response can be identified as a reduction in the tumor vascularity and in the amount of AV shunting. This method for evaluating tumor response is only utilized in those centers in which an arterial catheter has already been positioned for administration of chemotherapy. In all other patients, the information provided does not warrant the use of an invasive technique.[21,23]

MDP Technetium 99m Bone Scan. MDP technetium 99m bone scan has little role in evaluating response. Prior to therapy, there is normally an extended pattern of uptake, and correlation of overall uptake with tumor size is poor. Evaluation of response cannot, therefore, be accurate. An increase in uptake of radioisotope probably represents extension of the tumor and failed therapy. Reduction of uptake does not, however, correlate well, with response being inaccurate in 18 cases in one study.[24] In another study, evaluation of perfusion in blood pool images was found to be of no help, while evaluation of osseous phase images proved only 73 percent accurate in evaluating response to chemotherapy.[25] Another study suggests a good correlation between dynamic changes in MDP images and tumor response seen pathologically.[26] In another study, the ratio of uptake between gallium and technetium 99m MDP was utilized to evaluate response. A good chemotherapeutic response was diagnosed when the ratio of uptake of these two agents decreased.[8] Disadvantages of this technique are a relatively high radiation dose, relative nonspecificity, and the fact that the pretherapy uptake varies. For example, it is less with purely lytic lesions. Other experimental methods of evaluation of response, using radioisotopes, have been attempted. None have received routine clinical acclaim and they are not utilized in routine clinical practice.[24] One of these techniques involves intra-arterial infusion of MDP-labeled albumin macrospheres, with a good response being diagnosed by demonstration of decrease in tumor vascularity and intratumor shunts.[24]

CT. CT has been utilized effectively to evaluate tumor response to therapy. The CT criteria for response are summarized in Table 7–16. An excellent response is identified by demonstration of decrease in the soft-tissue mass, an increase in peripheral or central calcification, and a decrease in the extent of marrow abnormality. In 7 of 9 patients, there was excellent correlation between CT-predicted response following four courses of high-dose methotrexate and the histology of the tumor following resection on completion of the tumor therapy.[27] CT has been demonstrated to provide all the information needed for limb salvage surgery.[12]

MR. MR has been widely suggested to have a significant role in evaluation of response to chemotherapy (Fig. 7–20). There are, however, some conflicting results reported in the literature. In one study, it was felt that a decrease in size of the tumor correlated well with response to chemotherapy,[28] while in another study it was reported that a decrease in volume was seen in 73 percent of responders and 50 percent of nonresponders and that it was, therefore, not of great use.[25] Some of the studies do not clearly state whether the volume referred to is the entire tumor, including the bone component, or only the soft-tissue component. This may in part explain some of the conflicting results. My own belief is that one should consider only the volume of the extraskeletal soft-tissue component of the tumor when one is looking for a decrease in tumor size as an indicator of response to therapy. Some discrepancy is also reported in the results of utilization of changes in signal intensity to monitor therapy. One study[25] indicated that a reduction in signal intensity of the soft-tissue tumor on T2 weighted images was a fairly specific but not a very sensitive indicator of response. Enhancement with gadolinium-DTPA was a sensitive indicator of residual active tumor but a very nonspecific finding, as it could be seen with nontumor inflammatory and granulation tissue as well.[28] On dynamic images following gadolinium-DTPA administration, a reduction in the slope of intensity of change seen after chemotherapy had an 85 percent correlation with good tumor response.[25]

In another study of 38 patients treated with intra-arterial cisplatinum and systemic adriamycin, MR findings were correlated with pathology. MR was accurate in demonstrating progression or regression of tumor. The best MR pattern for prediction of greater than 90 percent necrosis of tumor was low signal intensity seen on both T1 and T2 weighted pulse sequences. Three patterns of alteration of signal intensity were identified. These were complex and their appearance did not correlate accurately with tumor response. Pathologically identified residual foci of tumor greater than 5 mm in diameter could usually be seen as areas of signal intensity equivalent to muscle on T1 and greater than muscle on T2 weighted pulse sequences. Most of the residual foci of tumor were thus identified, but the appearance was very nonspecific, as it could not differentiate tumor from identical-appearing areas of edema or granulation tissue. Residual foci of tumor less than 5 mm in diameter were often not seen on the MR images at all. A favorable response was usually accompanied by reduction in peritumor edema.[19,28] It is important, however, that the radiologist be aware of the route of administration of chemotherapy, as intra-arterial chemotherapy is toxic and causes significant edema in the muscles around the tumor, which must not be mistaken for failed response.[19] It is not surprising that the evaluation of signal intensity change in the tumor will yield some conflicting results. The tumors are complex areas of active tumor, granulation tissue, edema, hemorrhage, and residual blood products, including hemosiderin, necrotic cysts, and marrow infarct. With this complexity of histology it is unlikely that evaluation of signal intensity on MR alone will ever be found to provide consistent accurate prediction of tumor response to chemotherapy.

Tumor response to chemotherapy may be diagnosed on MR by a reduction in the size of the tumor mass, by a significant reduction in the signal intensity of the tumor on T2 weighted images, and by a return of bone marrow signal to normal. MR will never be able to accurately exclude the presence of small residual foci of active tumor in a background of largely necrotic tumor. Experimental MR phosphorus spectroscopy in 10 cases has demonstrated a correlation of tumor response with an increase in the phosphate peak and a decrease in the ATP and phosphomonoester peaks.[29] A potential advantage of this technique is that change may be detected as early as 48 hours after administration of chemotherapy.[29]

TABLE 7–16
CT Response to Preamputation Chemotherapy for Osteosarcoma[1]

Grade of CT Response	Criteria
Poor response	Increased bony destruction; increased soft-tissue mass; increased extent of marrow abnormality
No change	No significant interval change
Moderate response	Some decrease in soft-tissue mass; some increase in calcification
Excellent response	Marked decrease in soft-tissue mass; marked increase in peripheral or central calcification; decreased extent of marrow abnormality

Reference
1. Mail JT, Cohen MD, Mirkin LD, et al. Response of osteosarcoma to preoperative intravenous high-dose methotrexate chemotherapy: CT evaluation. AJR 1985;144:89–93.

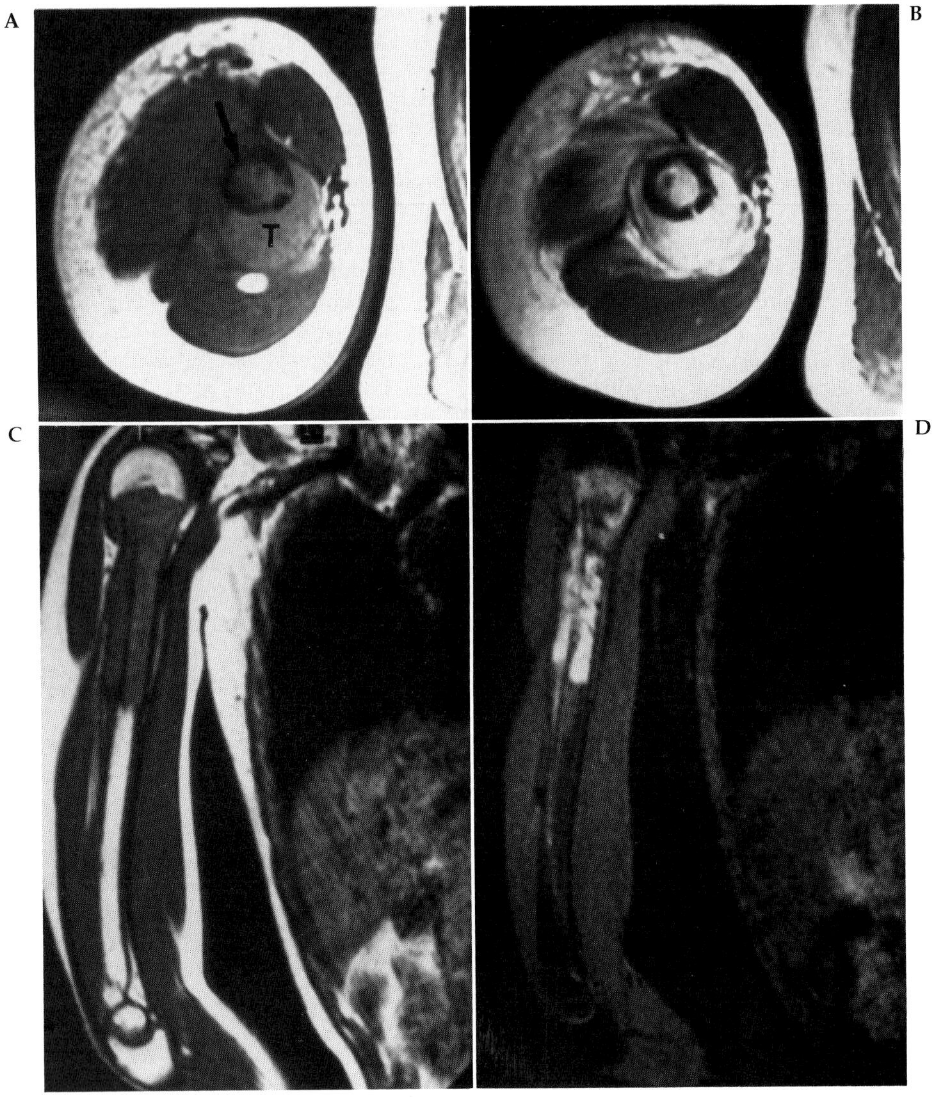

Figure 7–20. **Diagnosis: Osteosarcoma. Decrease in tumor size after chemotherapy.**
***A* and *B*, MR, T1 weighted images before and after gadolinium-DTPA administration. Before contrast administration, the tumor (*T*) is of slightly higher signal intensity than normal muscle. Signal intensity from bone marrow is low *(arrow)*. With gadolinium-DTPA administration both the soft tissue and marrow components of the tumor enhance. *C* and *D*, MR, T1 weighted and STIR images after chemotherapy. There has been significant reduction in the size of the tumor. There is very sharp demarcation between normal and abnormal bone marrow. This is helpful in planning local tumor resection.**

> *Comment:* CT and MR are the prime methods for evaluation of the response of the primary tumor mass to initial chemotherapy. Both modalities are reasonably accurate in detecting response but neither is completely accurate. When available, my own preference is to utilize MR rather than CT.

IMAGING PROTOCOLS

Initial Presentation. On initial presentation of a patient with osteosarcoma, aggressive imaging evaluation of the site of the primary disease and sites of potential metastasis must be performed. The specific appearance of the primary tumor on the various imaging studies has already been described. Imaging is asked to provide a differential diagnosis for the primary lesion, identify accurately spread of the tumor within the bone marrow space, and the soft tissues, and define its relationship to adjacent joints and critical structures such as major blood vessels and nerves. In terms of providing a differential diagnosis, the plain film radiograph is still excellent and probably better than other modalities. At the time of presentation, with clinical symptoms, the plain film radiograph will invariably be abnormal. Very occasionally, early subtle signs of tumor may be missed if they are not carefully looked for. Osteosarcoma usually spreads fairly extensively through the bone marrow of the affected bone. Both CT and MR are excellent for identification of this bone marrow spread,[30] with MR probably being given the advantage by most workers for absolute accuracy, but with CT (if performed properly) providing an accuracy quite adequate for surgical planning. Despite a few suggestions to the contrary, it is not believed that significant edema occurs in the bone marrow and correlations of pathological macroslides with imaging have been very close.[30] As mentioned, MR and CT are fairly equivalent for definition of marrow spread in the medullary cavity of the shaft of the bone. Within the trabecular bone of the epiphysis, MR is clearly superior to CT and, when available, should be utilized for evaluation of tumor spread within the epiphysis and its relationship to the joint surface. Because of its ability to image in multiple planes, MR is also better than CT for identification of invasion of the joint space by the tumor.

Accurate definition of the relationship of the soft-tissue component of the tumor to individual adjacent muscles is now of critical importance in planning limb salvage surgical procedures. Plain film radiograph is poor in this regard. CT is reasonably good, but MR is clearly the imaging modality of choice. There is academic debate as to the accuracy of MR in distinguishing the tumor margin from adjacent edema. Although the presence of edema might be suspected from its fluffy, ill-defined, and infiltrating outlines, it is probably wise to consider the entire area of abnormality demonstrated by MR as potential tumor and plan surgery accordingly.

Metastatic disease is not uncommon on initial diagnosis and, therefore, should be aggressively sought. Lung (Figs. 7–21, 7–22, 7–23, and 7–24) and bone (Fig. 7–25) are by far the most common sites of metastatic spread of osteosarcoma, and there is no argument that these two sites should be imaged, the lung with CT and the bones with MDP technetium 99m radioisotope scanning. Historically, metastasis might be expected in the lung in about 20 percent of patients presenting with osteosarcoma,[31] but more recent studies with improved imaging techniques will identify metastases in up to 40 percent of patients on initial diagnosis.[32] In one study of 111 patients, metastases were identified in 59 on initial presentation. Of these, 36 (61 percent) were in the lung alone, 11 (18 percent) in nonlung sites alone, and 12 (20 percent) involved both lung and extralung locations.[33] About half of the lung metastases will be bilateral. This does not matter, as CT scan routinely images both lungs.[34] Bone metastases, while not quite as common as metastases in the lung, do occur: They were reported in up to 10 percent of patients on initial presentation.[3] Of importance is the fact that bone metastases can occur independently of lung metastasis so that a negative chest CT cannot be utilized as reasoning to avoid performing a bone radioisotope scan.

In addition to lung and bone, metastases can occasionally be identified in a wide variety of organs, including the myocardium,[35] inferior vena cava,[10] kidneys[39] (see Fig. 7–10), liver,[36] brain[37] (Figs. 7–26 and 7–27), and lymph nodes[38] (Figs. 7–28 and 7–29). Each

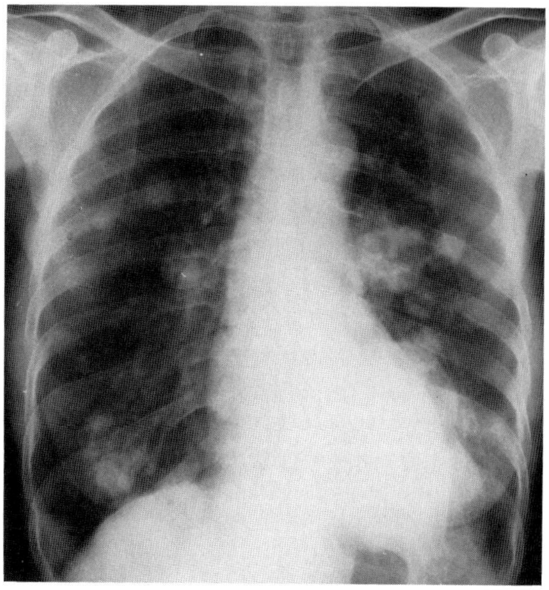

Figure 7–21. **Diagnosis: Metastases from osteosarcoma. Chest radiograph. Multiple lung metastatic lesions of varying size are identified. All are fairly well defined. Some of the lesions are very dense, indicating calcification. This is a not uncommon finding with osteosarcoma. (From Kumar R. Radiographic spectrum of osteogenic sarcoma. AJR 1987;148:767–772.)**

Figure 7–22. **Diagnosis: Osteosarcoma. Single calcified lung metastasis.**
Chest radiograph. There is a well-defined focal 1.5 cm lesion in the right lung. It is very dense, indicating the presence of calcium.

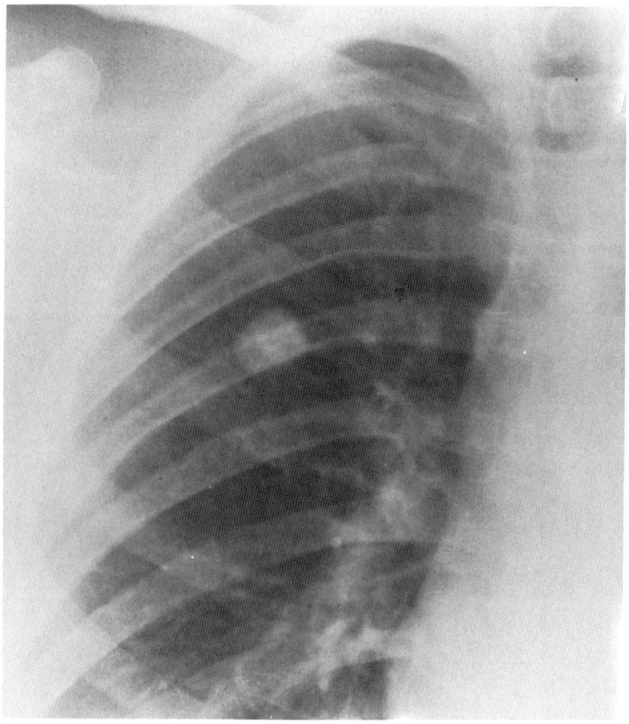

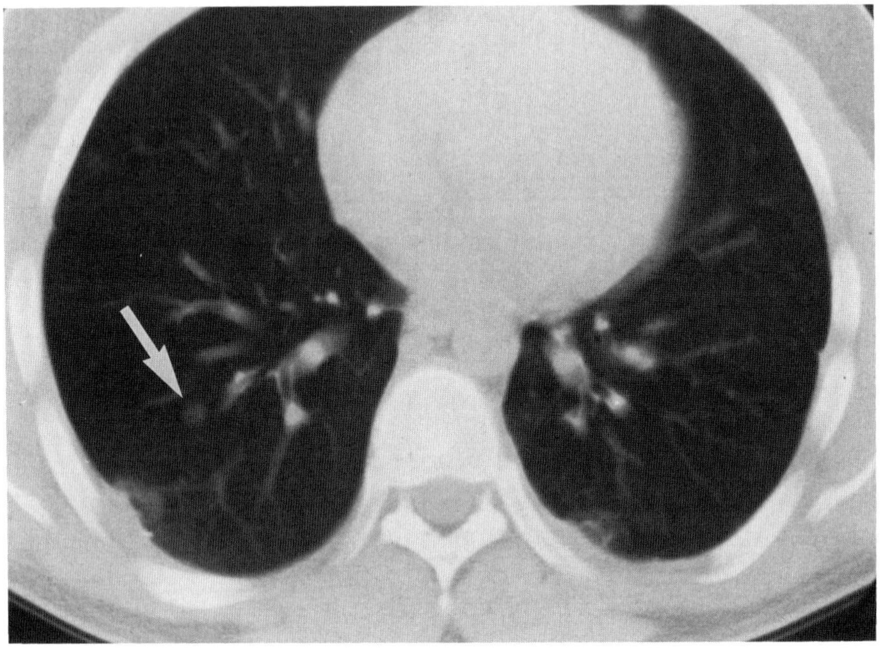

Figure 7-23. **Diagnosis: Osteosarcoma. Lung metastasis.**
CT. There is a well-defined round small metastatic lesion just under 1 cm in diameter in the right lower lobe *(arrow)*. It does not contain calcium and there are no specific diagnostic features.

and every one of these sites cannot be screened routinely in every patient. Fortunately, many metastases in these sites will be picked up by chest CT and bone radioisotope scan. The chest CT will include mediastinal lymph nodes, the heart and pericardium, and parts of the liver and kidneys. Uptake of MDP by metastases in sites other than the bone might draw attention to their presence. In the absence of symptoms, I would not recommend performing a routine head CT on any patient. It would not be unreasonable, however, particularly with primary tumors in the pelvis or leg, to extend the chest CT down to the iliac crests to include the entire abdomen. The yield from this would be small, but it might be particularly worthwhile in patients in whom no metastases have been identified on the bone scan or on the chest CT. If metastases have already been identified by these two modalities, the finding of additional lesions in the abdomen would have no impact on management.

Figure 7-24. **Diagnosis: Osteosarcoma. Calcified lung metastasis.**
CT. Heavily calcified single metastatic lesion is seen in the medial basal segment of the right lower lobe *(arrow)*.

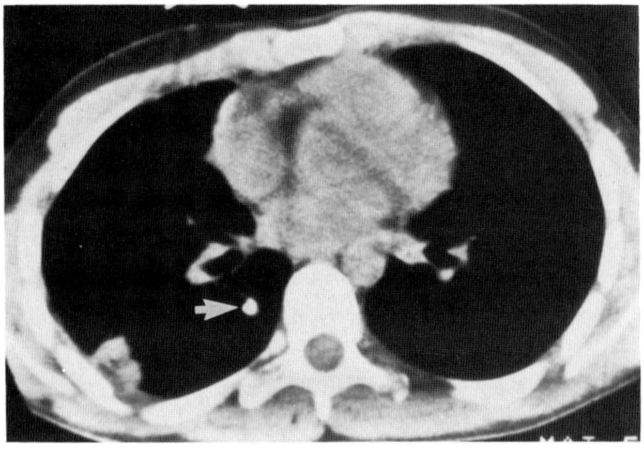

> *Comment:* For detection of metastases on initial presentation chest CT and bone MDP technetium 99m imaging should be performed. In selected cases, abdominal CT should be considered as well. Skip lesions will be identified by several modalities. The plain film radiographs, CT, MR, and radioisotope bone scans will all include the entire affected bone, and skip lesions should be looked for on all of these modalities. Plain film radiograph should be performed of any anatomical bone area in which there is a "hot spot" on the bone scan.

Follow-up Imaging. Follow-up imaging should be performed of the site of primary disease and at sites of potential metastases. As with other tumors, I strongly believe that it is no longer appropriate to lay down "menus" of required imaging modalities, at required sites, at specified times following the original diagnosis. Imaging needs to be *tailored* to the specific therapeutic protocols utilized by an individual institution and further modified by the specific needs of the individual patient. For example, the intensity of follow-up imaging of the site of the primary tumor must be based on the likelihood of local recurrence, which in turn depends on the chosen therapy. If amputation has been performed through the next most proximal joint, local recurrence is exceedingly rare at the surgical margin and aggressive

A B C

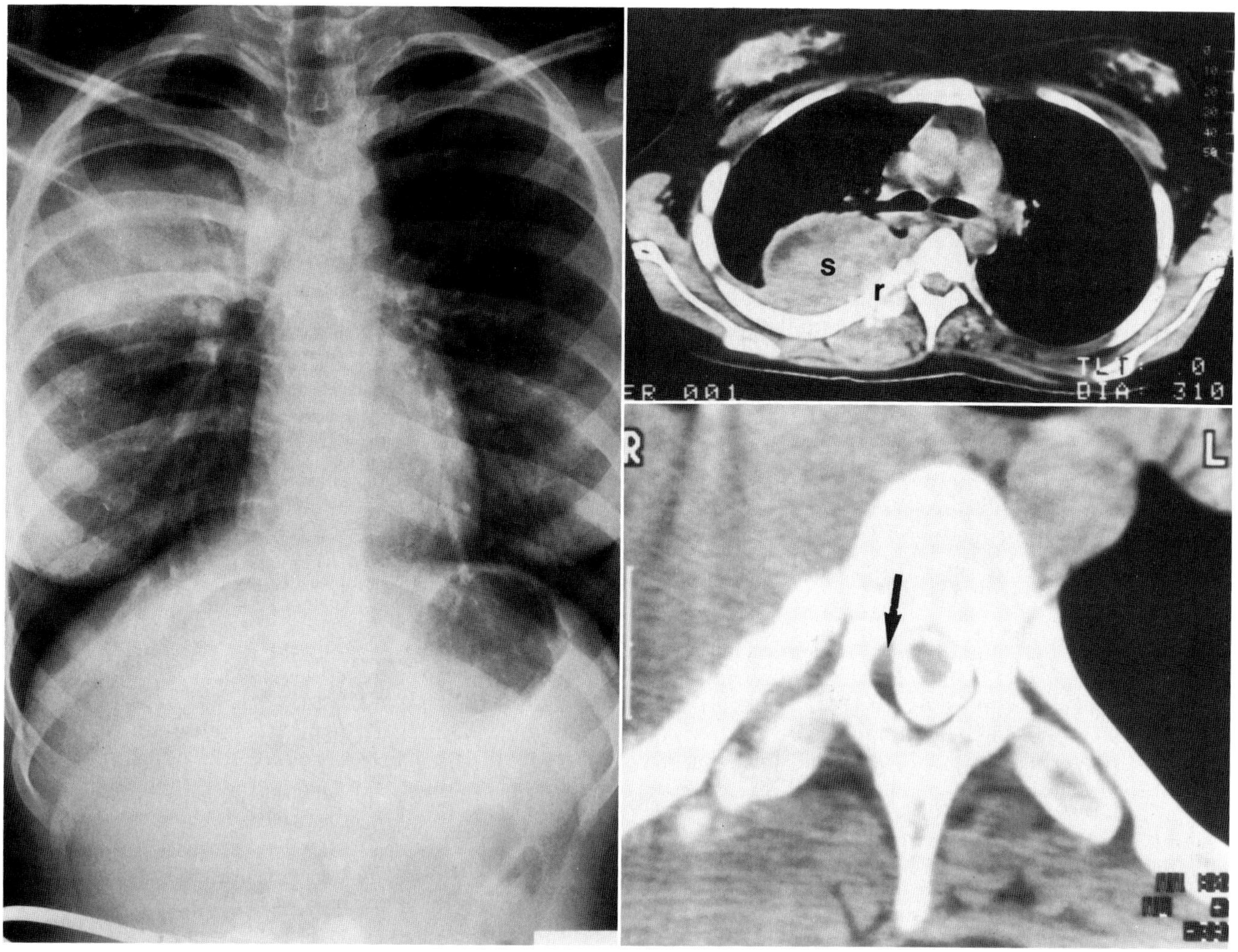

Figure 7–25. **Diagnosis: Osteosarcoma. Rib metastasis from a primary lesion in the femur. *A,* Chest radiograph. This shows a soft-tissue mass lesion in the right hemithorax. There is quite marked separation of adjacent ribs, indicating a posterior mediastinal location for the lesion. Specific rib destruction is very difficult to appreciate on this image. *B,* CT. This shows the lesion to be arising from the posterior aspect of a right-sided rib (*R*). There is a large soft-tissue component (*S*) to the lesion. *C,* CT image. The patient has been given intrathecal contrast. Extensive marginal cortical destruction of the rib and the transverse process of adjacent vertebra is identified on the right side. Extension of a soft-tissue component of the tumor into the spinal canal *(arrow)* can be seen.**

local imaging should not be performed. If amputation has been performed through the affected bone, local recurrence is more likely, particularly with the knowledge of the potential presence of tiny microscopic skip lesions proximal to the amputation. If local resection has been performed to permit limb salvage, the likelihood of local recurrence rises even further. In those patients in whom the primary tumor is in a location at which no surgery could be performed, the possibility of local recurrence is very high (even if there has been an excellent initial response to chemotherapy). Maximal imaging effort of the area of the primary tumor would obviously be performed in these patients.

The timing of follow-up studies should be maximal during the period when relapse is most likely. Most relapses occur within the first 2 years following diagnosis.[32]

Extensive imaging should be performed any time therapy is to be changed. This includes the insertion of a new therapy such as radiation therapy or surgery and also the stopping of any particular therapy. It is probably wise to perform studies no less frequently than every 3 months during the first 2 years. In the chest, it may be adequate not to perform CT on every occasion. For example, simple chest radiograph might be performed on some occasions when the results are not anticipated to cause an alteration in therapy. Similarly, at the site of the primary tumor, plain film radiograph rather than CT or MR could be used.

Planning of follow-up procedures should be influenced by the knowledge of the changing pattern and natural history of a disease process in response to therapy. For example, several studies suggest that nonlung metastases are becoming much more common in pa-

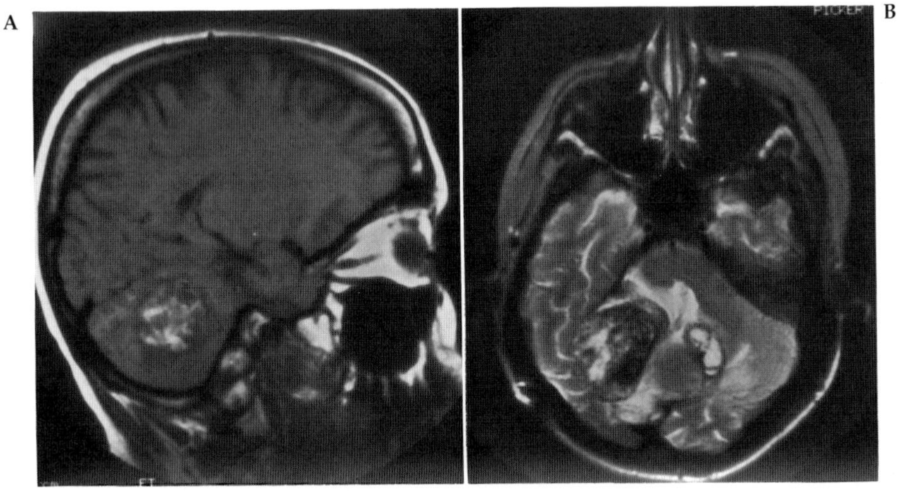

Figure 7–26. **Diagnosis: Osteosarcoma. Brain metastases. This is the same patient whose rib metastasis was illustrated in Figure 7–25.**
A **and** ***B,*** **MR, sagittal T1 and axial T2 weighted images. There is a fairly large lesion in the cerebellum. It is of mixed signal intensity on both pulse sequences. The high signal on the T1 weighted image and the areas of low signal on the T2 weighted image represent hemorrhage in this metastatic lesion.**

tients with osteosarcoma owing to prolonged survival. Previously, these had been reported in only up to 16 percent of cases, but more recent studies suggest that nonlung metastases can be found in up to 36 percent of patients.[6] In another study of 111 patients, lung was the only site of metastasis in 94 percent when the only treatment was surgery. In patients treated with surgery and chemotherapy, the lung was the only site of metastasis in only 45 percent of the patients.[33] Therefore, one must now be willing to use bone scans more frequently than previously and also to utilize CT scanning of other areas such as brain and abdomen, perhaps routinely, but certainly at the first sign of any clinical symptoms.

Figure 7–27. **Diagnosis: Osteosarcoma. Cerebral metastasis. CT after intravenous contrast administration. There is a large lesion in the occipital lobe *(arrows).* Calcification (*C*) is present in the lesion. This metastasis is causing mass effect.**

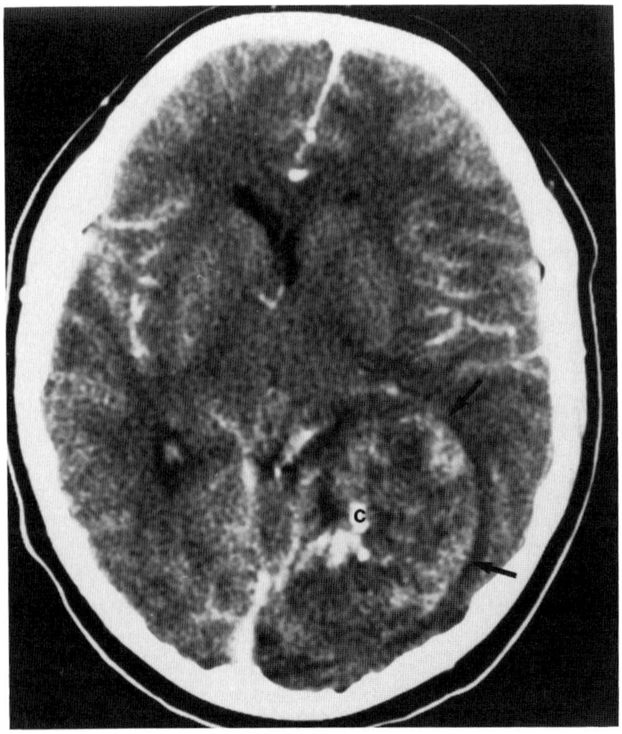

> *Comment:* Follow-up imaging for metastatic disease should rely predominantly on chest CT and MDP technetium 99m radioisotope bone scan. Frequency of study is not dogmatically recommended but should be tailored to patients' needs. Remember that with prolonged survival metastases in other sites are becoming more common.

Figure 7–28. **Diagnosis: Osteosarcoma. Calcified metastases to lymph nodes.**
CT. Heavily calcified metastatic lesions are well seen *(arrows).*

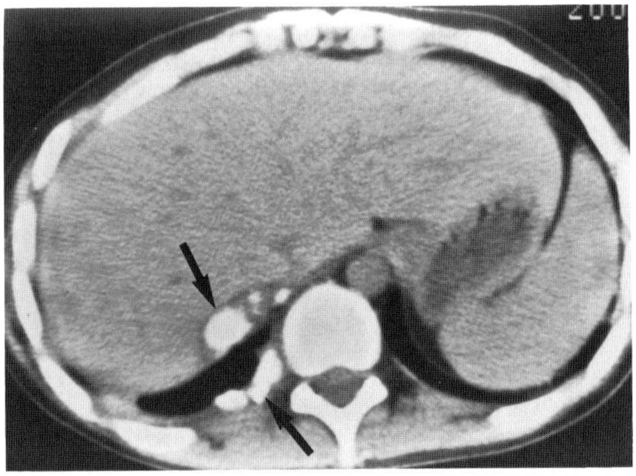

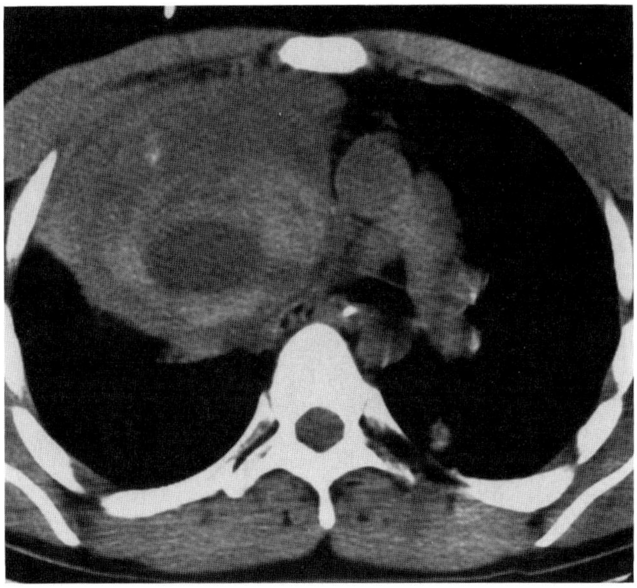

Figure 7-29. **Diagnosis: Osteosarcoma. Metastases to mediastinal lymph nodes.**
CT. A large mediastinal metastatic lesion is identified on the right side.

BIOPSY GUIDANCE

A final role of imaging in the initial evaluation of a newly presented tumor is to assist in determination of a biopsy site. Location of the biopsy site is important. It must be positioned so that the entire biopsy tract can be removed with subsequent surgical excision of the tumor.[40] Imaging, by identifying the soft-tissue component of the tumor, can help locate the biopsy site and provide the surgeon the shortest, most direct access to a potentially viable tumor.[40] Imaging-guided needle biopsies have been performed. In one study, it was reported that a yield of a diagnostic specimen could be obtained in 89 percent of patients.[21] In another study of 51 cases, 8 were completely nondiagnostic while in the other 43, the specimens could provide a diagnosis of malignancy but were inadequate for accurate characterization of the tumor as an osteosarcoma.[41] Because the histology of osteosarcoma is very varied, and because osteoid may be present in relatively small amounts, needle biopsy has no place in the diagnosis of these tumors. Osteoid must be identified on the tissue specimen to make the diagnosis of osteosarcoma and it might easily be missed with a needle biopsy.

References

1. Edeiken-Monroe B, Edeiken J, Jacobson HG. Osteosarcoma. Semin Roentgenol 1989;24:153–173.
2. deSantos LA, Edeiken B. Purely lytic osteosarcoma. Skeletal Radiol 1982;9:1–9.
3. Hudson TM, Schiebler M, Springfield DS, et al. Radiologic imaging of osteosarcoma: role in planning surgical treatment. Skeletal Radiol 1983;10:137–146.
4. Baro PR, Bastart FM, Bartrina JR, et al. Case report 529. Skeletal Radiol 1989;18:136–139.
5. Brown ML. The role of radionuclides in the patient with osteogenic sarcoma. Semin Roentgenol 1989;24:185–192.
6. Hopper KD, Moser RP, Haseman DB, et al. Osteosarcomatosis. Radiology 1990;175:233–239.
7. Vanel D, Henry-Amar M, Lumbroso J, et al. Pulmonary evaluation of patients with osteosarcoma: roles of standard radiography, tomography, CT, scintigraphy, and tomoscintigraphy. AJR 1984;143:519–523.
8. Yeh SDJ, Rosen G, Caparros B, et al. Semiquantitative gallium scintigraphy in patients with osteogenic sarcoma. Clin Nucl Med 1984;9:175–183.
9. Kern KA, Brunetti A, Norton JA, et al. Metabolic imaging of human extremity musculoskeletal tumors by PET. J Nucl Med 1988;29:181–186.
10. deSantos LA, Bernardino ME, Murray JA. Computed tomography in the evaluation of osteosarcoma: experience with 25 cases. AJR 1979;132:535–540.
11. Seeger LL, Eckardt JJ, Bassett LW. Cross-sectional imaging in the evaluation of osteogenic sarcoma: MRI and CT. Semin Roentgenol 1989;24:174–184.
12. Schreiman JS, Crass JR, Wick MR, et al. Osteosarcoma: role of CT in limb-sparing treatment. Radiology 1986;161:485–488.
13. Coffre C, Vanel D, Contesso G, et al. Problems and pitfalls in the use of computed tomography for the local evaluation of long bone osteosarcoma: report on 30 cases. Skeletal Radiol 1985;13:147–153.
14. Kornreich L, Grunebaum M, Ziv N, et al. Osteogenic sarcoma of the calvarium in children: CT manifestation. Neuroradiology 1988;30:439–441.
15. Kumar R, David R, Madewell JE, et al. Radiographic spectrum of osteogenic sarcoma. AJR 1987;148:767–772.
16. Beluffi G, Pazzaglia U, Mora R. Synchronous multicentric osteosarcoma. Pediatr Radiol 1983;13:292–293.
17. Ellis JH, Siegel CL, Martel W, et al. Radiologic features of well-differentiated osteosarcoma. AJR 1988;151:739–742.
18. Nurenberg P, Harms SE. Magnetic resonance imaging of musculoskeletal tumors. CRC 1988;28:331–338.
19. Pan G, Raymond AK, Carrasco CH, et al. Osteosarcoma: MR imaging after preoperative chemotherapy. Radiology 1990;174:517–526.
20. Carrasco CH, Charnsangavej C, Raymond AK, et al. Osteosarcoma: angiographic assessment of response to preoperative chemotherapy. Radiology 1989;170:839–842.
21. Carrasco CH, Charnsangavej C, Richli WR, et al. Osteosarcoma: interventional radiology in diagnosis and management. Semin Roentgenol 1989;24:193–200.
22. Smith J, Heelan RT, Huvos AG, et al. Radiographic changes in primary osteogenic sarcoma following intensive chemotherapy. Radiology 1982;143:355–360.
23. Chuang VP, Benjamin R, Jaffe N, Radiographic and angiographic changes in osteosarcoma after intraarterial chemotherapy. AJR 1982;139:1065–1069.
24. Brown ML. The role of radionuclides in the patient with osteogenic sarcoma. Semin Roentgenol 1989;24:185–192.
25. Erlemann R, Sciuk J, Bosse A, et al. Response of osteosarcoma and Ewing sarcoma to preoperative chemotherapy: assessment with dynamic and static MR imaging and skeletal scintigraphy. Radiology 1990;175:791–796.
26. Knop J, Delling G, Heise U, et al. Scintigraphic evaluation of tumor regression during preoperative chemotherapy of osteosarcoma. Correlation of ^{99m}Tc-methylene diphosphonate parametric imaging with surgical histopathology. Skeletal Radiol 1990;19:165–172.
27. Mail JT, Cohen MD, Mirkin LD, et al. Response of osteosarcoma to preoperative intravenous high-dose metho-

trexate chemotherapy: CT evaluation. AJR 1985;144:89–93.
28. Holscher HC, Bloem JL, Nooy MA, et al. The value of MR imaging in monitoring the effect of chemotherapy on bone sarcomas. AJR 1990;154:763–769.
29. Ross B, Helsper JT, Cox IJ, et al. Osteosarcoma and other neoplasms of bone. Magnetic resonance spectroscopy to monitor therapy. Arch Surg 1987;122:1464–1469.
30. Gillespy T, Manfrini M, Ruggieri P, et al. Staging of intraosseous extent of osteosarcoma: correlation of preoperative CT and MR imaging with pathologic macroslides. Radiology 1988;167:765–767.
31. Tebbi CK, Gaeta J. Osteosarcoma. Pediatr Ann 1988;17:285–299.
32. Dehner LP. Pediatric surgical pathology, 2nd ed. Baltimore: Williams & Wilkins, 1987:972–984.
33. Giuliano AE, Feig S, Eilber FR. Changing metastatic patterns of osteosarcoma. Cancer 1984;54:2160–2164.
34. Han M-T, Telander RL, Pairolero PC, et al. Aggressive thoracotomy for pulmonary metastatic osteogenic sarcoma in children and young adolescents. J Pediatr Surg 1981;16:928–933.
35. Watts FB, Zingas AP, Das L, et al. Computed tomographic diagnosis of an intracardiac metastasis from osteosarcoma. CT 1983;7:271–272.
36. Shapiro RS, Mendelson DS, Norton KI, et al. Case report: calcified liver metastases from osteosarcoma. CT: J Comput Tomogr 1988;12:196–198.
37. Danziger J, Wallace S, Handel SF, et al. Metastatic osteogenic sarcoma to the brain. Cancer 1979;43:707–710.
38. Dahlin DC, Unni KK. Osteosarcoma of bone and its important recognizable varieties. Am J Surg Pathol 1977;1:61–72.
39. Lockhart SK, Coan J, Jaffe N, et al. Osteosarcoma metastatic to the kidney. Clin Imag 1989;13:154–156.
40. Link MP, Eilber F. Osteosarcoma. In: Pizzo PA, Poplack DG, eds. Principles and practice of pediatric oncology. Philadelphia: JB Lippincott, 1989:689–711.
41. White VA, Fanning CV, Ayola AG, et al. Osteosarcoma and the role of fine needle aspiration. Cancer 1988; 62:1238–1246.

DIFFERENTIAL DIAGNOSIS

In the classic cases of osteosarcoma presenting around the knee joint, there is usually no difficulty in accurately suggesting the correct diagnosis from the plain film radiograph. There are, however, some pitfalls. Occasionally, other tumors, especially a Ewing sarcoma, may appear almost identical to a classic osteosarcoma. Osteosarcoma is very often not typical and the many various presentations of this tumor may be confused with other benign and malignant lesions. In almost every case, one can predict the presence of a malignant bone lesion on the plain film radiograph, but very occasionally, particularly with early, purely lytic lesions, the malignant tumor might be confused with a benign condition. The following are some of the other bone disorders that might be confused with an osteosarcoma.

1. Ewing sarcoma. Classically, this occurs in the mid shaft of a long bone and has more permeative destruction than osteosarcoma. It may, however, occur in the metaphysis. In the flat bones, it may be particularly difficult to differentiate Ewing sarcoma from osteosarcoma. The pattern of periosteal reaction is not particularly helpful. Both have large soft-tissue components. The absence of any calcification in the soft-tissue component of the tumor would strongly indicate a Ewing sarcoma, because matrix mineralization is common with osteosarcoma. Note, however, that occasionally dystrophic calcification may be seen in the soft-tissue component of a Ewing tumor, and in these situations biopsy might be required for differentiation.
2. Aneurysmal bone cyst and a giant cell tumor.[1] These may be difficult to differentiate from a purely lytic osteosarcoma or from a telangiectatic osteosarcoma. Cortical break and periosteal reaction might be present. A very large exophytic soft-tissue component is found with parosteal aneurysmal bone cyst, and these lesions may mimic parosteal osteosarcomas (Fig. 7–30).
3. Osteoid osteoma and Brody's abscess.[2] These may be confused with a densely blastic osteosarcoma. Neither has any significant soft-tissue component. CT should identify the nidus with osteoid osteoma and a cavity within the Brody's abscess.
4. Radiation osteitis.[3] This causes bone fragmentation, resorption, soft-tissue calcification, and bone sclerosis. An osteosarcoma developing within a region of radiation necrosis should be suggested by a sudden change in the appearance of the abnormality, new clinical symptoms, and the development of a soft-tissue mass.
5. Chondroblastoma.[4] These lesions may mimic a lytic osteogenic sarcoma. Up to 50 percent may have periosteal reaction. They are, however, usually thicker and more confluent than in osteosarcoma; there is no permeative bone destruction and no soft-tissue mass. They involve the epiphysis. A very unusual lytic osteosarcoma occurring in the epiphysis may be almost impossible to differentiate from a chondroblastoma.
6. Chondrosarcoma.[5] This tumor is much less common in children than osteosarcoma. The calcification in the soft tissues tends to be more granular and speckled than with osteosarcoma. On MR, the cartilage, which is much more mature than cartilage seen in osteosarcomas, may be extremely bright on T2 weighted images, suggesting the correct diagnosis.
7. Eosinophilic granuloma. This may mimic an osteosarcoma.
8. Callus.[6] Abundant callus, seen particularly in children with disorders such as osteogenesis imperfecta, might mimic a blastic osteosarcoma. A cortical break will be present. Osteosarcoma is suggested by the presence of spiculations in the periosteal reaction with the presence of a soft-tissue mass.
9. Healed infarct.[7] Again this might mimic a blastic osteosarcoma. Uptake of MDP may be minimal. There is no soft-tissue abnormality and no periosteal reaction.

References

1. deSantos LA, Edeiken B. Purely lytic osteosarcoma. Skeletal Radiol 1982;9:1–9.
2. Edeiken-Monroe B, Edeiken J, Jacobson HG. Osteosarcoma. Semin Roentgenol 1989;24:153–173.
3. Bragg DG, Shidnia H, Chu FCH, et al. The clinical and radiographic aspects of radiation osteitis. Radiology 1970;97:103–111.

A B C

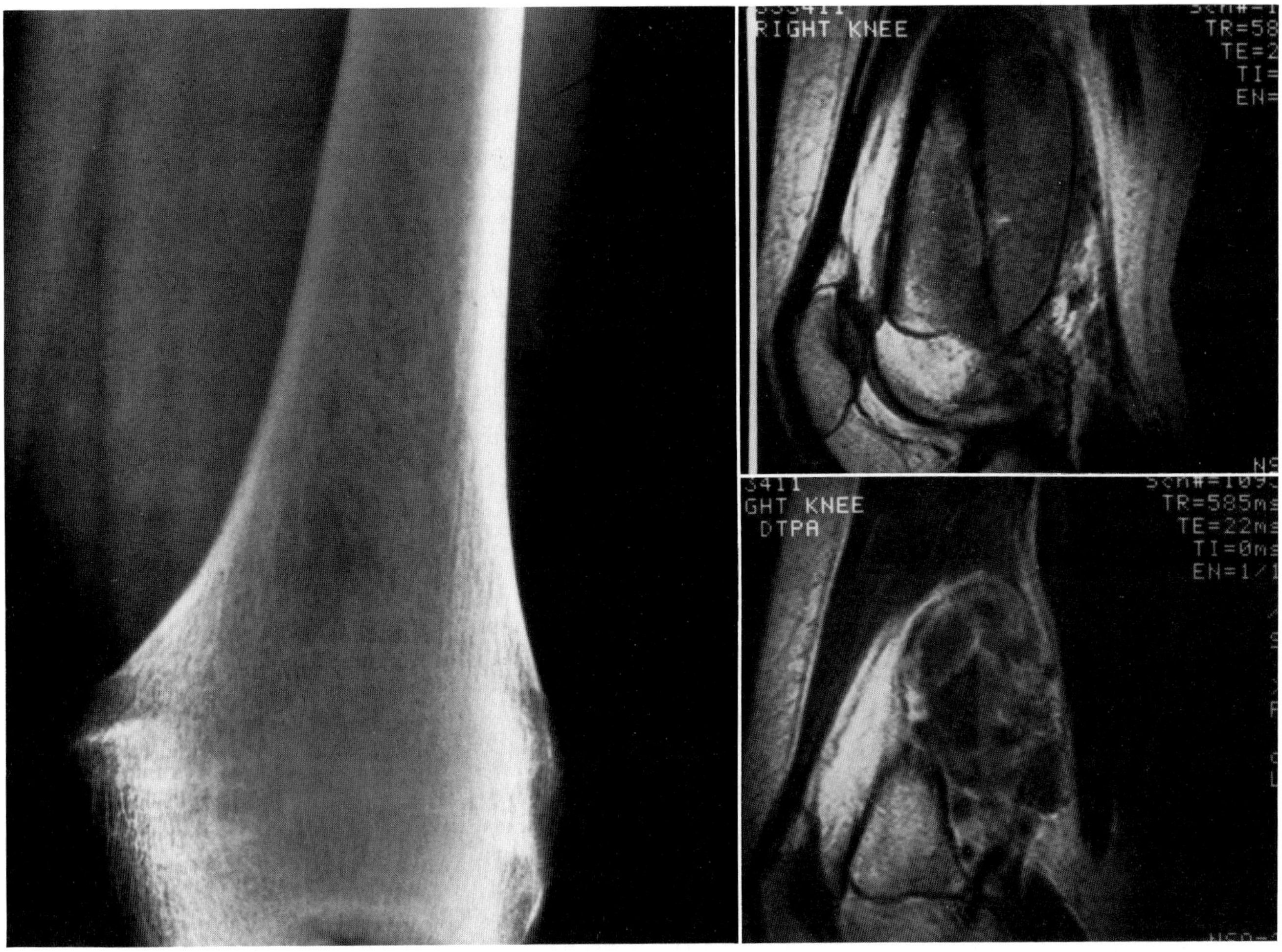

Figure 7-30. **Diagnosis: Parosteal aneurysmal bone cyst.**
A, **Plain film radiograph. This shows mottled lucencies in the distal femur suggestive of osteosarcoma.** ***B*** **and** ***C,*** **MR, T1 weighted images. The lesion has a very large soft-tissue component. Several fluid levels are identified. These should strongly suggest the diagnosis of aneurysmal bone cyst. The involvement of the bone marrow is indicated by decrease in signal intensity from the marrow.**

4. Brower AC, Moser RP, Kransdorf MJ. The frequency and diagnostic significance of periostitis in chondroblastoma. AJR 1990;154:309–314.
5. Cohen EK, Kressel HY, Frank TS, et al. Hyaline cartilage—origin bone and soft-tissue neoplasms: MR appearance and histologic correlation. Radiology 1988;167:477–481.
6. Reid BS, Hubbard JD. Osteosarcoma arising in osteogenesis imperfecta. Pediatr Radiol 1979;8:110–112.
7. Strecker W, Gilula LA, Kyriakos M. Case report 479. Skeletal Radiol 1988;17:220–225.

Therapy and Prognosis

Radiation therapy is of no use in the treatment of the primary lesion of osteosarcoma.[1,2] It is also of no use in the treatment of pulmonary metastases.[3] In one study of 53 patients with no metastases, whole lung radiation was used prophylactically. There was no difference between the treated patients and the controls with regard to subsequent development of lung metastases.[3] Surgery is important in the treatment of osteosarcoma. Prior to the 1970s, it was the only therapeutic modality utilized and the long-term survival was extremely poor, indicating that most patients have micrometastases at the time of presentation. In the past 10 or 15 years, significant changes have occurred in the surgical approach to osteosarcoma.

1. Surgery is usually utilized only after initial chemotherapy.
2. Because imaging can potentially identify all skip lesions, amputation surgery (for lesions in the distal part of a long bone) can now be performed through the shaft of the bone rather than through the more proximal joint. In all patients, this results in much greater preservation of limb function.[2]
3. Because imaging can accurately identify the marrow, the soft-tissue extent of tumor, and skip lesions,[4,5] limb salvage surgery with excision only of the tumor and adjacent tissues is being performed more frequently[1,6] (Fig.

A B C D, E

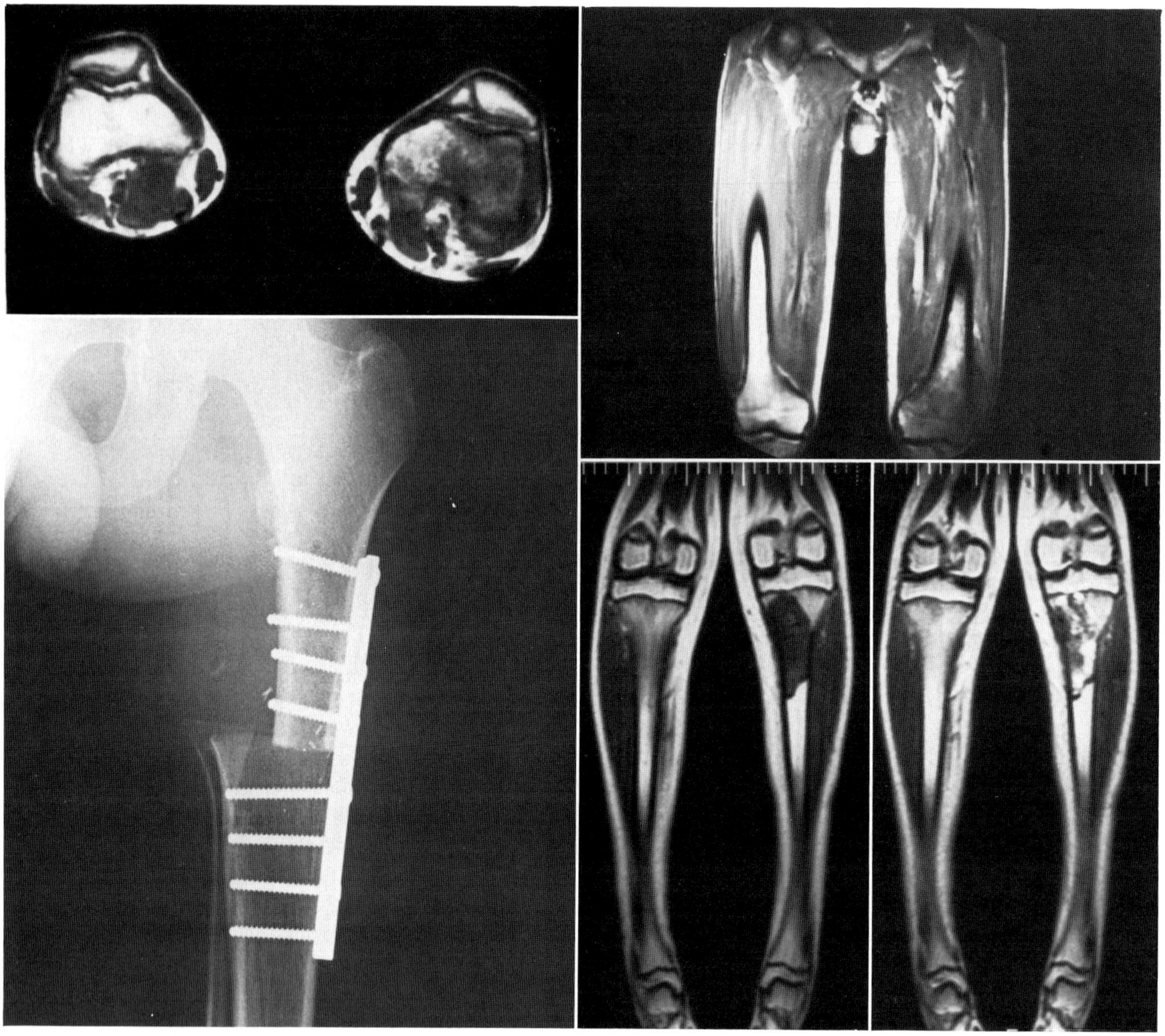

Figure 7-31. Diagnosis: Osteosarcoma. Planning of limb salvage surgery (2 cases). ***A*** and ***B***, MR images after chemotherapy. There is a lesion at the distal femur. Bone marrow abnormality involves the distal femur and the entire epiphysis. Because of the epiphyseal involvement and, therefore, close proximity of tumor to the joint, the surgical transection was through the proximal tibia and not through the knee joint. ***C***, Plain film radiograph after surgery. The distal femur and proximal tibia have been resected. The ends of the bones have been fused together. Note that the distal segment of the limb has been rotated through 180° so that the fibula now lies medially. This enables the residual ankle joint to function in the capacity of a knee, with the patient being given a more distal extension prosthesis. ***D*** and ***E***, Second case: Coronal T1 and T2 images. A tumor in the proximal tibia extends from the growth plate to the joint surface. Because of absence of joint involvement, the proximal resection can be done through the knee joint.

7–31). Patients must be old enough to have only minimal growth left on the opposite normal side (usually over the age of 14 to 15 years). A 1990 report gives equivalent prognosis for limb salvage versus amputation.[7]

4. In 1975, there was an early report suggesting that surgery to pulmonary metastases will improve prognosis.[8] In one study in 1981, 111 thoracotomies were performed in 57 children, with improved survival. Twenty-five of 57 were disease free 3 years following surgery.[9] In another study, it was concluded that aggressive surgical treatment of pulmonary metastasis could give up to 50 percent survival,[1] but patients must be carefully selected.[2] For example, the lungs should be the only site of metastatic disease, there must be no pleural or hilar involvement, and there must not be diffuse widespread

metastases.[7] Onset of the first detectable metastasis more than 1 year after initial diagnosis, the presence of less than 5 nodules, and complete resection of visualized nodules carries the best prognosis.[10] Obviously, imaging is extremely important in defining those patients suitable for surgical excision of pulmonary metastases.

Chemotherapy is responsible in large part for the improved survival of patients with osteosarcoma. This is because the vast majority do have micrometastasis at the time of presentation. Chemotherapy was introduced in the 1960s with progressive introduction of more effective agents. Agents utilized include adriamycin, methotrexate, cisplatinum, iphosphomide, bleomycin, actinomycin, and DTIC.[11] Combined chemotherapy is utilized in most cases. In one center, it is given intra-arterially, but this is not a widespread practice. Although one study suggested, even in the 1970s, that surgery was as effective as surgery plus chemotherapy,[1] virtually all of the other studies reported since then show an overwhelming improvement in survival that can be related to the use of chemotherapy. A wide variety of different chemotherapeutic protocols were utilized. There is no general agreement as to which is the best agent or for how long the therapy should be continued. Virtually all centers utilize initial chemotherapy prior to surgery. As previously indicated, the reasons for this are to identify favorable responders, to eliminate micrometastases, and to facilitate potential conservative surgery.[11,12]

The prognosis for osteosarcoma is summarized in Table 7–17, and the factors that have been identified that affect prognosis are summarized in Table 7–18. There is no doubt that the prognosis has improved from less than 20 percent to over 50 percent survival in the past 20 years. There is still, however, a significant variability in the reported survival. This can be explained by different study populations, histology, treatment protocols, follow-up time, and also (and very important) by the imaging techniques used. The importance of the application of modern imaging is stressed by two recent articles. In one study, it was reported that definition of the extent of involvement of the shaft of the long bone with marrow disease was important in terms of prognosis.[13] Patients with lung or bone metastases on presentation had over 60 percent of the marrow of the shaft of the affected bone abnormal. Patients who develop metastases on therapy had a mean of 39 percent of the shaft affected, while patients who never develop metastases had only 28 percent of the shaft affected. In another study of 23 patients, the accurate identification of skip lesions was a good predictor of prognosis.[14] Patients with skip lesions develop local recurrence in 50 percent of cases and distant metastases in 95 percent. Control patients with no skip lesions develop local recurrence in only 30 percent and distant metastases in 50 percent of cases.

References

1. Tebbi CK, Gaeta J. Osteosarcoma. Pediatr Ann 1988;17:285–299.
2. Link MP, Eilber F. Osteosarcoma. In: Pizzo PA, Poplack DG, eds. Principles and practice of pediatric oncology. Philadelphia: JB Lippincott, 1989:689–711.
3. Jones JC, Taylor WF, Wold LE. Effective whole lung irradiation in osteosarcoma treatment: appearance of bilateral breast cancer in long term survivors. Skeletal Radiol 1987;16:133–135.
4. Lindell MM, Shirkhoda A, Raymond AK, et al. Parosteal osteosarcoma: radiologic-pathologic correlation with emphasis on CT. AJR 1987;148:323–328.
5. Schreiman JS, Crass JR, Wick MR, et al. Osteosarcoma: role of CT in limb-sparing treatment. Radiology 1986;161:485–488.
6. Seeger LL, Eckardt JJ, Bassett LW. Cross-sectional imaging in the evaluation of osteogenic sarcoma: MRI and CT. Semin Roentgenol 1989;24:174–184.
7. Hudson M, Jaffe MR, Jaffe N, et al. Pediatric osteosarcoma: therapeutic strategies, results, and prognostic factors derived from a 10-year experience. J Clin Oncol 1990;18:1988–1997.
8. Beattie EJ, Martini N, Rosen G. The management of pulmonary metastases in children with osteogenic sarcoma with surgical resection combined with chemotherapy. Cancer 1975;35:618–621.
9. Han M-T, Telander RL, Pairolero PC, et al. Aggressive thoracotomy for pulmonary metastatic osteogenic sarcoma in children and young adolescents. J Pediatr Surg 1981;16:928–933.
10. Burk CD, Belasco JB, O'Neill JA, et al. Pulmonary metastases and bone sarcomas. Surgical removal of lesions ap-

TABLE 7–17
Prognosis of Osteosarcoma

Pre 1970	Surgery alone ≥80% mortality[1–6]
1980s	60% survival with operable primary and no lung metastases at diagnosis[2]
	85% survival in patients showing >90% necrosis of tumor in response to chemotherapy[4,7]
	Up to 70%[6] survival

References

1. Hayes FA, Smith EI. Neuroblastoma. In: Pizzo PA, Poplack DG, eds. Principles and practice of pediatric oncology. Philadelphia: JB Lippincott, 1989:607–622.
2. Stoker DJ. Management of bone tumours—the radiologist's role. Clin Radiol 1989;40:233–239.
3. Ayala AG, Ro JY, Raymond AK, et al. Small cell osteosarcoma. A clinicopathologic study of 27 cases. Cancer 1989;64:2162–2173.
4. Carrasco CH, Charnsangavej C, Richli WR, et al. Osteosarcoma: interventional radiology in diagnosis and management. Semin Roentgenol 1989;24:193–200.
5. Price CHG, Shuber K, Salzer-Kuntschik M, et al. Osteosarcoma in children. A study of 125 cases. J Bone Joint Surg 1975;57-B:341–345.
6. Tebbi CK, Gaeta J. Osteosarcoma. Pediatr Ann 1988;17:285–299.
7. Redmond OM, Stack JP, Dervan PA, et al. Osteosarcoma: use of MR imaging and MR spectroscopy in clinical decision making. Radiology 1989;172:811–815.

TABLE 7–18
Factors Affecting Prognosis in Osteosarcoma

Prognosis is worse with
- Proximally located lesions[1,2]
- Extensive local marrow abnormality[3]
- Skip metastases[4,5]
- Poor histologic response to chemotherapy[6,7]
- Males under 10 years old[8]
- Symptoms present for <2 months[8]
- Large tumor >15 cm in diameter[7,8]

Prognosis is better if
- There is good necrosis in response to initial chemotherapy[9,10]

References
1. Link MP, Eilber F. Osteosarcoma. In: Pizzo PA, Poplack DG, eds. Principles and practice of pediatric oncology. Philadelphia: JB Lippincott, 1989:689–711.
2. Bentzen SM, Poulsen HS, Kaae S, et al. Prognostic factors in osteosarcomas. A regression analysis. Cancer 1988;62:194–202.
3. Hermann G, Leviton M, Mendelson D, et al. Osteosarcoma: relation between extent of marrow infiltration on CT and frequency of lung metastases. AJR 1987;149:1203–1206.
4. Malawer MM, Dunham WK. Skip metastases in osteosarcoma: recent experience. J Surg Oncol 1983; 22:236–245.
5. Wuisman P, Enneking WF. Prognosis for patients who have osteosarcoma with skip metastasis. J Bone Joint Surg 1990;72:60–67.
6. Redmond OM, Stack JP, Dervan PA, et al. Osteosarcoma: use of MR imaging and MR spectroscopy in clinical decision making. Radiology 1989;172:811–815.
7. Hudson M, Jaffe MR, Jaffe N, et al. Pediatric osteosarcoma: therapeutic strategies, results, and prognostic factors derived from a 10-year experience. J Clin Oncol 1990;18:1988–1997.
8. Taylor WF, Ivins JC, Pritchard DJ, et al. Trends and variability in survival among patients with osteosarcoma: a 7-year update. Mayo Clin Proc. 1985;60:91–104.
9. Carrasco CH, Charnsangavej C, Richli WR, et al. Osteosarcoma: interventional radiology in diagnosis and management. Semin Roentgenol 1989;24:193–200.
10. Smith J, Heelan RT, Huvos AG, et al. Radiographic changes in primary osteogenic sarcoma following intensive chemotherapy. Radiology 1982;143:355–360.

pearing after adjuvant chemotherapy. Clin Orthoped Rel Res 1991;262:88–92.
11. Carrasco CH, Charnsangavej C, Richli WR, et al. Osteosarcoma: interventional radiology in diagnosis and management. Semin Roentgenol 1989;24:193–200.
12. Rosen G, Caparros B, Huvos AG, et al. Preoperative chemotherapy for osteogenic sarcoma: selection of postoperative adjuvant chemotherapy based on the response of the primary tumor to preoperative chemotherapy. Cancer 1982;49:1221–1230.
13. Hermann G, Leviton M, Mendelson D, et al. Osteosarcoma: relation between extent of marrow infiltration on CT and frequency of lung metastases. AJR 1987;149:1203–1206.
14. Wuisman P, Enneking WF. Prognosis for patients who have osteosarcoma with skip metastasis. J Bone Joint Surg 1990;72:60–67.

INTRAOSSEOUS WELL-DIFFERENTIATED OSTEOSARCOMA[1–5]

Intraosseous well-differentiated osteosarcoma accounts for approximately 1 percent of all osteosarcomas. It has a very low-grade histology. It usually occurs in the leg. The patients are usually slightly older than those with conventional osteosarcoma, with only 7 of 27 being under 20 years of age in one study.[5] Microscopically, the lesions are well differentiated with abundant osteoid.[5] Both histologically[5] and radiographically[2] a significant number of these lesions are initially called benign. They are true malignant lesions with a definite, although low, potential for metastasis. The radiographic findings in two series of patients are summarized in Table 7–19 (Fig. 7–32). There is some variation in appearance of these lesions. The differential diagnosis includes a giant cell tumor[5] and fibrous dysplasia.[2,4] The diagnosis of fibrous dysplasia is indicated by the presence of a sclerotic rim and the absence of any soft-tissue abnormality. Treatment of intraosseous low-grade osteosarcoma is widespread local resection. The prognosis in these lesions is excellent.

TABLE 7–19
Radiographic Findings in Intraosseous Well-Differentiated Osteosarcoma[1,2]

	Total No. of Cases (Reference)	
No. of Cases with	8[1]	18[2]
Poor margins	5	16
Sclerotic rim	0	4
Expansion	4	7
Cortical destruction	8	14
Size	All large	—
Metaphyseal	7	—
Soft-tissue mass	6	—
Mixed lytic and blastic	7	Most
Matrix mineralization	5	—
Periosteal reaction	2	—

References
1. Ellis JH, Siegel CL, Martel W, et al. Radiologic features of well-differentiated osteosarcoma. AJR 1988;151:739–742.
2. Unni KK, Dahlin DC, McLeod RA, et al. Intraosseous well-differentiated osteosarcoma. Cancer 1977;40:1337–1347.

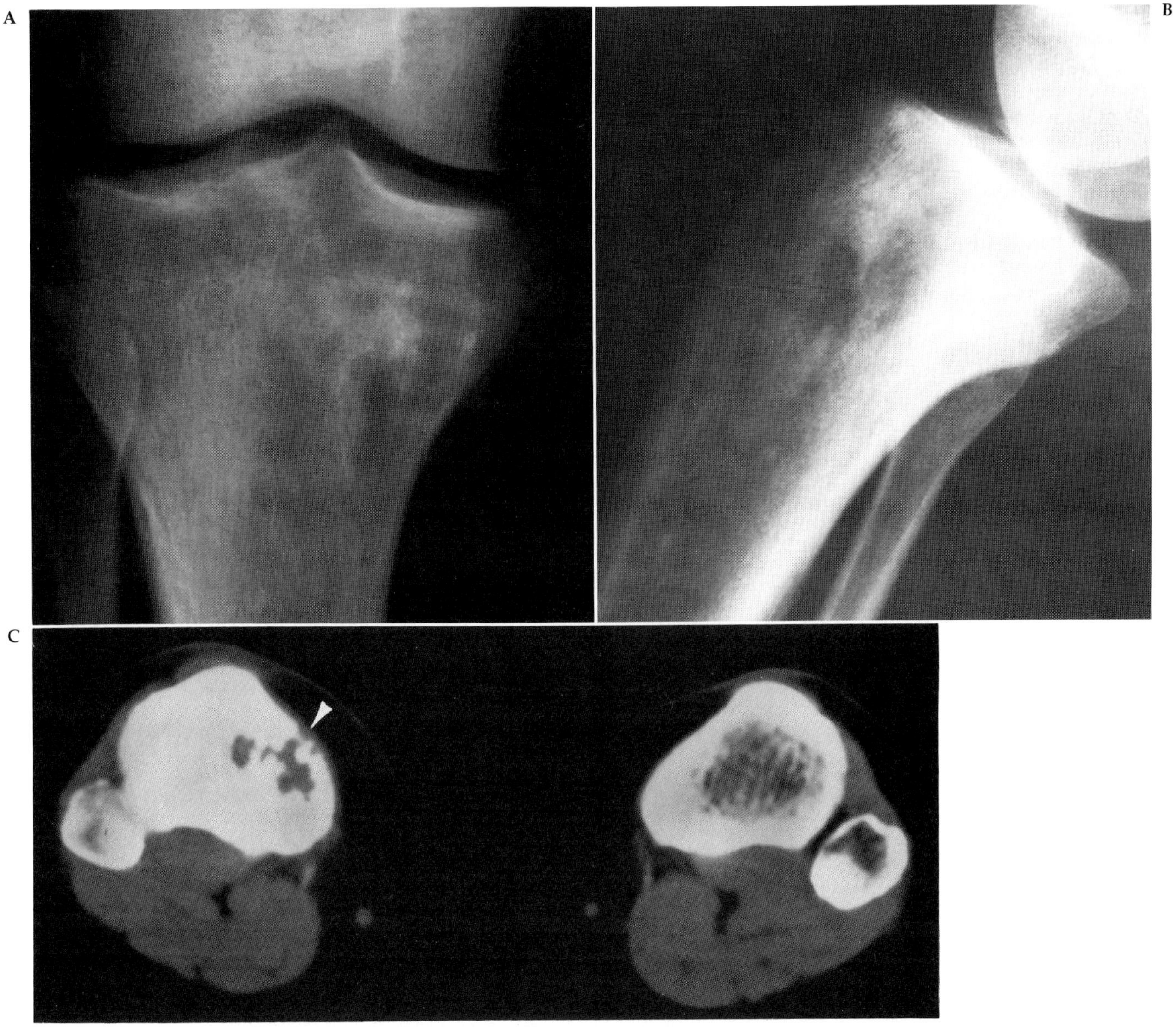

Figure 7-32. **Diagnosis: Well-differentiated intraosseous osteosarcoma.**
***A* and *B*, Plain film radiographs. There is a mixed mostly lytic eccentric lesion involving the right tibial metaphysis and epiphysis. The nonsclerotic margin is poorly defined. *C*, CT. This shows a cortical break *(arrow)*. The tumor is contained by periosteum. No extraosseous mass is present. (From Ellis JH. Radiological features of well differentiated osteosarcoma. AJR 1988;151:739–742.)**

References
1. Unni KK, Dahlin DC. Osteosarcoma: pathology and classification. Semin Roentgenol 1989;24:143–152.
2. Ellis JH, Siegel CL, Martel W, et al. Radiologic features of well-differentiated osteosarcoma. AJR 1988;151:739–742.
3. Dahlin DC, Unni KK. Osteosarcoma of bone and its important recognizable varieties. Am J Surg Pathol 1977;1:61–72.
4. Edeiken-Monroe B, Edeiken J, Jacobson HG. Osteosarcoma. Semin Roentgenol 1989;24:153–173.
5. Unni KK, Dahlin DC, McLeod RA, et al. Intraosseous well-differentiated osteosarcoma. Cancer 1977;40:1337–1347.

TELANGIECTATIC OSTEOSARCOMA[1–8]

Telangiectatic osteosarcomas account for about 2 to 3 percent of all osteosarcomas.[1] They are expansile medullary lesions. Histologically, they are quite cellular, with little matrix and only a small amount of osteoid.[3–5] They contain microscopic cysts and cavities with clot.[4] The age of patients is the same as seen with conventional osteosarcoma.[6] The lesions are found mainly in the metaphyses. The plain film imaging features of these tumors are described in Table 7–20 (Figs. 7–33 and 7–34). They are large expanding lytic areas with permeative margins. Parallel striations in these lesions have been described.[6] Pathologic fractures may be identified in up to 25 percent of patients.[1,2] Differential diagnosis includes aneurysmal bone cyst, giant-cell tumor, and eosinophilic granuloma[6,8–10] The lesions can look almost identical to an aneurysmal bone cyst. Careful attention to the interface of the lesion with normal bone will, however, usually identify a zone of permeative bone destruction with telangiectatic osteosarcoma. Reports of prognosis range from the same as conventional osteosarcoma[10] to much worse than conventional osteosarcoma.[1,3] Treatment is the same as with conventional osteosarcoma.

TABLE 7–20
Telangiectatic Osteosarcoma[1,2]

Almost completely lytic
Permeative margins
Large
Central or eccentric, usually in metaphysis
Periosteal reaction 12 of 14 cases
Cortical break 12 of 14 cases
Soft-tissue mass 12 of 14 cases

References
1. Edeiken-Monroe B, Edeiken J, Jacobson HG. Osteosarcoma. Semin Roentgenol 1989;24:153–173.
2. Vanel D, Tcheng S, Contesso G, et al. The radiological appearances of telangiectatic osteosarcoma. A study of 14 cases. Skeletal Radiol 1987;16:196–200.

References
1. Dehner LP. Pediatric surgical pathology, 2nd ed. Baltimore: Williams & Wilkins, 1987:972–984.
2. Vanel D, Tcheng S, Contesso G, et al. The radiological appearances of telangiectatic osteosarcoma. A study of 14 cases. Skeletal Radiol 1987;16:196–200.
3. Dahlin DC, Unni KK. Osteosarcoma of bone and its important recognizable varieties. Am J Surg Pathol 1977;1:61–72.
4. Unni KK, Dahlin DC. Osteosarcoma: pathology and classification. Semin Roentgenol 1989;24:143–152.
5. Tebbi CK, Gaeta J. Osteosarcoma. Pediatr Ann 1988;17:285–299.
6. Vanel D, Tcheng S, Contesso G, et al. The radiological appearances of telangiectatic osteosarcoma. A study of 14 cases. Skeletal Radiol 1987;16:196–200.
7. Edeiken-Monroe B, Edeiken J, Jacobson HG. Osteosarcoma. Semin Roentgenol 1989;24:153–173.
8. Gomes H, Menanteau B, Gaillard D, et al. Telangiectatic osteosarcoma. Pediatr Radiol 1986;16:140–143.
9. Kaufman RA, Towbin RB. Telangiectatic osteosarcoma simulating the appearance of an aneurysmal bone cyst. Pediatr Radiol 1981;11:102–104.

Figure 7–33. **Diagnosis: Telangiectatic osteosarcoma.**
***A* and *B*, Plain film radiographs. There is extensive permeative destruction involving the distal femur. (From Vanel D. The radiologic appearances of telangiectatic osteosarcoma. Skel Radiol 1987;16:196–200.)**

A

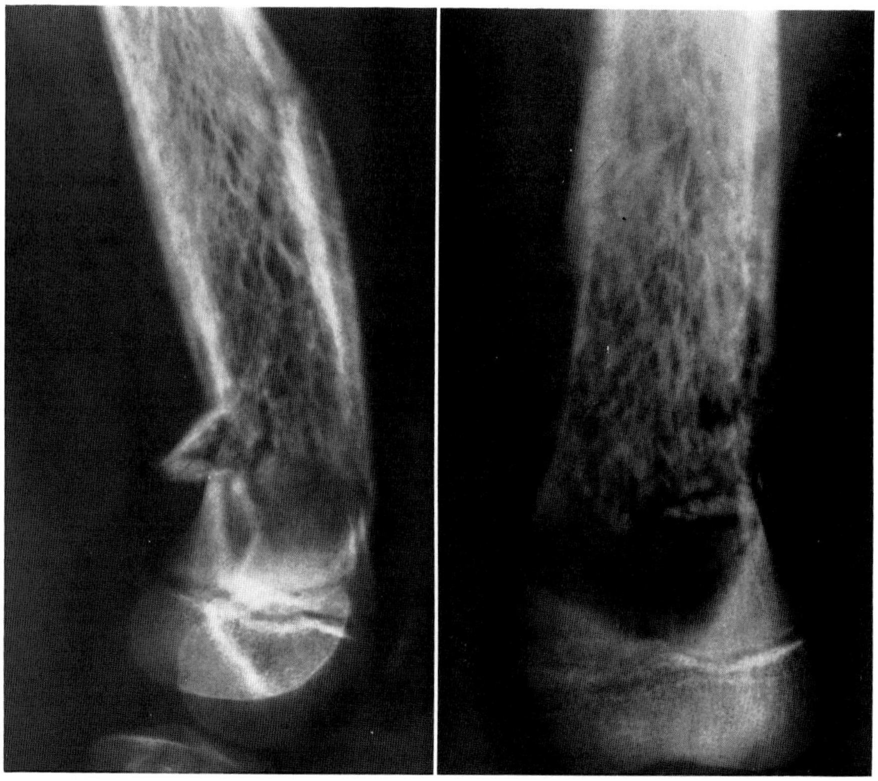

B

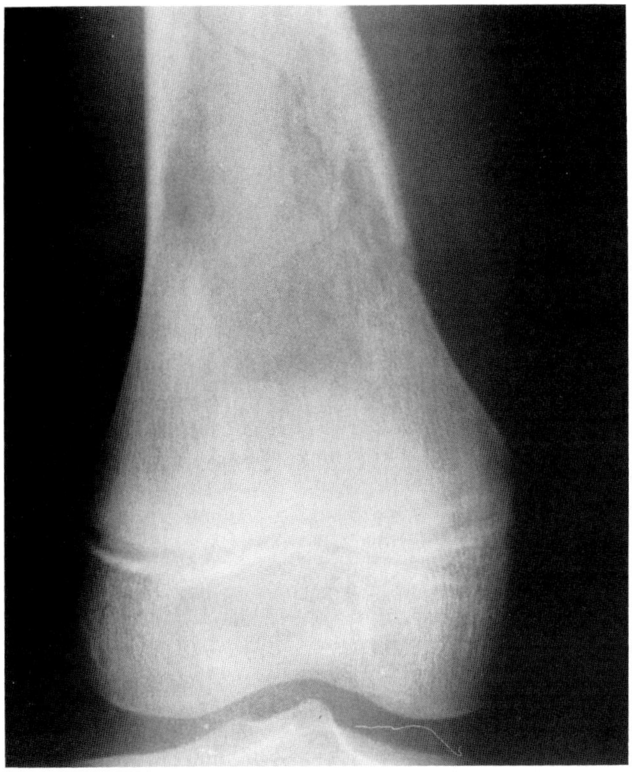

Figure 7-34. **Diagnosis: Telangiectatic osteosarcoma. Plain film radiograph. There is a large fairly homogenous area of lytic destruction of the distal femur with very poorly defined margins. (From Kumar R. Radiographic spectrum of osteogenic sarcoma. AJR 1987;148:767–772.)**

10. Link MP, Eilber F. Osteosarcoma. In: Pizzo PA, Poplack DG, eds. Principles and practice of pediatric oncology. Philadelphia: JB Lippincott, 1989:689–711.

SMALL CELL OSTEOSARCOMA[1–3]

Small cell osteosarcoma was first described in 1979 and represents about 4 percent of all osteosarcomas. The age of patients and anatomic location is the same as with conventional osteosarcoma. Histologically, these lesions show abundant small round cells[1] and may easily be misdiagnosed as a Ewing sarcoma or one of the other small round cell tumors. Careful evaluation will, however, show the presence of osteoid in all patients.[2] If only a needle biopsy is performed, the osteoid may be missed and an incorrect diagnosis made. The imaging appearance of these lesions is in general the same as for conventional osteosarcoma, although some will show unusually extensive spread of tumor along a long segment of the shaft of the bone.[3]

Radiographically, the differential diagnosis is the same as with conventional osteosarcoma. As mentioned, histologic diagnosis includes all of the round small cell sarcomas.[1] Prognosis for these lesions has been reported as being the same as[1] or slightly worse than[2] conventional osteosarcoma.

References

1. Ayala AG, Ro JY, Raymond AK, et al. Small cell osteosarcoma. A clinicopathologic study of 27 cases. Cancer 1989;64:2162–2173.
2. Bertoni F, Present D, Bacchini P, et al. The istituto Rizzoli experience with small cell osteosarcoma. Cancer 1989;64:2591–2599.
3. Edeiken J, Raymond AK, Ayala AG, et al. Small-cell osteosarcoma. Skeletal Radiol 1987;16:621–628.

PERIOSTEAL OSTEOSARCOMA[1–9]

Periosteal osteosarcoma is a broad-based lesion arising on the surface of a bone. The age of patients is similar to those with conventional osteosarcoma, most being seen in adolescence.[5] The area around the knee joint is the most common location; 80 percent of lesions are in the femur or tibia, with the tibia being more common than the femur. The lesions involve the diaphysis or diametaphyseal region of the bone.[3,5,8] Histologically, they show only moderate differentiation. Cartilage is the predominant tissue, with little osteoid being present.[4,8] There is some debate in the literature with regard to bone marrow involvement, with some authorities saying that the diagnosis should not be made if there is bone marrow abnormality. While this may be true of histology, care should be taken on imaging. For example, I believe that some reactive abnormality will be identified in the bone marrow with MR imaging, even if there is not actual tumor invasion of the marrow.

The lesions are sessile elliptical growths on the surface of the bone. The entire base of the soft-tissue component of the lesion is attached to the cortex by a broad base[6,10,11] (Table 7–21) (Fig. 7–35). The cortex is thickened and has an irregular margin. A periosteal reaction is usually present (Fig. 7–35). This is often seen as a spiculated reaction perpendicular to the shaft of the bone.[4,5,9] A soft-tissue component is almost always present. This is not lobulated and no daughter lesions are present.[4,11] Matrix mineralization is commonly present in the soft tissue. This characteristically is most dense close to the cortical surface and decreases toward the periphery of the lesion.[3] On CT, the findings are the same as those seen on the plain film. The soft-tissue component is better defined.[7]

The differential diagnosis includes Ewing sarcoma. This tumor may have a similar spiculated periosteal reaction. With Ewing sarcoma there is, however, always a large medullary component of the tumor, permeative destruction, and a large, noncalcified soft-tissue component.[3,10] Treatment of periosteal osteosarcoma is wide resection without chemotherapy.[12] Survival is better than with conventional osteosarcoma, up to 80 per-

TABLE 7-21
Differentiation of Periosteal and Parosteal Osteosarcoma

	Periosteal Osteosarcoma	Parosteal Osteosarcoma
Pedicle	No	Yes
Tendency to invade shaft	No	Yes
Most common site	Proximal tibia, diametaphysis	Distal femur, metaphysis
Periosteal reaction	Often present, often perpendicular spicules	Uncommon
Matrix mineralization	Decrease toward edges of lesion	Dense, homogeneous

cent.[4] It is not quite as good as that seen with parosteal osteosarcoma.[5]

References

1. Dehner LP. Pediatric surgical pathology, 2nd ed. Baltimore: Williams & Wilkins, 1987;972–984.
2. Unni KK, Dahlin DC. Osteosarcoma: pathology and classification. Semin Roentgenol 1989;24:143–152.
3. deSantos LA, Murray JA, Finklestein JB, et al. The radiographic spectrum of periosteal osteosarcoma. Radiology 1978;127:123–129.
4. Hall RB, Robinson LH, Malawar MM, et al. Periosteal osteosarcoma. Cancer 1985;55:165–171.
5. Dahlin DC, Unni KK. Osteosarcoma of bone and its important recognizable varieties. Am J Surg Pathol 1977;1:61–72.
6. deSantos LA, Edeiken B. Purely lytic osteosarcoma. Skeletal Radiol 1982;9:1–9.
7. Destouet JM, Gilula LA, Murphy WA. Computed tomography of long-bone osteosarcoma. Radiology 1979;131:439–445.
8. Schajowicz F, McGuire MH, Araujo ES, et al. Osteosarcomas arising on the surfaces of long bones. J Bone Joint Surg 1988;70-A:555–564.
9. Schreiman JS, Crass JR, Wick MR, et al. Osteosarcoma: role of CT in limb-sparing treatment. Radiology 1986;161:485–488.
10. Edeiken-Monroe B, Edeiken J, Jacobson HG. Osteosarcoma. Semin Roentgenol 1989;24:153–173.
11. Kumar R, David R, Madewell JE, et al. Radiographic spectrum of osteogenic sarcoma. AJR 1987;148:767–772.
12. Smith J, Heelan RT, Huvos AG, et al. Radiographic changes in primary osteogenic sarcoma following intensive chemotherapy. Radiology 1982;143:355–360.

Figure 7-35. **Diagnosis: Periosteal osteosarcoma. Plain film radiograph. The proximal humerus shows a broad-based sessile juxtacortical tumor arising from the shaft. Periosteal reaction along the bone cortex and irregular margins of the tumor are typical features. (From Kumar R. Radiographic spectrum of osteogenic sarcoma. AJR 1987;148:767-772.)**

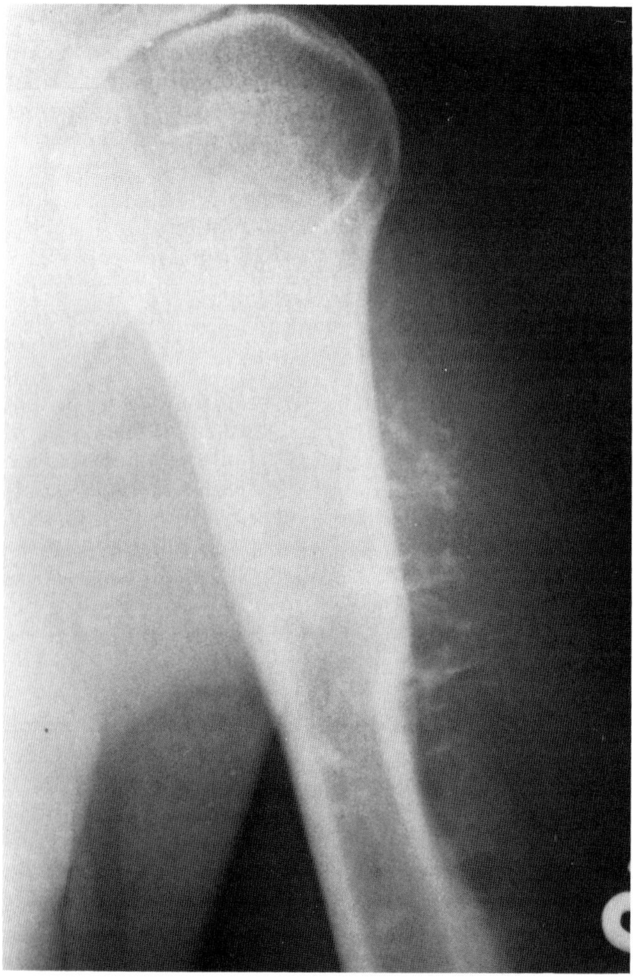

PAROSTEAL OSTEOSARCOMA[1–14]

Parosteal osteosarcoma is a well-differentiated tumor and accounts for about 3 percent of osteosarcomas. Patients are often slightly older than those with conventional osteosarcoma.[2,5–7] The lesions occur on the surface of the bone. The most common site is the posterior aspect of the distal femur[2] (Fig. 7–36). The lesions almost never occur in the spine or flat bones,[10] but have been described occasionally in the skull and facial bones[11] (Fig. 7–37). In the skull, they are round sessile masses with dense calcification, variable margins, and a cleft between the skull and the mass in up to 40 percent of cases.[12] Pathologically, they are low-grade well-differentiated lesions with well-formed bone and bland spindle cells.[4,6] They arise on the surface of the bone, grow slowly, and can become very big.[8] There is usually no periosteal reaction.[8] The lesions characteristically are

A B

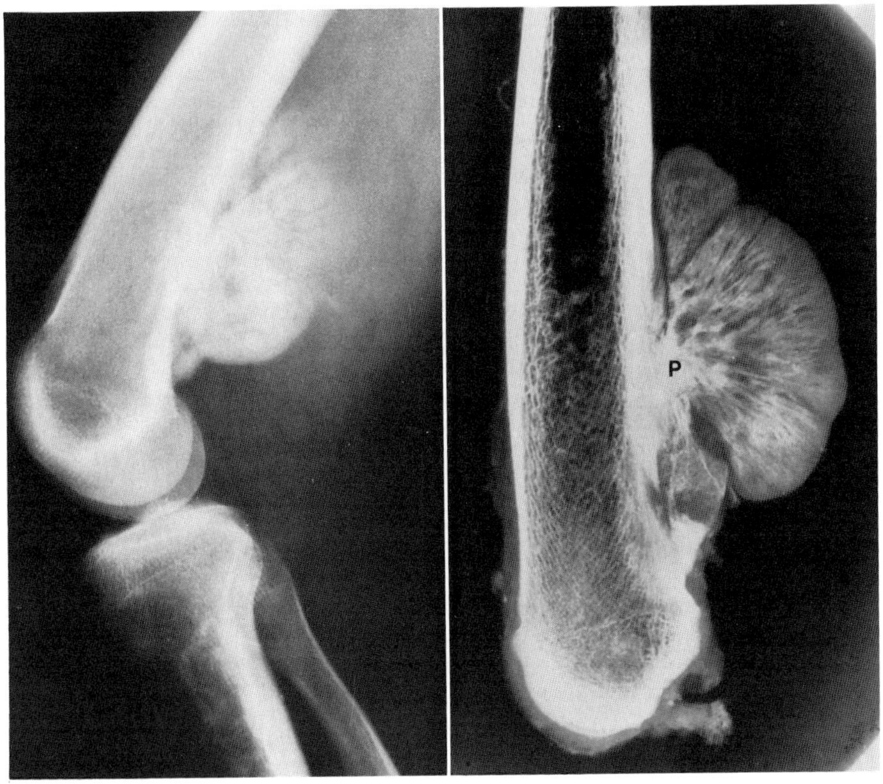

Figure 7–36. Diagnosis: Parosteal osteosarcoma.
A, Plain film radiograph. There is a juxtacortical pedunculated mushroomlike tumor of the bone surface with a smooth lobulated margin. It arises from the distal femur. There is a linear lucent line between the tumor and the bone cortex. There is dense central calcification of the tumor. ***B***, Radiograph of cut section through the tumor shows clearly the mushroom shape of the tumor with a narrow pedicle (*P*) and a clear lucent line between the rest of the tumor and the adjacent bone. (From Kumar R. Radiographic spectrum of osteogenic sarcoma. AJR 1987;148:767–772.)

Figure 7–37. Diagnosis: Parosteal osteosarcoma of the skull.
A, Skull radiograph. An extensive sclerotic lesion is seen overlying the occipital area. ***B***, CT. There is a heavily calcified lesion attached to the skull by a pedicle. The lesion has a mushroom shape with a lucent line *(arrow)* between part of the body of the lesion and the adjacent skull. (From Hinton CE. Parosteal osteosarcoma of the skull. Histopathology 1988;14:322–333.)

A B

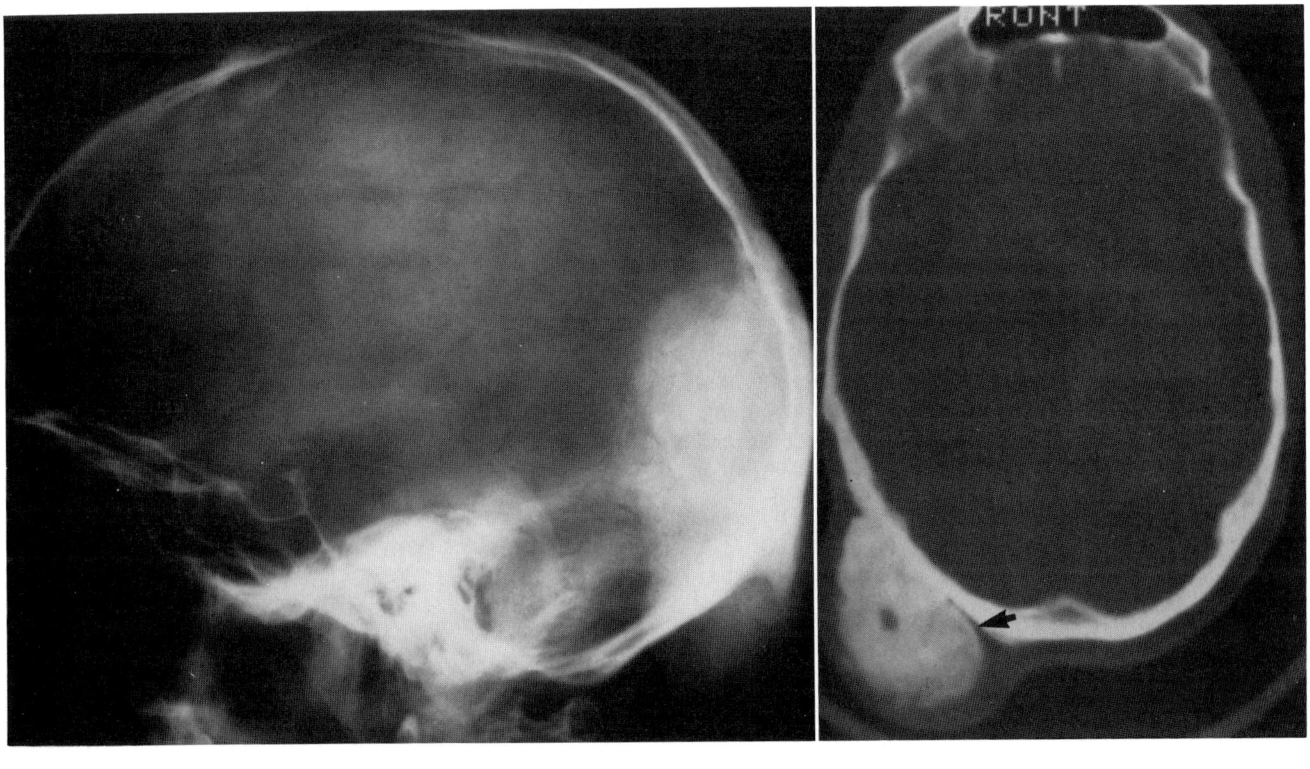

attached to the bone by a broad pedicle, with the more peripheral lesion expanding like a mushroom.[9] Because of the pedicle, there is a lucent cleavage between the expanded head of the lesion and the adjacent normal cortex. The lesions can become very large and tend then to encircle the shaft of the bone.[2,6,8] There is some debate with regard to medullary involvement. Several authorities state that the lesion never involves the medullary canal.[2] As with periosteal osteosarcoma I believe that MR will show at least some minimal reactive change in the bone marrow in a significant number of patients. The large lesions tend to have a lobular appearance and may in some cases show the presence of satellite daughter lesions.[13] Matrix mineralization is diffuse, dense, and homogeneous.[6,13] CT shows the very dense large mass with the pedicle attaching it to the adjacent bone.[11]

Differential diagnosis includes osteochondroma, myositis, calcified hematoma, exuberant callus, parosteal aneurysmal bone cyst.[9,10,14] With osteochondroma the medullary cavity can be seen extending into the lesion.[10] Myositis tends to be less heavily calcified in the center of the lesion.[9,10] Aneurysmal bone cyst has no calcification and may have fluid/fluid levels. Treatment of the lesions is surgical excision and prognosis is excellent,[2,7] being better than with any other type of osteosarcoma.

References

1. Schreiman JS, Crass JR, Wick MR, et al. Osteosarcoma: role of CT in limb-sparing treatment. Radiology 1986;161:485–488.
2. Dahlin DC, Unni KK. Osteosarcoma of bone and its important recognizable varieties. Am J Surg Pathol 1977;1:61–72.
3. deSantos LA, Edeiken B. Purely lytic osteosarcoma. Skeletal Radiol 1982;9:1–9.
4. Unni KK, Dahlin DC. Osteosarcoma: pathology and classification. Semin Roentgenol 1989;24:143–152.
5. Dehner LP. Pediatric surgical pathology, 2nd ed. Baltimore: Williams & Wilkins, 1987;972–984.
6. Lindell MM, Shirkhoda A, Raymond AK, et al. Parosteal osteosarcoma: radiologic-pathologic correlation with emphasis on CT. AJR 1987;148:323–328.
7. Schajowicz F, McGuire MH, Araujo ES, et al. Osteosarcomas arising on the surfaces of long bones. J Bone Joint Surg 1988;70-A:555–564.
8. Tebbi CK, Gaeta J. Osteosarcoma. Pediatr Ann 1988;17:285–299.
9. Kumar R, David R, Madewell JE, et al. Radiographic spectrum of osteogenic sarcoma. AJR 1987;148:767–772.
10. Edeiken-Monroe B, Edeiken J, Jacobson HG. Osteosarcoma. Semin Roentgenol 1989;24:153–173.
11. Hinton CE, Turnbull AE, O'Donnell HDT, et al. Parosteal osteosarcoma of the skull. Histopathology 1988;14:322–323.
12. Kumar R, Moser RP, Madewell JE, et al. Parosteal osteogenic sarcoma arising in cranial bones: clinical and radiologic features in eight patients. AJR 1990;155:113–117.
13. deSantos LA, Murray JA, Finklestein JB, et al. The radiographic spectrum of periosteal osteosarcoma. Radiology 1978;127:123–129.
14. Moser RP, Madewell JE. An approach to primary bone tumors. Radiol Clin N Am 1987;25:1049–1093.

HIGH-GRADE SURFACE OSTEOSARCOMA

High-grade surface osteosarcoma is a conventional type of osteosarcoma, differing only in its location. It lies predominantly on the surface rather than within the bone itself. Patients may be slightly younger than those with conventional osteosarcoma. The tumor's location is commonly in the diaphysis.[1] Treatment and prognosis are the same as for conventional osteosarcoma. Occasionally, these lesions may become heavily mineralized and may mimic parosteal osteosarcoma.[1] There is some confusion with regard to terminology in these patients. Some would call them a heavily mineralized high-grade surface osteosarcoma,[1] while other workers prefer to call them dedifferentiated parosteal osteosarcomas, claiming they occur in about 10 percent of all patients with parosteal sarcoma.[2] In the lesions, imaging features that suggest the presence of poorly differentiated (high-grade) tissue are deep-seated lucencies seen on plain film or CT lying within the predominantly calcified tumor matrix.

References

1. Schajowicz F, McGuire MH, Araujo ES, et al. Osteosarcomas arising on the surfaces of long bones. J Bone Joint Surg 1988;70-A:555–564.
2. Unni KK, Dahlin DC. Osteosarcoma: pathology and classification. Semin Roentgenol 1989;24:143–152.

EXTRAOSSEOUS OSTEOSARCOMA[1–4]

Extraosseous osteosarcoma is of little interest to the pediatric radiologist. It is a soft-tissue sarcoma that contains osteoid and, therefore, is classified as osteosarcomas.[1–4] Bone is not involved. The lesions occur almost entirely in adults, with most patients being over 50 years of age.[2,3] They can occur at any site, but are most common in the thigh. Approximately 10 percent of patients have received previous radiotherapy to the affected area.[1] Mortality is very high.

References

1. Edeiken-Monroe B, Edeiken J, Jacobson HG. Osteosarcoma. Semin Roentgenol 1989;24:153–173.
2. Stark P, Smith DC, Watkins GE, et al. Primary intrathoracic extraosseous osteogenic sarcoma: report of three cases. Radiology 1990;174:725–726.
3. Sordillo PP, Hajdu SI, Magill GB, et al. Extraosseous osteogenic sarcoma. A review of 48 patients. Cancer 1983;51:727–734.
4. Batsakis JG, Manning JT. Soft tissue tumors: unusual forms. Otolaryngol Clin N Am 1986;19:659–683.

EWING SARCOMA

Epidemiology

Ewing sarcoma is the second most common malignant bone tumor in children, accounting for approximately 35 percent of such tumors. There are no known causative factors and very few associated congenital anomalies.[1] The tumor is more common in males than females. It is particularly unusual in being extremely rare in black persons.[2] The overall incidence is about 1.7 cases per million children under the age of 15 years per year.[1] The age of peak incidence is between 10 and 15 years[2]; it is reported as having a median age of 11 years in one study[3] and a mean of 14 years in another.[4] A 1965 review of 720 cases reported an average age of 18 years.[5] Ewing sarcoma can occur in very young children, with several reports of its presence under the age of 2 years.[2,6–9] It has been reported in children as young as 3 months of age.[8]

References
1. Miser JS, Triche TJ, Pritchard DJ, et al. Ewing's sarcoma and the nonrhabdomyosarcoma soft tissue sarcomas of childhood. In: Pizzo PA, Poplack DG, eds. Principles and practice of pediatric oncology. Philadelphia: JB Lippincott, 1989:659–688.
2. Kissane JM, Askin FB, Foulkes M, et al. Ewing's sarcoma of bone: clinicopathologic aspects of 303 cases from the intergroup Ewing's sarcoma study. Hum Pathol 1983;14:773–779.
3. Brown AP, Fixsen JA, Plowman PN. Local control of Ewing's sarcoma: an analysis of 67 patients. Br J Radiol 1987;60:261–268.
4. Dehner LP. Pediatric surgical pathology, 2nd ed. Baltimore: Williams & Wilkins, 1987:993–998.
5. Falk S, Alpert M. The clinical and roentgen aspects of Ewing's sarcoma. Am J Med Sci 1965;250:44–60.
6. Kozlowksi K, Beluffi G, Masel J, et al. Primary vertebral tumours in children. Report of 20 cases with brief literature review. Pediatr Radiol 1984;14:129–139.
7. Dahlin DC, Coventry MB, Scanlon PW. Ewing's sarcoma. A critical analysis of 165 cases. J Bone Joint Surg 1961;43-A:185–195.
8. Green DM, Marinello MJ, Fisher J, et al. Ewing's sarcoma of the scapula with metastases to the lung and eye. Am J Pediatr Hematol/Oncol 1986;8:134–143.
9. Sherman RS, Soong KY. Ewing's sarcoma: its roentgen classification and diagnosis. Radiology 1956;66:529–539.

Pathology

Ewing's sarcoma arises in the medullary cavity of bone. Macroscopically, the tumor infiltrates the bone marrow, permeates into the cortex through the periosteum and into the soft tissues. A soft-tissue mass is very common.[1,2] The soft-tissue mass tends to be particularly large in patients with rib or pelvic primaries, and in these sites it is usually larger than in the limbs.[3] Microscopically, the tumors characteristically are made up of small, undifferentiated round cells, although larger cells are frequently identified.[1] The cell of origin is not known. Primitive mesenchymal cells and neural cells have been suggested[1]; current thought favors origin from a neural cell. Histologically, the differential diagnosis includes other small-cell tumors, and because there is an absence of specific tumor markers for Ewing sarcoma, the final diagnosis is often made by excluding other small round-cell tumors.[1] The specific features differentiating Ewing sarcoma from primitive neuroectodermal tumor (PNET) are described in detail in the section dealing with this latter tumor.

Ewing sarcoma can be found in virtually any bone of the body (Table 7–22). There is quite good uniformity in the data presented by the five different studies cited in Table 7–22. The femur and pelvis are the most common sites of Ewing sarcoma. The next most common locations are the tibia, fibula, and humerus. Spine involvement occurs in between 6 and 10 percent of patients.[2,4–6] Ribs are involved in between 6 and 10 percent of patients,[7] and the skull in up to 3 percent of patients. Although classically described as a lesion of the diaphysis, Ewing sarcoma is more frequently located in the diametaphyseal region of the bone[8] and can be confined to the metaphysis.[8]

TABLE 7–22
Anatomic Location of Ewing Sarcoma

Site (Percentage of Cases)	No. of Cases (Reference)				
	303[1]	140[2]	165[3]	111[4]	836[5]
Femur	20	17	28	33	22
Pelvis	12	18	16	17	19
Tibia	10	?	8	7	11
Fibula	12	?	7	7	9
Humerus	10	16	8	7	10
Spine	6	10	?	?	7
Rib	6	10	?	?	6
Skull	3	?	2	?	2

References
1. Kissane JM, Askin FB, Foulkes M, et al. Ewing's sarcoma of bone: clinicopathologic aspects of 303 cases from the intergroup Ewing's sarcoma study. Hum Pathol 1983;14:773–779.
2. Wilkins RM, Pritchard DJ, Burgert EO, et al. Ewing's sarcoma of bone. Experience with 140 patients. Cancer 1986;58:2551–2555.
3. Dahlin DC, Coventry MB, Scanlon PW. Ewing's sarcoma. A critical analysis of 165 cases. J Bone Joint Surg 1961;43-A:185–195.
4. Sherman RS, Soong KY. Ewing's sarcoma: its roentgen classification and diagnosis. Radiology 1956;66:529–539.
5. Dehner LP. Pediatric surgical pathology, 2nd ed. Baltimore: Williams & Wilkins, 1987:993–998.

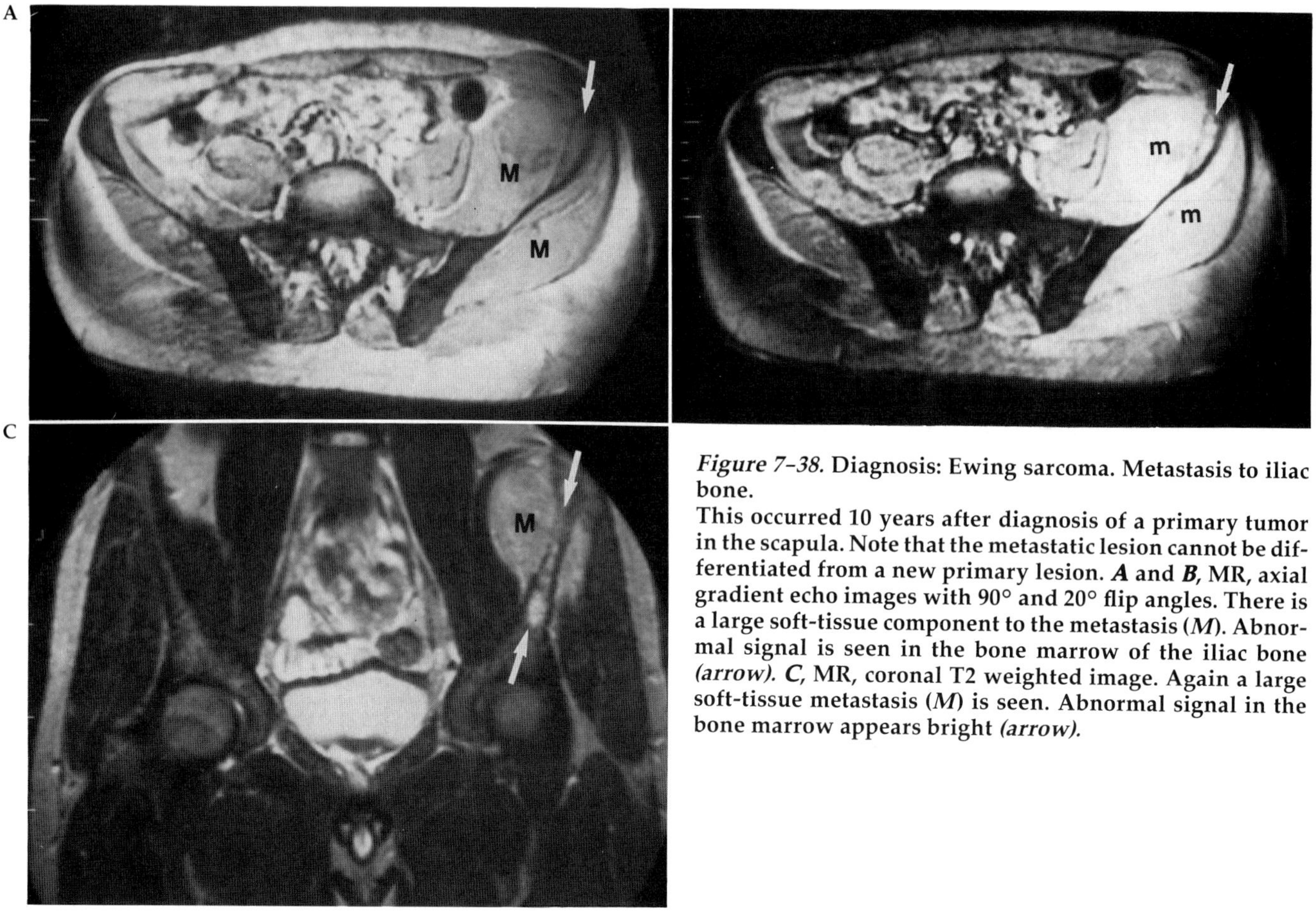

Figure 7–38. **Diagnosis: Ewing sarcoma. Metastasis to iliac bone.**

This occurred 10 years after diagnosis of a primary tumor in the scapula. Note that the metastatic lesion cannot be differentiated from a new primary lesion. *A* and *B*, MR, axial gradient echo images with 90° and 20° flip angles. There is a large soft-tissue component to the metastasis (*M*). Abnormal signal is seen in the bone marrow of the iliac bone *(arrow)*. *C*, MR, coronal T2 weighted image. Again a large soft-tissue metastasis (*M*) is seen. Abnormal signal in the bone marrow appears bright *(arrow)*.

Metastases are quite commonly identified at the time of diagnosis. Micrometastases are certainly present in almost all patients. Without systemic therapy, and with only local therapy to the primary tumor, 90 percent of patients will eventually develop metastases.[1] Metastases that can be identified by imaging on initial presentation are said to occur in between 15 and 50 percent of patients.[1] They were described in 13 of 76 patients and 35 of 140 patients[2] in two reported studies. By far the most common location for the metastases are the lung, bone, or both of these sites (Table 7–23). From an imaging viewpoint it is important to note that the metastases can occur either in the lung or bone or in both locations[2,9] (Figs. 7–38 and 7–39). Metastases can occur in other sites. Of these, lymph nodes are the most common[3] (Fig. 7–40). Other described metastatic sites include the pleura vessels[5] (Fig. 7–41) and central nervous system[1,5,10–12] (Fig. 7–42). The incidence of metastases at diagnosis is dependent on the anatomic location of the primary tumor. In one study of 107 patients, metastases were identified on initial presentation in 40 percent of those with truncal primaries and 25 percent of those with the primary tumor in the arm or leg. In another study, metastases were found in only 8 percent of patients in whom the primary tumor was located in the hands or feet.[13]

Pathological fracture may occur; it was present in 16 percent of 140 patients.[2]

The mean total tumor volume in one study of 47 patients was 886 cc.[14]

Extraskeletal Ewing sarcoma is described as a soft-tissue tumor, not involving bone, with a histology identical to that of bone Ewing tumor.[15,16] The site of the tumor is commonly in the paravertebral area, chest wall, or legs.[15,17] In 22 cases, the size ranged from 2 to 20

TABLE 7–23
Ewing Sarcoma: Location of Metastases Present at Initial Diagnosis in 47 Cases[1]

Site	No. of Cases
Lung alone	25
Bone alone	16
Both lung + bone	6

Reference
1. Wilkins RM, Pritchard DJ, Burgert EO, et al. Ewing's sarcoma of bone. Experience with 140 patients. Cancer 1986;58:2551–2555.

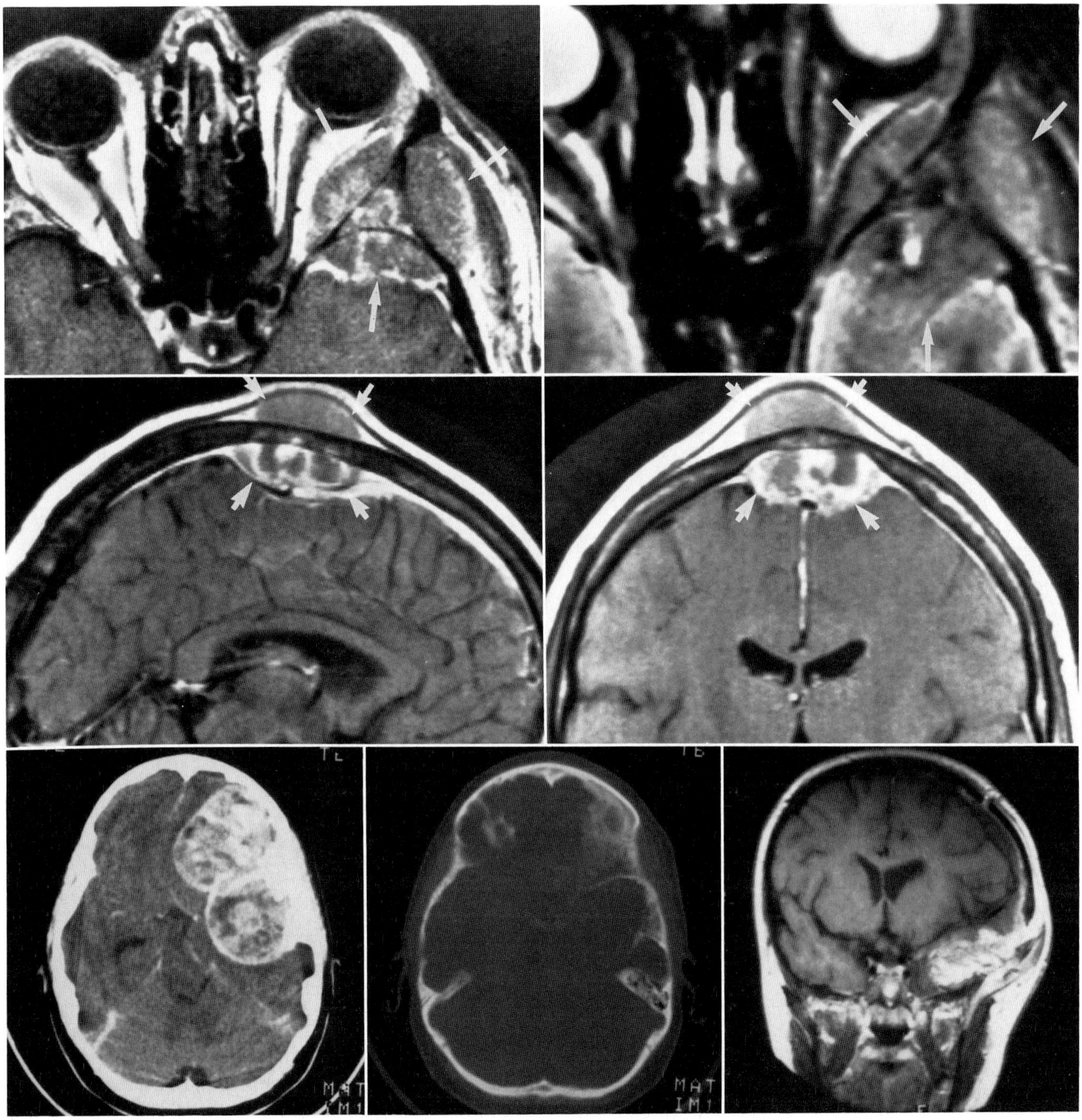

Figure 7-39. Diagnosis: Ewing sarcoma (2 cases).
(1) Skull metastases (***A*** through ***D***). (2) Skull primary (***E*** through ***G***). ***A*** and ***B***, Case 1, MR images. There is a large metastatic lesion *(arrows).* It involves the lateral wall of the left orbit, extends laterally into the soft tissues, medially into the orbit, and posteriorly into the middle cranial fossa. ***C*** and ***D***, Case 1, MR, sagittal and coronal images. There is a large metastasis *(arrows)* to the skull apex with soft-tissue extension both into the soft tissues of the skull and into the extradural space. ***E*** and ***F***, Case 2, CT shows destruction of bone and a large soft-tissue mass. ***G***, Case 2, MR, T1 weighted image with gadolinium-DTPA. The soft-tissue mass enhances.

A B

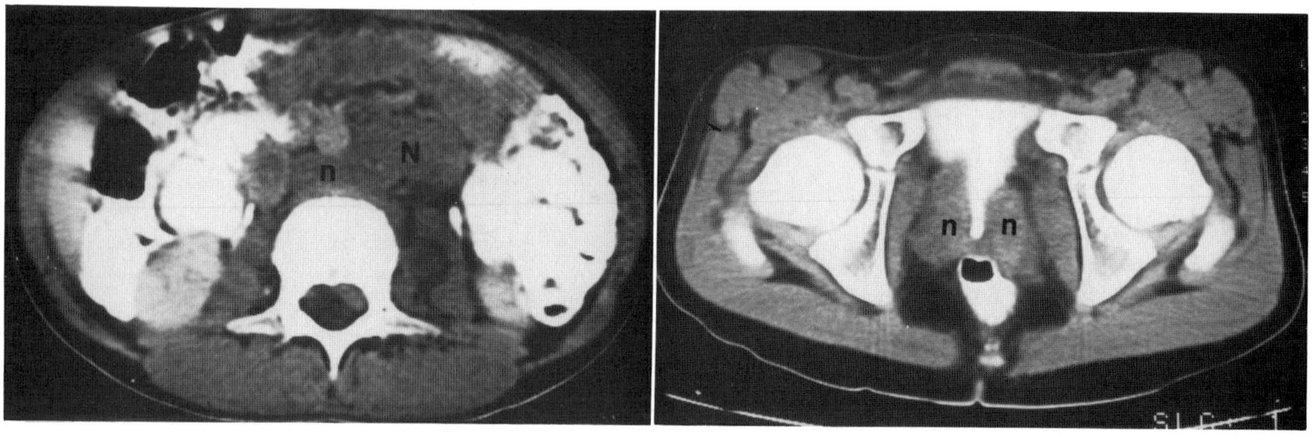

Figure 7-40. **Diagnosis: Ewing sarcoma. Pelvic lymph node metastases.**
***A* and *B*, CT images through the abdomen and pelvis. Multiple enlarged lymph nodes (*N*) are seen.**

cm.[16] There can be a dumbbell extension from paravertebral tumors into the extradural space of the spinal canal.[18] There is a considerable controversy regarding the true existence of these lesions and the most prevalent current view would tend to deny their existence,[19] believing that most of the tumors that are called extraskeletal Ewing sarcoma are in fact either primitive neuroectodermal tumors or poorly differentiated rhabdomyosarcomas.

> *Comment:* Compared to osteosarcoma, Ewing sarcoma shows more variation in age of patient and site of presentation.

References

1. Miser JS, Triche TJ, Pritchard DJ, et al. Ewing's sarcoma and the nonrhabdomyosarcoma soft tissue sarcomas of childhood. In: Pizzo PA, Poplack DG, eds. Principles and practice of pediatric oncology. Philadelphia: JB Lippincott, 1989:659–688.
2. Wilkins RM, Pritchard DJ, Burgert EO, et al. Ewing's sarcoma of bone. Experience with 140 patients. Cancer 1986;58:2551–2555.
3. Brown AP, Fixsen JA, Plowman PN. Local control of Ewing's sarcoma: an analysis of 67 patients. Br J Radiol 1987;60:261–268.
4. Kissane JM, Askin FB, Foulkes M, et al. Ewing's sarcoma of bone: clinicopathologic aspects of 303 cases from the intergroup Ewing's sarcoma study. Hum Pathol 1983;14:773–779.
5. Dehner LP. Pediatric surgical pathology, 2nd ed. Baltimore: Williams & Wilkins, 1987:993–998.
6. Pilepich MV, Vietti TJ, Nesbit ME, et al. Ewing's sarcoma of the vertebral column. Int J Radiat Oncol Biol Phys 1981;7:27–31.
7. Levine E, Levine C. Ewing tumor of rib: radiologic find-

Figure 7-41. **Diagnosis: Ewing sarcoma spread into inferior vena cava.**
***A* and *B*, MR, coronal T1 and sagittal T2 weighted images. A large mass of tumor is well identified in the inferior vena cava *(arrow)*. This extension was the result of direct growth from adjacent metastasis in lymph nodes (*N*).**

A B

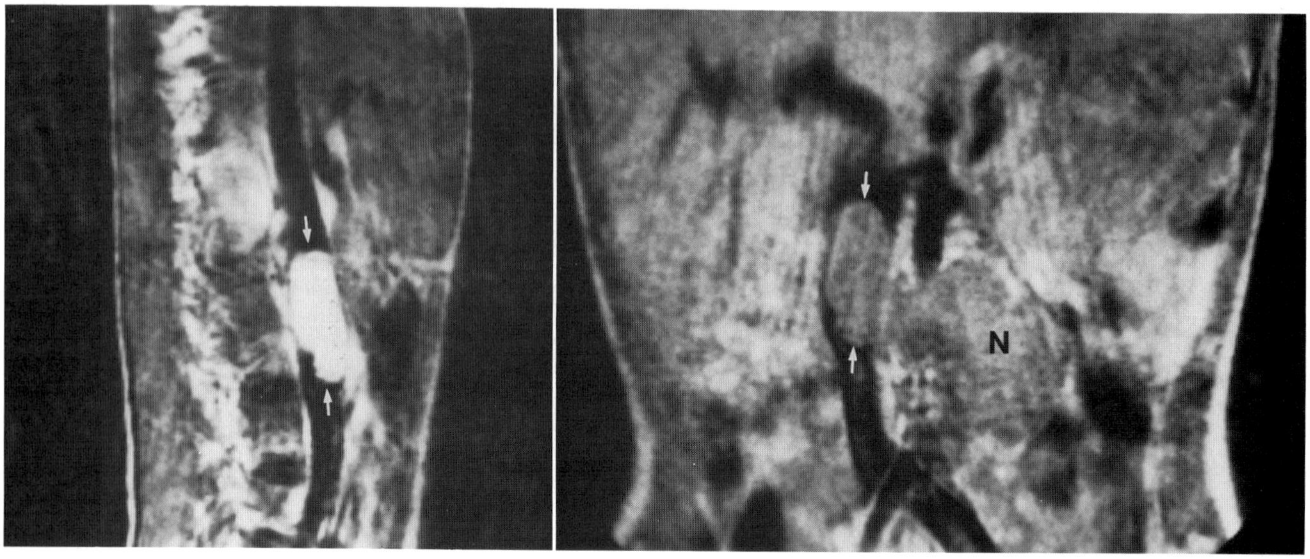

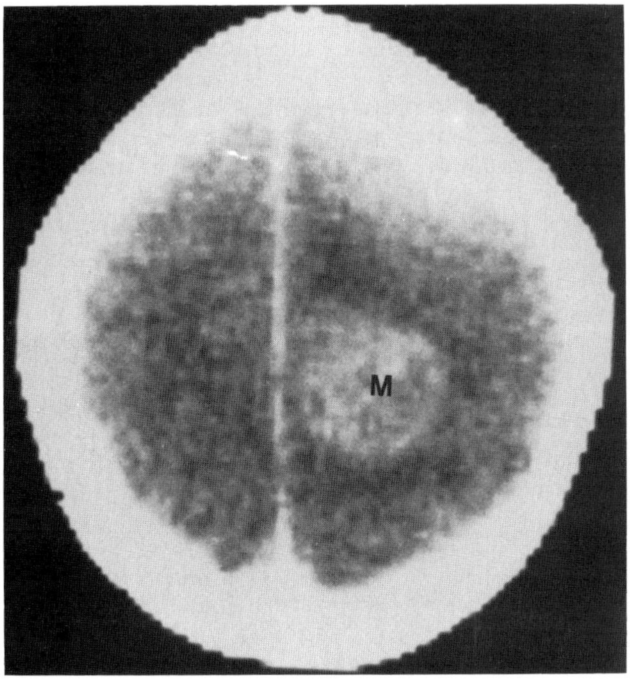

Figure 7-42. **Diagnosis: Ewing sarcoma. Brain parenchymal metastasis.**
CT after intravenous contrast administration. A large moderately well-defined enhancing metastasis (*M*) is seen in the brain parenchyma on the left side.

ings and computed tomography contribution. Skeletal Radiol 1983;9:227–233.
8. Reinus WR, Gilula LA. Radiology of Ewing's sarcoma: intergroup Ewing's sarcoma study (IESS). RadioGraphics 1984;4:929–944.
9. Miser JS, Kinsella TJ, Triche TJ, et al. Preliminary results of treatment of Ewing's sarcoma of bone in children and young adults: six months of intensive combined modality therapy without maintenance. J Clin Oncol 1988;6:484–490.
10. O'Connor MI, Pritchard DJ. Ewing's sarcoma. Prognostic factors, disease control, and the reemerging role of surgical treatment. Clin Orthoped Rel Res 1991;262:78–87.
11. Mineura K, Yasuda T, Suda Y, et al. Ewing's sarcoma with intracranial metastasis presenting depressed cerebral blood flow and metabolism in the contralateral gray matter. Comput Med Imag Graph 1989;13:185–190.
12. Green DM, Marinello MJ, Fisher J, et al. Ewing's sarcoma of the scapula with metastases to the lung and eye. Am J Pediatr Hematol/Oncol 1986;8:134–143.
13. Reinus WR, Gilula LA, Shirley SK, et al. Radiographic appearance of Ewing sarcoma of the hands and feet: report from the intergroup Ewing sarcoma study. AJR 1985;144:331–336.
14. Sailer SL, Harmon DC, Mankin HJ, et al. Ewings sarcoma: surgical resection as a prognostic factor. Int J Oncol Biol Phys 1988;15:43–57.
15. Chen KTK, Padmanabhan A. Extraskeletal Ewings sarcoma. J Surg Oncol 1983;23:70–72.
16. O'Keeffe F, Lorigan JG, Wallace S. Radiological features of extraskeletal Ewing sarcoma. Br J Radiol 1990;63:456–460.
17. Shirkhoda A, Peuchot M. Extraosseous Ewing's sarcoma computed tomography evaluation before and after chemotherapy. Clin Imag 1989;13:142–146.
18. Tefft M, Vawter GF, Mitus A. Paravertebral "round cell" tumors in children. Radiology 1969;92:1501–1504.
19. Triche TJ, Cavazzana AO. Pathology in pediatric oncology. In: Pizzo PA, Poplack DG, eds. Principles and practice of pediatric oncology. Philadelphia: JB Lippincott 1989:93–125.

Clinical Presentation

Pain, with or without the presence of a mass, is a common presenting symptom in Ewing sarcoma. This finding is similar to that in osteosarcoma. Pain is present in over 85 percent of patients.[1,2] A soft-tissue mass may be felt in between 40 to 61 percent of patients[1,2] and is more likely to be detected with peripheral than centrally located primary tumors. Unlike osteosarcoma patients, Ewing sarcoma patients frequently have systemic symptoms at the time of presentation.[3] These symptoms include fatigue, malaise, anemia, weight loss, poor appetite, local warmth over the tumor, and fever.[3,4] The erythrocyte sedimentation rate (ESR) and white blood cell counts may be elevated. These findings, together with fever, may incorrectly suggest the diagnosis of infection in some patients. In one series, there was fever in 27 percent, elevation of white cell count in 43 percent, and an increase in ESR in 30 percent.[5] Of interest is the complete absence of systemic findings in patients with the rare hand or foot primary tumor location.[6] This may be because these locations result in earlier diagnosis of the tumor. Patients with primary tumors in the spine may present with severe neurological symptoms such as weakness and loss of bowel or bladder control.[7]

Comment: Ewing sarcoma is not infrequently misdiagnosed and treated as osteomyelitis.

References

1. Munoz A, Madero L, Amaya J, et al. Local control and survival of Ewing's sarcoma in children with radiotherapy and chemotherapy without radical surgery. Acta Oncol 1989;28:245–248.
2. Wilkins RM, Pritchard DJ, Burgert EO, et al. Ewing's sarcoma of bone. Experience with 140 patients. Cancer 1986;58:2551–2555.
3. Miser JS, Triche TJ, Pritchard DJ, et al. Ewing's sarcoma and the nonrhabdomyosarcoma soft tissue sarcomas of childhood. In: Pizzo PA, Poplack DG, eds. Principles and practice of pediatric oncology. Philadelphia: JB Lippincott, 1989;659–688.
4. Dahlin DC, Coventry MB, Scanlon PW. Ewing's sarcoma. A critical analysis of 165 cases. J Bone Joint Surg 1961;43-A:185–195.
5. Falk S, Alpert M. The clinical and roentgen aspects of Ewing's sarcoma. Am J Med Sci 1965;250:44–60.
6. Reinus WR, Gilula LA, Shirley SK, et al. Radiographic appearance of Ewing sarcoma of the hands and feet: report from the intergroup Ewing sarcoma study. AJR 1985;144:331–336.
7. Kozlowski K, Beluffi G, Masel J, et al. Primary vertebral

tumours in children. Report of 20 cases with brief literature review. Pediatr Radiol 1984;14:129–139.

Imaging Studies

IMAGING BY MODALITY

Plain Film Radiograph. The plain film radiographic findings in Ewing sarcoma show a significant variation (Table 7–24).[1,2] The appearance varies from patient to patient for any one particular anatomic location and also varies depending on the anatomic location. The location of the tumor within the long bones is summarized in Table 7–25. The most common location for the tumor in the long bones is in the metadiaphysis.[1] The classic appearance of Ewing sarcoma in the long bone is of a symmetric (medullary origin) lesion with permeative bone destruction, a laminated periosteal reaction, and a soft-tissue mass.[1,2] There is lacelike cortical destruction without a focal break in the cortex. The many variations on this typical theme include an unusual location within the bone and asymmetric positioning, spiculated periosteal reaction, focal cortical destruction, areas of sclerosis, punched out areas of lysis, bone expansion, and soft-tissue calcification[1,2] (Figs. 7–43 and 7–44).

In the ribs, there is often bone expansion with extensive lysis. Sometimes the abnormality may be subtle.[3] Rib lesions frequently have a large soft-tissue component.[4] Periosteal reaction is frequently absent.[1,2] Pleural implants are seen in up to 25 percent of cases.[5]

In the flat bones, such as the scapula (Fig. 7–45) and pelvis (Fig. 7–46), there is usually a large area of abnormality, which may be lytic, blastic, or mixed. Soft-tissue masses are usually very prominent. Areas of sclerosis within the bone are more common in the flat bones than

TABLE 7–24
Ewing Sarcoma: Plain Film Radiographic Findings in 373 Cases[1]

Specific Finding	Percentage
Soft-tissue mass	80
Permeative destruction	76
Laminated periosteal reaction	56
Sclerosis in the tumor	39
Spiculated periosteal reaction	27
Cortical thickening	21
Cortical break	19
Purely lytic component	19
Pathologic fracture	15
Cystic component	12
Bone expansion	13
Soft-tissue calcification	9
Honeycomb appearance	6
Well marginated	6
Vertebral planes	6

Reference
1. Reinus WR, Gilula LA. Radiology of Ewing's sarcoma: Intergroup Ewing's Sarcoma Study. RadioGraphics 1984;4:929–944.

TABLE 7–25
Location of Ewing Sarcoma in Long Bones[1]

Location	No. of Cases
Epiphysis	1
Metaphysis	11
Metadiaphysis	121
Diaphysis	73

Reference
1. Reinus WR, Gilula LA. Radiology of Ewing's sarcoma: Intergroup Ewing's Sarcoma Study. RadioGraphics 1984;4:929–944.

Figure 7-43. **Diagnosis: Ewing sarcoma of radius. There is permeative destruction of the distal radius with no significant periosteal reaction.**

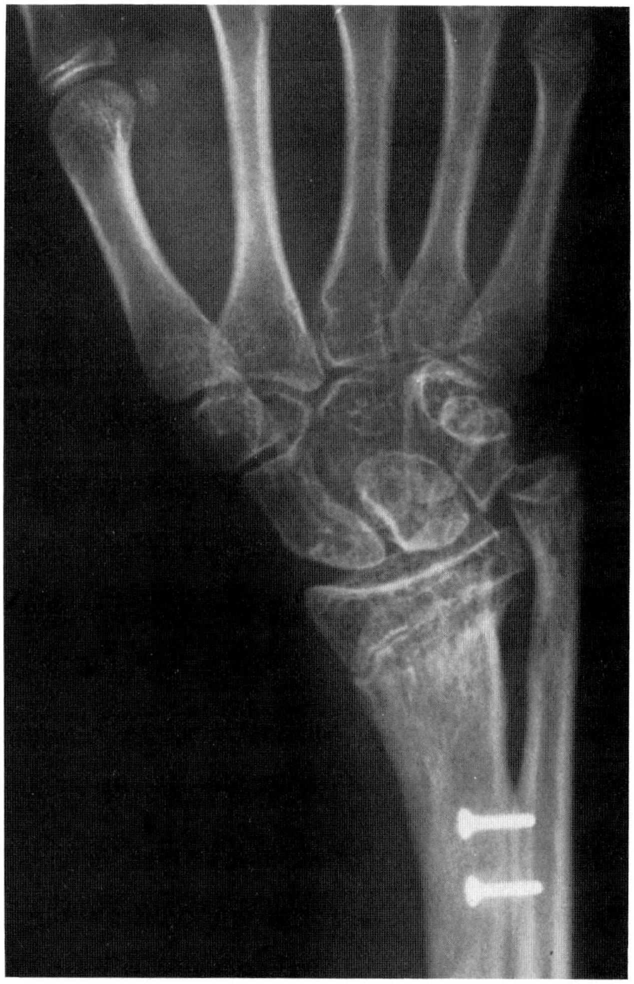

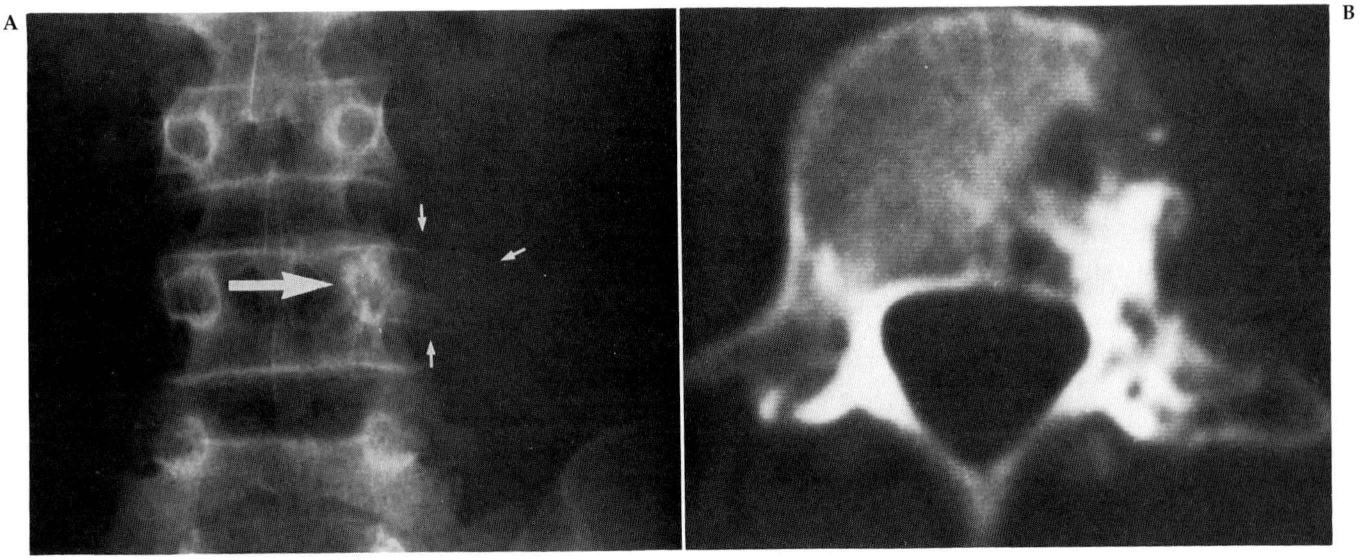

Figure 7-44. Diagnosis: Ewing sarcoma of the spine.
A, Plain film radiograph. The pedicle of the fourth lumbar vertebra *(large arrow)* shows lack of sharp definition of outline together with areas of destruction and sclerosis. The transverse process *(small arrows)* is expanded, with suggestion of some destruction. ***B***, CT. This shows destruction involving the right quarter of the body of the fourth lumbar vertebra, the pedicle, and the transverse process. The transverse process is expanded. There is sclerosis, seen particularly in the region of the pedicle and the medial part of the transverse process.

Figure 7-45. Diagnosis: Ewing sarcoma of the scapula. There is a large lesion involving the lateral part of the scapula including the glenoid. Permeative destruction is identified. The lesion has no sharp margins. A Codman type of periosteal reaction is present *(arrow).*

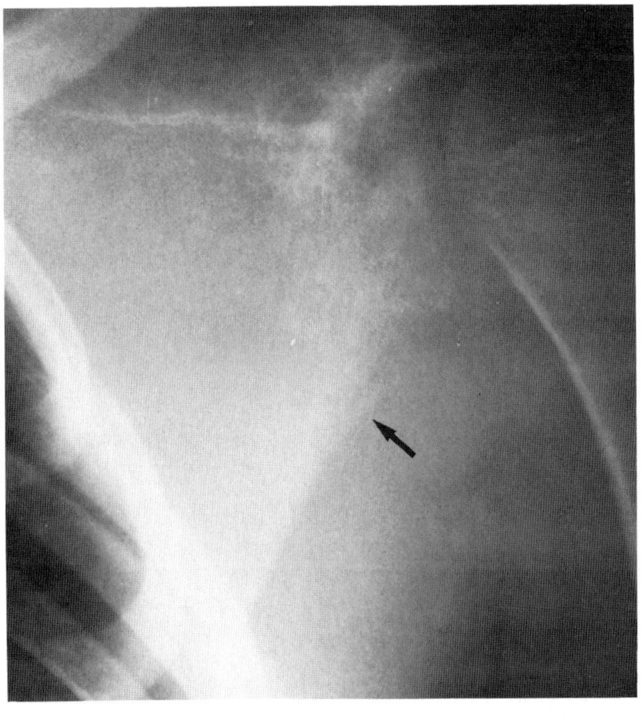

in the long bones, having been identified in 38 percent of patients in one series.[6]

In the hands and feet (Figs. 7–47 and 7–48), the tumors resemble Ewing sarcoma in other sites in that there is permeative destruction (75 percent), soft-tissue mass (77 percent), and areas of sclerosis (42 percent). Periosteal reaction (8 percent) is much less common than in most other sites. Bone expansion (33 percent), pathological fractures (34 percent), and sclerotic margins (17 percent) are all more common findings than in other anatomic locations.[7,8]

Sclerosis in Ewing sarcoma is the result of periosteal new bone formation, endosteal new bone formation, or areas of bone necrosis with new bone formation on the surface of the necrotic bone[6] (Fig. 7–49). Unlike osteosarcomas and chondrosarcomas, the soft-tissue matrix of Ewing sarcoma does not produce calcium.

Identification of a spontaneously occurring pneumothorax in a patient with Ewing sarcoma almost invariably indicates the presence of an underlying pulmonary metastasis even if it cannot be identified on the radiographs.[9]

On plain film radiographs, Ewing sarcoma is unique in that bone metastatic lesions resemble the primary bone tumor.[10]

Healing of Ewing sarcoma is identified by solidification of the periosteal reaction, which becomes confluent and incorporates into the adjacent cortex.[11] The cortex reconstitutes and the permeative bone destruction resolves. The soft-tissue component of the tumor decreases in size.[11] The appearance of tumor response on the plain film radiograph occurs much later than can be identified with CT or MR imaging. Because many pa-

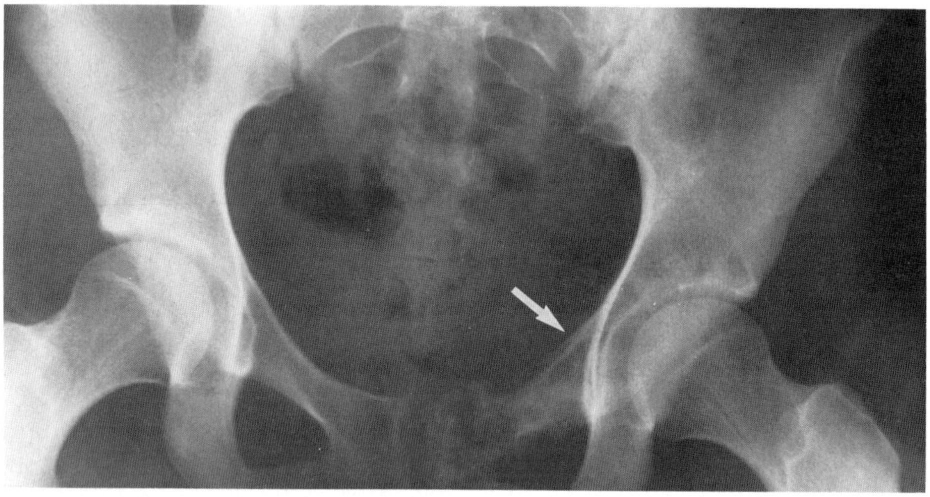

Figure 7-46. Diagnosis: Ewing sarcoma of the pubic bone.
There is a large lesion of the left pubic bone. It involves the symphysis and both the superior and inferior pubic rami. There is expansion with predominantly mottled destruction and a small amount of sclerosis. A periosteal reaction is present *(arrow).*

Figure 7-47. Diagnosis: Ewing sarcoma of the hand. Two cases.
A, Plain film radiograph. The entire first metacarpal is affected. There is extensive destruction, with a permeative appearance, together with some sclerosis. ***B,*** There is a predominantly lytic lesion in the distal end of the first phalanx of the fourth finger. This is causing some bone expansion. A large soft-tissue mass is also present. (From Kozlowski K. Primary bone tumors of the hand. Pediatr Radiol 1988;18:140–148.)

A B

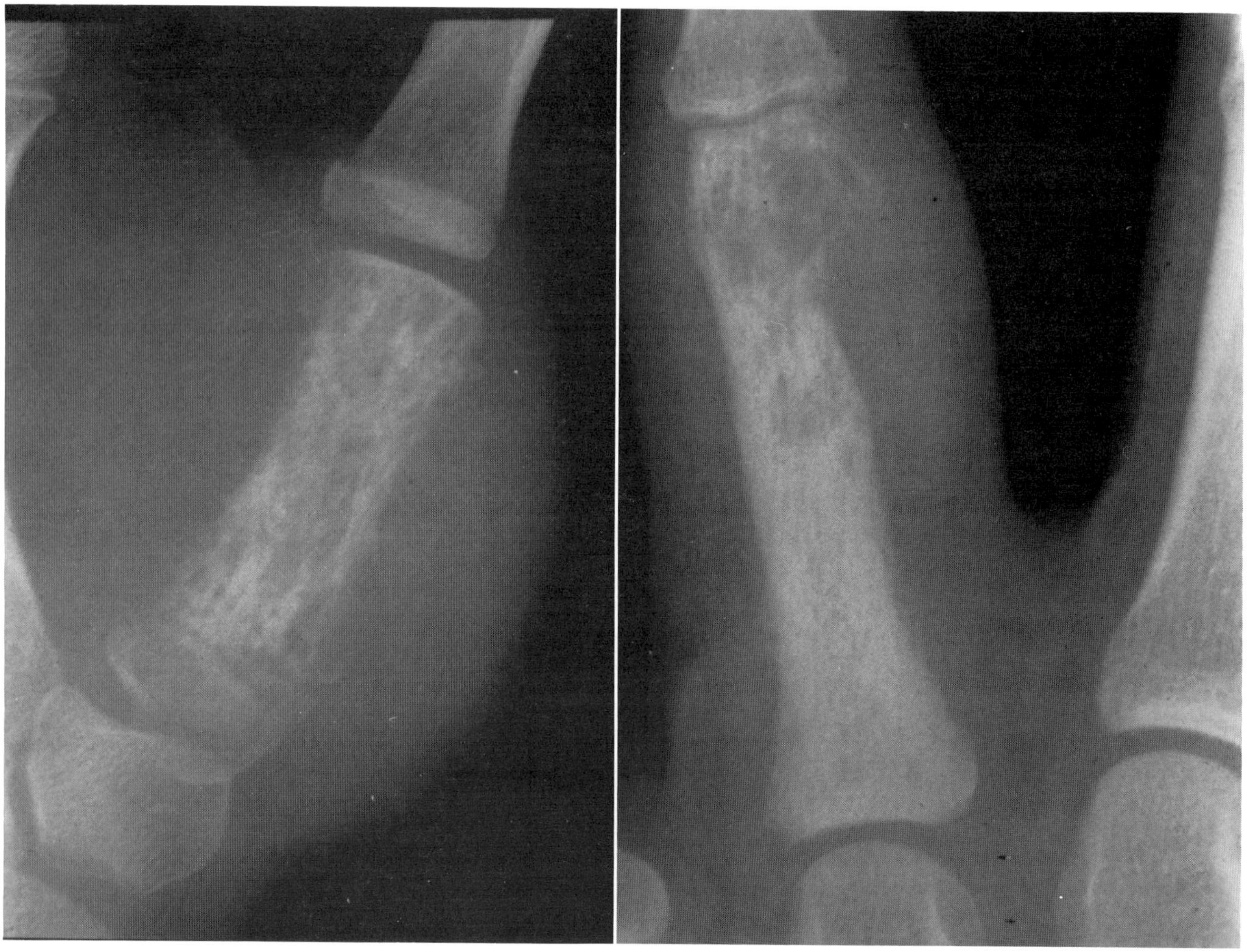

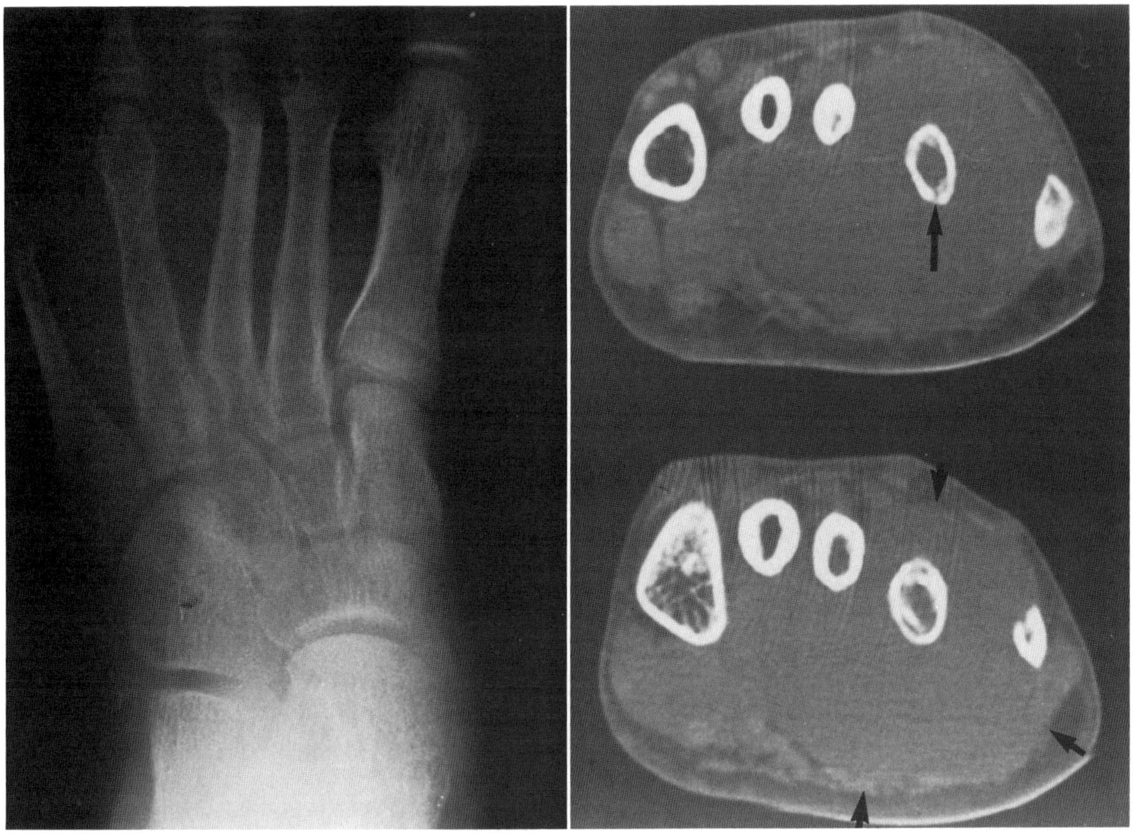

Figure 7–48. **Diagnosis: Ewing sarcoma of the foot.**
A, **Plain film radiograph. There is subtle but definite permeative destruction of the distal two-thirds of the fourth metatarsal. A large soft-tissue mass is present, displacing the third and fifth metatarsal. *B,* CT. This shows mild expansion of the fourth metatarsal *(large arrow),* with cortical thinning and destruction. No significant periosteal reaction is present. A very large soft-tissue mass *(small arrows)* is present. (From Leeson MC. Ewing's sarcoma of the foot. Foot and Ankle 1989;10:147–151.)**

tients are treated with radiotherapy, the signs of radionecrosis may be present as well.

> *Comment:* Plain film radiographs are very valuable in evaluating Ewing sarcoma.

Technetium 99m MDP. Nuclear medicine evaluation of Ewing sarcoma is done with technetium 99m MDP. This shows intense uptake of the isotope in the tumor. The appearance is completely nonspecific. Decrease in uptake will occur in response to therapy, but the absolute correlation in an individual patient is not accurate enough to utilize bone scanning routinely to evaluate response to therapy. Metastatic bone lesions are identified as hot spots. This is the modality of choice for seeking such metastases.[4,12]

CT. CT is widely used in the evaluation of Ewing sarcoma. It is used to study the primary tumor and to evaluate the lung for pulmonary metastases. It may also be utilized for detection of lymph node metastases in other sites.

As early as 1978 CT, in 9 cases, was reported as providing more information than plain film radiographs.[12] It was superior to the plain film for visualization of cortical destruction (see Figs. 7–44 and 7–48), marrow and soft-tissue spread (Fig. 7–48), and had a greater potential for evaluation of response to therapy. These findings have been confirmed in other series with larger numbers of patients.[14,15] Compared with the plain films, these studies have indicated that CT is not of great help in the initial differential diagnosis. It has consistently been better in identifying bone marrow and soft-tissue tumor and has resulted in alteration of therapy in up to as many as 50 percent of patients.[16] The various bony changes described for plain film radiographs can all be identified on the CT images (Fig. 7–44). Response to therapy is indicated by reduction in size of the tumor consolidation and thickening of the periosteal reaction and eroded cortex.[16] A persistent bone marrow abnormality may be seen even with a good response.[16] This probably represents tumor necrosis, fibrosis, or both.

One difficulty with CT imaging is that although there will usually be significant reduction in the size of the soft-tissue tumor mass in response to chemotherapy and radiation therapy, this soft-tissue mass will frequently not completely resolve. This is particularly true in the flat bones, but it may also be seen at other sites.

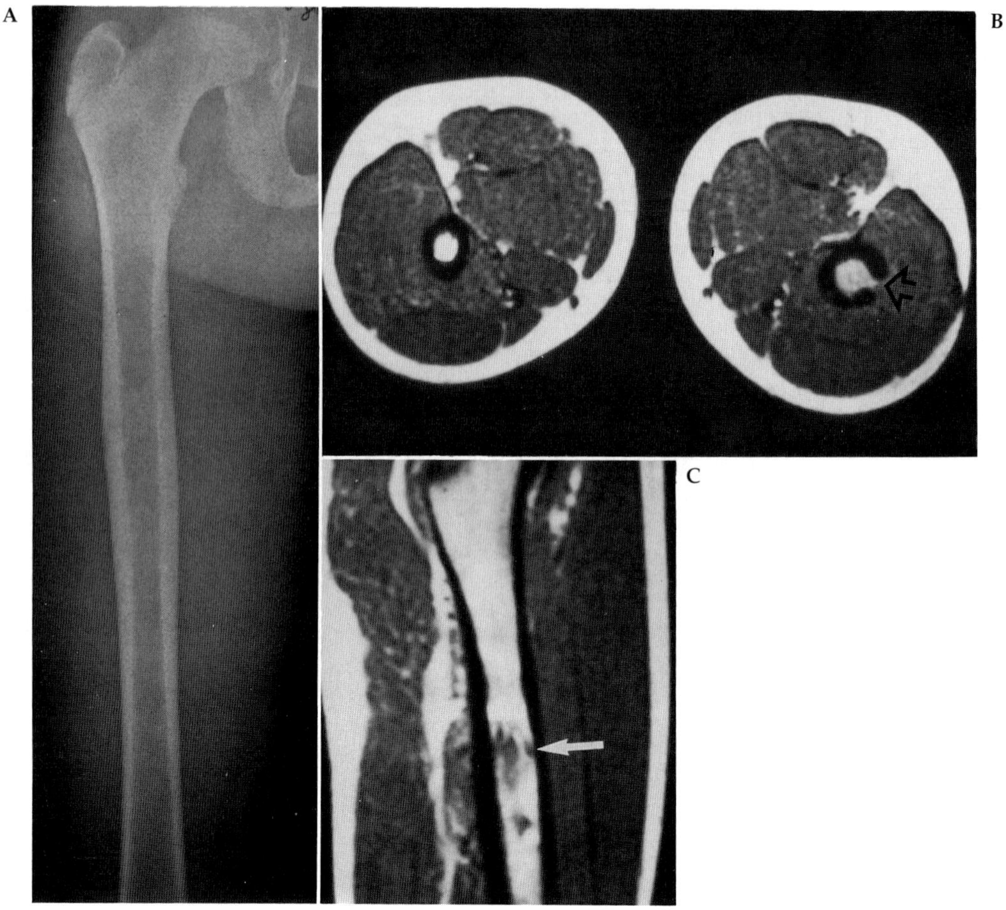

Figure 7-49. **Diagnosis: Ewing sarcoma.**
This tumor is unusual in being predominantly sclerotic. *A*, Plain film radiograph. There is cortical thickening of the diaphysis of the right femur, with no significant elevated periosteal reaction identified. *B* and *C*, MR, T1 weighted images. The cortical thickening is seen as an increase in the width of the cortex, which contains no signal. The high signal seen in the cortex *(open arrow)* on the axial image is the result of a biopsy. Signal reduction in the marrow *(arrow)* indicates the presence of tumor.

CT cannot accurately resolve the problem of deciding whether or not residual active tumor is present in the small remaining soft-tissue mass. Even needle biopsy may not resolve this problem, since the small sample obtained could easily miss tumor. Obviously an increase in size of the soft-tissue tumor with sequential follow-up studies does indicate the presence of active tumor.

In a study of 22 cases of extraosseous Ewing sarcoma, CT showed the masses well. They were of lower intensity than adjacent muscle and showed variable enhancement with intravenous contrast injection[17] (Fig. 7–50).

CT of the chest should be performed utilizing 1 cm thick contiguous slices. The administration of intravenous contrast is not required for detection of lung metastases. I do not routinely utilize contrast, but if there is suspicion of hilar or mediastinal lymph node disease, I would go back and repeat images through this region with a bolus of intravenous contrast. Imaging of the primary tumor site should be carried out using slice thickness no greater than 1 cm. For small tumors thinner slices may be obtained. Contiguous slices should be done. Visualization of the soft-tissue component of the tumor might be improved by intravenous injection of contrast, but there are no reported studies comparing CT images obtained with and without contrast administration. Since skip lesions have not been reported with Ewing sarcoma, it may be adequate to terminate scanning when two or three slices (adjacent to the tumor) have been obtained that appear completely normal. It is probably not necessary to continue to scan the entire affected bone.

Surgical resection of Ewing sarcoma is not performed nearly as aggressively as with osteogenic sarcoma, and the requirements for delineation of precise relationships of the tumor to adjacent soft tissue, joints, and blood vessels is not as demanding. Obviously, in those few patients in whom resection is to be performed, these questions are still of vital importance. Recent improvements in the chemotherapy for metastatic disease is causing renewed enthusiasm for surgical resection of the primary tumor.

In some specific situations, CT is particularly helpful

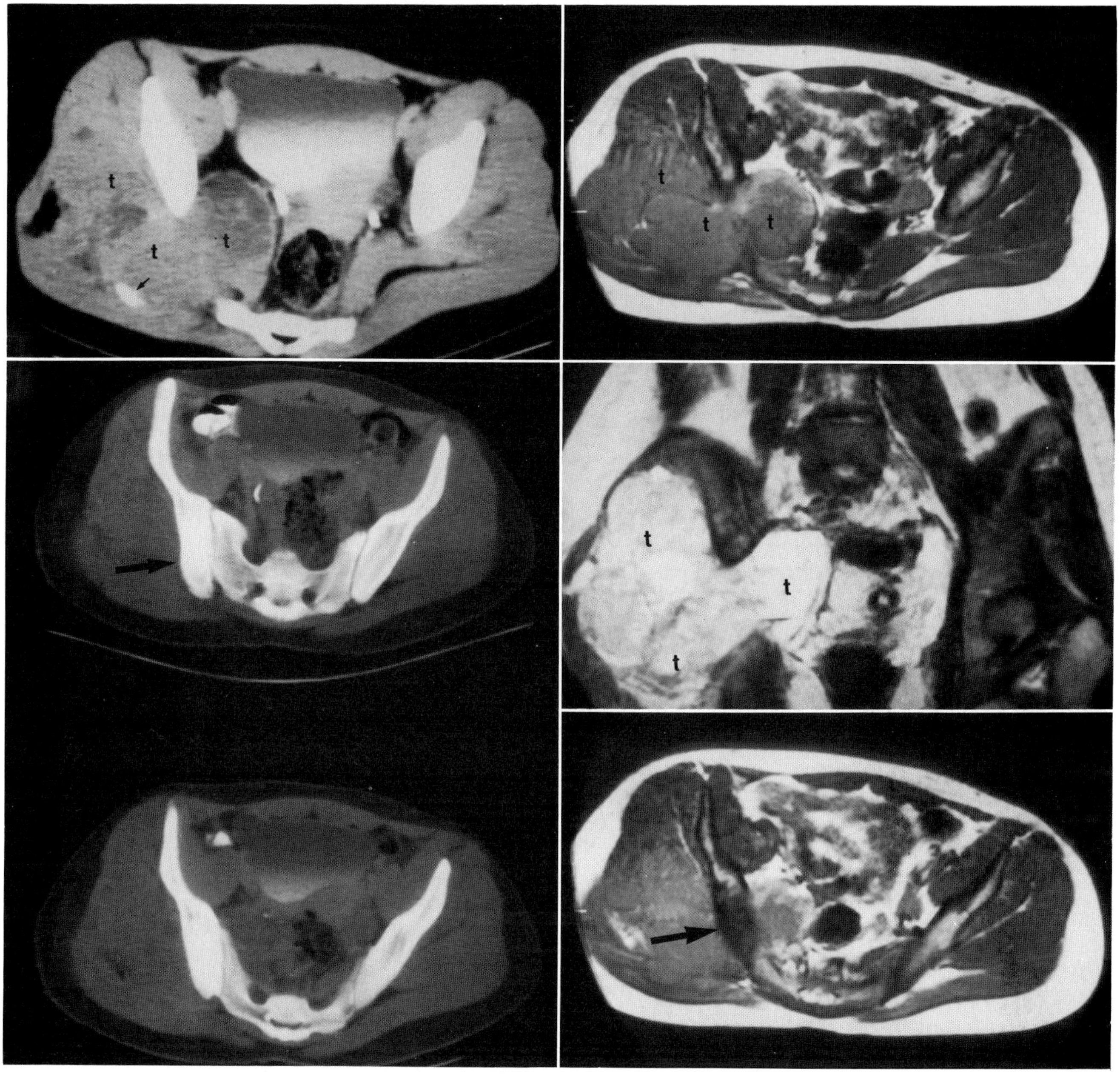

Figure 7–50. Diagnosis: Extraosseous Ewing sarcoma.
There is a very large bilobed soft-tissue mass extending through the notch between the iliac bone and sacrum. It is causing a secondary sclerotic reaction in adjacent bone. ***A***, CT. This shows the large bilobed tumor mass (*T*). A small area of calcification is present *(arrow).* Note that laterally it is difficult to define a plane separating tumor from adjacent normal muscle. ***B*** and ***C***, MR, axial T1 and coronal T2 weighted images. The tumor (*T*) is of similar intensity to muscle on the T1 weighted image but much brighter than muscle on the T2 weighted image. Note that the calcium seen on the CT image is more difficult to appreciate on the MR picture. The margins of the tumor are, however, much better defined on the T2 weighted MR image than on the CT. ***D*** and ***E***, Axial CT and T1 weighted MR images showing reactive sclerosis in the posterior aspect of the iliac bone. This is seen as increased density on the CT image and decreased signal in the marrow, with expansion of the cortex on the MR image *(arrows).*

(Fig. 7–51). For example, in those rare Ewing sarcomas arising in the skull or facial bones, plain film radiography is particularly poor at defining the extent of the tumor. CT will accurately show the local invasion of the bone. It will show areas of bone destruction better than MR (Fig. 7–51). It will show soft-tissue extent of the tumor extremely well, but probably not as well as MR. In one patient with a large destructive facial Ewing sarcoma,[18] CT was able to define the tumor well. In this patient, there was marked homogeneous increase in attenuation following contrast administration. CT was able to follow this lesion and demonstrate complete resolu-

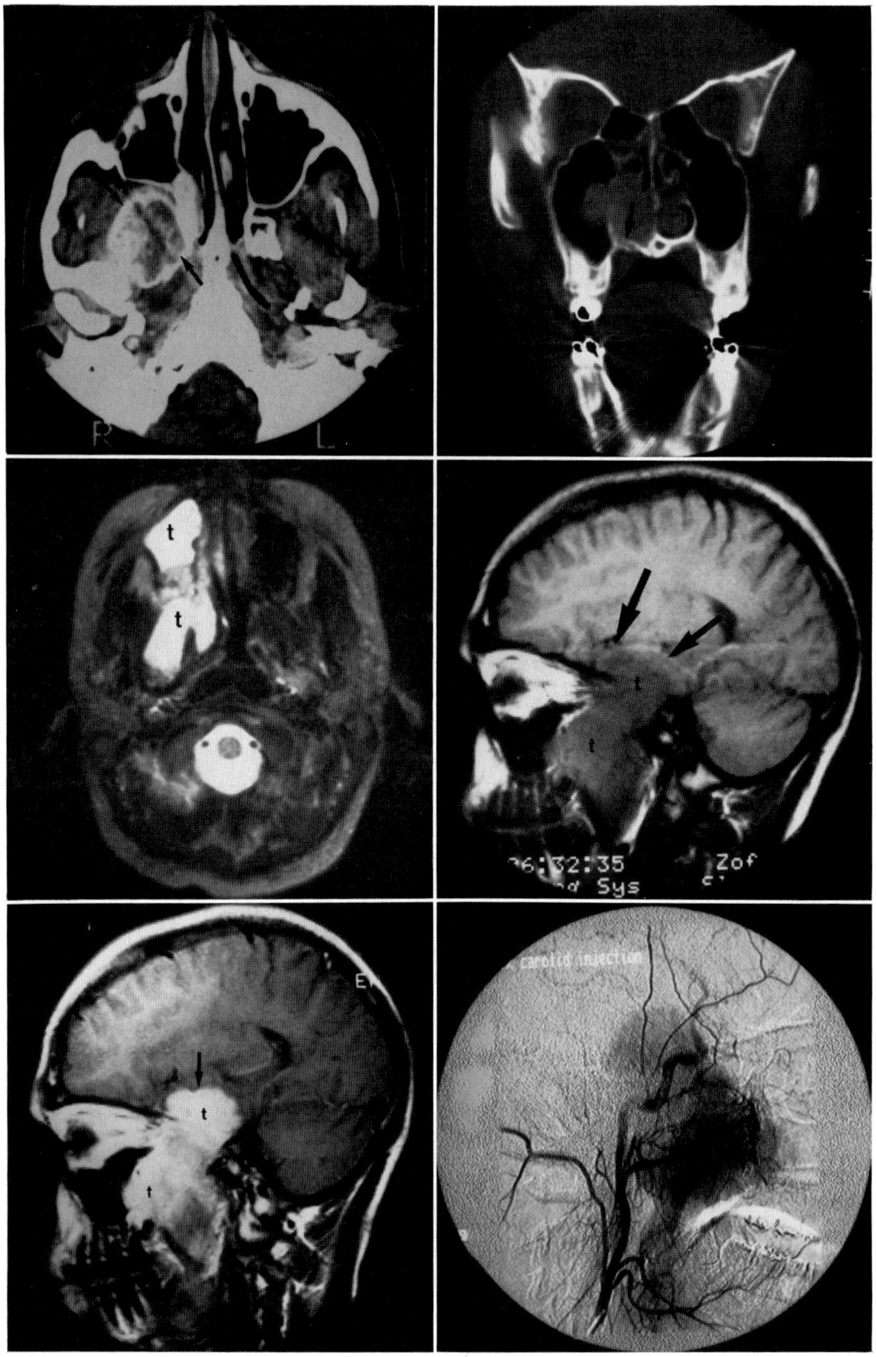

Figure 7-51. Diagnosis: Facial Ewing sarcoma.

There is a large tumor involving the nose, maxillary sinus, and pterygoid region. There is extension into the temporal fossa. CT shows areas of bone destruction better than MR. MR T2 weighted images define the margins of the tumor to best advantage. Sagittal MR images are best for appreciating the extent of the soft-tissue component of the tumor. *A* and *B*, Axial and coronal CT images. At these levels tumor is seen in the pterygoid regions, nose, and maxillary sinus. Areas of bone destruction are clearly identified *(arrows)*. *C* through *E*, Axial T2, sagittal T1, and sagittal T1 (after gadolinium-DTPA) weighted images. These show the soft-tissue component of the tumor well (*T*). The bone destruction can be inferred but not clearly defined. The sagittal images show the extension into the temporal fossa *(arrows)*. *F*, Angiogram. This shows marked increase in vascularity of the tumor with an intense tumor blush.

tion with chemotherapy and radiation therapy. In the ribs, CT is very helpful for predicting surgical resectability.[3]

CT is not utilized routinely for the evaluation of bone metastases, but either CT or MR is particularly helpful with metastatic lesions to the head. This is because these lesions frequently have a large intracranial soft-tissue component,[19–21] and CT has accurately identified the extent of the soft-tissue component of these lesions.[19–21] In very rare cases of brain metastases, these lesions may be identified with CT.[22] In one patient, such a metastasis showed ring enhancement following intravenous contrast injection. CT has not been compared with MR. CT may occasionally provide information that is confusing. In two patients, one with an occipital bone metastasis and one with a primary tumor in the spine, large areas of calcification were identified in the soft-tissue component of the tumor. The presence of this calcium suggested matrix mineralization and, therefore, a diagnosis of osteosarcoma. The calcification, as these were Ewing tumors, was probably dystrophic calcification occurring in necrotic tumor.[19,23]

MR. Magnetic resonance imaging has been utilized to evaluate Ewing sarcoma.[24,25] In one study of 9 patients, MR was superior to CT for definition of the soft-tissue and bone-marrow extent of the tumor. It was not as good as CT for identification of bone destruction and periosteal formation[24] (Figs. 7–51 and 7–52). In another study of 27 patients, MR was better than CT for identification of soft-tissue spread, bone-marrow spread, and the relationship of the tumor to the epiphysis.[25] Following nonsurgical therapy, it was equivalent to CT for identification of the size of the residual soft-tissue mass.[25] In most patients, the periosteal reaction can be identified with high-resolution MR, but perhaps not as clearly as on the plain film or CT. The soft-tissue and marrow components of the tumor have signal intensity consistent with prolongation of T1 and T2 relaxation times (Figs. 7–50 and 7–52). Marrow disease is best identified on T1 weighted images, appearing as decreased signal compared to normal marrow (see Fig. 7–49). Soft-tissue tumor is best seen on T2 weighted images where the tumor is of higher signal than adjacent muscle (Figs. 7–50, 7–51, 7–53, and 7–54). Contrast between tumor and normal muscle was found to be greatest with T2 spin echo pulse sequences and better than with gadolinium-DTPA enhanced T1 weighted images or gradient echo images with 20° flip angles.[26] On T1 pulse sequences, the change in signal in marrow and soft tissues in response to therapy is variable. In the determination of tumor activity in residual soft-tissue masses, MR is perhaps a little better than CT, but it still does not provide the required information in many patients.

A favorable tumor response to chemotherapy or radiation therapy is indicated by reduction in the size of the soft-tissue tumor.[25] A reduction in the signal intensity on T2 images is probably also an indication of response, but response can occur without alteration of signal. In a residual soft-tissue mass, a high signal intensity on T2 weighted images can be seen from reactive inflammation or from tumor and thus cannot be used to differentiate these two conditions. A low signal intensity on T2 weighted images probably indicates fibrosis and not tumor. Gadolinium-DTPA has not proved helpful, in a few patients, in differentiating necrosis and fibrosis from active tumor.[25]

> *Comment:* MR and CT provide complementary information. In a residual mass, neither can accurately differentiate tumor from fibrosis.

IMAGING PROTOCOLS

Imaging of the patient on initial presentation of Ewing sarcoma and on follow-up requires the use of multiple imaging modalities and a thorough understanding of the pathologic behavior of this tumor. As with other tumors, it is no longer appropriate to make generalized recommendations for all patients with Ewing sarcoma. The type of study and the frequency of repetition on follow-up will depend on the specific therapeutic protocols being utilized by an individual institution. It will also depend on the site of the primary tumor. For example, if the location is such that an initial complete resection of tumor is performed, localized imaging follow-up will need to be much less intense than for patients in whom surgical excision has not been performed.

The biologic behavior of Ewing sarcoma in different locations varies and this information too needs to be reflected in imaging decisions. For example, in one study of 107 children,[27] it was found that lung and bone metastases could be present on initial presentation from either truncal or extremity primary tumors. The incidence of lung and bone metastases was similar when the primary tumor was in an extremity. When the primary tumor was located in the trunk (spine or pelvis), the number of patients with lung metastases was less than 50 percent of those with bone metastases. This behavior difference, depending on the location of the primary tumor, was also seen with regard to development of metastases on follow-up. In patients with primary truncal lesions, 90 percent of metastases discovered on follow-up occurred during the first two years, compared to only 70 percent of metastases in those patients with extremity lesions. These findings would mean that surveillance for development of metastasis should be continued beyond two years for patients with an extremity primary but perhaps not beyond this time period (as the yield will be very low) in patients with a truncal primary. In an Intergroup Ewing's Study reported in 1985, 62 patients with nonmetastatic primaries of the pelvis were followed. Thirty-four percent had no recurrence. Local (in 27 percent of patients) or metastatic (in 61 percent of patients) recurrence occurred with a mean time to relapse of 92 weeks.[28] (Some patients had local and metastatic recurrence.)

Another finding that will influence imaging is that the local failure rate is much greater in those patients

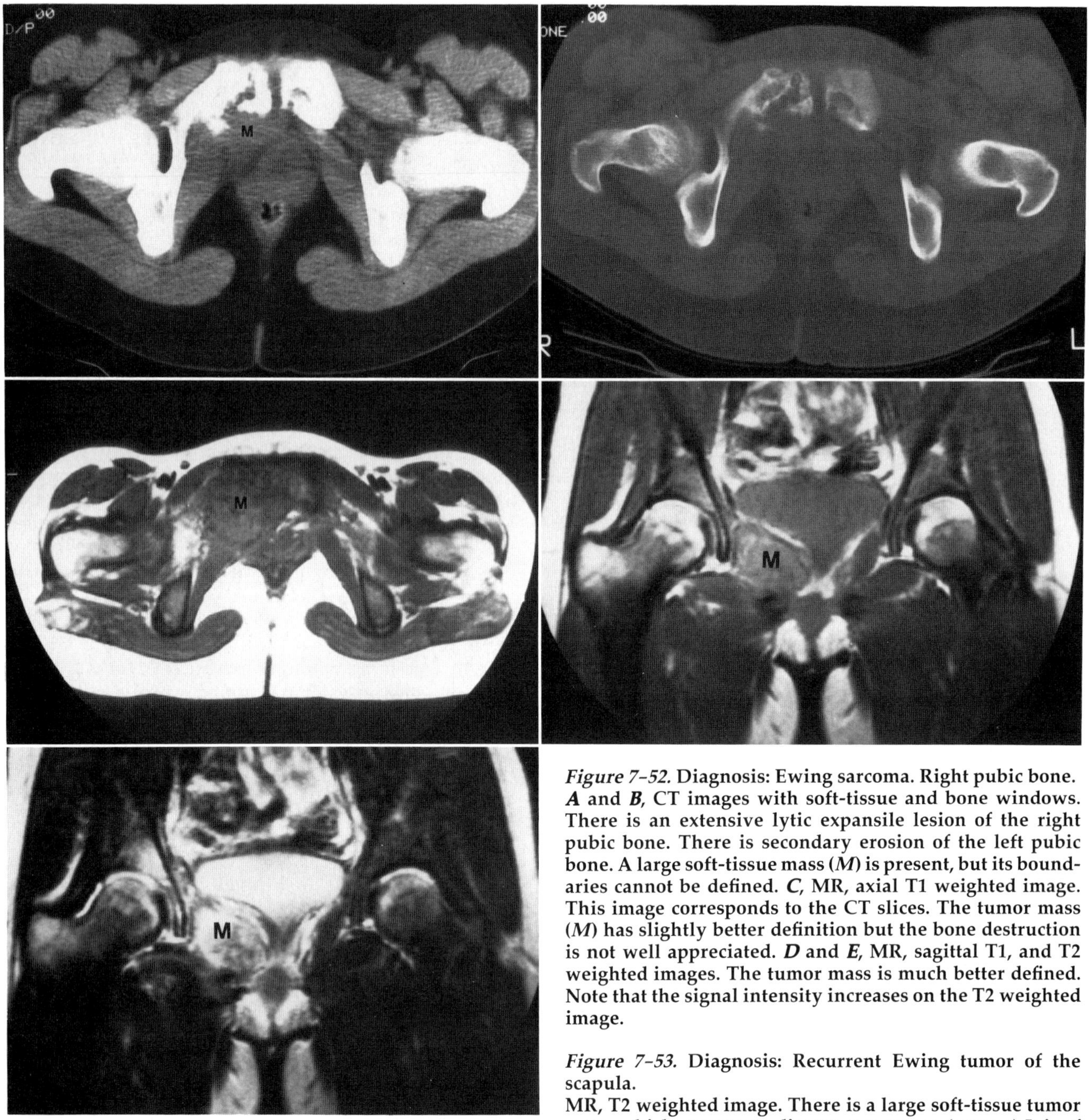

Figure 7-52. **Diagnosis: Ewing sarcoma. Right pubic bone. *A* and *B*, CT images with soft-tissue and bone windows. There is an extensive lytic expansile lesion of the right pubic bone. There is secondary erosion of the left pubic bone. A large soft-tissue mass (*M*) is present, but its boundaries cannot be defined. *C*, MR, axial T1 weighted image. This image corresponds to the CT slices. The tumor mass (*M*) has slightly better definition but the bone destruction is not well appreciated. *D* and *E*, MR, sagittal T1, and T2 weighted images. The tumor mass is much better defined. Note that the signal intensity increases on the T2 weighted image.**

Figure 7-53. **Diagnosis: Recurrent Ewing tumor of the scapula.**
MR, T2 weighted image. There is a large soft-tissue tumor mass, which represents disease recurrence *(arrows).* It is of very bright signal on this T2 weighted image and sharply defined. Note the marked decrease in size of the left hemithorax caused by radiation therapy many years previously.

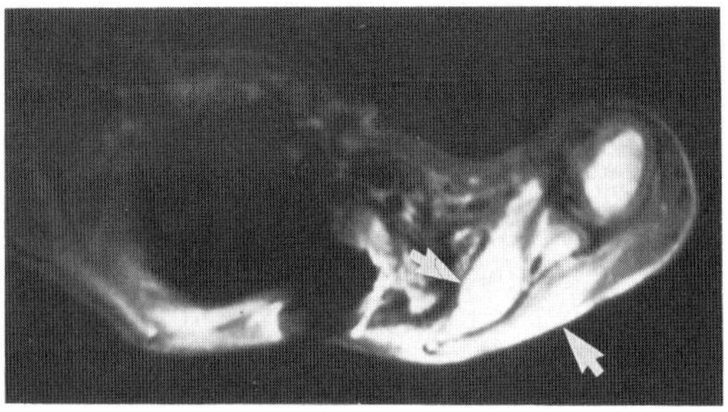

with a soft-tissue mass at diagnosis than in those patients in whom the tumor is confined to bone.[29] This means that imaging intensity needs to be greatest in those patients in whom a soft-tissue mass has been identified. Studies of relapse patterns also should influence imaging decisions. Obviously, before basing imaging decisions on such studies, one must be aware that the particular relapse pattern is occurring in a patient population receiving similar treatment to that in the radiologist's own institution. In one study reported in 1989 with patients receiving combined modern therapy with chemotherapy, radiation therapy and surgery re-

A B C D, E

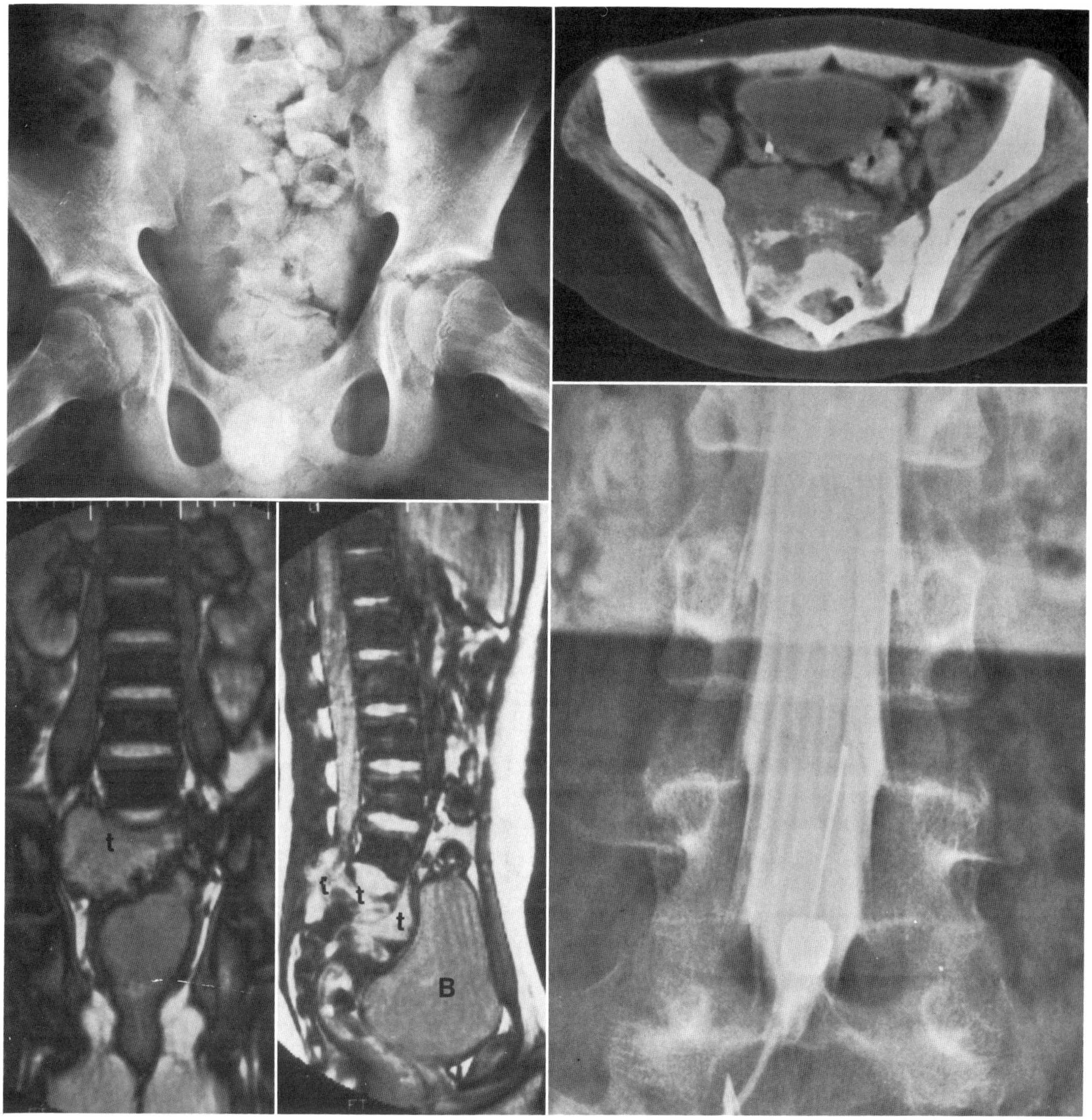

Figure 7–54. **Diagnosis: Ewing sarcoma of the sacrum. Advantages of the MR imaging. *A*, Plain film radiograph. This shows extensive destruction of the lateral part of the sacrum on the right side. *B*, CT. This shows sacral destruction with a soft-tissue tumor mass (*T*). *C*, Myelogram. This shows block of flow of contrast inferiorly, but does not define the extent of the abnormality causing the obstruction. *D* and *E*, MR, coronal and sagittal spin density images. These show the soft-tissue component of the tumor (*T*). Note the tumor anterior to the sacrum, penetrating through the sacrum, and extending inferiorly and superiorly in the spinal canal. The total extent of the lesion is beautifully demonstrated on the sagittal image. The bladder (*B*) is distended because of neurologic involvement.**

lapse occurred in 7 of 27 patients. The relapse was in bone only in 3 patients, lung only in 3 patients, and in both in 1 patient. The median time to relapse was 19 months. Although the numbers in this study are small, they indicate that one cannot survey only the lung with follow-up. One could do this if lung metastases always occurred before bone metastases, but this is not the case. The mean time to relapse is 19 months, which means surveillance for metastatic disease must be continued for a time period longer than this. Other studies provide similar important information; 24 of 47 patients relapsing on therapy had local relapse in 8 months and metastatic relapse in 16 months.[30] Not all of the patients with local relapse had metastatic disease. The implications from this study are that in patients in whom the local tumor has not been resected, imaging attention must be paid to the local tumor site, as one-third of relapses occurred here. Another study looked at the problem of late local recurrence. Reports from this study and a review of the literature indicated that recurrence beyond 3 years could occur in between 7 and 38 percent of patients,[31] again indicating the need for extended surveillance. In a collaborative European study of patients treated between 1981 and 1985, relapse occurred in 39 of 93 patients. The relapse was confined to the site of the primary tumor in 12 patients and was metastatic in 28. Metastatic disease was twice as common in lung as in bone.[32]

A study reported in 1987[33] evaluated local relapse following chemotherapy and radiation therapy, with or without surgery, in 60 cases. Local relapse occurred in 69 percent of cases with pelvic primary, 47 percent with rib primary, and 15 percent with limb primary. The local relapse could occur alone or with metastases. The median time to local relapse was 27 months for the limbs and 6 months for the rib and pelvis. In another study reported in 1986, intensive chemotherapy and radiation therapy got apparent complete remission in 28 of 30 patients. Fourteen of these later relapsed locally and of these 10 had metastases as well.

All of this information may seem overwhelming and confusing, but it does attempt to put recommendations for imaging onto some kind of scientific rather than empirical basis. It is important to stress that imaging protocols must change as therapy changes, as response to therapy changes, and as imaging technology changes.

Comment:

Plain film radiographs should always be utilized for evaluation of the site of primary tumors. Others studies may be performed as well.

MDP bone scan should be utilized for detection of bone metastases.

CT scanning should be used for evaluation of the primary tumor, the lung for metastases, and for the skull (if bone metastases are identified on MDP scan).

MR, when available, should be utilized for evaluation of the primary tumor (see Fig. 7–54). Its value will be greatest in two situations. These are immediately prior to any planned surgical resection of the tumor and in helping to determine the presence or absence of viable tumor in a residual soft-tissue mass. Whether MR should be performed routinely at other times, or only following CT in these two specific situations, is not known. For research reasons I would perform MR routinely at least on initial diagnosis and at the end of chemotherapy.

Follow-up imaging should routinely include the lungs, bones, and local site of tumor (unless it is completely surgically removed).

Imaging surveillance should continue for at least 2 years and probably longer than this, in some patients.

Imaging should be done in all areas of potential metastases on initial presentation, and at any time therapy is altered. Follow-up imaging each year should occur probably no less frequently than every 3 months. At times when therapeutic changes are not anticipated, chest radiograph rather than chest CT and plain film radiograph of the primary tumor rather than CT may prove adequate.

Imaging should be performed at any time in any location should new clinical symptoms develop.

No adequate information is available to make recommendation for image screening for lymph node metastases. At a minimum I think it is reasonable to perform abdominal CT when the primary tumor is in the pelvis or legs, particularly if metastases have not been identified by bone scan or lung CT.

More intensive imaging should be given to areas of known tumor, in order to follow their resolution.

References

1. Reinus WR, Gilula LA. Radiology of Ewing's sarcoma: Intergroup Ewing's Sarcoma Study (IESS). RadioGraphics 1984;4:929–944.
2. Sherman RS, Soong KY. Ewing's sarcoma: its roentgen classification and diagnosis. Radiology 1956;66:529–539.
3. Levine E, Levine C. Ewing tumor of rib: radiologic findings and computed tomography contribution. Skeletal Radiol 1983;9:227–233.
4. Kozlowski K, Campbell J, Morris L, et al. Primary rib tumours in children (report of 27 cases with short literature review). Australas Radiol 1989;33:210–222.
5. Wilkins RM, Pritchard DJ, Burgert EO, et al. Ewing's sarcoma of bone. Experience with 140 patients. Cancer 1986;58:2551–2555.
6. Shirley SK, Gilula LA, Siegal GP, et al. Roentgenographic-pathologic correlation of diffuse sclerosis in Ewing sarcoma of bone. Skeletal Radiol 1984;12:69–78.
7. Reinus WR, Gilula LA, Shirley SK, et al. Radiographic appearance of Ewing sarcoma of the hands and feet: report from the Intergroup Ewing Sarcoma Study. AJR 1985;144:331–336.
8. Kozlowski K, Azouz EM, Campbell J, et al. Primary bone tumours of the hand. Report of 21 cases. Pediatr Radiol 1988;18:140–148.
9. Singer J, Sundaram M, Naunheim K. Failure of standard imaging techniques in the staging of Ewing sarcoma. J Bone Joint Surg 1989;71-A:775–780.
10. Plowman PN. Bone metastases from Ewing's sarcoma radiologically recapitulate the features of a primary Ewing's tumour. Clin Radiol 1989;40:498–500.
11. Taber DS, Libshitz HI, Cohen MA. Treated Ewing sarcoma: radiographic appearance in response, recurrence, and new primaries. AJR 1983;140:753–758.
12. Carlson DH, Simon H. Uptake of ^{99m}Tc-methylene diphosphonate in a case of extraskeletal Ewing's sarcoma. Clin Nucl Med 1979;4:203–207.
13. Berger PE, Kuhn JP. Computed tomography of tumors of the musculoskeletal system in children. Radiology 1978;127:171–175.
14. Brown KT, Kattapuram SV, Rosenthal DI. Computed tomography analysis of bone tumors: patterns of cortical destruction and soft tissue extension. Skeletal Radiol 1986;15:448–451.
15. Vanel D, Contesso G, Couanet D, et al. Computed tomography in the evaluation of 41 cases of Ewing's sarcoma. Skeletal Radiol 1982;9:8–13.

16. Strege DW, Hanel DP, Vogler C, et al. Ewing sarcoma in a phalanx of an infant's finger. J Bone Joint Surg 1989;71-A:1262–1264.
17. O'Keeffe F, Lorigan JG, Wallace S. Radiological features of extraskeletal Ewing sarcoma. Br J Radiol 1990;63:456–460.
18. Williams MP, Husband JE, McElwain TJ. Role of computed tomography scanning in the management of Ewing's sarcoma. Med Pediatr Oncol 1989;17:414–417.
19. Freeman MP, Currie CM, Gray GF, et al. Ewing sarcoma of the skull with an unusual pattern of reactive sclerosis: MR characteristics. J Comput Assist Tomogr 1988;12:143–146.
20. Taets ven Amerongen AHM, Kaiser MC, de Waal FC. Metastatic Ewing's sarcoma to the skull: CNS involvement excluded by MRI. Pediatr Radiol 1987;17:242–243.
21. Turoff NB, Becker M, Lewis M. Ewing's sarcoma: unusual presentation delineated by computerized tomography. J Bone Joint Surg 1978;60:1109–1111.
22. Mineura K, Yasuda T, Suda Y, et al. Ewing's sarcoma with intracranial metastasis presenting depressed cerebral blood flow and metabolism in the contralateral gray matter. Comput Med Imag Graph 1989;13:185–190.
23. Weinstein JB, Siegel MJ, Griffith RC. Spinal Ewing sarcoma: misleading appearances. Skeletal Radiol 1984;11:262–265.
24. Boyko OB, Cory DA , Cohen MD, et al. MR imaging of osteogenic and Ewing's sarcoma. AJR 1987;148:317–322.
25. Frouge C, Vanel D, Coffre C, et al. The role of magnetic resonance imaging in the evaluation of Ewing sarcoma. Skeletal Radiol 1988;17:387–392.
26. Erleman R, Vassallo P, Bongartz G, et al. Musculoskeletal neoplasm: fast low-angle shot MR imaging with and without Gd-DTPA. Radiology 1990;176:489–495.
27. Dwyer AJ, Glaubiger DL, Ecker JG, et al. The radiographic follow-up of patients with Ewing sarcoma: a demonstration of a general method. Radiology 1982;145:327–331.
28. Evans R, Nesbit M, Askin F, et al. Local recurrence, rate and sites of metastases, and time to relapse as a function of treatment regimen, size of primary and surgical history in 62 patients presenting with non-metastatic Ewing's sarcoma of the pelvic bones. Int J Radiat Oncol Biol Phys 1985;11:129–136.
29. Mendenhall CM, Marcus RB, Enneking WF, et al. The prognostic significance of soft tissue extension in Ewing's sarcoma. Cancer 1983;51:913–917.
30. Bao BN, Hayes FA, Thompson EI, et al. Chest wall resection for Ewing's sarcoma of the rib: an unnecessary procedure. Ann Thorac Surg 1988;46:40–44.
31. Sailer SL, Harmon DC, Mankin HJ, et al. Ewings sarcoma: surgical resection as a prognostic factor. Int J Oncol Biol Phys 1988;15:43–57.
32. Jurgens H, Exner U, Gadner H, et al. Multidisciplinary treatment of primary Ewing's sarcoma of bone. Cancer 1988;61:23–32.
33. Brown AP, Fixsen JA, Plowman PN. Local control of Ewing's sarcoma: an analysis of 67 patients. Br J Radiol 1987;60:261–268.

Differential Diagnosis

In those patients in whom a Ewing sarcoma has a classic appearance, the correct diagnosis can usually be strongly suggested from the imaging study. The marked variation of appearance of Ewing sarcoma results, however, in a large differential diagnosis for many patients. A few of the abnormalities to be considered in the differential diagnosis are:

Radiation osteitis (Fig. 7–55). Changes of radiation osteitis show permeative destruction and later sclerosis with a narrow transition zone, absent periosteal reaction (in the absence of a fracture), no soft-tissue mass, and lack of progression with time.[1] True tumor recurrence in patients who have received radiation for Ewing sarcoma is suggested by an alteration in the above pattern, particularly in patients with new clinical symptoms.[1]

Stress fracture.[2,3] Stress fractures can occasionally be confused with Ewing sarcoma. They typically will show a continuous periosteal reaction, no soft-tissue tumor, and no bone destruction. There is minimal hyperemia on the first phase of a bone scan (unlike Ewing sarcoma,

Figure 7–55. **Diagnosis: Radiation osteitis.**
This is the same patient illustrated in Figure 7–43. The original lesion was treated with radiation and chemotherapy. This image is obtained 6 years later. There is extensive patchy change in the distal radius with a predominantly sclerotic reaction. Early recurrent tumor would be extremely difficult to identify.

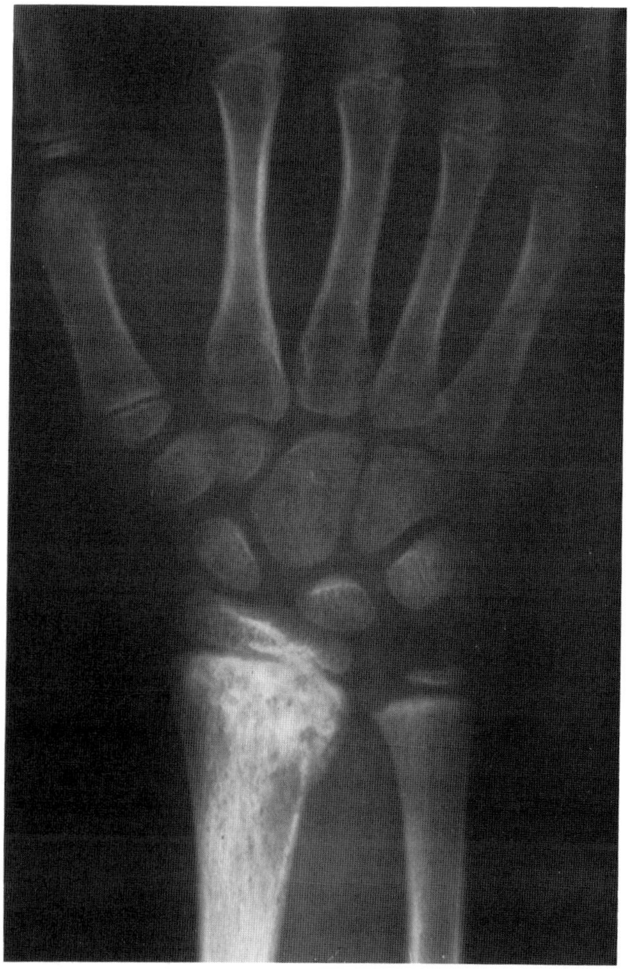

which is more intense) and the delayed bone scan shows eccentric cortical uptake not as intense as with typical Ewing tumor. A fracture line may be seen and when present is good evidence of a stress fracture. CT may be required to identify the fracture line. It is important not to mistake a nutrient vessel for a fracture (comparison with the opposite normal side is helpful). The bone marrow can be abnormal with a stress fracture and the finding of marrow abnormality, therefore, does not help in the differential diagnosis.

Aneurysmal bone cyst. An aneurysmal bone cyst can easily be confused with a Ewing or osteogenic sarcoma. MR is most helpful in identifying fluid levels, which strongly suggest the correct diagnosis (Fig. 7–56).

Other small round cell tumors. Small, round-cell tumors may cause problems in differential diagnosis, particularly to the pathologist.

Osteomyelitis. Osteomyelitis can cause particular difficulty, especially as some patients with Ewing sarcoma may have a fever, local warmth, and an elevated blood white cell count.[4,5] With infection, periosteal reaction is usually laminar, the bone destruction less, the soft-tissue abnormality smaller and much less sharply defined than with Ewing sarcoma.

Eosinophilic granuloma.[5] In some patients, it may not be possible to differentiate eosinophilic granuloma from a Ewing sarcoma without biopsy.

Primitive neuroectodermal tumor. The differential diagnosis between primitive neuroectodermal tumor and Ewing sarcoma is discussed in detail in the section relating to primitive neuroectodermal tumor.

References

1. Paling MR, Herdt JR. Radiation osteitis: a problem of recognition. Radiology 1980;137:339–342.
2. Davies AM, Carter SR, Grimer RJ, et al. Fatigue fractures of the femoral diaphysis in the skeletally immature simulating malignancy. Br J Radiol 1989;62:893–896.
3. Davies AM, Evans N, Grimer RJ. Fatigue fractures of the proximal tibia simulating malignancy. Br J Radiol 1988;61:903–908.
4. Miser JS, Triche TJ, Pritchard DJ, et al. Ewing's sarcoma and the nonrhabdomyosarcoma soft tissue sarcomas of childhood. In: Pizzo PA, Poplack DG, eds. Principles and practice of pediatric oncology. Philadelphia: JB Lippincott, 1989:659–688.
5. Dahlin DC, Coventry MB, Scanlon PW. Ewing's sarcoma. A critical analysis of 165 cases. J Bone Joint Surg 1961;43-A:185–195.

Therapy and Prognosis

A number of factors affecting prognosis in Ewing sarcoma have been identified. These are summarized in Table 7–26. One of the most important of these is the location of the primary tumor. Tumors located in the pelvis have a particularly poor prognosis. Metastatic disease on initial presentation is also associated with a very poor prognosis. It should be noted that some of the factors indicated in Table 7–26 will change as therapeutic approaches change. Also some of the studies on which the statements are based were not blind, random studies. For example, the study indicating a more favorable response with complete surgical resection may well have shown this result because the more favorable tumors were resected. A 1991 review believes that when local control by surgical excision is possible, prognosis is improved.[1]

There is no doubt that the overall prognosis in Ewing sarcoma has improved in the past 20 years. Prior to

Figure 7-56. **Diagnosis: Aneurysmal bone cyst in 2 different patients.**
A**, Plain film radiograph. This shows extensive destruction of the superior ramus of the pubic bone. There is a large soft-tissue mass, the margins of which are indicated by an arrow. The initial radiographic diagnosis was Ewing sarcoma. The initial biopsy diagnosis was telangiectatic osteosarcoma. The lesion was, in fact, an aneurysmal bone cyst.** ***B*****, Axial MR image. This is another patient with a right-sided aneurysmal bone cyst. The presence of multiple fluid levels** ***(arrows)*** **strongly suggests the correct diagnosis and differentiates this from other pelvic tumors with bone destruction and large soft-tissue abnormality.**

A

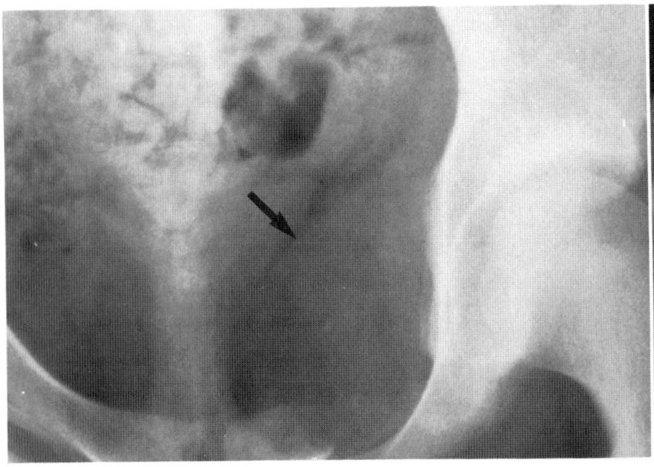

B

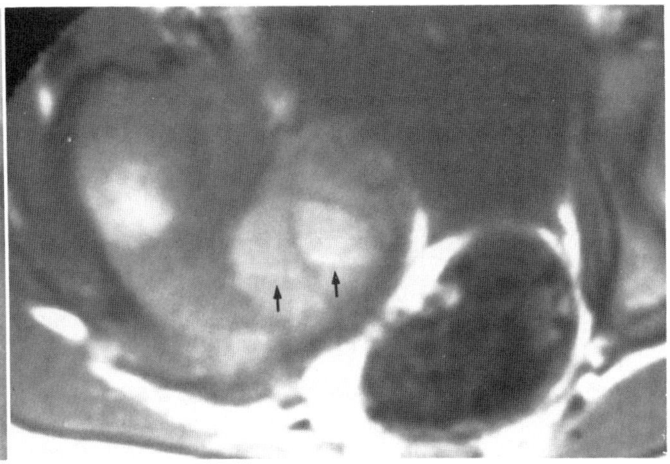

TABLE 7-26

Factors Affecting Prognosis in Ewing Sarcoma

Worse prognosis
- Metastases on initial presentation[1-4]
- Bone metastases rather than lung metastases[1,2]
- Primary tumor in axial skeleton, especially pelvis[1,3,5]
- Tumor volume >100 ml (17% vs. 78% 3-year survival if volume <100 ml)[1,4]
- Poor histologic response to initial chemotherapy[4]

Better prognosis
- Complete surgical resection (74% 5-year survival with resection and 34% without resection)[3,6]
- Primary tumor in hands or feet[7,8]
- No soft-tissue component to the primary tumor[9]

References

1. Miser JS, Triche TJ, Pritchard DJ, et al. Ewing's sarcoma and the nonrhabdomyosarcoma soft tissue sarcomas of childhood. In: Pizzo PA, Poplack DG, eds. Principles and practice of pediatric oncology. Philadelphia: JB Lippincott, 1989:659–688.
2. Miser JS, Kinsella TJ, Triche TJ, et al. Preliminary results of treatment of Ewing's sarcoma of bone in children and young adults: six months of intensive combined modality therapy without maintenance. J Clin Oncol 1988;6:484–490.
3. Sailer SL, Harmon DC, Mankin HJ, et al. Ewings sarcoma: surgical resection as a prognostic factor. Int J Oncol Biol Phys 1988;15:43–57.
4. Jurgens H, Exner U, Gadner H, et al. Multidisciplinary treatment of primary Ewing's sarcoma of bone. Cancer 1988;61:23–32.
5. Kissane JM, Askin FB, Foulkes M, et al. Ewing's sarcoma of bone: clinicopathologic aspects of 303 cases from the intergroup Ewing's sarcoma study. Hum Pathol 1983;14:773–779.
6. Wilkins RM, Pritchard DJ, Burgert EO, et al. Ewing's sarcoma of bone. Experience with 140 patients. Cancer 1986;58:2551–2555.
7. Reinus WR, Gilula LA, Shirley SK, et al. Radiographic appearance of Ewing sarcoma of the hands and feet: report from the intergroup Ewing sarcoma study. AJR 1985;144:331–336.
8. Leeson MC, Smith MJ. Ewing's sarcoma of the foot. Foot & Ankle 1989;10:147–151.
9. Mendenhall CM, Marcus RB, Enneking WF, et al. The prognostic significance of soft tissue extension in Ewing's sarcoma. Cancer 1983;51:913–917.

1970 the survival rate, independent of location, was less than 15 percent[2] (Table 7–27). More recent studies indicate that in patients without metastases on initial presentation overall survival can be expected to be between about 50 and 60 percent, with survival higher in certain specific subgroups of patients.

Therapy for Ewing sarcoma involves surgical procedures, chemotherapy, and radiation therapy.

Unlike osteosarcoma, Ewing sarcoma is very sensitive to radiation therapy and a good local response can be achieved in most patients.[2] Unfortunately, most patients have micrometastasis at the time of diagnosis, so that chemotherapy is required as well as radiation therapy. In addition to achieve local tumor control, very high doses of radiation therapy are required and this may cause significant local deformity and loss of function. Current protocols tend to use initial chemotherapy to shrink the tumor, followed by radiation therapy. This reduces the size of the radiation field. Radiation will be utilized initially in patients with severe symptomatic disease, particularly involving spinal cord compression. Radiation therapy may also be utilized to alleviate pain in metastatic foci of tumor. Imaging is particularly important for the radiotherapist, as accurate delineation of tumor extent by CT, MR, or both helps to ensure that the total tumor is included in the radiation field while helping to minimize radiation to normal tissue.

Surgery was at one time the major therapy for Ewing sarcoma. It was ineffective for two reasons. First, most patients will have micrometastases at the time of presentation. Second, the anatomic location of many Ewing sarcomas means a complete surgical resection is impossible, or even when performed is significantly disfiguring. Present thinking is that amputation is not favored, is never done in the arm, and is done in the leg only in selected patients. Surgery is important in initial diagnosis of the tumor as biopsy is required. Needle biopsy does not provide adequate tissue and open biopsy must be done.[2] Imaging is important in identifying the most direct route to the soft-tissue component of the

TABLE 7-27

Prognosis for Ewing Sarcoma[1-3]

Local therapy alone (pre-1970)
- <15% survival[1]

107 cases 1964–1977
- 35% 5-year survival

Nonmetastatic at diagnosis
- Distal lesions
  - 60–70% 3-year survival[1]
- Proximal (axial) lesions
  - 30–35% 3-year survival[1]
- 1981–1985 study
  - >50% 5-year survival[2]
- Intergroup Ewing's studies
  - 1970s, 56% 3-year survival[1]
  - 1989, 74% alive at 17–80 months[3]

References

1. Miser JS, Triche TJ, Pritchard DJ, et al. Ewing's sarcoma and the nonrhabdomyosarcoma soft tissue sarcomas of childhood. In: Pizzo PA, Poplack DG, eds. Principles and practice of pediatric oncology. Philadelphia: JB Lippincott, 1989:659–688.
2. Jurgens H, Exner U, Gadner H, et al. Multidisciplinary treatment of primary Ewing's sarcoma of bone. Cancer 1988;61:23–32.
3. Munoz A, Madero L, Amaya J, et al. Local control and survival of Ewing's sarcoma in children with radiotherapy and chemotherapy without radical surgery. Acta Oncol 1989;28:245–248.

tumor. Patients are then treated initially with chemotherapy followed by radiation therapy. Subsequent decision whether or not to attempt surgical resection is based on the location of the tumor and the potential loss of function with surgical excision. In sites at which a bone may be sacrificed without causing significant loss of function, e.g., in the fibula, complete surgical excision of the tumor will be performed. In most patients, the primary tumor is, however, not completely excised. Surgery plays no role in the treatment of metastases. In one study of 19 patients, lung metastatic nodules were surgically resected without any improvement in patient prognosis.[3]

Chemotherapy has improved dramatically in the past 20 years. Active agents include cyclophosphamide, doxorubicin, iphosphomide, etoposide, vincristine actinomycin, and bifluorouracil.[2] The early studies with modern chemotherapy were done by the first Intergroup Ewing's Study Group.[2] The results of this large study in patients without original metastatic disease showed that combined chemotherapy was better than a single agent, that doxorubicin improved survival, and that proximally located primary tumors had a worse prognosis than peripheral tumors. The second intergroup study showed that more intensive chemotherapy was of further benefit in patients without metastases on initial presentation. Since then several large studies have shown that varying chemotherapy can result in effective local control and prolonged remissions with reduction in those patients getting metastases. The most recent approach seems to be to utilize initial intensive chemotherapy.[4–6] This enables the initial response of the tumor to chemotherapy to be determined in most patients. This is then followed by local radiation therapy, and, as discussed above, surgical resection in a few selected patients. The objects of this approach are to minimize severe local handicap. Even with this approach local relapse and metastatic relapse still occur, unfortunately.

> *Comment:* Overall prognosis for Ewing sarcoma is still only moderately good.

References

1. O'Connor MI, Pritchard DJ. Ewing's sarcoma. Prognostic factors, disease control, and the reemerging role of surgical treatment. Clin Orthoped Rel Res 1991;262:78–87.
2. Miser JS, Triche TJ, Pritchard DJ, et al. Ewing's sarcoma and the nonrhabdomyosarcoma soft tissue sarcomas of childhood. In: Pizzo PA, Poplack DG, eds. Principles and practice of pediatric oncology. Philadelphia: JB Lippincott, 1989:659–688.
3. Lanza LA, Miser JS, Pass HI, et al. The role of resection in the treatment of pulmonary metastases from Ewing's sarcoma. J Thorac Cardiovasc Surg 1987;94:181–187.
4. Miser JS, Kinsella TJ, Triche TJ, et al. Preliminary results of treatment of Ewing's sarcoma of bone in children and young adults: six months of intensive combined modality therapy without maintenance. J Clin Oncol 1988;6:484–490.
5. Munoz A, Madero L, Amaya J, et al. Local control and survival of Ewing's sarcoma in children with radiotherapy and chemotherapy without radical surgery. Acta Oncol 1989;245–248.
6. Bao BN, Hayes FA, Thompson EI, et al. Chest wall resection for Ewing's sarcoma of the rib: an unnecessary procedure. Ann Thorac Surg 1988;46:40–44.

ADAMANTINOMA[1,2]

Twenty to 25 percent of adamantinoma occurs in children. The youngest reported child is 8 years of age. Over 80 percent occur in the mid shaft of the tibia, where they are identified as a region of multicystic lucency with a periosteal reaction. The appearance on CT and MR is not known. Approximately 15 to 20 percent will show metastases to lymph nodes or lung. Treatment is by wide local excision.

References

1. Spjut HJ, Ayala AG. Skeletal tumors in children and adolescents. Hum Pathol 1983;14:628–642.
2. Dehner LP. Pediatric surgical pathology, 2nd ed. Baltimore: Williams & Wilkins, 1987:1005–1006.

ALVEOLAR SOFT-PART SARCOMA

Alveolar soft-part sarcoma gets its name from its microscopic appearance. It occurs in the age range from 1 to 30 years[1] and is most common in adolescents.[2] The tumor is more common in females than males. In some reports, there is a 2:1 right-sided preference.

The location of the tumor is varied. Approximately one-quarter occur in the head and neck,[3] with this location being more common in children than adults.[1] In the head and neck, the tongue and orbit are favored locations.[1,3,4] Other sites include the limbs.[3,4] Pathologically, these are low-grade, slow-growing soft-tissue tumors with a varied reported incidence of metastases.[3] They are very vascular lesions with early vessel invasion.[3] The cell of origin is not known.[1] Sites of metastasis include lung and bone.[3]

Clinically, the tumors present as slow-growing painless masses.[5] On imaging, they may not be identified on plain film radiograph. Calcification and destruction of adjacent bones may occasionally be identified.[3] On CT scan, they are seen as focal well-defined soft-tissue masses with marked enhancement following contrast administration. Large draining veins may frequently be seen.[3] The MR appearance of these lesions is of a nonspecific soft-tissue mass with signal intensity consistent with prolonged T1 and T2 relaxation times as compared to muscle.[3]

The treatment of these lesions is mainly surgical resection[1] and the prognosis is reasonably good, with an

80 percent 2-year survival.[5] The prognosis is better in children than in adults, in the orbit compared to other locations in the head, and in the head compared to an extremity.[6]

References

1. Simmons WB, Haggerty HS, Ngan B, et al. Alveolar soft part sarcoma of the head and neck. A disease of children and young adults. Int J Pediatr Otorhinolaryngol 1989;17:139–153.
2. Batsakis JG, Manning JT. Soft tissue tumors: unusual forms. Otolaryngol Clin N Am 1986;19:659–683.
3. Lorigan JG, O'Keeffe FN, Evans HL, et al. The radiologic manifestations of alveolar soft-part sarcoma. AJR 1989;153:335–339.
4. Rubinstein MI, Drake AF, McClatchey KD. Alveolar soft part sarcoma of the nasal cavity: report of a case of a review of the literature. Laryngoscope 1988;98:1246–1250.
5. Miser JS, Triche TJ, Pritchard DJ, et al. Ewing's sarcoma and the nonrhabdomyosarcoma soft tissue sarcomas of childhood. In: Pizzo PA, Poplack DG, eds. Principles and practice of pediatric oncology. Philadelphia: JB Lippincott, 1989:659–688.
6. Stringel G, Shandling B, Mancer K, et al. Lipoblastoma in infants and children. J Pediatr Surg 1982;17:277–280.

CHONDROSARCOMA

Epidemiology

Chondrosarcomas are rare in children. Less than 10 percent occur in the pediatric age group. When they do occur in children, it is usually after the age of 10 years.[1–3]

Pathology

The tumors may arise from bone or occur in the soft tissues.[1,2,4] Most of the nonosseous tumors are mesenchymal chondrosarcomas.[1] These mesenchymal chondrosarcomas can rarely arise from the dura, in which case they can grow into large intradural mass, with cord compression.[5] Most, but not all, of the pediatric chondrosarcomas arise de novo and not in a preexisting bone lesion.[6] In one study of 12 chondrosarcomas in children, 10 arose de novo and 2 in an osteochondroma.[7] In another study of chondrosarcomas in 47 children aged between 3 and 16 years, 12 arose in preexisting lesions. Seven of these were solitary osteochondromas, 3 were osteochondromas in patients with multiple lesions, 1 arose in an enchondroma, and 1 in a site of previous radiation therapy.[8] In another study of 12 patients aged between 6 and 20 years,[9] 1 chondrosarcoma arose in an area of previous radiation therapy and 1 in an osteochondroma. The tumors contain hyaline cartilage. They are often lobulated.[1] Calcification is common. Most of the lesions show a low-grade (well-differentiated) histology. In the study of 47 children,[8] 39 had a low-grade histology, only 1 had a high-grade (poorly differentiated) histology, and 7 had an intermediate histology. In this series, metastases were identified in none of the 47 children. The chondrosarcomas, therefore, tend to be well-differentiated tumors with a propensity for local invasion, and metastasis is uncommon.

Clinical Presentation

Clinical signs and symptoms are nonspecific. Pain and a mass lesion are the most common complaints.[9,10] Rarely, other unusual syndromes occur. One 14-year-old child had chondrosarcoma that produced large amounts of heparin, causing coagulation problems. These reversed following resection of the tumor.[11] The diagnosis of chondrosarcoma in a preexisting osteochondroma may be difficult. Signs suggestive of malignancy are an expansion of the cartilaginous cap, rapid change in the appearance of the lesion, or the new development of pain.

Imaging Studies

The radiographic appearance of these lesions varies, with a spectrum ranging from quite benign to malignant. Skeletal lesions occur most commonly in the ribs, skull, and spine and extraskeletal tumors mainly in the head and neck.[12] Calcification, when present, tends to have a granular, stippled appearance unlike that seen with matrix mineralization in osteosarcoma[6,11,12] (Fig. 7–57). The tumors can be quite large[6] (Fig. 7–58). They may occur centrally (Fig. 7–59) or eccentrically (Fig. 7–60) within the bone.[1] Pathological fractures can occur.[7] On plain film radiographs, the lesions may appear lytic[7] or moth eaten,[13] and may have cortical destruction[13] (Fig. 7–59). As previously mentioned, calcification is seen within the soft-tissue parts of the tumor. Chondrosarcomas are not uncommon in the facial area in children.[10] Most tend to occur around the nose, sinuses, and mandible.[10] Other common sites include the pelvis.[9] In the spine, in one study of 10 patients, the lesions all demonstrated cortical destruction with poor margins; a soft-tissue mass was present in 9, and characteristic calcification in 7. Three of the 10 patients had a pathological fracture and invasion of the adjacent vertebra was identified in 7 of 10.[14] On MR, chondrosarcomas with hyaline cartilage can often be differentiated from cartilaginous osteosarcomas, because the latter have a more immature cartilage that does not cause as bright a signal on T2 weighted images[13] (Fig. 7–58). CT shows large, well-defined, lobulated, calcified masses with varying bone changes (Fig. 7–57).

Therapy and Prognosis

Treatment is surgical excision. The prognosis has been reported as ranging from poor[6] to good[8] and depends largely on the histologic differentiation of the primary

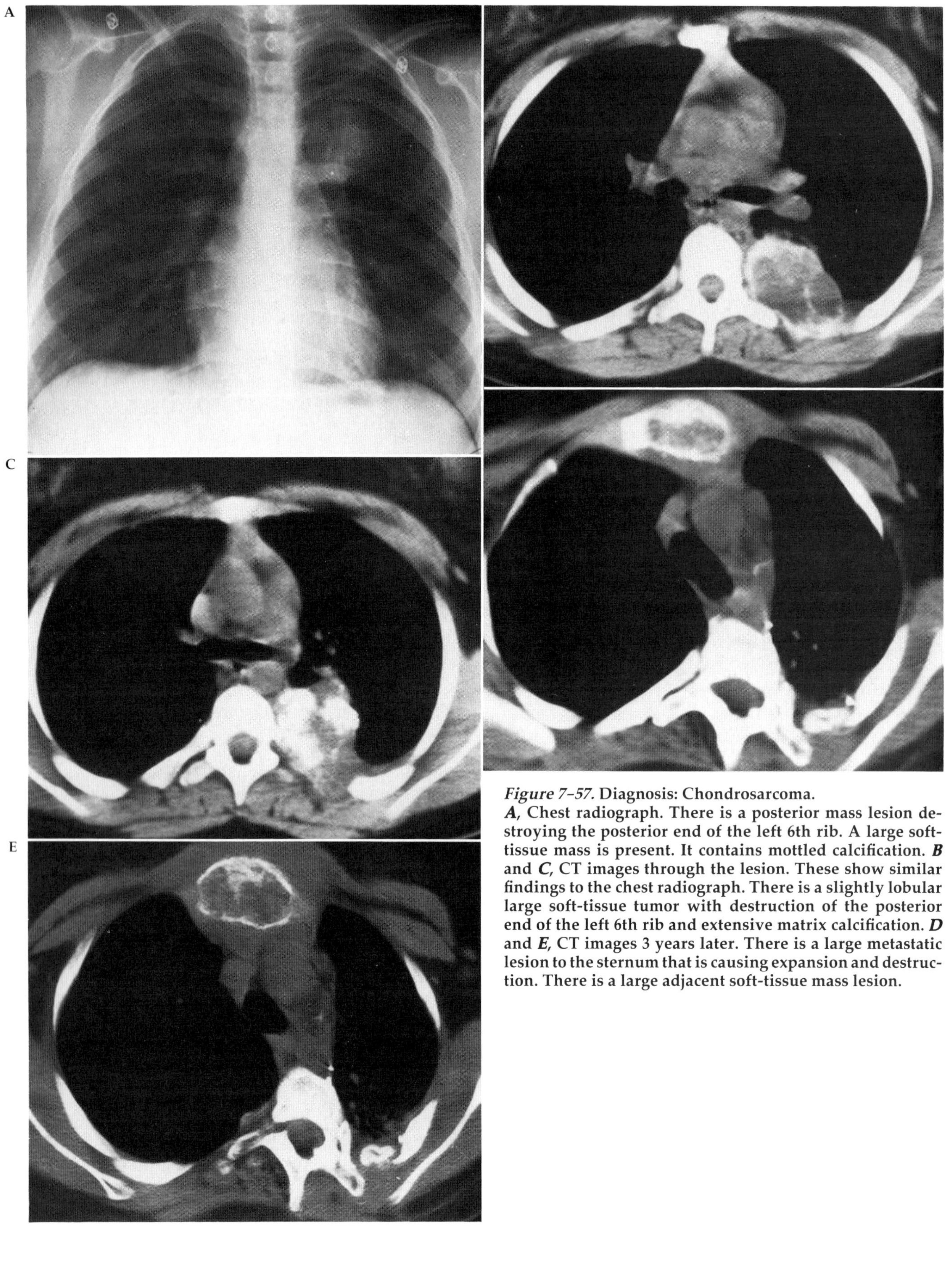

Figure 7–57. Diagnosis: Chondrosarcoma.
A, Chest radiograph. There is a posterior mass lesion destroying the posterior end of the left 6th rib. A large soft-tissue mass is present. It contains mottled calcification. ***B*** and ***C***, CT images through the lesion. These show similar findings to the chest radiograph. There is a slightly lobular large soft-tissue tumor with destruction of the posterior end of the left 6th rib and extensive matrix calcification. ***D*** and ***E***, CT images 3 years later. There is a large metastatic lesion to the sternum that is causing expansion and destruction. There is a large adjacent soft-tissue mass lesion.

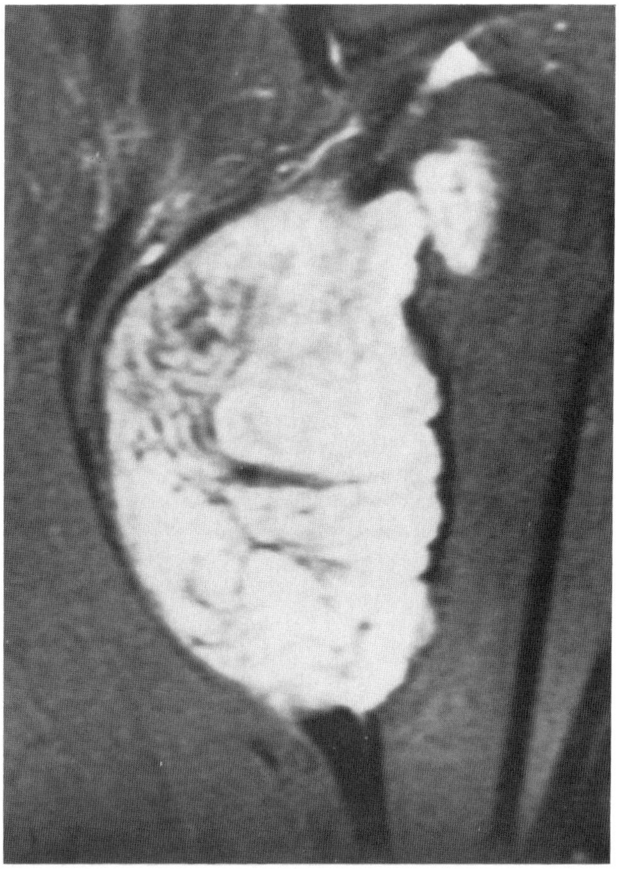

Figure 7-58. Diagnosis: Chondrosarcoma.
MR, T2 weighted image. There is a gigantic tumor arising eccentrically from the lateral aspect of the right femur. The epiphysis is involved. The very bright signal on this T2 weighted image is caused by the presence of extensive hyaline cartilage within the tumor. This is a fairly characteristic appearance. (From Cohen E. Hyaline cartilage origin. Bone and soft tissue neoplasms. Radiology 1988;167:477–481.)

Figure 7-59. Diagnosis: Chondrosarcoma.
A and ***B***, Plain film radiographs in frontal view and with external rotation. There is a lytic lesion in the region of the femoral neck extending into the greater trochanter. The lesion is lobulated. The zone of transition is narrow. There is a pathological fracture through the lesion *(arrow)*. (From Herman G. Case report 541. Skel Radiol 1989;18:241–244.)

A B

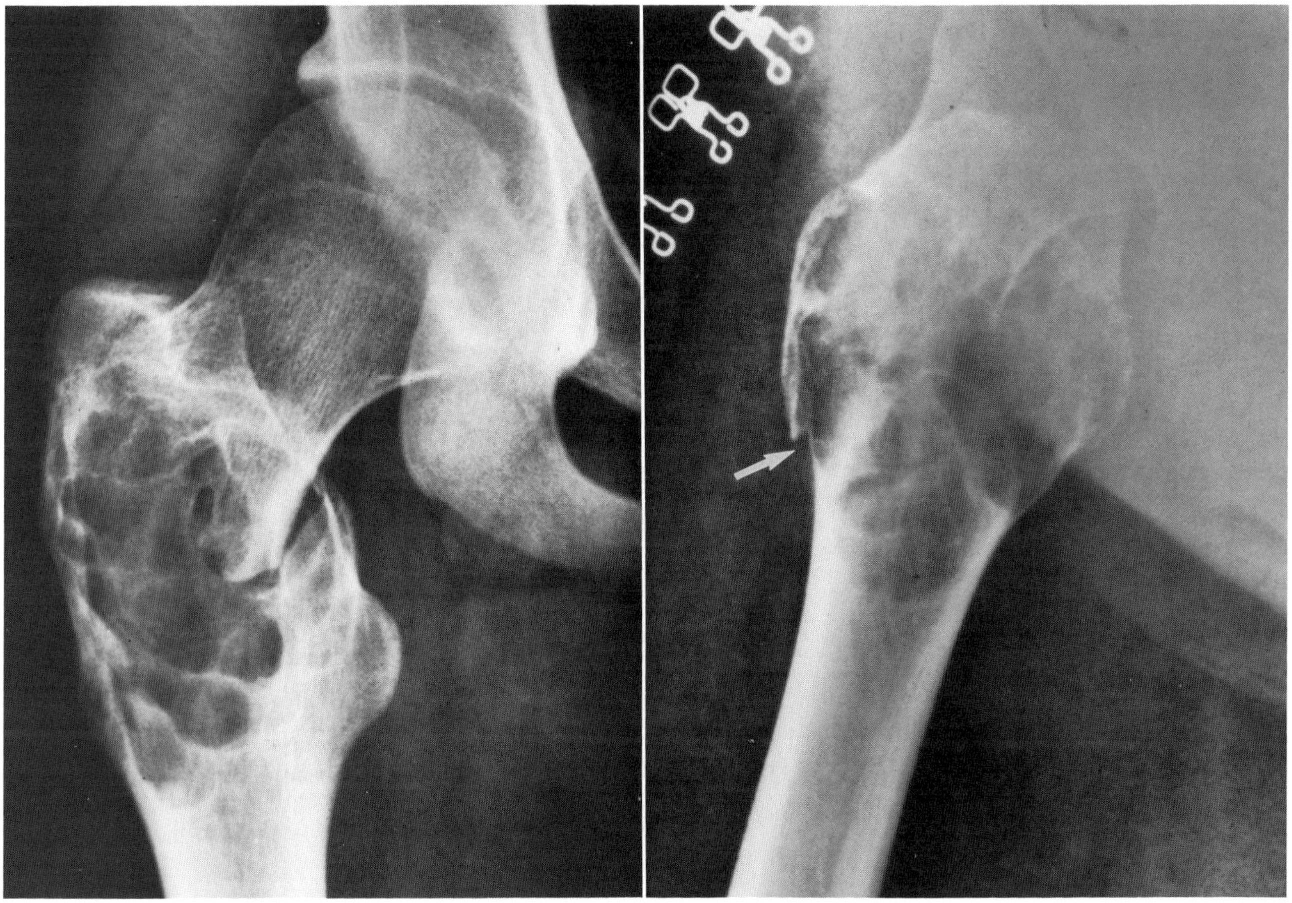

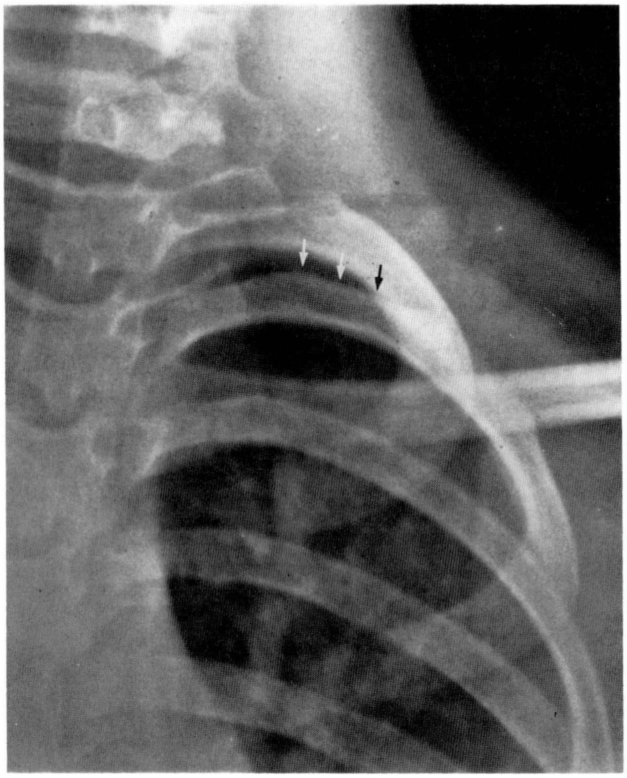

Figure 7-60. **Diagnosis: Chondrosarcoma of left second rib. There is an eccentric lesion arising from the superior aspect of this rib. The abnormality is subtle but distinct destruction of the superior margin of the segment of the involved rib is identified *(arrows).***

tumor. Metastases were not identified in one study of 47 children.[8] In another study of 12 children, metastases occurred on 6 occasions, to the lung in 4 and to bone in 2.[9]

Comment: Chondrosarcomas are usually low-grade lesions. They do occur in children. The best therapy is complete resection. Imaging, particularly MR and CT, are extremely important in defining accurately the total extent of the lesion prior to surgical resection.[16]

References

1. Spjut HJ, Ayala AG. Skeletal tumors in children and adolescents. Hum Pathol 1983;14:628–642.
2. Jakacki R, Knisely A. Chondrosarcoma. Med Pediatr Oncol 1990;18:61–63.
3. Dehner LP. Pediatric surgical pathology, 2nd ed. Baltimore: Williams & Wilkins, 1987:986–990.
4. Hachitanda Y, Tsuneyoshi M, Daimaru Y, et al. Extraskeletal myxoid chondrosarcoma in young children. Cancer 1988;61:2521–2526.
5. Lorigan JG, Libshitz HI, Peuchot M. Radiation-induced sarcoma of bone: CT findings in 19 cases. AJR 1989;153:791–794.
6. Moser RP, Madewell JE. An approach to primary bone tumors. Radiol Clin N Am 1987;25:1049–1093.
7. Hermann G, Wagner LD, Klein MJ, et al. Skeletal Radiol 1989;18:241–244.
8. Young CL, Sim FH, Unni KK, et al. Case report 559. Skeletal Radiol 1989;18:403–405.
9. Aprin H, Risenborough EJ, Hall JE. Chondrosarcoma in children and adolescents. Clin Orthop Rel Res 1982;166:226–232.
10. Meyer C, Hauck KW, Gonzalez C. Chondrosarcoma of the facial skeleton in a child. Otolaryngol 1989;101:591–594.
11. Kaufman RA, Towbin RB, Ball WS, et al. Pediatric case of the day. RadioGraphics 1987;7:597–598.
12. Hernandez R, Heidelberger KP, Poznanski AK. Case report 63. Skeletal Radiol 1978;3:61–63.
13. Laissy JP, Guillon F, Chesneau AM, et al. Chondromyxosarcoma: a rare form of bone neoplasm in children. Pediatr Radiol 1987;17:429–431.
14. Shives TC, McLeod RA, Unni KK, et al. Chondrosarcoma of the spine. J Bone Joint Surg 1989;71:1158–1165.
15. Nurenberg P, Harms SE. Magnetic resonance imaging of musculoskeletal tumors. CRC 1988;28:331–338.
16. Sen CN, Sekhar LN, Schramm VL, et al. Chordoma and chondrosarcoma of the cranial base: an 8-year experience. Neurosurgery 1989;25:931–941.

CLEAR CELL SARCOMA[1]

Clear cell sarcoma is a soft-tissue malignant tumor. In one study of 27 patients, 11 were under the age of 20 years. The tumor occurs in close association with tendons and aperneurosis and is especially common in the hands and feet. Histologic diagnosis is made by identification of a clear cytoplasm. Local recurrence is common following surgical resection and local lymph node metastasis may occur. Distant metastases are rare. Imaging shows a nonspecific soft-tissue mass. Treatment is surgical excision.

Reference

1. Eckardt JJ, Pritchard DJ, Soule EH. Clear cell sarcoma. A clinicopathologic study of 27 cases. Cancer 1983;52:1482–1488.

FIBROSARCOMA[1–4]

Fibrosarcoma can occasionally occur in children. Most cases occur under the age of 2 years (even in the newborn) and there is an additional peak in the age range 10 to 15 years.[4] In children, 70 percent of the lesions occur in the limbs. They grow rapidly and may metastasize. In one study, late metastases developed in 2 of 8 patients.[1] Radiographically, plain film findings are predominantly of a destructive bone lesion that appears lucent and large adjacent soft-tissue mass.[4]

The differential diagnosis includes aggressive fibromatosis, myositis, and nodular fasciitis. Treatment is wide surgical excision. Local recurrence can occur repeatedly for many years.[4]

References
1. Spjut HJ, Ayala AG. Skeletal tumors in children and adolescents. Hum Pathol 1983;14:628–642.
2. Salloum E, Flamant F, Caillaud JM, et al. Diagnostic and therapeutic problems of soft tissue tumors other than rhabdomyosarcoma in infants under 1 year of age: a clinicopathological study of 34 cases treated at the Institut Gustave-Roussy. Med Pediatr Oncol 199018:37–43.
3. Miser JS, Triche TJ, Pritchard DJ, et al. Ewing's sarcoma and the nonrhabdomyosarcoma soft tissue sarcomas of childhood. In: Pizzo PA Poplack DG, eds. Principles and practice of pediatric oncology. Philadelphia: JB Lippincott, 1989:659–688.
4. Faure C, Gruner M, Boccon-Gibod L. Case report 149. Skeletal Radiol 1981;6:208–211.

HEMANGIOPERICYTOMA

Epidemiology

Hemangiopericytoma was first described in 1942.[1] It can occur in adults or children.[2] Approximately 10 to 15% of these tumors occur in children,[3] and boys are more commonly affected than girls.[3] When hemangiopericytomas occur in children, they are frequently congenital.[4]

Pathology

Hemangiopericytomas arise from pericytes. These cells normally form the outer layer of all capillaries and are contractile.[1–3,5] There is marked variability in the histologic appearance[4] and the lesions may be benign or malignant. It is frequently difficult to predict the degree of malignancy from the microscopic evaluation. In general, congenital hemangiopericytomas are more likely to be benign.[3,4,6] They can occur anywhere in the body, including bone, soft tissue, or organs.[7] In infants, they are often subcutaneous, this being the finding in 6 cases.[6] They may show very rapid growth.[6] About one-half of all the lesions occur in the extremities.[1,2,5] The head and neck, in children, are also not uncommon locations, being found in 11 of 31 children in one study.[4] Metastases most commonly go to lung.[1] The next most common site is bone.[2,3,8] Primary tumors in the abdomen may metastasize to the liver.[2]

Clinical Presentation

The clinical presentation is very varied and depends to a large extent on the anatomic location of the tumor. For example, soft-tissue tumors present as painless masses.[5] Pain in all locations is rare.[1,4] In the thorax, the lesions may cause tracheal compression and respiratory distress.[3] Occasional cases are reported as presenting with hypoglycemia.

Imaging Studies

Plain film radiograph of bone, when involved, shows a predominantly lytic and nonspecific abnormality.[5] Soft-tissue tumors may be seen as nonspecific masses. Ultrasound in 9 patients reported in 2 studies[5,8] showed the lesions to be cystic, mixed, or solid. Even the solid lesions had relatively low echoes. The lesions are all heterogeneous in appearance and always have well-defined margins.

CT in 3 patients showed tumors with well-defined margins. The lesions generally enhance with contrast apart from central areas of necrosis.[8] They are located in any part of the body. Calcification may be present.[5] It tends to be speckled.[11] The reported incidence of calcification ranges from 1 to 70 percent.[8] MR imaging has been reported as showing some increased signal intensity compared to muscle on T1 weighted images and more marked increased signal intensity on T2 weighted images. The appearance is nonspecific. CT identified calcification in one lung metastasis in an adult.[9] Angiography when performed shows a very classic appearance[5,10] with radially arranged branching of the feeder vessels inside the tumor and a persistent uniform blush (Fig. 7–61).

Differential Diagnosis

Differential diagnosis includes any soft-tissue malignancy. Histologically, glomus tumor and angioma may look similar and need to be excluded.[1]

Therapy and Prognosis

Treatment is by wide local resection[1] and careful follow-up for development of metastases.

Figure 7–61. **Diagnosis: Hemangiopericytoma. Angiogram. A small lesion is identified. It overlies the left clavicle. There is an abundance of abnormal vessels seen within the tumor *(arrows)*. These are arranged in a fairly classic radial pattern.**

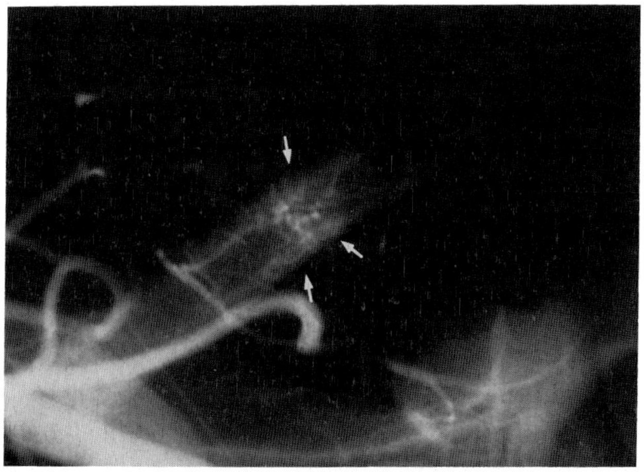

References
1. Pitluk HC, Conn J. Hemangiopericytoma. Am J Surg 1979;137:413–417.
2. Auguste L-J, Razack MS, Sako K. Hemangiopericytoma. J Surg Oncol 1982;20:260–264.
3. Atkinson JB, Mahour GH, Isaacs H, et al. Hemangiopericytoma in infants and children. A report of six patients. Am J Surg 1984;148:372–377.
4. Kauffman SL, Stout AP. Hemangiopericytoma in children. Cancer 1960;13:695–699.
5. Grant EG, Gronvall S, Sarosi TE, et al. Sonographic findings in four cases of hemangiopericytoma. Correlation with computed tomographic, angiographic, and pathologic findings. Radiology 1982;142:447–451.
6. Salloum E, Flamant F, Caillaud JM, et al. Diagnostic and therapeutic problems of soft tissue tumors other than rhabdomyosarcoma in infants under 1 year of age: a clinicopathological study of 34 cases treated at the Institut Gustave-Roussy. Med Pediatr Oncol 1990;18:37–43.
7. Moser RP, Madewell JE. An approach to primary bone tumors. Radiol Clin N Am 1987;25:1049–1093.
8. Lorigan JG, David CL, Evans HL, et al. The clinical and radiologic manifestations of hemangiopericytoma. AJR 1989;153:345–349.
9. Alpern MB, Thorsen MK, Kellman GM, et al. CT appearance of hemangiopericytoma. J Comput Assist Tomogr 1986;10:264–267.
10. Yaghmai I. Angiographic manifestations of soft-tissue and osseous hemangiopericytomas. Radiology 1978; 126:653–659.

LIPOSARCOMA

Liposarcoma is a very rare tumor in children. In a report of one case and a review of 56 other cases in the literature, the tumor was described, in children, to have age peaks at 1 and 13 years. Two-thirds of the patients were male. Liposarcomas are most common in the extremities, with 50 percent of tumors occurring in this location. Ten percent are mediastinal. Imaging, particularly CT and MR, show soft-tissue tumors in which the presence of fat can be accurately determined. Treatment is surgical excision. Local recurrence is common. The overall prognosis is good.[1,2]

References
1. Castleberry RP, Kelly DR, Wilson ER, et al. Childhood liposarcoma. Report of a case and review of the literature. Cancer 1984;54:579–584.
2. Chung EB, Enzinger FM. Benign lipoblastomatosis. An analysis of 35 cases. Cancer 1973;32:482–492.

LIPOBLASTOMATOSIS[1–3]

Lipoblastomatosis does occur in children, who are almost always young, with 88 percent of 35 patients being under 3 years of age. In a literature review of 56 patients,[1] all were under the age of 8 years. Most of the tumors are found in the extremities.[1,3] Fifty-five percent occur under the age of 1 year. They are three times more common in males than females.[3] The tumors tend to recur locally but metastases are extremely rare. Two-thirds are well circumscribed and superficial, and one-third tend to be more diffuse and infiltrating and lie deeper within the soft tissues.[1] Histologically, the tumors arise from embryonal fat. They can grow very rapidly. Imaging identifies a soft-tissue tumor mass, which may be well or poorly defined (Figs. 7–62 and 7–63). CT and MR will both accurately identify fat within the tumor (Figs. 7–62 and 7–63). Calcification does not occur.[3]

Treatment is surgical excision. Recurrence, if it occurs, usually does so within a year. Prognosis is very good.

References
1. Chung EB, Enzinger FM. Benign lipoblastomatosis. An analysis of 35 cases. Cancer 1973;32:482–492.
2. Goslee L, Clermont V, Bernstein J, et al. Superficial connective tissue tumors in early infancy. A study of fibromatosis and lipoblastomatosis. J Pediatr 1964;65:377–387.
3. Stringel G, Shandling B, Mancer K, et al. Lipoblastoma in infants and children. J Pediatr Surg 1982;17:277–280.

Figure 7-62. **Diagnosis: Lipoblastoma.**
MR, T1 weighted image. There is a large tumor mass *(arrows)* adjacent to the lower femur. The entire lesion contains patchy areas of very high signal intensity consistent with the presence of fat. (Although hemorrhage may give a similar bright signal, it would not be expected to have such a diffusely nodular appearance.)

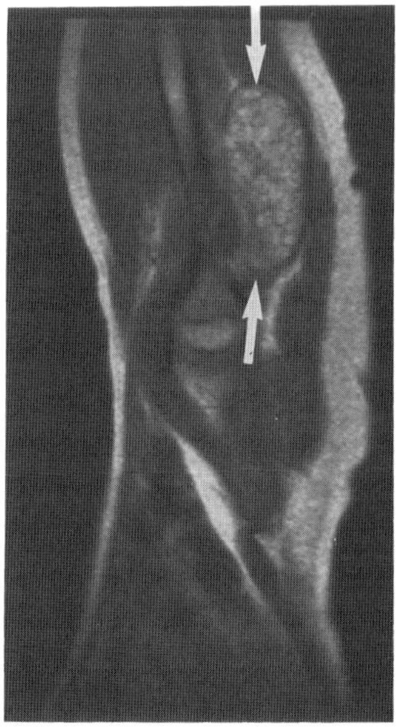

A

B

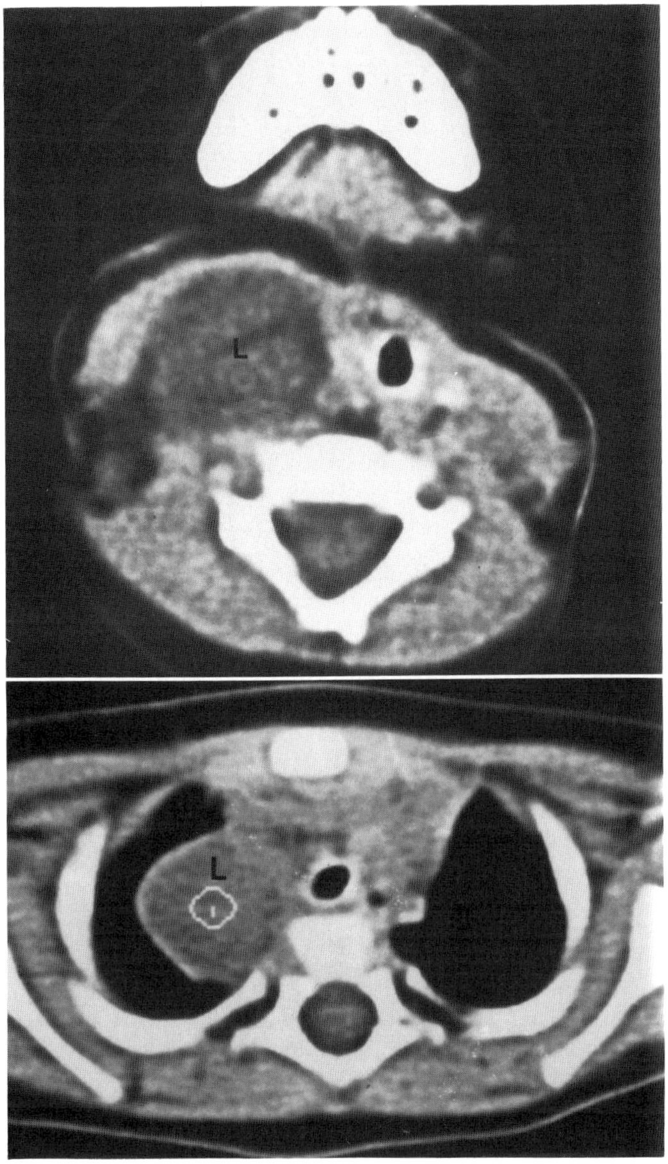

Figure 7-63. **Diagnosis: Lipoblastoma.**
***A* and *B*, CT images through the neck and upper thorax. There is a large well-defined lipoblastoma (*L*). It is displacing the trachea in the neck. The density is less than that of muscle but greater than that of subcutaneous fat. The reason the density is not the same as subcutaneous fat is that in addition to containing fat the tumor had a mucoid matrix. This lesion could easily be mistaken for a cystic hygroma.**

MALIGNANT FIBROUS HISTIOCYTOMA[1–6]

Twenty-five percent of malignant fibrous histiocytoma tumors are found in children. Most occur in adolescents, with a mean age of about 13 years.[1] They can, however, occur at any age, having been identified in the newborn. They may be found within bone or in the soft tissues. Histologically, they can contain fibrogenic cells and cells that resemble histiocytes.[1,4]

If metastases occur, the lung is the most common site. Metastases have also been identified in bone, lymph nodes, and liver.[5,6]

In the bone, the metaphyses around the knee are the most common sites.[3,4] The tumor is seen as a lytic lesion involving the medulla, cortex, and soft tissue. In one study, there was no soft-tissue calcification and no periosteal reaction,[3] while in another study, periosteal reaction was identified in 5 of 20 patients. There is a fairly wide spectrum of appearance on plain film radiograph.

In the soft tissue, the tumors are seen as nodular subcutaneous masses that are frequently hemorrhagic. On CT or MR imaging, they are seen as nonspecific soft-tissue tumor masses with a nonhomogeneous appearance because of hemorrhage (Figs. 7–64 and 7–65). The prognosis seems to be varied.

References

1. Enzinger FM. Angiomatoid malignant fibrous histiocytoma. A distinct fibrohistiocytic tumor of children and young adults simulating a vascular neoplasm. Cancer 1979;44:2147–2157.
2. Spjut HJ, Ayala AG. Skeletal tumors in children and adolescents. Hum Pathol 1983;14:628–642.
3. Dehner LP. Pediatric surgical pathology, 2nd ed. Baltimore: Williams & Wilkins, 1987:905, 1002.
4. Dahlin DC, Unni KK, Matsuno T. Malignant (fibrous) histiocytoma of bone—fact or fancy? Cancer 1977;39:1508–1516.
5. Raney RB, Allen A, O'Neill J, et al. Malignant fibrous histiocytoma of soft tissue in childhood. Cancer 1986;57:2198–2201.
6. Feldman F, Norman D. Intra- and extraosseous malignant histiocytoma (malignant fibrous xanthoma). Radiology 1972;104:497–508.

MELANOTIC NEUROECTODERMAL TUMOR[1–5]

Melanotic neuroectodermal tumors are rare, occurring in the head and neck and less commonly in the genitals.[1,2,5] They arise from neural crest cells.[5] They may occur around the maxilla but are most typically located in the region of the anterior fontanelle,[3,4] where they invade bone and dura. They cause expansion of the diploic space of the bone and they then spread into the soft tissues. Plain film may show a spiculated periosteal reaction perpendicular to the bone with some destruction; adjacent sutures may be wide and sclerotic. CT and MR will show the soft-tissue component of the tumor mass.[5] CT in one case showed a dense extradural mass, with homogenous enhancement; the tumor extended

A B

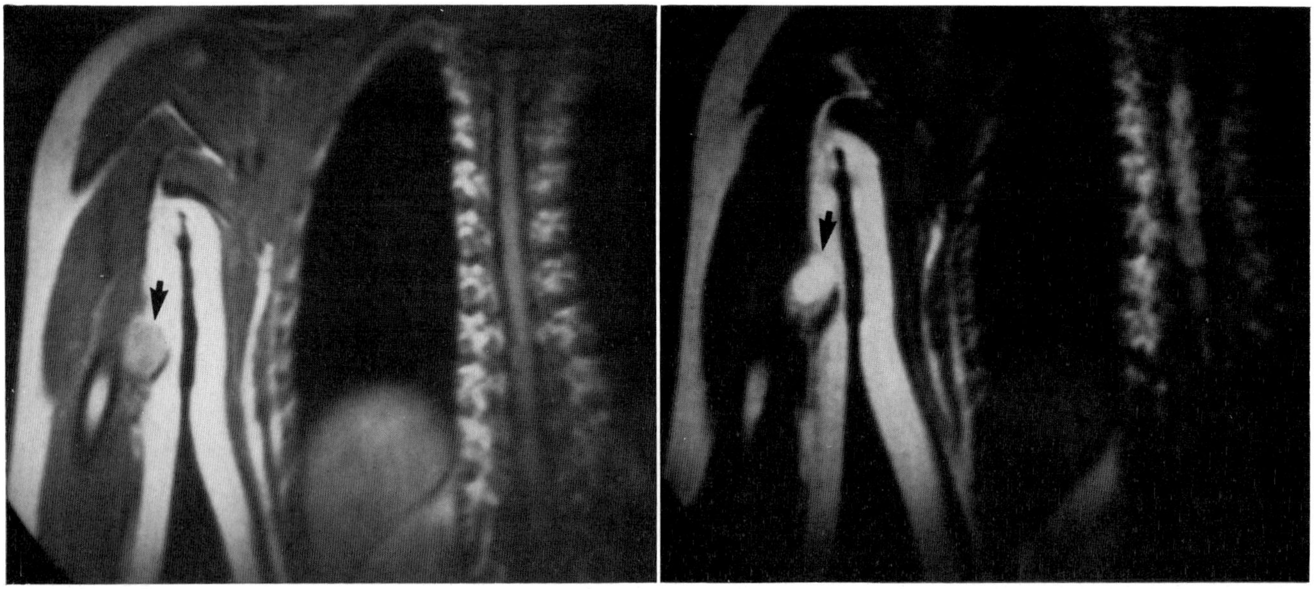

Figure 7-64. **Diagnosis: Malignant fibrous histiocytoma.**
***A* and *B*, MR, coronal spin density and T2 weighted images. There is a soft-tissue mass on the medial aspect of the right upper arm *(arrows)*. It is of moderate signal intensity on the spin density image. On the T2 weighted image the center of the lesion is much brighter than the rim, possibly indicating the presence of hemorrhage.**

into the anterior fontanelle and the adjacent sutures were wide and sclerotic.[5] MDP bone scan will be "hot."[5] Treatment is surgical excision. These tumors tend to recur locally and may not metastasize. In a review of 110 cases, local recurrence was common, but no metastasis occurred.[3]

References

1. Arthur RJ, Brunelle F. Computerised tomography in the evaluation of expansile lesions arising from the skull vault in childhood—a report of 5 cases. Pediatr Radiol 1988;18:294–301.
2. Dehner LP. Pediatric surgical pathology, 2nd ed. Baltimore: Williams & Wilkins, 1987:913, 1066.
3. Bignold LP, Nicks R. Melanotic neuroectodermal tumour of infancy arising in anterior fontanelle. Pathology 1980;12:473–477.
4. Gilmore RL, Mealey J. Melanotic neuroectodermal tumor involving the cranium in infancy. J Neurosurg 1972;36:507–511.
5. Atkinson GO, Davis PC, Patrick LE, et al. Melanotic neuroectodermal tumor of infancy. MR findings and a review of the literature. Pediatr Radiol 1989;20:20–22.

MESENCHYMOMA (Mesenchymal Hamartoma)

Mesenchymoma is, strictly speaking, a benign tumor but is included because it may mimic malignancy. The tumor always arises in the chest wall.[1–4] It is a congenital tumor of mesenchymal origin.[2,6] Histologically, the tumor has two or more cell types, all of mesenchymal origin. Symptoms are the detection of a chest wall mass, chest deformity, or respiratory distress. In one series, 5 of 9 patients had dyspnea.[3]

Chest radiograph shows a very large mass that can fill an entire hemithorax. The lesions are usually fairly well defined.[6] Calcification can usually be identified within the mass,[2] and it was identified in 8 of 9 patients in one series.[3] Rib abnormality is always present and tumor usually affects several ribs[3,4] (Fig. 7–66). The ribs are deformed and some may be destroyed.[3,4] The tumors are usually single, but there is one report of two separate lesions occurring in the same patient, one of 7 cm diameter and one of 2 cm diameter.[7] CT shows a large soft-tissue mass with calcium: cystic areas with fluid levels may be identified. MR similarly will show these findings and may characterize the presence of blood within the lesion. The destruction and displacement of the ribs will be better identified on CT than MR. MDP study performed in one patient with two tumors showed uptake of the radioisotope in bone and in the soft-tissue component of both tumors.[5] The differential diagnosis includes chest wall masses in the soft tissues (desmoid, hamartoma, hemangioma, hygroma, synovioma, mesenchymoma, rhabdomyosarcoma), ribs (sarcoma, histiocytosis, metastasis, osteochondroma), or extrapleural tissues (mesenchymoma, rhabdomyosarcoma, chloroma, lymphoma).[8] These tumors do not metastasize and treatment is local resection.

References

1. Schlesinger AE, Smith MB, Genez BM, et al. Chest wall mesenchymoma (hamartoma) in infancy. CT and MR findings. Pediatr Radiol 1989;19:212–213.

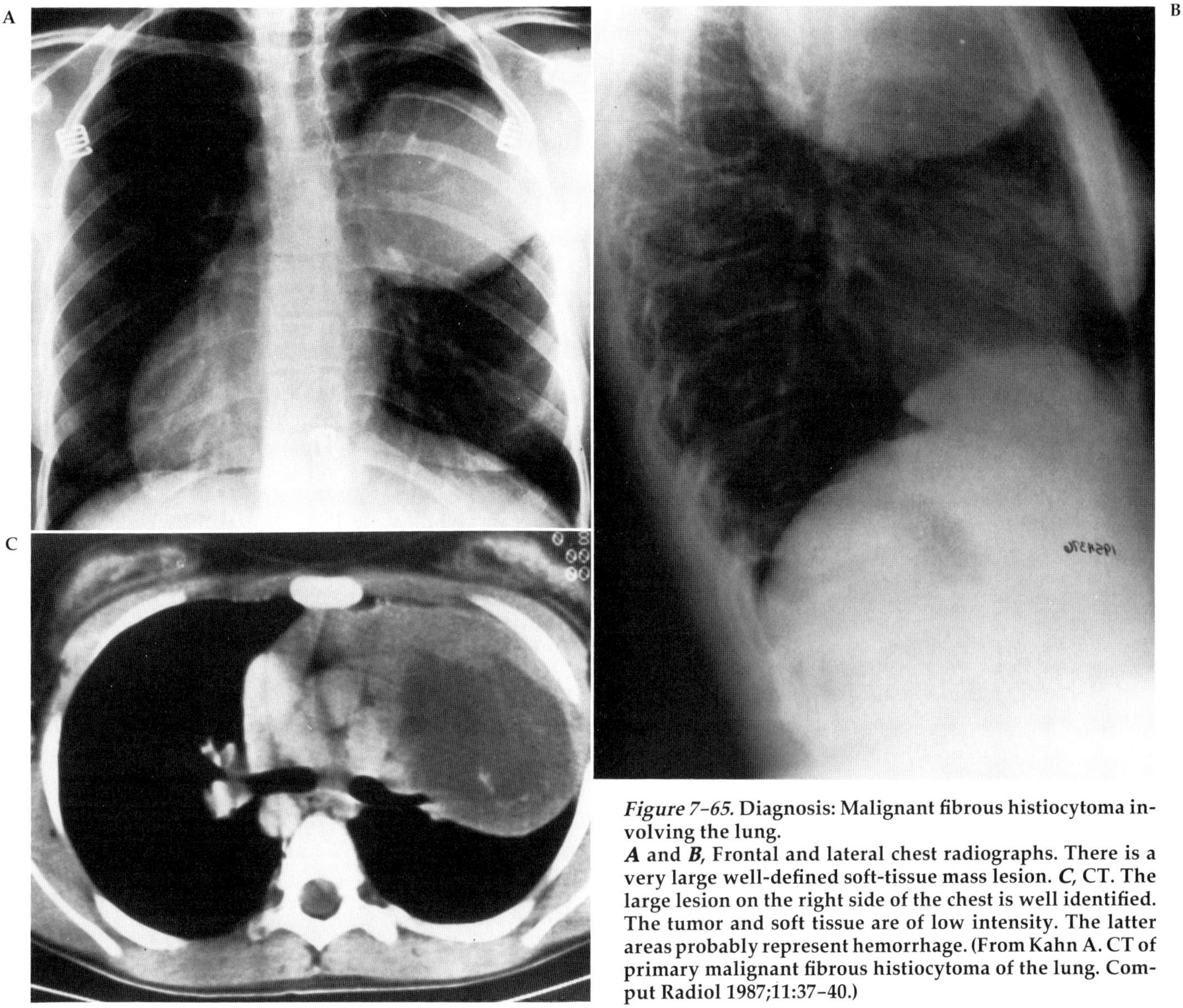

Figure 7-65. **Diagnosis: Malignant fibrous histiocytoma involving the lung.**
A **and** ***B*****, Frontal and lateral chest radiographs. There is a very large well-defined soft-tissue mass lesion.** ***C*****, CT. The large lesion on the right side of the chest is well identified. The tumor and soft tissue are of low intensity. The latter areas probably represent hemorrhage. (From Kahn A. CT of primary malignant fibrous histiocytoma of the lung. Comput Radiol 1987;11:37–40.)**

2. Blumenthal BI, Capitanio MA, Queloz JM, et al. Intrathoracic mesenchymoma. Observations in two infants. Radiology 1972;104:107–109.
3. McLeod RA, Dahlin DC. Hamartoma (mesenchymoma) of the chest wall in infancy. Radiology 1979;131:657–661.
4. Oakley RH, Carty H, Cudmore RE. Multiple benign mesenchymomata of the chest wall. Pediatr Radiol 1985;15:58–60.
5. Miser JS, Kinsella TJ, Triche TJ, et al. Treatment of peripheral neuroepithelioma in children and young adults. J Clin Oncol 1987;5:1752–1758.
6. Dehner LP. Pediatric surgical pathology, 2nd ed. Baltimore: Williams & Wilkins, 1987:924.
7. Bignold LP, Nicks R. Melanotic neuroectodermal tumour of infancy arising in anterior fontanelle. Pathology 1980;12:473–477.
8. Franken EA, Smith JA, Smith WL. Tumors of the chest wall in infants and children. Pediatr Radiol 1977;6:13–18.

PRIMITIVE NEUROECTODERMAL TUMOR (PNET)

PNETs of the central nervous system are discussed in Chapter 8. This section discusses PNETs in all other locations.

Epidemiology

In various series, the mean age of patients with PNET has been reported as 14½ years,[1] 9 years,[2] 14 years,[3,4] and 15 years.[5] Different series have reported the tumor being more common in females[1] or more common in males.[4,5]

A B

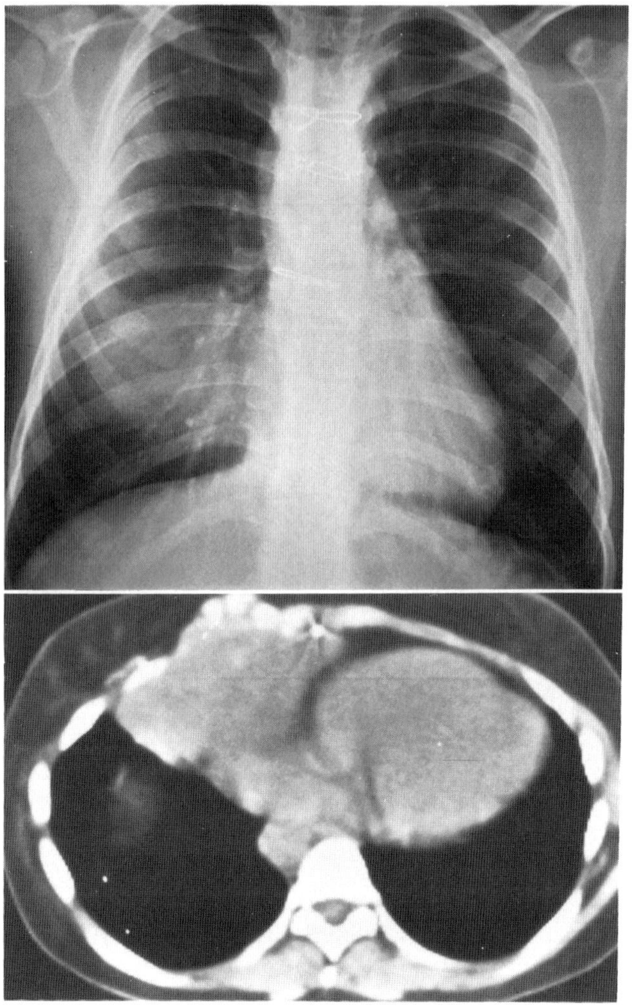

Figure 7-66. **Diagnosis: Mesenchymoma.**
***A*, Chest radiograph. There is a nonspecific mass lesion overlying the right lower chest. The patient had had prior surgery for an unassociated congenital heart lesion. *B*, CT. This shows a moderate-sized mass lesion involving the anterior lower right rib ends, with several ribs deformed and destroyed.**

Pathology

The tumor can occur in bones or soft tissues. The tumors are undifferentiated small round cell sarcomas. The lesions must be differentiated from other tumors with small round cells, including neuroblastoma, rhabdomyosarcoma, lymphoma, and Ewing sarcoma. The greatest difficulty arises in differentiating these tumors from Ewing sarcoma. Table 7–28 summarizes the most important differentiating features. PNETs have a pattern of lobular rosettes on light microscopy,[4–7] and show the presence of neural elements (granules, tubules, and phlegmons) on electron microscopy,[4–6,8,9] and of neuron specific enolase within the tumor cells.[4,6] Ewing sarcoma demonstrates none of these features.

TABLE 7–28
Differences between PNET and Ewing Sarcoma

	PNET	Ewing
Lobular rosettes	Yes	No
Presence of neural elements on electron microscopy	Yes	No
Presence of neuron specific enolase in tumor cells	Yes	No

Triche[7] introduces a very helpful concept and states that Ewing sarcoma and PNET represent two ends of a spectrum of peripheral neural tumors. He believes that Ewing sarcoma also arises from a neural cell. At one end of the spectrum Ewing sarcoma is the most undifferentiated of the tumors. PNET lies at the other end of the spectrum. While most of the tumors have features permitting easy characterization as either Ewing or PNET, he emphasizes that a number of tumors will show features of both and suggests that these be called atypical Ewing sarcoma.[7] He also believes that many so-called nonosseous Ewing tumors are probably PNETs (or undifferentiated rhabdomyosarcomas). Neuroepitheliomas are also probably PNETs. Metastases occur to lung, bone, marrow, liver, adrenal, sympathetic chain, brain, and other sites.[10,11] "Askin" tumors are PNETs involving the chest wall.

Clinical Presentation

The symptoms from PNET vary depending mainly on its location. In the limbs, the soft-tissue tumors may present as a mass, which can frequently be quite large. These tumors can occur in any site. They have been described in the arm,[11] leg,[6] thorax,[1] abdomen or pelvis,[4] or in the psoas muscle.[12] When they occur in bone, the leg is the most common location,[5] followed by the pelvis and humerus. Large chest lesions may cause cough or dyspnea.[8,13] Systemic symptoms including fever and weight loss are not uncommon, occurring in up to 55 percent of patients.[5]

Imaging Studies

Plain film radiographs may or may not show soft-tissue lesions in the limbs. In the chest, large masses are seen in the chest wall, with an intra- or extrathoracic component[1] (Figs. 7–67 and 7–68). An associated pleural effusion is often present and the tumor may extend into the pleura.[1] The underlying lung may be collapsed or even invaded by the tumor.[1] Rib destruction occurred in 5 of 20 patients and mediastinum or hilar lymph node involvement was identified in 2 of 20 patients.[1] In another series of chest wall lesions, periosteal reaction in

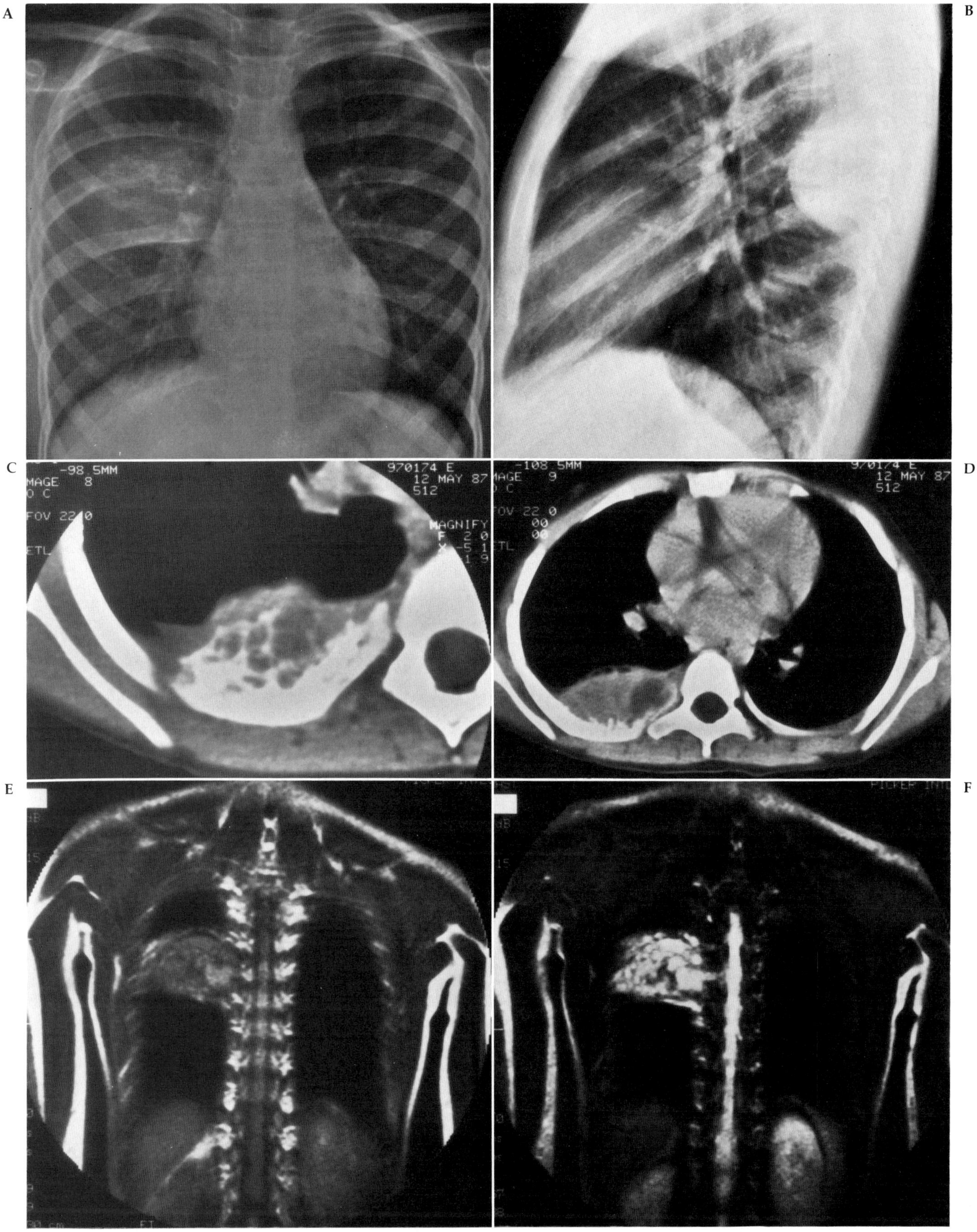

Figure 7–67. Diagnosis: Primitive neuroectodermal tumor of chest (Askin tumor).
A and ***B***, PA and lateral radiograph. The frontal view shows extensive destruction of the posterior aspect of the right 6th rib with an adjacent soft-tissue mass lesion. On the lateral film, the soft-tissue component of the tumor appears well defined. ***C*** and ***D***, CT scan through the tumor. The tumor is causing expansion and destruction of the rib. There is a moderate-sized soft-tissue component to the tumor. ***E*** and ***F***, MR, T1 and T2 weighted images. The tumor is of similar intensity to muscle on T1 and very bright on T2 weighted images. The very nonhomogeneous appearance of the lesion is caused by the extensive calcification scattered throughout it.

A B C D

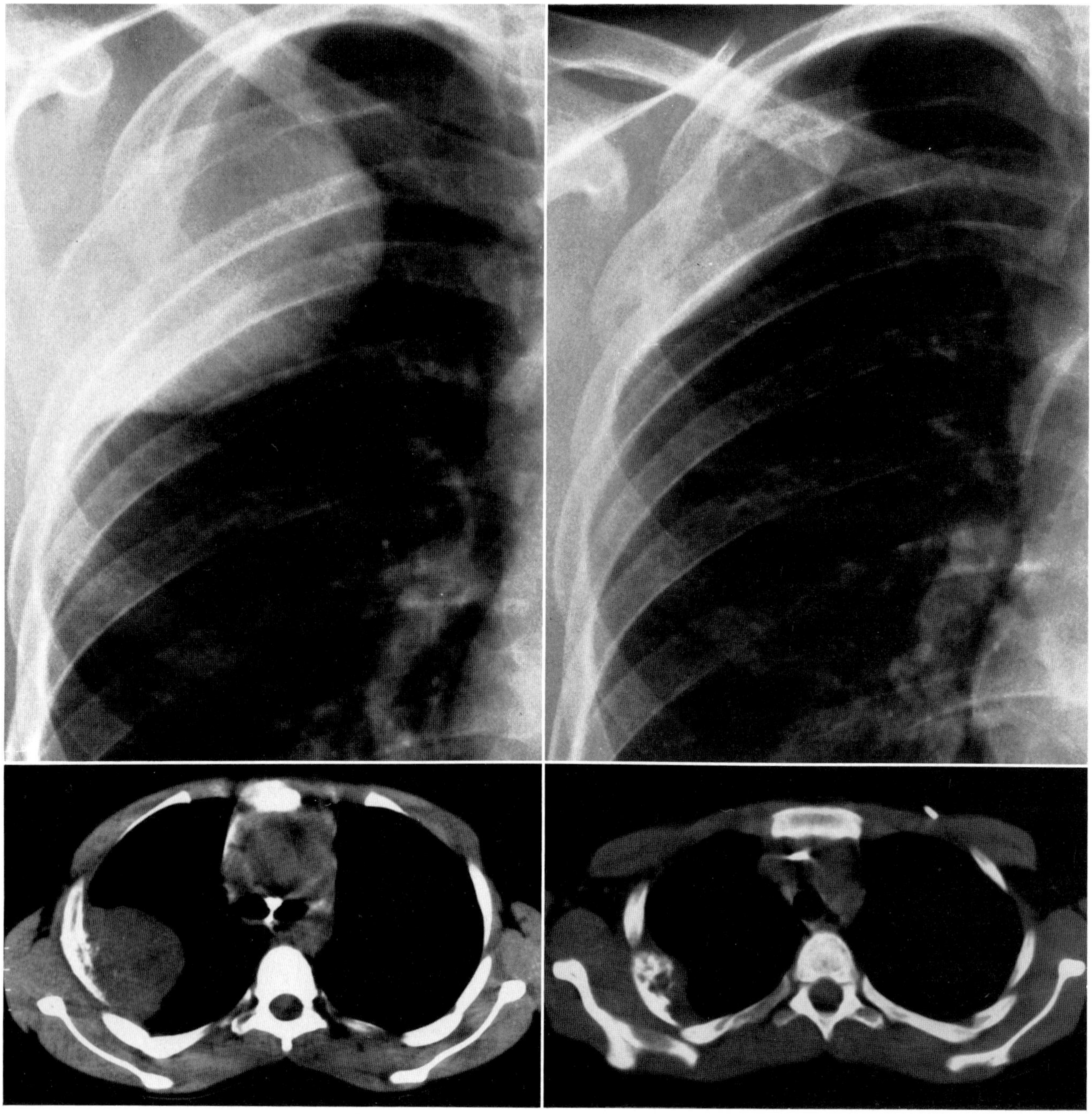

Figure 7-68. **Diagnosis: Primitive neuroectodermal tumor of rib. Response to chemotherapy. *A* and *B*, Chest radiograph and CT. These show a lesion causing destruction of the posterolateral aspect of the right third rib. There is a large soft-tissue component to the tumor. *C* and *D*, Chest radiograph and CT following chemotherapy. There is marked reduction in the size of the soft-tissue component. The areas of rib destruction show a more homogenous consolidated appearance.**

the rib was identified in 4 of 5 patients. An MDP bone scan was positive in 3 of 5 patients. Calcification was identified in none of the 5 tumors. In 10 patients with chest wall tumors, rib changes were seen in 6 and pleural changes in 2.[10] Plain film radiographs in the long bones or flat bones show lesions similar to Ewing sarcoma, with a tendency to appear at the more aggressive end of the spectrum of Ewing sarcoma. In one series of 13 patients,[5] aggressive lesions were identified in the metaphysis or diaphysis with poor margins. Cortical destruction in 11 of 13, periosteal reaction in 12 of 13, and soft tissue mass in 13 of 13 were common findings. Calcification was seen in the soft-tissue component in only 1 of 13 tumors. Bone sclerosis was identified in only 2 of the 13 patients (Fig. 7–69). Pathological fracture occurred in 4 of the 13.[5] Findings on CT and MR of bone lesions reflect the abnormalities described on the plain film, with the tumors appearing similar to Ewing sarcoma (Figs. 7–69, 7–70, 7–71, 7–72, and 7–73). They cannot be differentiated from Ewing sarcoma by imaging. In the face and head, the tumors have large soft-tisse components and cause extensive destruction of bone. PNETs can occur in the soft tissues with no bone involvement (Figs. 7–74 and 7–75).

Metastases are not uncommon. In one series of 26 patients, metastases were identified in the lung (10), lymph nodes (8) (Fig. 7–75), liver (3), and bone (3)[4] Figs. 7–76 and 7–77). In another study,[1] bone metastases were present in 5 of 6 patients on initial diagnoses and node metastases in 1 patient.[6] In two other series, metastases were present on initial diagnosis in 11 of 26 patients[4] and 7 of 13 patients.[5] From all of the studies, metastases seem to be most common in the lung and bone (as with Ewing sarcoma), with lymph nodes being the next most common site. On rare occasions, metastases may also be identified in the liver[5,11] and in the brain.[11] Tumor recurrence after initial therapy may be either local or metastatic.[11]

Differential Diagnosis

The differential diagnosis includes Ewing sarcoma, neuroblastoma, rhabdomyosarcoma, and lymphoma[1] (Table 7–29).

Therapy and Prognosis

Treatment is the same as for Ewing sarcoma, with chemotherapy and radiation therapy, plus surgery when possible. The prognosis in all reported series is extremely poor, with less than 20 percent survival of 20 patients,[1] 1 survival in 14 patients,[6] 1 survival in 10 patients,[14] 9 survivals in 26 patients,[4] and 1 survival in 13 patients.[5]

References

1. Askin FB, Rosai J, Sibley RK, et al. Malignant small cell tumor of the thoracopulmonary region in childhood. A distinctive clinicopathologic entity of uncertain histogenesis. Cancer 1979;43:2438–2451.
2. Batsakis JG, Manning JT. Soft tissue tumors: unusual forms. Otolaryngol Clin N Am 1986;19:659–683.
3. Auguste L-J, Razack MS, Sako K. Hemangiopericytoma. J Surg Oncol 1982;20:260–264.
4. Marina NM, Etcubanas E, Parham DM, et al. Peripheral primitive neuroectodermal tumor (peripheral neuroepithelioma) in children. A review of the St. Jude experience and controversies in diagnosis and management. Cancer 1989;64:1952–1960.
5. Rousselin B, Vanel D, Terrier-Lacombe MJ, et al. Clinical and radiologic analysis of 13 cases of primary neuroectodermal tumors of bone. Skeletal Radiol 1989;18:115–120.
6. Llombart-Bosch A, Lacombe MJ, Peydro-Olaya A, et al. Malignant peripheral neuroectodermal tumours of bone other than Askin's neoplasm: characterization of 14 new cases with immunohistochemistry and electron microscopy. Virchows Archiv A Pathol Anat Histopathol 1988;412:421–430.
7. Triche TJ, Cavazzana AO. Pathology in pediatric oncology. In: Pizzo PA, Poplack DG, eds. Principles and practice of pediatric oncology. Philadelphia: JB Lippincott, 1989:93–125.
8. Bourque MD, Di Lorenzo M, Collin P-P, et al. Malignant small-cell tumor of the thoracopulmonary region: "Askin Tumor." J Pediatr Surg 1989;24:1079–1083.
9. Linnoila RI, Tsokos M, Triche TJ, et al. Evidence for neural origin and PAS-positive variants of the malignant small cell tumor of thoracopulmonary region ("Askin Tumor"). Am J Surg Pathol 1986;10:124–133.
10. Fink IJ, Kurtz DW, Cazenave L, et al. Malignant thoracopulmonary small-cell ("Askin") tumor. AJR 1985;145:517–520.
11. Voss BL, Pysher TJ, Humphrey GB. Peripheral neuroepithelioma in childhood. Cancer 1984;54:3059–3064.
12. Shamberger RC, LaQuaglia MP. Resection of a tumor of the psoas muscle. J Pediatr Surg 1989;24:933–935.
13. Castleberry RP, Kelly DR, Wilson ER, et al. Childhood liposarcoma. Report of a case and review of the literature. Cancer 1984;54:579–584.
14. Llombart-Bosch A, Terrier-Lacombe J, Peydro-Olaya A, et al. Peripheral neuroectodermal sarcoma of soft tissue (peripheral neuroepithelioma): a pathologic study of ten cases with differential diagnosis regarding other small, round-cell sarcomas. Hum Pathol 1989;20:273–280.

TABLE 7–29
Small Round Cell Tumors Involving Bone

Ewing sarcoma
PNET
Small cell osteosarcoma
Mesenchymal chondrosarcoma
Lymphoma
Rhabdomyosarcoma
Neuroblastoma

PERIPHERAL NEUROEPITHELIOMA

Peripheral neuroepithelioma should probably be included as a part of primitive neuroectodermal tumor. In one reported series[1] of 17 patients, all had a translocation between the number 11 and 22 chromosome. The location of the primary tumor was chest wall (12), pelvis (3) and extremity (2). Fifteen of these 17 tumors were stage III or IV. Metastases occurred to the bone (6), bone marrow (5), lung (3), and lymph nodes (2). Metastases to multiple sites were present in 6 patients. The patients were treated with intensive chemotherapy and radiation therapy. Sixteen of the 17 patients went into complete remission, but 6 subsequently relapsed.

Reference

1. Oakley RH, Carty H, Cudmore RE. Multiple benign mesenchymomata of the chest wall. Pediatr Radiol 1985;15:58–60.

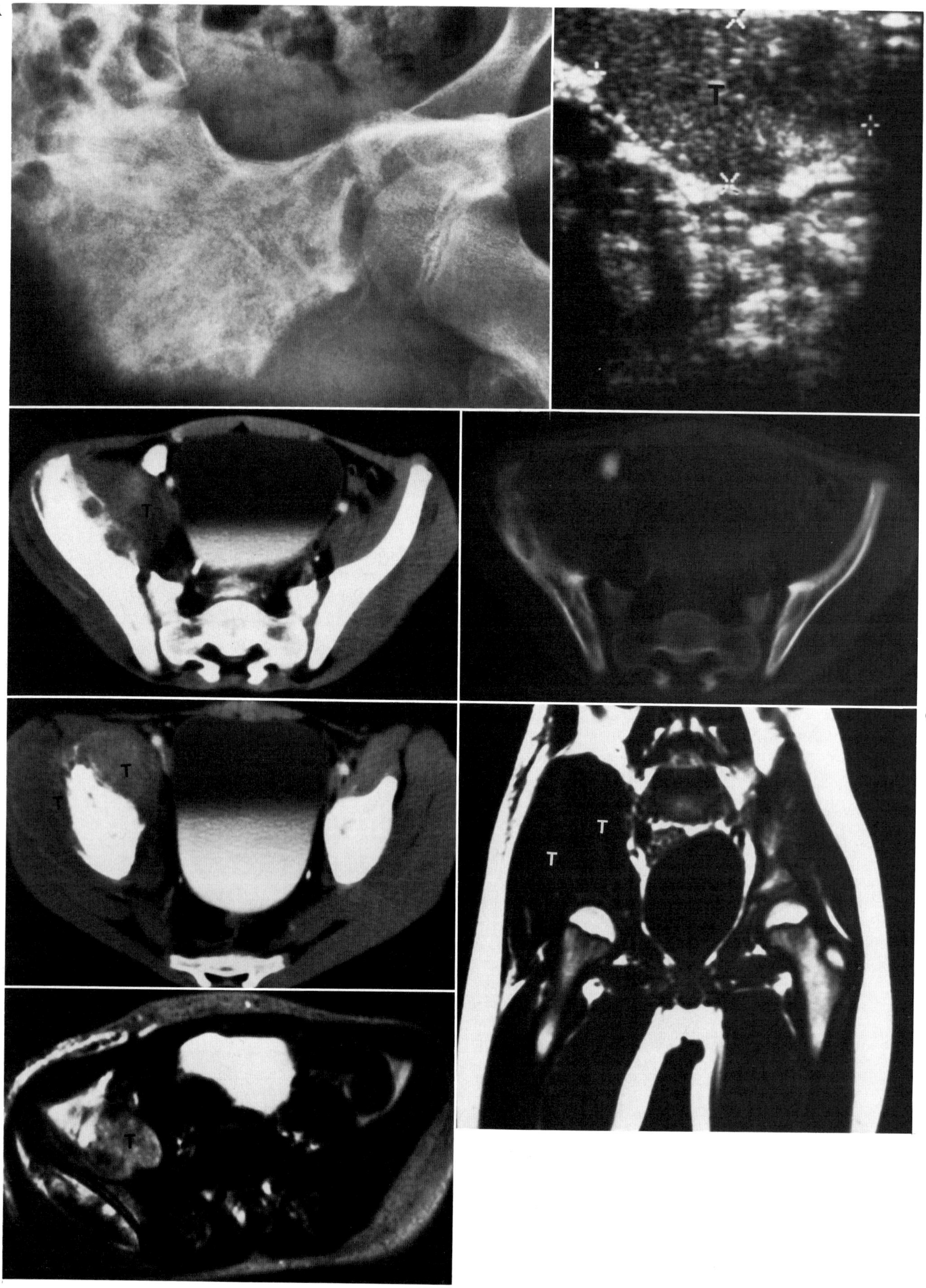

Figure 7-69. Diagnosis: Primitive neuroectodermal tumor of the right iliac bone.
A, Plain film radiograph. There is extensive mottled sclerosis, with some destruction, involving almost the entire right iliac. ***B,*** Ultrasound. This shows well a large soft-tissue mass (*T*) but does not identify clearly its relationship to adjacent structures. ***C*** through ***E,*** CT images with soft-tissue and bone windows. These show an extensive expanding sclerotic destructive lesion of the right iliac bone with a large soft-tissue mass (*T*) lying both medially and laterally. ***F,*** MR, axial T2 weighted image. The soft-tissue component of the tumor (*T*) is of bright signal intensity. Some bright signal is seen in the marrow space because of tumor infiltration. The extensive low signal in the marrow space is caused by the sclerotic tumor. ***G,*** MR, coronal T1 weighted image. There is very low signal from the iliac bone and the adjacent soft-tissue tumor. *T* = soft tissue component of tumor.

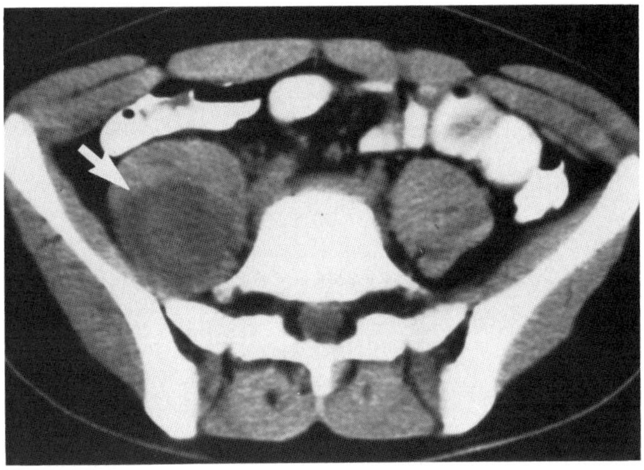

Figure 7-70. Diagnosis: Primitive neuroectodermal tumor of the psoas muscle.
CT. There is a large well-defined soft-tissue tumor *(arrow)* lying in the posterior part of the right psoas muscle. (From Schamberger RC. Resection of a tumor of the psoas muscle. J Pediatr Surg 1989;24:933–935.)

Figure 7-71. Diagnosis: Primitive neuroectodermal tumor of soft tissues. There is no bone involvement.
MR, T1 weighted image after gadolinium-DTPA administration. There is a moderately well-defined tumor (*T*) involving the trapezius erector spinae and rhomboid muscles on the right side. The bone was not involved.

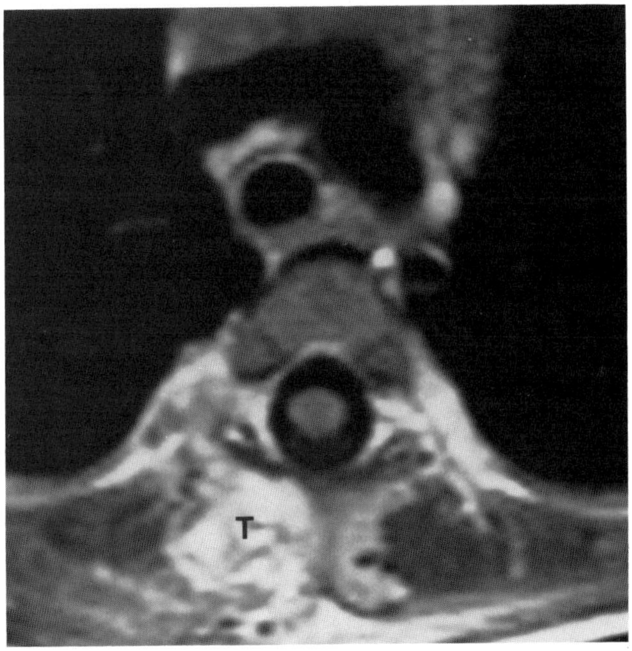

SYNOVIAL CELL SARCOMA

Synovial cell sarcoma is more common in adults than children, with approximately 30 percent of all cases occurring in patients under the age of 20 years.[1,2]

Histologically, these lesions arise from a multipotential mesenchymal cell and not from mature synovium. They are, therefore, not in contact with joints or bursa,[3] but tend to occur close to articular surfaces, bursa, or tendon sheaths. Most occur in the peripheral extremities,[2,3] with 70 percent of lesions below the elbow or knee.[2] The leg is a more common site than the arm.[1] Grossly, the tumors may have areas of hemorrhage or necrosis and frequently have areas of cystic, mucoid material. Microscopically, the tumors are diagnosed by a characteristic biphasic appearance. The two cell types identified are a stromal spinal cell and an epithelioid cell.[2] When both of these cell types are present, this biphasic appearance is diagnostic of synovial cell sarcoma. Controversy exists regarding the diagnosis when only a single (monophasic) cell is identified.

Symptoms are usually a painless soft-tissue mass.[2] Little or no abnormality may be detected on plain film radiograph.

CT will show a soft-tissue mass in most patients. Calcification may be identified in up to 30 percent of cases. In one study of 10 patients evaluated with MR,[3] the signal characteristics of the tumor were found to be similar to muscle on T1 weighted images. There was increase in signal intensity on T2 weighted images. Seven of the 10 lesions were homogeneous, 6 were lobulated, and 8 had sharp margins. Most lay deep in the soft tissue. One tumor invaded the adjacent femoral vein. Very occasionally the presence of mucoid material will result in two clearly different compartments to the tumor (Fig. 7–78).

In most patients, the findings on CT and MR are nonspecific and the histologic diagnosis cannot be suggested from the imaging.

Treatment is surgical excision. Overall prognosis is at least 50 percent survival.[2] Survival is increased in patients with a small-size tumor, younger patients, and in patients with a predominantly epithelioid histology.[1]

References

1. Miser JS, Triche TJ, Pritchard DJ, et al. Ewing's sarcoma and the nonrhabdomyosarcoma soft tissue sarcomas of childhood. In: Pizzo PA, Poplack DG, eds. Principles and practice of pediatric oncology. Philadelphia: JB Lippincott, 1989:659–688.

A B C

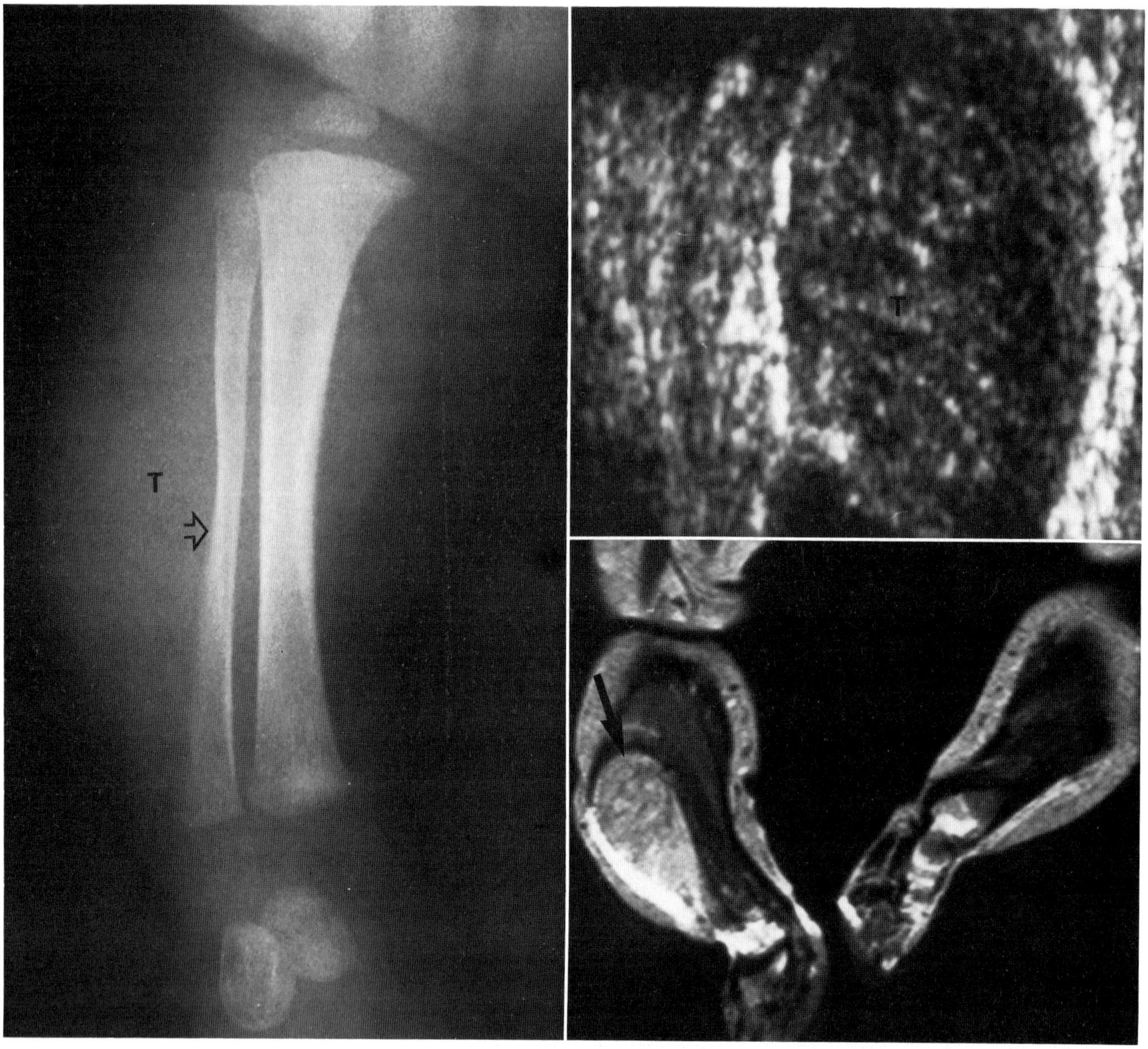

Figure 7–72. Diagnosis: Primitive neuroectodermal tumor of soft tissues without bone involvement. ***A***, Radiograph of the lower leg. There is a large soft-tissue tumor mass (*T*). There is secondary scalloping of the fibula *(open arrows)*. ***B***, Ultrasound. This shows a nonspecific solid soft-tissue tumor mass (*T*). ***C***, MR, T2 weighted image. The tumor mass *(arrows)* is well defined. It is of bright signal intensity on this T2 weighted image. The appearance is nonspecific.

2. Mackenzie DH. Synovial sarcoma. A review of 58 cases. Cancer 1966;19:169–175.
3. Mahajan H, Lorigan JG, Shirkhoda A. Synovial sarcoma: MR imaging. Mag Reson Imag 1989;7:211–216.

METASTASES

Table 7–30 lists pediatric tumors that may metastasize to bone. Most of the tumors produce lytic-type lesions

TABLE 7–30
Pediatric Tumors that Can Metastasize to Bone

Neuroblastoma
Clear cell Wilms tumor
Rhabdomyosarcoma
Retinoblastoma
Ewing sarcoma
Osteosarcoma
Lymphoma
Medulloblastoma

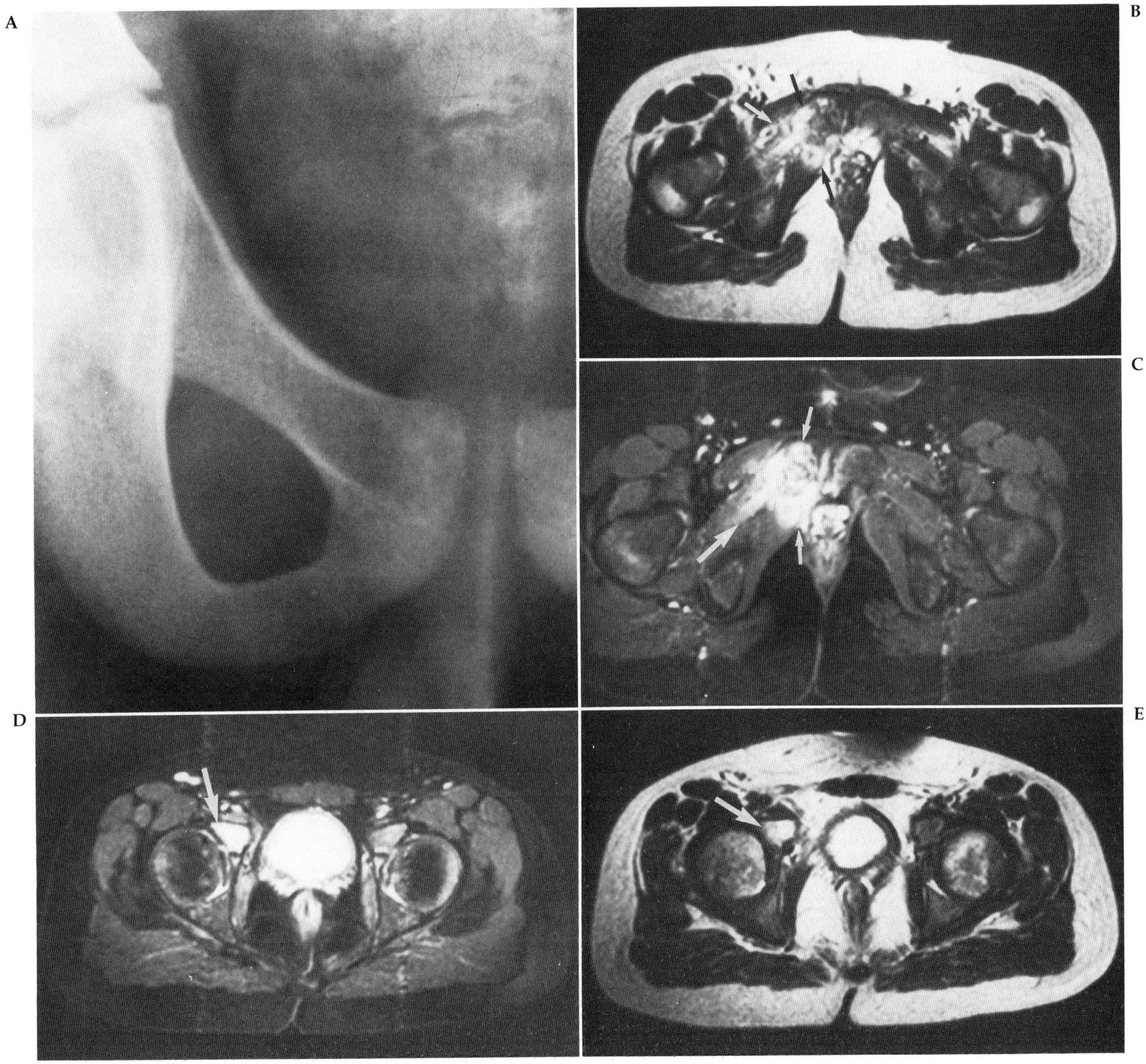

Figure 7–73. Diagnosis: Primitive neuroectodermal tumor of the pubic bone.
A, Plain film radiograph. This shows subtle lucencies in the medial aspect of the public bone. ***B*** and ***C***, MR, T2 and STIR images through the pubic bone at the level of the symphysis. There is a moderate-sized abnormality involving the bone and adjacent soft tissues *(arrows)*. The lesion is somewhat unusual in that the soft-tissue component is poorly defined. ***D*** and ***E***, MR, T2 and STIR pulse sequences obtained at the level of the hip joint. Both images show very strong signal intensity *(arrows)* in the bone marrow of the pubic bone adjacent to the hip joint. This indicates tumor infiltration extensively throughout the entire pubic bone. This extent of tumor spread, on the MR images, is far greater than might be predicted from the plain film radiograph. These findings are important in planning any potential surgical excision of the tumor.

with no periosteal reaction, though some may produce a periosteal reaction. Many do not have a significant soft-tissue component, but some, particularly neuroblastoma and Ewing sarcoma, may have a large soft-tissue component. Blastic metastases are most likely to be caused by medulloblastoma, osteosarcoma, or retinoblastoma. Neuroblastoma metastases may sometimes have blastic areas. Ewing sarcoma is unusual in that the metastases very frequently look like a primary Ewing tumor.

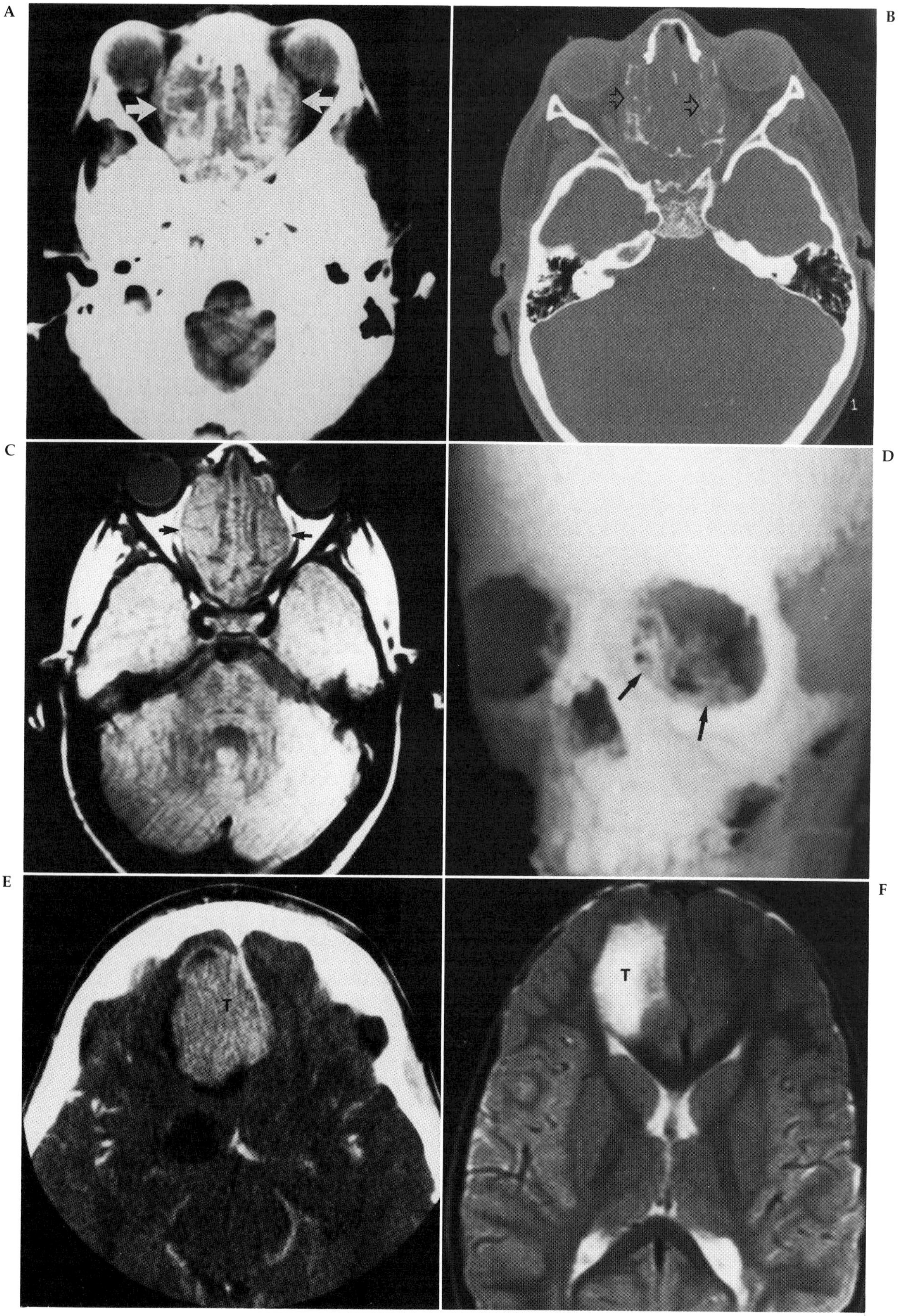
A
B
C
D
E
T
F
T

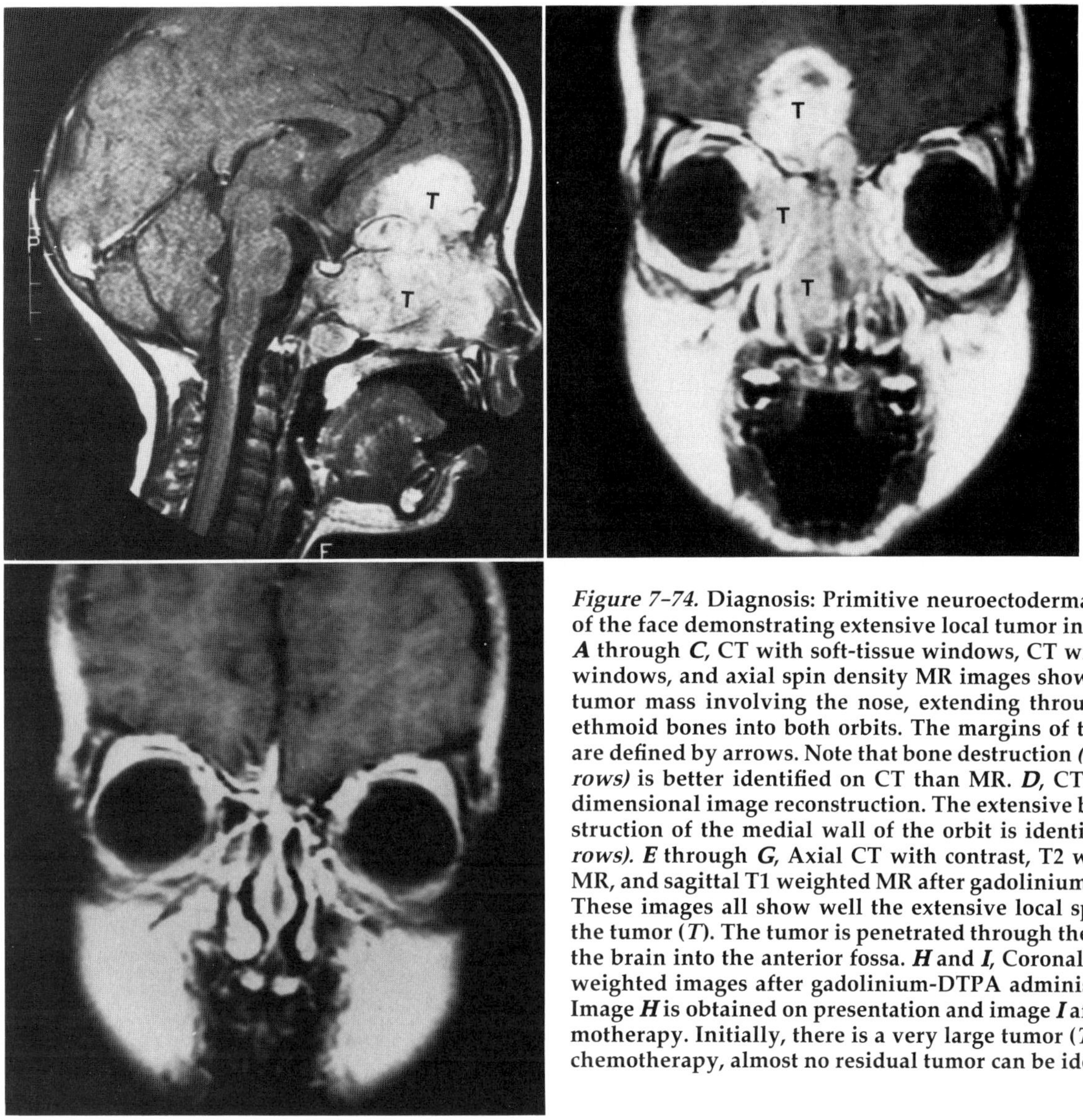

Figure 7-74. Diagnosis: Primitive neuroectodermal tumor of the face demonstrating extensive local tumor invasion. ***A*** through ***C,*** CT with soft-tissue windows, CT with bone windows, and axial spin density MR images show a large tumor mass involving the nose, extending through both ethmoid bones into both orbits. The margins of the mass are defined by arrows. Note that bone destruction *(open arrows)* is better identified on CT than MR. ***D,*** CT. Three-dimensional image reconstruction. The extensive bony destruction of the medial wall of the orbit is identified *(arrows).* ***E*** through ***G,*** Axial CT with contrast, T2 weighted MR, and sagittal T1 weighted MR after gadolinium-DTPA. These images all show well the extensive local spread of the tumor (*T*). The tumor is penetrated through the base of the brain into the anterior fossa. ***H*** and ***I,*** Coronal MR, T1 weighted images after gadolinium-DTPA administration. Image ***H*** is obtained on presentation and image ***I*** after chemotherapy. Initially, there is a very large tumor (*T*). After chemotherapy, almost no residual tumor can be identified.

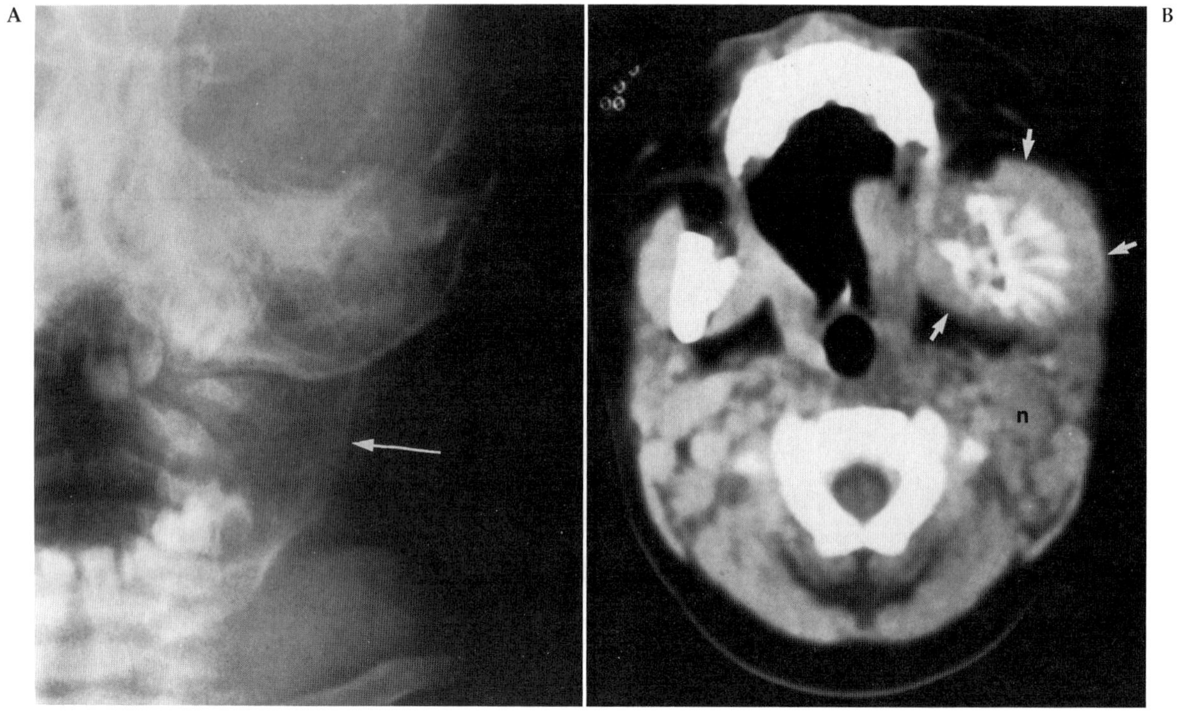

Figure 7-75. Diagnosis: Primitive neuroectodermal tumor of the mandible with local lymph node metastasis.
A, Plain film radiograph. There is destruction of the ramus of the mandible *(arrow)*. ***B***, CT. There is expansion and destruction of the ramus of the mandible. There is a spiculated pattern to the remaining bone. There is a moderate soft-tissue tumor mass surrounding the bone *(arrows)*. Local lymph node metastasis (*N*) is present.

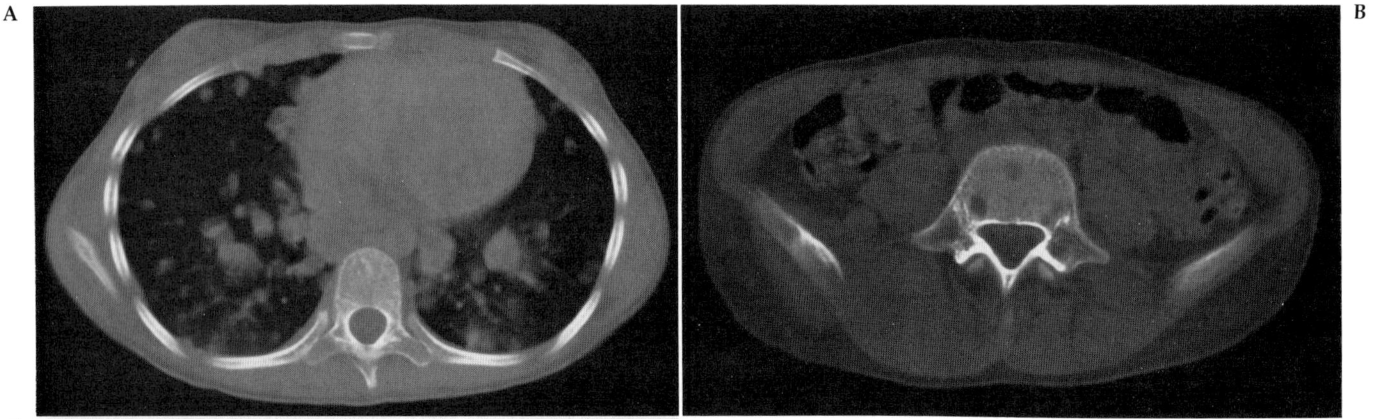

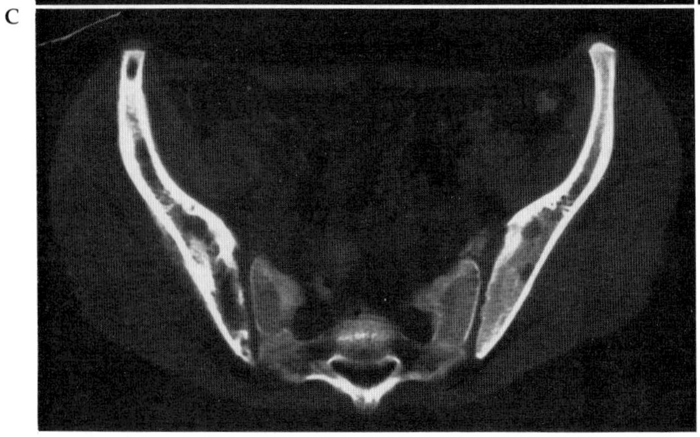

Figure 7-76. Diagnosis: Primitive neuroectodermal tumor. Metastases to lung and bone.
A, CT scan of chest. Widespread nodular metastases are present in both lung fields. ***B*** and ***C***, CT images of the lower spine and pelvis. Multiple sharply defined, punched-out lytic lesions are identified.

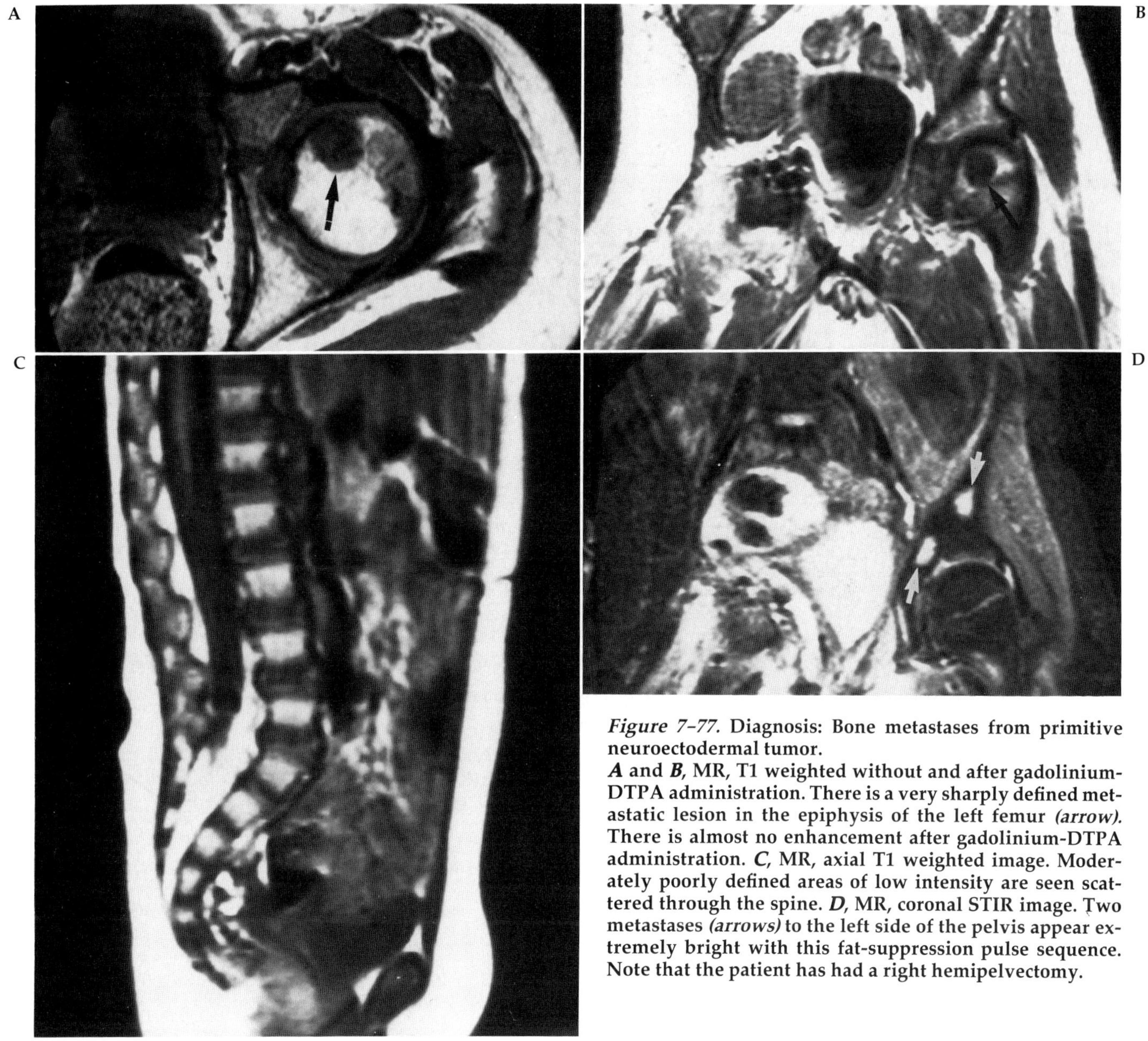

Figure 7–77. Diagnosis: Bone metastases from primitive neuroectodermal tumor.
A and ***B***, MR, T1 weighted without and after gadolinium-DTPA administration. There is a very sharply defined metastatic lesion in the epiphysis of the left femur *(arrow).* There is almost no enhancement after gadolinium-DTPA administration. ***C***, MR, axial T1 weighted image. Moderately poorly defined areas of low intensity are seen scattered through the spine. ***D***, MR, coronal STIR image. Two metastases *(arrows)* to the left side of the pelvis appear extremely bright with this fat-suppression pulse sequence. Note that the patient has had a right hemipelvectomy.

A C

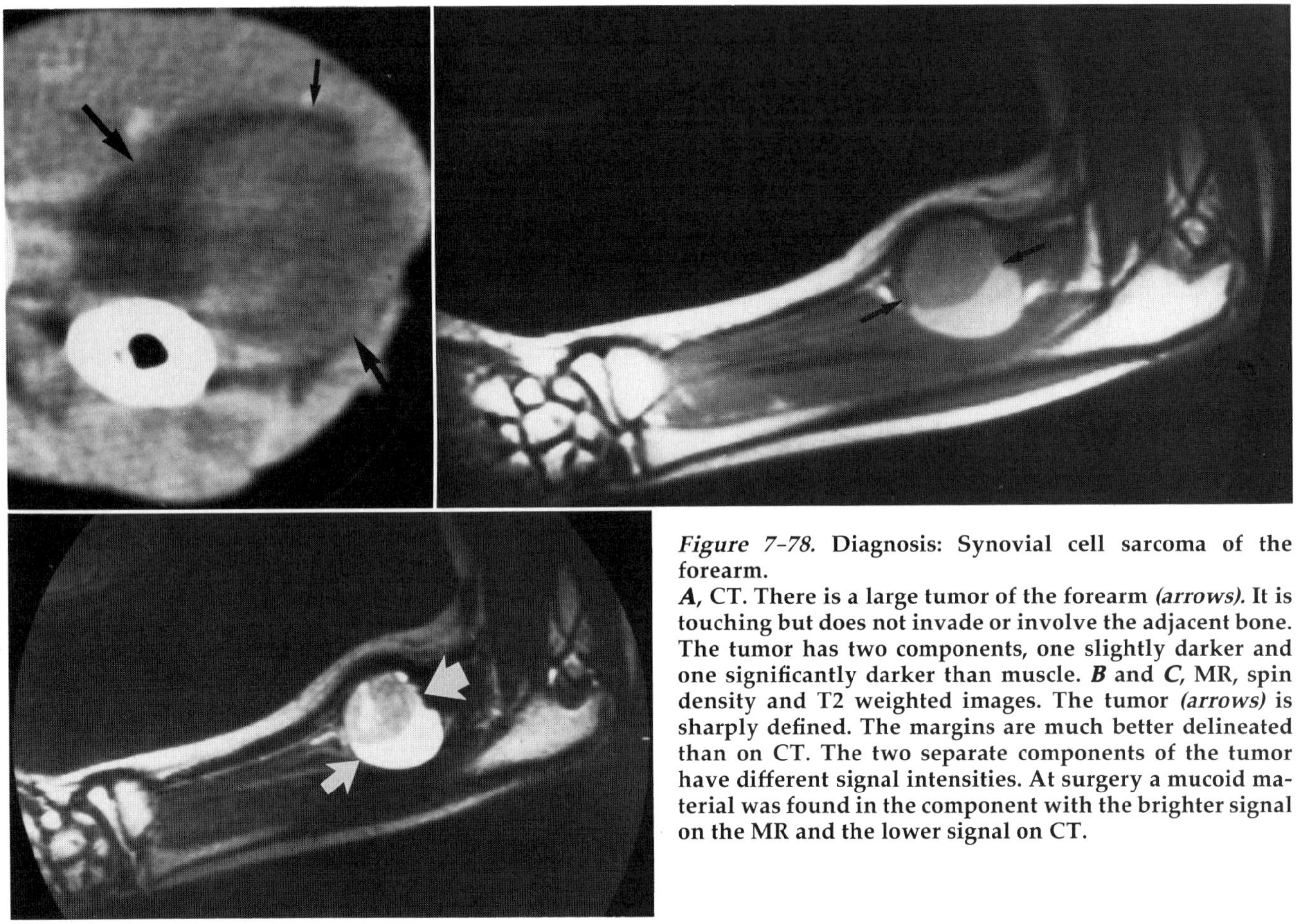

B

Figure 7–78. Diagnosis: Synovial cell sarcoma of the forearm.
A, CT. There is a large tumor of the forearm *(arrows).* It is touching but does not invade or involve the adjacent bone. The tumor has two components, one slightly darker and one significantly darker than muscle. ***B*** and ***C***, MR, spin density and T2 weighted images. The tumor *(arrows)* is sharply defined. The margins are much better delineated than on CT. The two separate components of the tumor have different signal intensities. At surgery a mucoid material was found in the component with the brighter signal on the MR and the lower signal on CT.

CHAPTER

8 CENTRAL NERVOUS SYSTEM TUMORS

Tumors of the central nervous system (CNS) in children are extremely important, because they represent the most common solid tumors in childhood. The incidence of brain tumors in children is about 24 per million children under the age of 15 years per annum,[1] which means that approximately 1,200 new cases are seen in the United States each year.[1–3] These tumors are completely different from brain tumors in adults: For example, their location is commonly in the posterior fossa[4] (Table 8–1).

Etiology and Epidemiology

There are very few factors that can be identified as contributing to the etiology of brain tumors in children. There is a high incidence of gliomas, particularly of the visual tracts in children with neurofibromatosis.[1,5] Patients with von Hippel-Lindau syndrome have an increased incidence of many tumors, of which hemangioblastoma of the cerebellum and hemangioma of retina are the only two likely to be seen in children.[1,6] Pineoblastoma has a very high association with bilateral retinoblastomas.[1,5] Low-grade gliomas have occasionally been identified in patients with tuberosclerosis.[1] Children with rhabdoid tumors of the kidney have a small incidence of associated second primary tumors in the central nervous system.[1,5]

TABLE 8–1
Anatomic Location of CNS Tumors in Children[1]

Location	Percentage
Posterior fossa	60
Supratentorial	
Hemispheres	25
Midline	15

Reference
1. Walker RW, Allen JC. Pediatric brain tumors. Pediatr Ann 1983;12:383–391.

Pathology

The classification of CNS tumors is an area of significant controversy,[7,8] which is way beyond my ability to resolve. Many of the tumors have commonly accepted names that have become established over the years. I use these as the basis for describing the CNS tumors in this chapter (Table 8–2). This somewhat simplistic classification is reasonably adequate when viewed from an imaging perspective. Primitive neuroectodermal tumor (PNET) is a term used to describe a variety of intracranial tumors arising from a poorly differentiated primitive cell. While tumors such as medulloblastoma, pinealoblastoma, ependymoma, and retinoblastoma are in fact primitive neuroectodermal tumors, I shall continue to use the more common name for these tumors and reserve the term PNET to describe a group of undifferentiated tumors occurring predominantly in the cerebral hemispheres. This includes all tumors previously termed intracerebral neuroblastoma. Another difficulty arises with regard to the definition of glioblastoma. Some treat this as a separate tumor, while others consider it as a grade IV astrocytoma. I take the latter approach. The terms low-grade and high-grade are frequently used in the description of CNS tumors. Low-grade tumors are the most differentiated and, therefore, most benign looking on microscopy. High-grade tumors are more malignant and poorly differentiated. The tumors are usually described on a scale of I to IV with grade I being the most low grade and IV the most high grade.

Although brain tumors can be divided into benign and malignant on their histologic appearance, this subdivision is not nearly as good a predictor of behavior and prognosis as it is with tumors in other parts of the body. For one reason the prognosis, both in terms of morbidity and mortality for many of the brain tumors, depends as much on its anatomic location as its histologic appearance. A small brain tumor, in a critical location in the brain, can be devastating, while in other areas a very large tumor may produce minimal symptoms and not be life threatening. In addition, very few brain tumors metastasize outside the central nervous system, regardless of their microscopic appearance. In

TABLE 8–2
Classification of Brain Tumors

Tumors of neuroepithelial tissue
Astrocytoma
Oligodendroglioma
Ependymoma
Pineal cell tumors
Pineoblastoma
Pineocytoma
Ganglioglioma
Poorly differentiated
Medulloblastoma
Retinoblastoma
PNET
Tumors of meningeal tissue
Meningioma
Tumors of germ cells
Germinoma
Embryonal carcinoma
Choriocarcinoma
Teratoma
Other Tumors
Craniopharyngioma
Chordoma
Choroid plexus papilloma
Lymphoma
Metastases

one large study,[9] 21 of 917 (2 percent) children with brain tumors demonstrated extracranial metastases. Three-quarters of these tumors were medulloblastoma, so that with the exception of medulloblastoma, extracranial metastases from brain tumors are exceedingly rare.[9]

There are few markers that are helpful in the evaluation of brain tumors. Estimation of concentration of beta human choriogonadotropin and alpha-fetoprotein in the cerebrospinal fluid is helpful in the diagnosis of pineal region germ cell tumors. Estimation of cerebrospinal fluid polyamine levels can be used to monitor recurrence of some tumors. Levels are elevated with recurrence of medulloblastoma, PNET, and some germinomas.[2,10]

Clinical Presentation

Clinical symptoms from most brain tumors are relatively nonspecific and often occur late so that there is frequently a delay in making the diagnosis. The most common symptom of a brain tumor is headache. Because brain tumors are rare and headaches are common, this early symptom may frequently be ignored for months or years before investigation is initiated. This is true of other symptoms such as vomiting and behavior disturbance, which may also be ignored. Some symptoms do not manifest themselves because they occur in very young children. For example, in a young child of 2 to 3 years of age, a mild loss of visual acuity is very difficult to detect and will usually go unnoticed. The most common symptoms of brain tumors are those due to an elevation of intracranial pressure caused either by mass effect from the tumor itself or more commonly secondary hydrocephalus. This produces headache, vomiting, visual disturbance, alteration in behavior, and alteration in intellectual ability. Depending on location, more focal symptoms will occur earlier or later. Infratentorial tumors will cause ataxia, nystagmus, problems with gait, and eventually focal abnormalities owing to involvement of the cranial nerves. Supratentorial tumors may cause proptosis, loss of visual acuity, reduction in visual fields, convulsions, hemiparesis, abnormalities of eye movement, behavior and intellectual problems.[1,5] Spinal seeding of tumors may cause weakness, loss of urinary control, or sensory problems[1,5] (Table 8–3).

Imaging Studies

Imaging is essential in the evaluation, diagnosis, and monitoring of therapy for pediatric cranial tumors. Computed tomography (CT) and magnetic resonance (MR) dominate the imaging of intracranial tumors. In the past 15 years, there has been a complete and dramatic change in imaging of brain tumors. Previous imaging, including air ventriculography, was invasive and relatively poor for the demonstration and characterization of disease. These studies are no longer done. Plain film radiographs, which were frequently performed in the past and which may still be positive in a number of patients, should no longer be routinely performed, since the information they provide is readily obtained from CT and MR. With the exception of experimental studies with PET scanning, brain isotope scans are seldom performed. A new agent, Tc hexakis, showed uptake in one patient with a brain stem glioma.[11] Angiography, which was frequently utilized to identify and characterize tumors, is now seldom performed. In the posterior fossa, the only indication for angiography is further evaluation of vascular malformations.[12] For supratentorial lesions angiography may be performed to aid in the diagnosis of vascular malformations and to demonstrate the vascular supply and location of other tumors prior to surgical resection.[3] With continued improvements in

TABLE 8–3
Primary CNS Tumors that Spread via Cerebrospinal Fluid into Subarachnoid Space[1]

Medulloblastoma
Ependymoma
PNET
Germinoma
High-grade astrocytoma
Malignant choroid plexus papilloma
Pineoblastoma

Reference
1. Kun LE, D'Souza B, Tefft M. The value of surveillance testing in childhood brain tumors. Cancer 1985;56:1818–1823.

MR, it is expected that the utilization of angiography will continue to decline.

CT has been utilized since the 1970s and MR since the 1980s. An early study in 1984 of 25 children with brain tumors was one of the first to show some superiority for MR over CT.[13] For many children it has now become possible to define the specific advantages and disadvantages of CT and MR. CT is clearly better than MR for demonstration of calcium or areas of bone destruction. Identification of calcium is particularly important in differential diagnosis of many of the brain tumors and this advantage of CT is significant. CT has also been better than MR for demonstration of meningeal deposits of tumor through cerebrospinal fluid spread. Recent utilization of gadolinium-DTPA has greatly improved the ability of MR to demonstrate such tumors, and this advantage of CT may no longer exist. In some patients, CT may also be better for characterizing a lesion as cystic. In complex tumors with areas of hemorrhage, or when unusual fluids fill cysts, this may sometimes be difficult on MR. The advantages of MR are its ability to better define the extent and margins of tumors in many cases. In some children, MR will define an actual tumor when CT has only shown secondary mass effect. The ability of MR to image in multiple planes is also sometimes helpful for better definition of the extent of tumor. MR is superior to CT for demonstration of intracranial vessels and can better show the relationship of tumor to major arteries and veins.

With regard to technique, initial CT scans should always be performed with and without the utilization of intravenous contrast. On the precontrast scan, calcification and the intensity of the tumor are useful for differential diagnosis. The pattern and amount of enhancement following intravenous contrast is similarly helpful. MR images should be obtained in at least two imaging planes. For midline lesions the sagittal plane is particularly helpful. For laterally placed lesions coronal imaging is useful, permitting comparison of both sides. Axial images should probably be done in all patients because of our familiarity with anatomy in this plane and also to facilitate comparisons with CT images. It is also becoming apparent that the utilization of T1 gadolinium-DTPA enhanced images is helpful in a large number of patients. This permits improved contrast between tumor and normal tissues with retention of excellent normal anatomy. In addition, it permits differentiation of tumor from cerebrospinal fluid, which may be difficult on T2 weighted images in which both many tumors and cerebrospinal fluid appear of bright signal.[14]

One advantage of gadolinium-DTPA is that the degree of enhancement may help differentiate benign from malignant lesions. In tumors in which there is patchy enhancement with gadolinium-DTPA, it is suggested that this may be helpful in guiding biopsy, with tumor most likely to be found in areas showing enhancement.[15] One study suggests that gadolinium-DTPA should not be used if both the precontrast T1 and T2 weighted images are negative. In this study, gadolinium-DTPA showed no tumor in patients with negative precontrast images.[15]

When either CT or MR is performed, the following questions need to be answered.

- Location of tumor?
- Size of tumor?
- Definition of tumor margins?
- Intensity of tumor before and after contrast administration?
- Homogeneity of tumor and internal structure, including necrosis, hemorrhage, cyst formation and calcification?
- Local effects on surrounding tissues, edema, and metastases?

CT and MR are extremely good for identification of a variety of brain tumors. In a few cases, imaging can suggest a very specific histologic diagnosis. It is extremely important to note that in many cases imaging cannot differentiate between tumor types nor can it always differentiate between tumor and other pathology. Other problems imaging encounters are in differentiating edema from tumor and in differentiating residual tumor from residual necrosis and fibrosis.[2] Imaging may also not be helpful in differentiating benign from malignant tumors. In one study of 60 patients with thalamic tumors, the degree of enhancement was found not to be a predictor of malignancy.[16] In another study of supratentorial lesions, it was found that imaging showed an overlap, but that malignancy was strongly suggested by the appearance of an irregular tumor shape, irregular edema, a lateral location, and ring enhancement (Table 8–4).

Questions have to be answered regarding the choice of modality and timing of studies in patients with suspected or known brain tumors. In patients with suspected brain tumors, the radiologist is extremely reliant on the clinical acumen and skill of clinical colleagues. Obviously, all children with headaches cannot receive a CT and MR scan. The clinician must carefully evaluate each patient with clinical symptoms relating to the central nervous system, knowing that brain tumors can occasionally be the cause. The age of the patient (tumors occur frequently in young children), the persistence and nature of the nonspecific symptoms, the presence or absence of focal neurological signs, the presence of high risk factors (e.g., neurofibromatosis), or prior skull radiation will all guide the clinician by raising the level of suspicion to a threshold sufficient to order imaging studies. For the initial study, the trend is moving toward MR when this is available. A review in 1989 stated a preference for MR over CT for all brain tumors.[17] As previously discussed, it is probably prudent to perform CT on the initial presentation in addition to MR particularly if any abnormality is detected on the MR scan. This is especially true if there is any doubt as to the specific diagnosis after evaluation of the MR images. If the screening MR is negative, CT will not, I believe, add any useful information.

Long-term follow-up studies either with CT or MR will be needed for many years in patients surviving with brain tumors. Criteria for response and relapse are more difficult to define for the CNS tumors than for any other

TABLE 8–4
Difficulties in Differentiation of Benign and Malignant Brain Tumors[1]

Qualitative CT Signs in 49 Supratentorial Primary Tumors in Children

		Benign (n=38)	Malignant (n=11)
Tumor shape	Spherical	27	
	Irregular	11	11
Calcification		18	3
Cyst formation		7	1
Central lucency		13	9
Perifocal edema		8	10
Tumor attenuation on the plain CT	Hypodense	9	—
	Isodense	9	—
	Hyperdense	8	4
	"Mixed"	12	7
Contrast			
No Enhancement		5	—
Enhancement	Slight	7	2
	Moderate	14	6
	Strong	11	3
	Homogeneous	18	2
	Inhomogeneous	14	9

Reference

1. Pedersen H, Gjerris F, Klinken L. Malignancy criteria in computed tomography of primary supratentorial tumors in infancy and childhood. Neuroradiology 1989;31:24–28.

tumor.[18] If residual tumor is suspected following surgery, it may be advantageous to perform CT or MR within a few days of the surgery. It has been suggested that focal enhancement with intravenous iodinated contrast for CT or gadolinium-DTPA for MR occurring in the first few days after surgery represents residual tumor.[3] Such enhancement occurring more than 5 days after surgery may represent breakdown of the blood brain barrier and surgical edema. In the longer term, it may sometimes be difficult to differentiate tumor from edema, ischemia, necrosis, gliosis, or encephalomalacia. These may look similar on CT and may all have features of prolonged T1 and T2 relaxation time on MR. In differentiating these, contrast-enhanced CT is probably better than MR without contrast enhancement.[19] Recent utilization of gadolinium-DTPA, however, shows good results for MR compared to contrast-enhanced CT.[20] Enhancing tumor is usually lobular and focal. Surgical margins are usually linear and decrease with time. Abscesses usually show a thin rim of enhancement, as do resolving clots. Focal radiation therapy necrosis may be impossible to diffferentiate from residual tumor with either enhanced CT or enhanced MR imaging.[21]

Detection of CSF spread of tumors has traditionally been performed with myelography (see Table 8–3).[22] For areas of suspicion or doubt the myelographic information can be supplemented by doing a CT scan while the contrast is still present in the subarachnoid space. Carefully performed state-of-the-art MR will replace myelography with or without CT for the detection of spinal seeding from intracranial tumor. MR imaging needs to be performed with gadolinium-DTPA enhancement. A 1991 study in 17 children concluded that gadolinium-DTPA enhanced MR was superior for delineating spinal cord nodules and coating with tumor; CT with myelography was superior for nerve root sleeve filling defects.[23] All patients with positive CT with myelography had some subarachnoid tumor seen on MR.[23] Further work comparing myelography and MR needs to be performed.

Differential Diagnosis

The differential diagnosis of intracranial tumors is very large and includes infection and inflammatory processes, developmental mass lesions, extension into the cranium of tumors arising in the bones of the skull or growing through these bones, hematoma, and vascular malformation. Some of these differentiations may be quite difficult; for example, a hemorrhagic tumor may look very similar to a vascular malformation on MR.[24]

Therapy and Prognosis

Therapy of brain tumors is difficult and prognosis has not been good. Some of the problems with brain tumor therapy are summarized in Table 8–5. Combinations of surgery, chemotherapy, and radiation therapy are utilized for treating most patients. Recent trends with each of these three modalities are attempting to improve prognosis and limit side effects.

With radiation therapy, CT, MR, and treatment simulators are being used to better plan treatment fields to include all of the tumor and limit radiation to normal brain.[3] The extent of radiation used depends on the tumor type. Local radiation is used for low-grade gliomas, supratentorial ependymomas, craniopharyngiomas, and meningiomas. Whole brain radiation is utilized for most children with lymphoma and grade III or IV astrocytoma (high grade). Whole brain and spinal cord irradiation is utilized for medulloblastomas, PNETs, germ cell tumors, infratentorial ependymomas, and pinealoblastomas.[5] Trials are being performed to decrease side effects by increasing the frequency and decreasing the dose of radiation given at each treatment session. A good response to radiation therapy does require utilization of high doses.[25]

Chemotherapy, which traditionally has been very ineffective, has shown some improvements, with, for example, one new regime utilizing a combination of 8 different drugs.[3] A 1990 study of carboplatinum in 95 children with brain tumors showed a significant effect in some children, including 6 of 19 children with medulloblastoma.[26]

Surgery has been greatly aided by refined surgical techniques and improved information provided the surgeon by very accurate CT and MR imaging. A few tumors, such as low-grade cerebellar astrocytomas, can be excised and cured with resection alone. For most other tumors it is becoming accepted that aggressive debulking will prolong survival. Intraoperative ultrasound is being used to help evaluate the tumor extent during surgery. Lasers and ultrasound fragmentation are being used to break up tumor and aid in removal. Biopsies are done of almost all tumors with the possible exception of pontine and optic nerve gliomas, where in many cases the diagnosis is made from imaging and clinical findings. Operative mortality and morbidity has decreased significantly in recent years.[3]

Long-term side effects are as important as survival in children with brain tumors. Though many children may survive, the quality of life may not be desirable. Handicaps may result from the direct effect of the tumor itself on adjacent brain structures, complications of surgery, chemotherapy, or radiation therapy. Aggressive surgical debulking of tumors will of necessity result in some local morbidity. The severity of this will vary depending on the tumor location. Chemotherapy may cause brain side effects. For example, in one study of 8 children with a mean age of 14 years given intravenous methotrexate for nonneurological tumors, MR showed abnormality in 4 patients. The abnormalities included chronic edema, multifocal white matter necrosis, and brain atrophy.[1,27] Following cranial radiation therapy a somnolence syndrome including lethargy and headache is seen in about 6 to 8 weeks.[1,5] It is believed to be caused by temporary demyelinization and lasts for only a few weeks. After 6 months, many other effects may be identified due to radiation. Clinically, there may be decrease in patient's IQ and memory ability, there may be endocrine dysfunction from irradiation of the pituitary, and there is a significant increase of second brain tumors following cranial radiation.[5,27,28] When children are imaged following radiation therapy, abnormalities may be identified. In one study, CT scans of 49 children who had received cranial radiation identified atrophy in 51 percent, calcification in 28 percent, and white matter abnormality in 26 percent. The calcification was commonly in the gray/white matter junction or less commonly in the basal ganglia.[29] In this study, 73 percent of the 49 children had at least one abnormality not at the site of the primary tumor.[29]

TABLE 8-5
Problems with Therapy of Brain Tumors

Each type is rare, so experience is limited
Anatomic location precludes resection in many cases
Very slow-growing tumors do not respond well to radiation or chemotherapy
Drugs may not cross the blood–brain barrier
Tumors occur in young children, whose brains are very sensitive to radiation

Before moving on to discuss the specific intracranial tumors individually, mention should be made of one specific group of patients, namely those under the age of 1 year. Tumors in this age group are being diagnosed with increasing frequency, probably as a result of more widespread use of cranial ultrasound in young infants and antenatally. These tumors account for up to 8 percent of all pediatric brain tumors.[30] The pathology and imaging appearance of any particular tumor are the same as in older children.[30] The types of tumor found and the symptoms are, however, completely different. Because of the expansibility of the head, the most common symptom is that of a rapidly increasing occipitofrontal head circumference.[30] Other symptoms include drowsiness, failure to thrive, altered behavior, and convulsions.[30–32] These tumors are often large at the time they are detected. Ultrasound in this age group is excellent for initial imaging.[33]

Two-thirds of all the tumors in children under the age of 1 year are benign.[31] The specific tumor depends on the age of the patient. Tumors occurring at or close to birth are most likely to be germ cell tumors.[31,34,35] Later in the first year of life, gliomas, medulloblastomas, choroid plexus papillomas, and other tumors become more common.[30,31,36] Craniopharyngiomas can also occasionally occur under the age of 1 year.[34] The other unusual feature of brain tumors under the age of 1 is that over 60 percent are supratentorial in location.[30,32] In a review of 45 intracranial tumors diagnosed under the age of 2 months, two-thirds were found to be supratentorial.[37] Of these, 12 were teratomas, 8 PNETs, 13 astrocytoma (including 4 glioblastomas), 4 medulloblastomas, and 3 choroid plexus papillomas.[37] CT in 24 cases showed a large heterogenous mass with marked hydrocephalus. The features were nonspecific for any particular tumor. MR in 5 cases and ultrasound in 4 cases similarly showed large masses with hydrocephalus and a variable appearance to the tumor.[37] Imaging defined the tumor extent well, but except for the presence of calcification in teratomas and dense uniform enhancement after contrast injection with choroid plexus papillomas was rarely able to suggest the correct diagnosis. Symptoms included an increasing head circumference in 28 children, abnormal signs relating to the orbit in 7, vomiting in 5, and convulsions in 3.[37] Mortality is usually high.[31,32]

Some of the likely anatomic locations of the various tumors are summarized in Table 8–6.

TABLE 8–6

Tumor Types by Common Locations[1,2]

Extradural mass
- Spread from primary bone tumor in skull
- Spread from metastases to skull, e.g., neuroblastoma
- Invasion through skull of extracranial tumor, e.g., rhabdomyosarcoma, lymphoma
- Soft-tissue component of dermoid

Suprasellar tumors[1,2]
- Craniopharyngioma
- Glioma—chiasm, hypothalamus
- Germ cell tumor

Tumors likely to involve ventricles
- Choroid plexus papilloma
- Ependymoma
- Pineal tumors
- Medulloblastoma

Posterior fossa
- Medulloblastoma
- Glioma
- Ependymoma

References

1. Scott EW, Mickle JP. Pediatric diencephalic gliomas—a review of 18 cases. Pediatr Neurosci 1987;13:225–232.
2. Chang T, Teng MMH, Guo W-Y, et al. CT of pineal tumors and intracranial germ-cell tumors. AJNR 1989;10:1039–1044.

References

1. Walker RW, Allen JC. Pediatric brain tumors. Pediatr Ann 1983;12:383–391.
2. Davis P. Tumors of the brain. In: Cohen MD, Edwards MK, eds. Magnetic resonance imaging of children. Philadelphia: BC Decker, 1990:155–220.
3. Finlay JL, Goins SC. Brain tumors in children. I. Advances in diagnosis. Am J Pediatr Hematol/Oncol 1987;9:246–255.
4. Ebner F, Ranner G, Slavc I, et al. MR findings in methotrexate-induced CNS abnormalities. AJR 1989;153:1283–1288.
5. Heideman RL, Packer RJ, Albright LA, et al. Tumors of the central nervous system. In: Pizzo PA, Poplack DG, eds. Principles and practice of pediatric oncology. Philadelphia: JB Lippincott, 1989:505–553.
6. Sato Y, Waziri M, Smith W, et al. Hippel-Lindau disease: MR imaging. Radiology 1988;166:241–256.
7. Hammond D. Comments on the clinical investigation of brain tumors in children. Cancer 1985;56:1890–1893.
8. Rorke LB, Gilles FH, Davis RL, et al. Revision of the World Health Organization Classification of brain tumors for childhood brain tumors. Cancer 1985;56:1869–1886.
9. Campbell AN, Chan HSL, Becker LE, et al. Extracranial metastases in childhood primary intracranial tumors. Cancer 1984;53:974–981.
10. Kun LE, D'Souza B, Tefft M. The value of surveillance testing in childhood brain tumors. Cancer 1985;56:1818–1823.
11. O'Tuama LA, Parkard AB, Treves ST. SPECT imaging of pediatric brain tumor with hexakis (methoxyisobutylisonitrile) technetium (I). J Nucl Med 1990;31:2040–2041.
12. Naidich TP, Zimmerman RA. Primary brain tumors in children. Semin Roentgenol 1984;19:100–114.
13. Peterman SB, Steiner RE, Bydder GM. Magnetic resonance imaging of intracranial tumors in children and adolescents. AJNR 1984;5:703–709.
14. Dietrich RB, Lufkin RB, Kangarloo H, et al. Head and Neck MR imaging in the pediatric patient. Radiology 1986;159:769–776.
15. Elster AD, Rieser GD. GD-DTPA-enhanced cranial MR imaging in children: initial clinical experience and recommendations for its use. AJR 1989;153:1265–1268.
16. Bernstein M, Hoffman HJ, Halliday WC, et al. Thalamic tumors in children: long-term follow-up and treatment guides. J Neurosurg 1984;61:649–656.
17. Lukin R. Neuroimaging: 1990. Semin Roentgenol 1989;24:218–230.
18. Zeltzer PM, Friedman HS, Norris DG, et al. Criteria and definitions for response and relapse in children with brain tumors. Cancer 1985;56:1824–1826.
19. Davis PC, Wichman RD, Takei Y, et al. Primary cerebral neuroblastoma: CT and MR findings in 12 cases. AJNR 1990;11:115–120.
20. Dickman CA, Rekate HL, Bird CR, et al. Unenhanced and gadolinium-DTPA-enhanced MR imaging in postoperative evaluation in pediatric brain tumors. J Neurosurg 1989;71:40–53.
21. Bird CR, Drayer BP, Medina M, et al. Gd-DTPA-enhanced MR imaging in pediatric patients after brain tumor resection. Radiology 1988;169:123–126.
22. Stanley P, Suminski N. The incidence and distribution of spinal metastases in children with posterior fossa medulloblastomas. Am J Pediatr Hematol/Oncol 1988;10:283–287.
23. Kramer ED, Rafto S, Packer RJ, et al. Comparison of myelography with CT follow-up versus gadolinium MRI for subarachnoid metastatic disease in children. Neurology 1991;41:46–50.
24. Sze G, Krol G, Olsen WL, et al. Hemorrhagic neoplasms: MR mimics of occult vascular malformations. AJR 1987;149:1223–1230.
25. Bloom HJG, Glees J, Bell J. The treatment and long-term prognosis of children with intracranial tumors: a study of 610 cases, 1950–1981. Int J Radiation Oncol Biol Phys 1990;18:723–745.
26. Gaynon PS, Ettinger LJ, Baum ES, et al. Carboplatin in

childhood brain tumors. A Children's Cancer Study Group Phase II trial. Cancer 1990;66:2465–2469.
27. Finlay JL, Goins SC. Brain tumors in children. III. Advances in chemotherapy. Am J Pediatr Hematol/Oncol 1987;9:264–271.
28. Freeman MP, Kessler RM, Allen JH, et al. Craniopharyngioma: CT and MR imaging in nine cases. J Comput Assist Tomogr 1987;11:810–814.
29. Davis PC, Hoffman JC Jr, Pearl GS, et al. CT evaluation of effects of cranial radiation therapy in children. AJR 1986;147:587–592.
30. Ambrosino MM, Hernanz-Schulman M, Genieser NB, et al. Brain tumors in infants less than a year of age. Pediatr Radiol 1988;19:6–8.
31. Radkowski MA, Naidich TP, Tomita T, et al. Neonatal brain tumors: CT and MR findings. J Comput Assist Tomogr 1988;12:10–20.
32. Jooma R, Hayward RD, Grant DN. Intracranial neoplasms during the first year of life: analysis of one hundred consecutive cases. Neurosurgery 1984;14:31–41.
33. Chuang S, Harwood-Nash D. Tumors and cysts. Neuroradiology 1986;28:463–475.
34. Hurst RW, McIlhenny J, Park TS, et al. Neonatal craniopharyngioma: CT and ultrasonographic features. J Comput Assist Tomogr 1988;12:858–861.
35. Uken P, Sato Y, Smith W. MR findings of malignant intracranial teratoma in a neonate. Pediatr Radiol 1986;16:504–505.
36. Qing-cheng X, Pei-yu P, Yu-shan Y, et al. A survey of 790 cases of astrocytoma. Clin Neurol Neurosurg 1990;92:27–33.
37. Buetow PC, Smirniotopoulos JG, Done S. Congenital brain tumors: a review of 45 cases. AJR 1990;155:587–593.

CHORDOMA

Epidemiology

Chordomas are very rare tumors in children, usually being found in adults.[1]

Pathology

Chordomas arise from notochordal remnants.[2] They are slow-growing tumors, with only very rare cases of metastases being described.[2] They can cause extensive local invasion and bone destruction.[2,3] One-third of the tumors are intracranial, usually in the clivus, with most of the rest being in the sacrococcygeal region.[1,3] Very rare cases have been described in association with tuberosclerosis.[1] A review of 35 children with chordoma indicated that the pathology showed large areas of mucin and gelatinous material, with hemorrhage and necrosis being common.[4] Unlike as in adults, two-thirds of chordomas in children are found in the skull.[6] In very young children, less than 3 years of age, a high percentage of chordomas extend through the foramen magnum. Metastases are much more common, being present in 4 of 8 children under the age of 5 years. They go to the lung but also to unusual sites such as the adrenal and heart.[4]

Clinical Presentation

Symptoms are nonspecific and are caused by mass effect. Clinical signs include raised intracranial pressure, cranial nerve palsies (especially diplopia and tongue weakness), pyramidal tract signs, headache, and sometimes quadriparesis.[4]

Imaging Studies

In the skull, CT shows a mass with its epicenter in the clivus. There is frequently extensive local invasion,[2] including sella and sphenoid.[4] On CT, the mass shows enhancement with injection of intravenous contrast.[3] The enhancement is usually homogeneous.[1,3] On MR, the lesions are well defined and have signal characteristics consistent with prolonged T1 and T2 relaxation times, usually appearing relatively dark on T1 and bright on T2 weighted images. They can be extremely bright on T2 weighted images.[3] In one patient, MR showed homogeneous signal on T1 and T2 weighted images. The signal on T2 ranged from moderate to bright.[4] MR was particularly helpful in showing the epicenter of the lesion being related to clivus, thus suggesting the correct diagnosis.[4] Very occasionally, hemorrhage will cause bright areas to be seen on T1 weighted images.[3] Both CT and MR identify the tumor margins well.[3,5] Bone destruction is better shown on the CT scan. Local effects such as backward displacement of the basilar artery are sometimes better shown with MR.

Therapy and Prognosis

Only surgery is effective, with poor response to radiation or chemotherapy. The prognosis in children is poor, with 6 of 29 patients reviewed dying.[6]

References

1. Shroeder BA, Wells RB, Starshak RJ, et al. Clivus chordoma in a child with tuberous sclerosis: CT and MR demonstration. J Comput Assist Tomogr 1987;11:195–197.
2. Brooks LJ, Afshani E, Hidalgo C, et al. Clivus chordoma with pulmonary metastases appearing as failure to thrive. Am J Dis Child 1981;135:713–715.
3. Oot RF, Melville GE, New PFJ, et al. The role of MR and CT in evaluating clival chordomas and chondrosarcomas. AJR 1988;151:567–575.
4. Sze G, Krol G, Olsen WL, et al. Hemorrhagic neoplasms: MR mimics of occult vascular malformations. AJR 1987;149:1223–1230.
5. Bernstein M, Hoffman HJ, Halliday WC, et al. Thalamic tumors in children: long-term follow-up and treatment guides. J Neurosurg 1984;61:649–656.
6. Matsumoto J, Towbin RB, Ball WS Jr. Cranial chordomas in infancy and childhood. A report of two cases and review of the literature. Pediatr Radiol 1989;20:28–32.

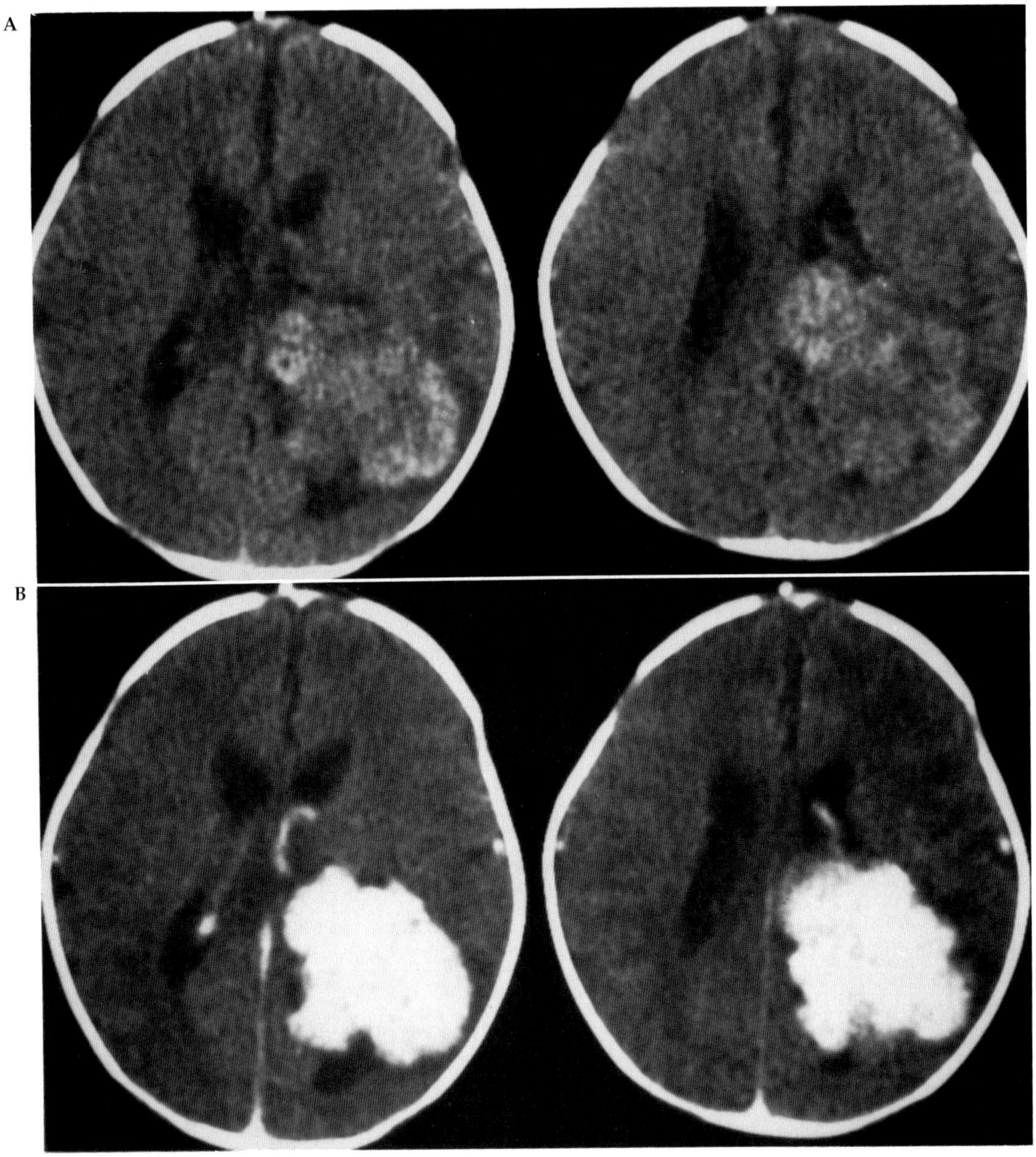

Figure 8–1. **Diagnosis: Benign choroid plexus papilloma of the left lateral ventricle. 11-day-old girl. *A,* CT. Axial image. There is a large lobulated partially calcified hyperdense mass that is related to dilated choroidal vessels. The mass expands the ventricle and extends into the surrounding parenchyma. *B,* CT after intravenous contrast administration. There is marked enhancement from the tumor. (From Radkowski MA. Neonatal brain tumors: CT and MR findings. J CAT 1988;12:10–20.)**

CHOROID PLEXUS PAPILLOMA

Epidemiology

Choroid plexus papillomas are rare tumors, accounting for less than 1 percent of all pediatric CNS tumors.[1,2] Fifty percent will occur under the age of 10 years and 20 percent under the age of 1 year.[2]

Pathology

Most choroid plexus papillomas are benign, with between 10 and 20 percent being malignant.[1,2] The likelihood of malignancy is increased in very young children. In children, 80 percent of the lesions will be found in the lateral ventricles (Fig. 8–1) (in adults the fourth ventricle is the most common site), with 4 percent occurring in the third and 16 percent in the fourth ventricle[1,2] (Fig. 8–2). The tumors are irregular, having a cauliflower-like

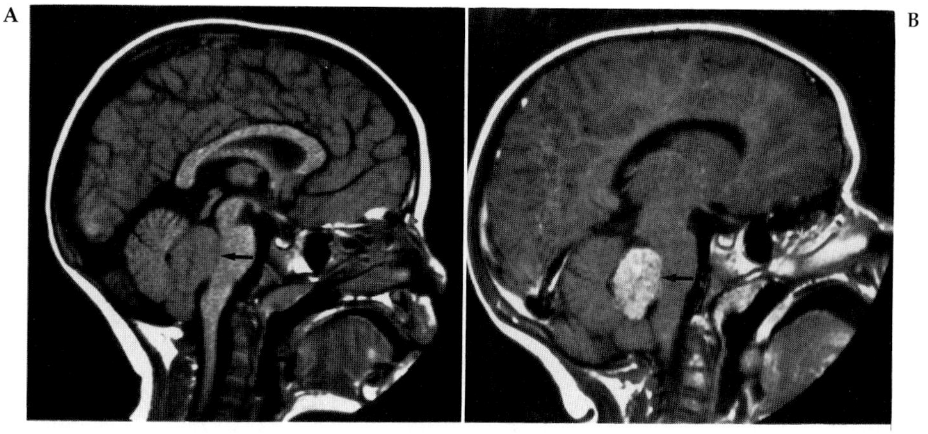

Figure 8–2. **Diagnosis: Choroid plexus papilloma.**
***A* and *B*, Sagittal T1 weighted MR images before and after administration of gadolinium-DTPA. There is a well-defined mass lesion *(arrows)* lying in the fourth ventricle. There is bright patchy enhancement following gadolinium-DTPA administration. Dark areas on both pulse sequences probably represent flow voids from large vessels lying within the tumor.**

appearance.[1] They are frequently attached to the normal choroid by a pedicle and can move around in the cerebrospinal fluid.[1] Calcification is usually reported as being a rare finding, but in one study was identified in 4 of 5 patients.[3] They may spread through the ventricular foramina. Hydrocephalus is common (Fig. 8–1). It is believed to result mainly from overproduction of cerebrospinal fluid with or without the presence of obstruction.[1] Cerebrospinal fluid dissemination of the tumor occurs when the histology is malignant.[2]

Clinical Presentation

Symptoms are extremely nonspecific and are usually those of raised intracranial pressure.[1]

Imaging Studies

Investigations reveal a mass lesion with its epicenter in the choroid. Hydrocephalus is usually identified. CT usually shows a well-defined mass lesion in the lateral ventricle with some increased attenuation prior to contrast injection and moderate to marked uniform enhancement following contrast administration[1,3] (see Fig. 8–1). These findings are fairly characteristic. On MR, well-marginated lobulated lesions are again seen (see Fig. 8–2). They may engulf the normal choroid.[1] Signal intensity is intermediate on T1 weighted images and intermediate or increased on T2 weighted images. They enhance with gadolinium-DTPA. All patients show some signal voids on both pulse sequences because of flow through enlarged vessels (Fig. 8–2) or occasionally clot. Some increased signal in the periventricular tissues is often seen on T2 weighted images. This is most likely caused by transependymal fluid resorption and not tumor.[1] Gadolinium-DTPA is helpful in identifying residual postoperative tumor (Fig. 8–3).

Spread of tumor through the ventricular foramina seen on either imaging modality strongly suggests the diagnosis of choroid plexus papilloma. Irregular margins and a nonhomogeneous internal structure are signs suggesting malignancy.[1]

Angiography shows a very vascular tumor. It is sometimes performed to show the location of the vascular pedicle prior to surgery.[4]

Differential Diagnosis

Differential diagnosis includes vascular malformations, astrocytoma, ependymoma, cysticercosis, medulloblastoma, cysts, and hemangioma.[1,2]

Therapy and Prognosis

Surgical resection is curative for most choroid plexus papilloma. The few tumors that are malignant do not respond well to any therapy.[2]

References
1. Coates TL, Hinshaw DB, Peckman N, et al. Pediatric choroid plexus neoplasma: MR, CT, and pathologic correlation. Radiology 1989;173:81–88.
2. Davis P. Tumors of the brain. In: Cohen MD, Edwards MK, eds. Magnetic resonance imaging of children. Philadelphia: BC Decker, 1990:155–220.
3. Radkowski MA, Naidich TP, Tomita T, et al. Neonatal brain tumors: CT and MR findings. J Comput Assist Tomogr 1988;12:10–20.
4. Heideman RL, Packer RJ, Albright LA, et al. Tumors of the central nervous system. In: Pizzo PA, Poplack DG, eds. Principles and practice of pediatric oncology. Philadelphia: JB Lippincott, 1989:505–553.

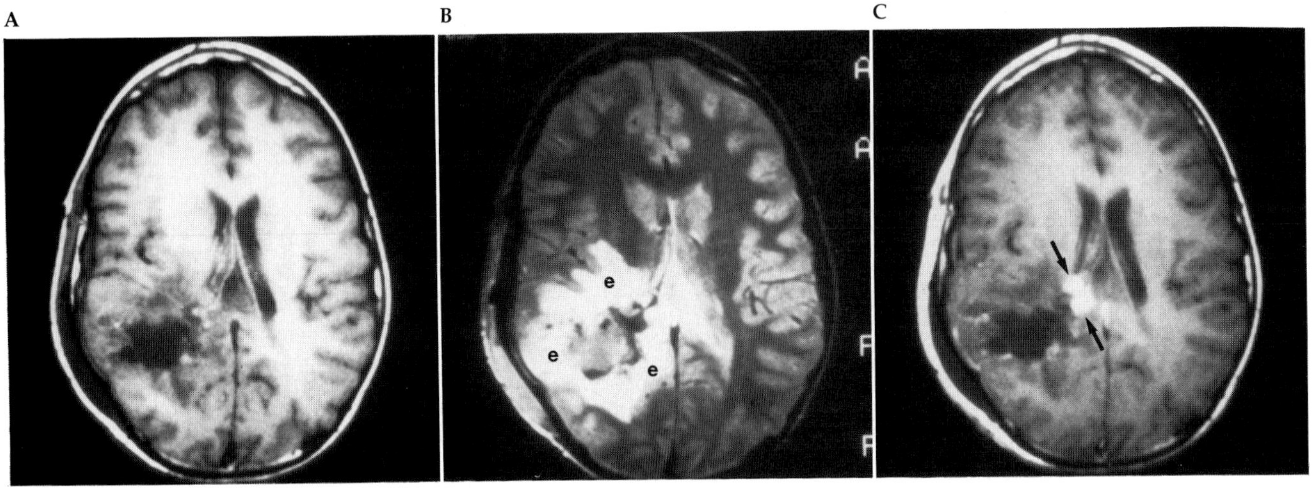

Figure 8–3. **Diagnosis: Residual choroid plexus carcinoma. Images obtained 3 days after resection of the main tumor mass.**
***A*, MR, T1 weighted noncontrast image. The area of resection is seen adjacent to the atrium of the right lateral ventricle. *B*, MR, T2 weighted noncontrast image. There is high signal intensity from edema (*E*) surrounding the tumor bed and decreased signal intensity at the margins of the resection secondary to hemorrhage. *C*, MR, T1 weighted image after gadolinium-DTPA. Two nodules of enhancing residual tumor tissue are identified at the inframedial margin of resection *(arrows)*. This was confirmed by surgery.**

CRANIOPHARYNGIOMA

Epidemiology

Craniopharyngiomas account for 50 percent of sellar and suprasellar region mass lesions in children. They represent between 5 and 10 percent of all pediatric intracranial tumors.[1] They are rarely reported in the newborn[2] and are unusual under the age of 2 years.[3] The peak incidence is between 6 and 12 years of age, with a median of about 8 years.[1,3]

Pathology

Craniopharyngiomas are benign, slow-growing tumors that arise from Rathke pouch remnants.[4] Most of the tumors arise in the suprasellar area, but they frequently spread to involve the sella as well. In one study, both the sella and suprasellar area were involved in 15 of 21 patients. Very rarely craniopharyngiomas can arise in the infrasellar region, usually in the sphenoid sinus[5] (Fig. 8–4). The tumors are usually moderate to large and occasionally can be gigantic.[6] The margins are usually smooth, well defined, and lobulated.[3] The tumors usually contain large multiple cysts and appear predominantly cystic or mixed solid and cystic[3,4] (Figs. 8–5 and 8–6). The cysts can contain cholesterol or hemorrhage. Calcification is extemely common, being present in 16 of 22 patients in one study[5] and being reported as occurring in between 70 to 90% of patients overall.[5] The tumors grow and compress adjacent structures. There is usually tight adherence between the tumor margins and adjacent tissues, which can cause difficulty during surgical removal.[3] Upward growth can cause obstruction of the third ventricle.[7] Forward growth can involve the optic chiasm. In 3 patients with giant tumors, the growth extended down to the level of the foramen magnum in 2 and upward and laterally into the lateral ventricle in one patient.[6] Metastases do not occur. Compared to adults, craniopharyngiomas in children tend to show more calcium, more cysts, and to be larger.[5]

Clinical Presentation

Headache, caused by a rise in cranial pressure, is the most common symptom. It is often overlooked and may be present for many years before the tumor is diagnosed.[5] Other symptoms include visual disturbance from involvement of the optic chiasm or endocrine malfunction from involvement of the pituitary gland.[1,3,5,8]

Imaging Studies

Skull radiograph is not needed if CT scan is performed, but it may frequently be done. Prior to availability of CT imaging, skull radiograph was extremely useful for diagnosis of craniopharyngioma. On the skull radiograph, enlargement of the sella turcica is seen in 45 percent of patients and calcification in between 50 and 80 percent.[3,8] Some abnormality on the skull radiograph was identified in 21 of 22 patients.[5] Abnormalities in the sella include increase in size, abnormal shape, abnormal

A

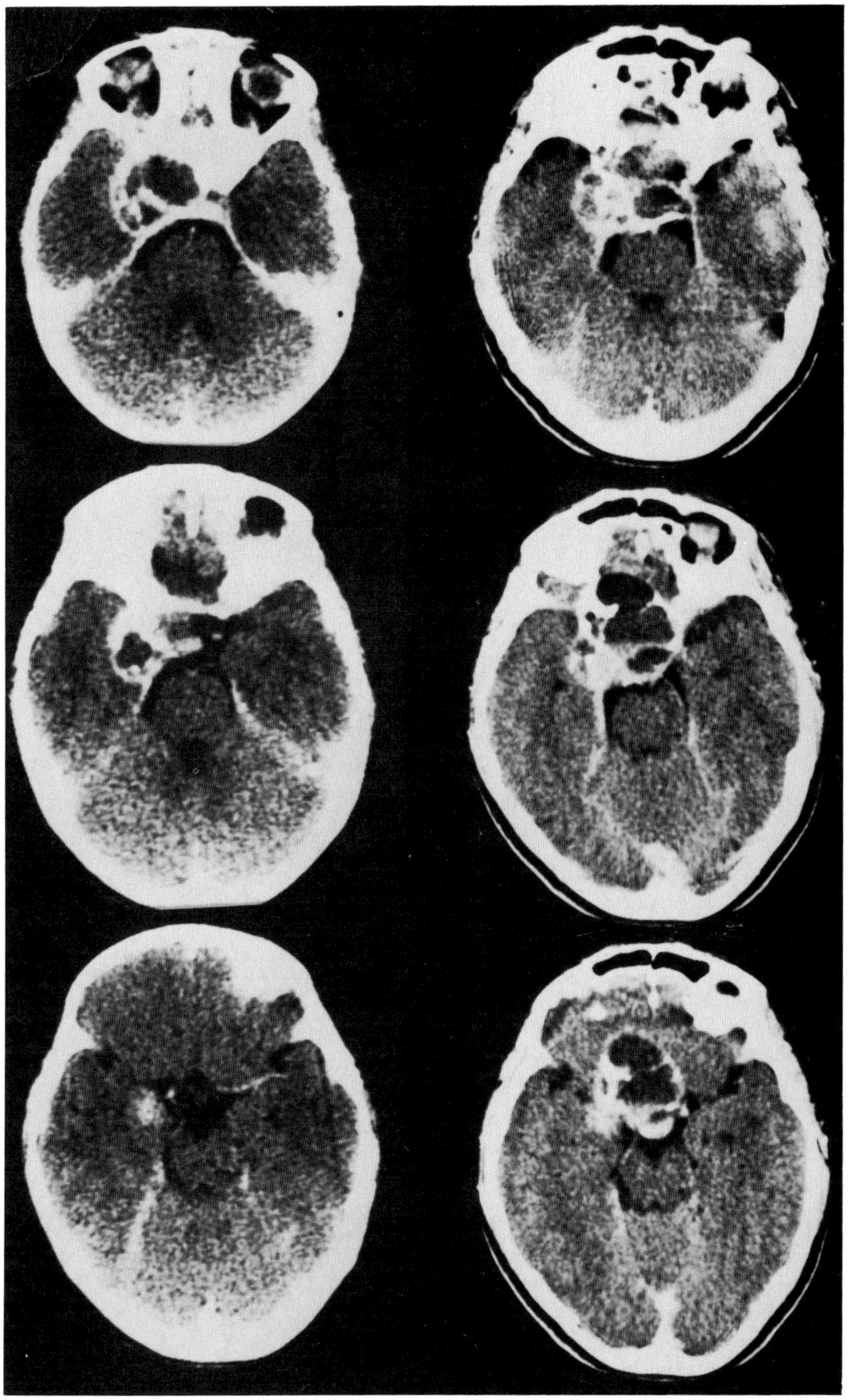

Figure 8–4. Diagnosis: Infrasellar craniopharyngioma.
A, Series of CT images. The three left images were obtained on initial presentation. The right images were obtained 3 months later and show enlargement of the lesion. There is a mass involving the right sphenoid sinus with extension into the ethmoid sinuses and right cavernous sinus. There are multilobulated cysts with contrast enhancement of the rim. There is also a soft-tissue component to the abnormality. ***B** (next page),* MR, sagittal images. The left two images are T1 weighted and the right two images T2 weighted. The cystic components of the tumor are bright on T1 and T2 weighted images. The bright signal on the T1 weighted images is caused by hemorrhage or the presence of protein. (From Akimura T. Infrasellar craniopharyngioma. Neuroradiology 1989;31:180–183.)

Figure 8–4, B

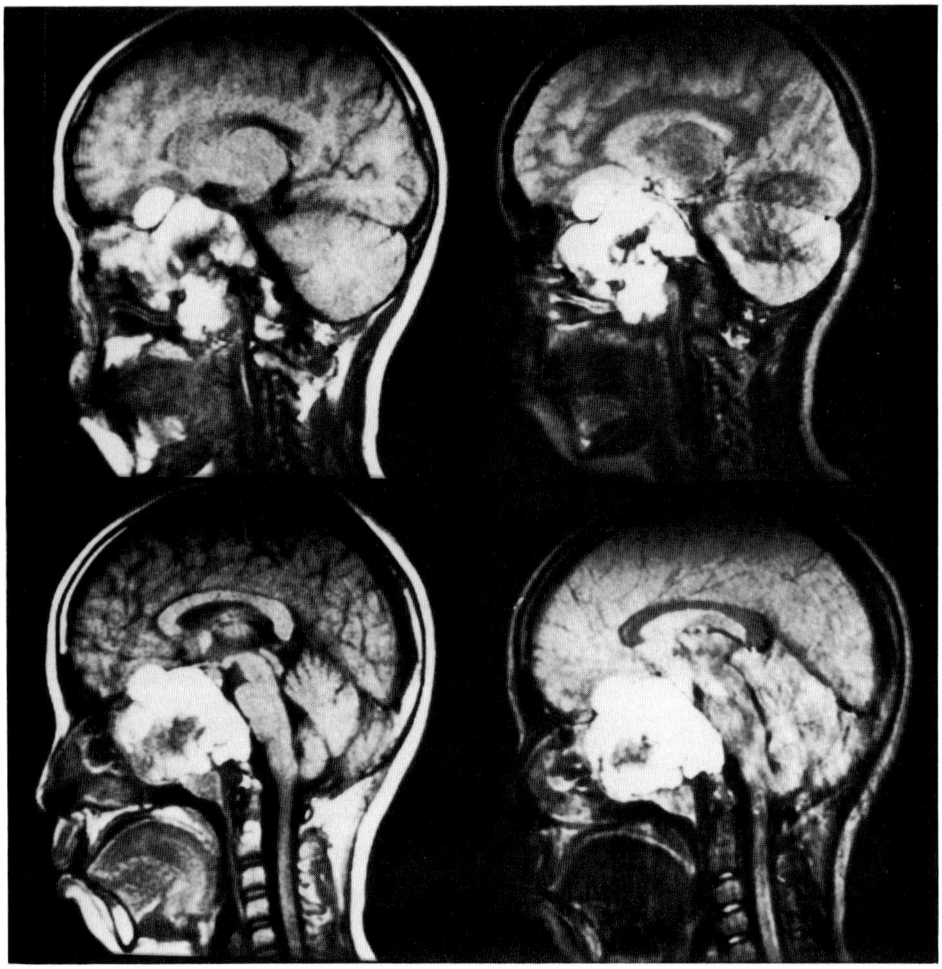

contour to the floor, sclerosis of the floor, and erosion of the dorsum sellae.[5]

The most typical appearance on CT is of a large mass lesion in the suprasellar region involving the sella, with multiple cysts (see Fig. 8–5) and calcification. In some patients, the cysts may not appear of low intensity but may show increased signal intensity because of the presence of high protein concentration.[9] The tumors are always in the midline. CT will show spread of tumor in all directions. On MR imaging, a midline mass is again seen. Calcification is not well identified unless very large (see Fig. 8–6). Cyst characterization may be difficult and signal intensity is very variable on T1 weighted images. This is because the cysts may contain protein, blood, and cholesterol, all of which may cause high signal on T1 weighted images.[1,4,8–11] The cysts are always bright on T2 weighted images but may not be particularly different from solid parts of the tumor.[10] Coronal and sagittal images are particularly helpful in showing the inferior extent of the tumor (Figs. 8–5 and 8–6). Overall the extent of the tumor is better identified on MR than CT.[11] CT is more helpful than MR for making the specific diagnosis because of its better ability to demonstrate calcium and characterize the cysts.[8,10,11] For follow-up imaging only MR is required.[8,11]

Differential Diagnosis

Differential diagnosis includes germ cell tumors and gliomas. Other cystic tumors, such as epidermoid and arachnoid cysts, are usually simpler and more well defined, do not contain calcium, and do not have complex material present within the cyst. A Rathke pouch cyst is a congenital mucoid cyst. It has no calcification and no soft-tissue component. It may occur in or above the sella. Because of the mucoid material, it appears very bright on T1 weighted images and slightly less bright on T2 weighted MR images.[12]

Therapy and Prognosis

There is considerable debate regarding two therapeutic regimes. These are radical surgery versus tumor debulking and radiation therapy.[3] About 80 percent of tumors may initially be believed to be resectable, but about 20 percent of these will recur. Recurrence may be late (2 to 5 years or more), so that imaging needs to be continued for many years. If a postoperative CT or MR shows no visible tumor after surgery, the likelihood of recurrence

A

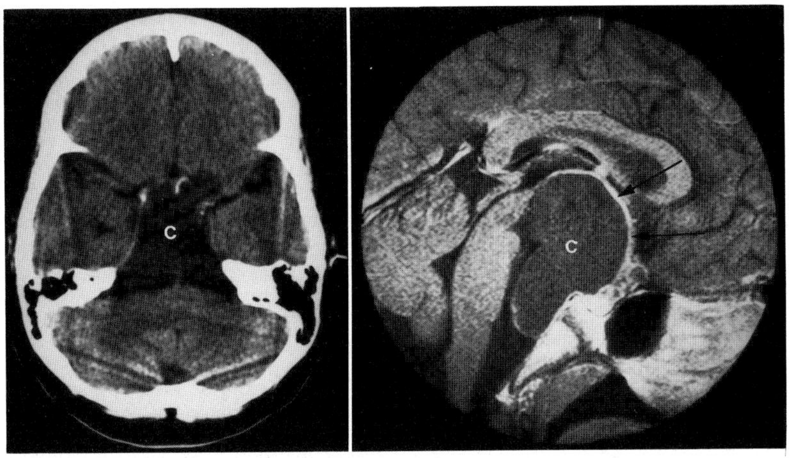

B

Figure 8-5. **Diagnosis: Craniopharyngioma.**
***A,* CT. There is a large cystic mass (*C*) extending down in front of the clivus. *B,* MR, sagittal T1 weighted image after administration of gadolinium-DTPA. There is a large cystic suprasellar lesion demonstrating peripheral enhancement *(arrows).* The mass extends down inferiorly adjacent to the clivus and displaces the brain stem and pons posteriorly.**

is reduced. MR is particularly helpful in planning the surgical approach (e.g., involvement of the pituitary fossa may alter the surgical approach) or in determining resectability (e.g., by demonstrating involvement of the cavernous sinus).[8] Chemotherapy has no role in the treatment of craniopharyngioma. Overall survival is good, over 80 percent, but complications such as visual or endocrine disturbance may persist even if the tumor has been successfully treated. The prognosis is worse if the tumor cannot be resected or if the patient is under the age of 5 years.[3]

Figure 8-6. **Diagnosis: Craniopharyngioma.**
***A,* MR, axial T2 weighted image. Cystic components (*C*) of the craniopharyngioma appear very bright. There is a septum of soft tissue between them. A fluid level *(arrow)* within one of the cysts is probably caused by hemorrhage within it. *B,* MR, T1 weighted image with gadolinium-DTPA. There is a large mass arising in the suprasellar region and extending superiorly and posteriorly. It is causing posterior displacement of the brain stem (*B*). A large part of the mass is of low intensity and appears to be cystic (*C*). The rest of the mass *(arrows)* shows patchy enhancement from the gadolinium-DTPA. Low-intensity areas within the region of enhancement probably represent calcification.**

A

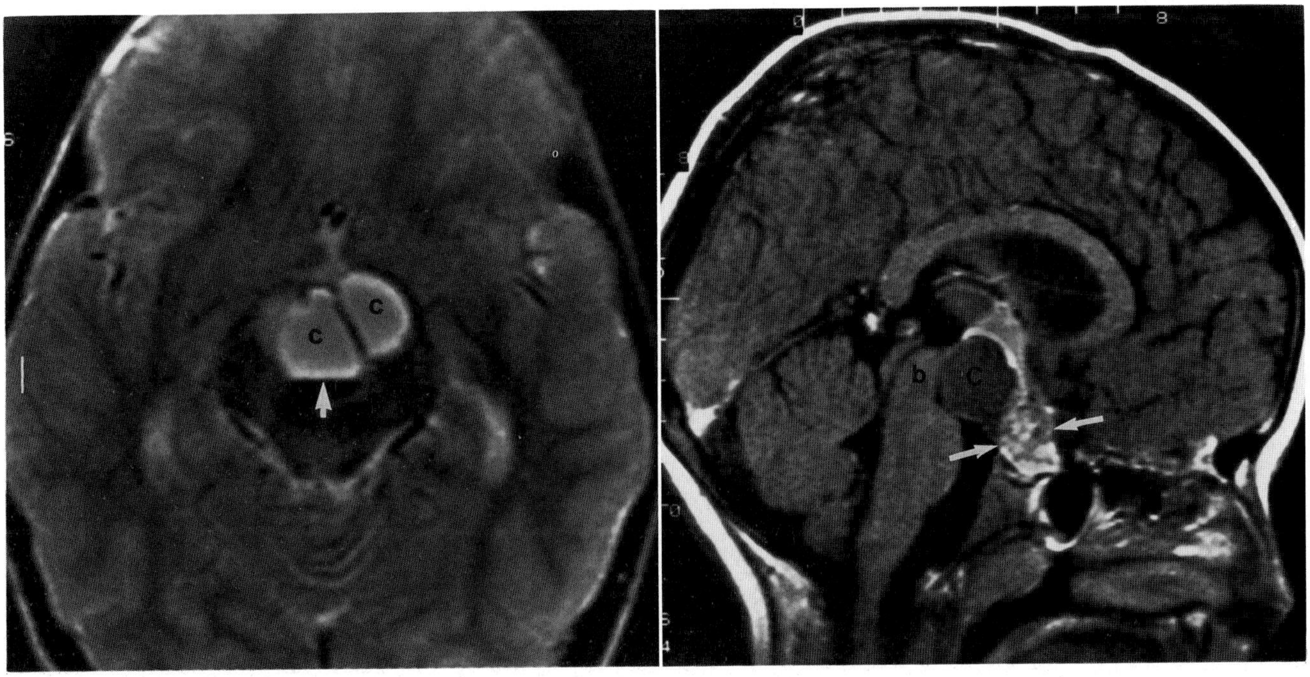

B

References

1. Davis P. Tumors of the brain. In: Cohen MD, Edwards MK, eds. Magnetic resonance imaging of Children. Philadelphia: BC Decker, 1990:155–220.
2. Hurst RW, McIlhenny J, Park TS, et al. Neonatal craniopharyngioma: CT and ultrasonographic features. J Comput Assist Tomogr 1988;12:858–861.
3. Heideman RL, Packer RJ, Albright LA, et al. Tumors of the central nervous system. In: Pizzo PA, Poplack DG, eds. Principles and practice of pediatric oncology. Philadelphia: JB Lippincott, 1989:505–553.
4. Akimura T, Kameda H, Abiko S, et al. Infrasellar craniopharyngioma. Neuroradiology 1989;31:180–183.
5. Sorva R, Jaaskinen J, Heiskanen O. Craniopharyngioma in children and adults. Acta Neurochir 1987;89:3–9.
6. Wechsler-Jentzsch K, Witt JH, Fitz CR, et al. Unresectable gliomas in children: tumor-volume response to radiation therapy. Radiology 1988;169:237–242.
7. Finlay JL, Goins SC. Brain tumors in children. I. Advances in diagnosis. Am J Pediatr Hematol/Oncol 1987;9:246–255.
8. Pusey E, Kortman KE, Flannigan BD, et al. MR of craniopharyngiomas: tumor delineation and characterization. AJR 1987;149:383–388.
9. Young SC, Zimmerman RA, Nowell MA, et al. Giant cystic craniopharyngiomas. Neuroradiology 1987;29:468–473.
10. Freeman MP, Kessler RM, Allen JH, et al. Craniopharyngioma: CT and MR imaging in nine cases. J Comput Assist Tomogr 1987;11:810–814.
11. Pusey E, Kortman KE, Flannigan BD, et al. MR of craniopharyngiomas: Tumor delineation and characterization. AJNR 1987;8:439–444.
12. Towbin RB, Ball WS, Kaufman RA. Pediatric case of the day. RadioGraphics 1987;7:385–395.

EPENDYMOMA

Epidemiology

Ependymomas account for about 10 percent of intracranial tumors in children.[1–3] The sex incidence is approximately equal. The peak incidence is in the age range of 1 to 6 years.[2–4]

Pathology

Ependymomas arise from mature ependymal cells, usually from the cells lining the ventricles or the spinal canal.[4,5] They can sometimes arise from the rest of the ectopic cells in the white matter of the frontal or parietal lobes.[4] In children, between 60 and 80 percent are reported to lie in the posterior fossa, below the tent.[3,4,6] A small percentage will arise in the spinal cord. The tumors are moderately encapsulated and may contain hemorrhage and necrosis.[3] Calcification is fairly common, seen in about 50 percent, with cysts being present in up to 70 percent.[4] Local growth can demonstrate extensive infiltration.[4,6] In the posterior fossa, the tumor grows into the fourth ventricle. It may grow into the choroid plexus. It may penetrate the cerebellar hemispheres or grow through the foramina of Luschka and Magendie into the cisterna magna and even down into the spinal canal.[4] Cerebrospinal fluid dissemination can occur.[5,6] These tumors may be malignant. Malignancy is more likely in tumors above the tentorium and in tumors occurring in young patients.[5] About 60 percent of supratentorial tumors will be high grade. In children under the age of 2, over 90 percent of tumors are in the posterior fossa.[4]

Clinical Presentation

Signs of ependymoma are very nonspecific. They include signs of raised intracranial pressure. Supratentorial tumors may cause convulsions. Infratentorial tumors may cause pyramidal signs, ataxia, or cranial nerve abnormality.[3]

Imaging Studies

These tumors have a very varied appearance, reflecting the common findings of hemorrhage, necrosis, and cysts, and the infiltrative growth pattern[4] (Figs. 8–7 and 8–8). On CT, the most common appearance is that of an isodense or hypodense mass[5,7] on the precontrast im-

Figure 8–7. **Diagnosis: Ependymoma.**
MR, T1 weighted image after gadolinium-DTPA administration. There is a mass lesion present in the right CP cistern. There is gadolinium-DTPA enhancement of the lesion in a heterogeneous fashion. There is compression of the adjacent pons with slight rotation. There is also probably invasion of the pons.

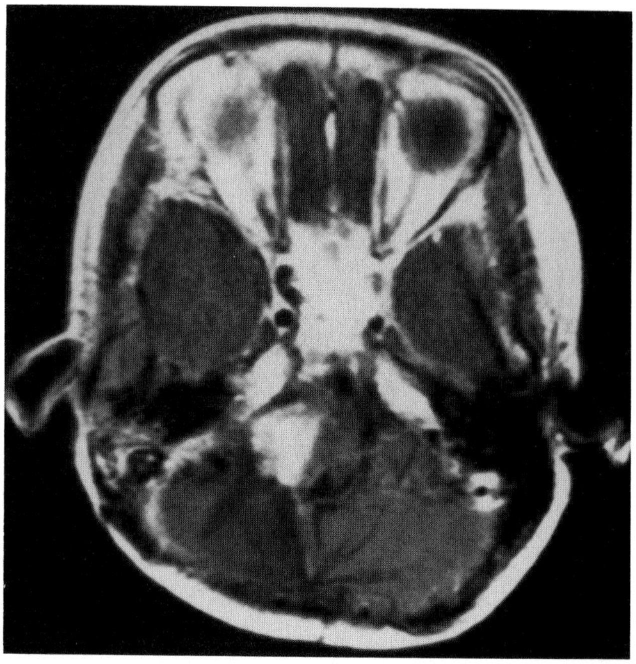

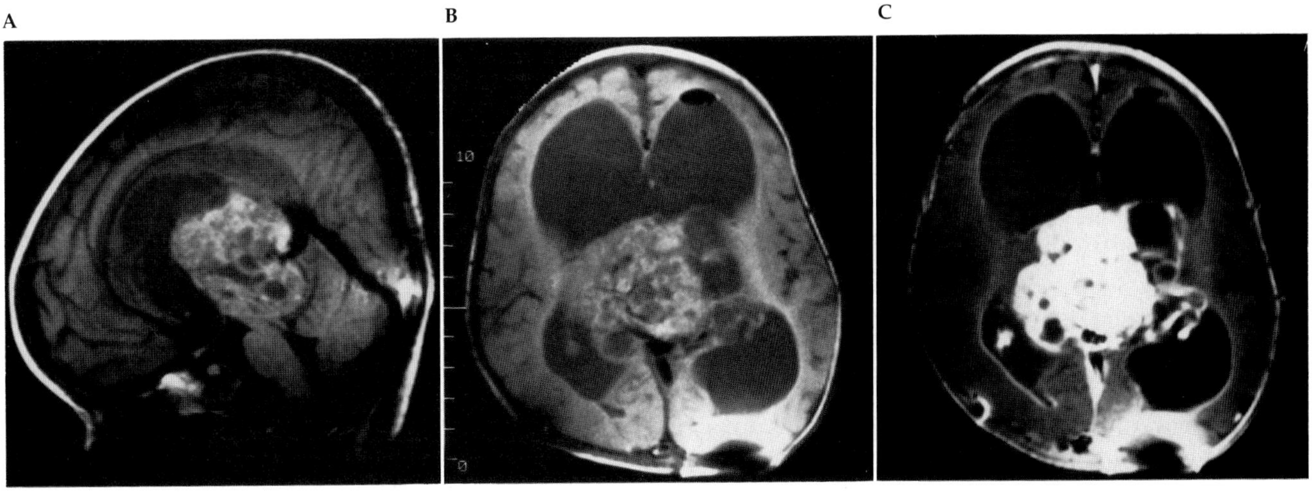

Figure 8-8. **Diagnosis: Ependymoma of the pineal region.**
***A* and *B*, MR, T1 weighted images. There is a very large complex cystic solid mass seen to be arising in the region of the pineal gland. There is marked hydrocephalus. *C*, MR, T1 weighted after gadolinium-DTPA administration. There is marked enhancement of the tumor.**

ages, with moderate enhancement following intravenous contrast injection. Calcification is common. The tumors are located in the posterior fossa, in the region of the fourth ventricle, with extension into the cisterns and cerebral pontine angle and through the foramina of the fourth ventricle.[4,5,7] Their epicenter is usually midline. Hydrocephalus may be present. The MR appearance is nonspecific, with variable signal intensity on T2 and T1 weighted images.[6,7] The tumors are heterogeneous. Calcification, which helps in the differentiation of fourth ventricle ependymoma from medulloblastoma, is not seen in most MR images.[5] MR shows the local spread and extent of the tumor better than CT.[5] Imaging of the meninges must be performed in all cases. In the cranium, this is probably best done with contrast-enhanced MR. There is debate as to the relative advantages or disadvantages of contrast-enhanced MR versus contrast-enhanced CT for evaluation of the spine. One or both of these studies needs to be performed.[4]

Differential Diagnosis

Supratentorial lesions have a large differential diagnosis, including glioma, PNET, and choroid plexus papilloma. In the posterior fossa, it may be difficult to differentiate ependymoma from midline astrocytoma. The epicenter of the ependymoma relates to the fourth ventricle, whereas the astrocytoma may be more posterior in the vermis. Ependymoma can be differentiated from medulloblastoma by the presence of calcium, the very inhomogeneous enhancement, cysts, and extrusion through the foramina of the fourth ventricle.

Therapy and Prognosis

The main form of treatment is surgical resection. This may be achieved with supratentorial lesions, but for the more common infratentorial lesions it is usually impossible to excise the lesion completely.[3,5] All patients receive radiation therapy. Prophylactic radiation to the spine may be given for high-grade tumors.[3] Overall survival is poor, reported in the range of 20 to 30 percent.[2,5] It may approach 50 percent for favorable tumors, which are low grade and have no cerebrospinal fluid spread. Prognosis also tends to be better for primary tumors occurring in the spine.[3] Some response to chemotherapy can be detected, but the overall efficacy of chemotherapy for treatment of ependymoma is not known.[2,3]

References

1. Campbell AN, Chan HSL, Becker LE, et al. Extracranial metastases in childhood primary intracranial tumors. Cancer 1984;53:974–981.
2. Walker RW, Allen JC. Pediatric brain tumors. Pediatr Ann 1983;12:383–391.
3. Heideman RL, Packer RJ, Albright LA, et al. Tumors of the central nervous system. In: Pizzo PA, Poplack DG, eds. Principles and practice of pediatric oncology. Philadelphia: JB Lippincott, 1989:505–553.
4. Naidich TP, Zimmerman RA. Primary brain tumors in children. Semin Roentgenol 1984;19:100–114.
5. Davis P. Tumors of the brain. In: Cohen MD, Edwards MK, eds. Magnetic resonance imaging of children. Philadelphia: BC Decker, 1990;155–220.
6. Gusnard DA. Cerebellar neoplasms in children. Semin Roentgenol 1990;25:263–278.
7. Zimmerman RA. Pediatric supratentorial tumors. Semin Roentgenol 1990;25:225–248.

ESTHESIONEUROBLASTOMA

Esthesioneuroblastoma tumors are also called olfactory neuroblastoma.

Epidemiology

These are very uncommon tumors in children. There are peaks in teenage years and later adulthood,[1] with a total of less than 20 percent occurring under the age of 20.[2]

Pathology

The tumors probably arise from olfactory epithelium close to the cribriform plate.[3–5] They are primitive neuroectodermal tumors.[3] They are slow growing and mainly demonstrate local invasion, including the base of the skull and the cranium.[4] They can grow into the orbit and cause proptosis.[4] Metastases are uncommon, occurring in less than 20 percent of patients. They are usually local to lymph nodes[1,2] and rarely to the lung.

Clinical Presentation

The tumors are slow growing and often present very late. Symptoms include nasal obstruction and epistaxis, which are present in about three-quarters of all patients.[2,6] Other symptoms may include proptosis.[4] VMA excretion in the urine is usually normal.[1]

In a large review of 97 patients, nodal metastases were identified in 11 and lung metases in one.[6]

Imaging Studies

CT shows the presence of an enhancing mass lesion centered in the roof of the nose. There may be extensive local spread, including the cranium, orbit, and sinuses. Intracranial spread is seen in about 20 percent of cases.[7] Bone destruction is well identified.[7] Orbital spread was identified in 17 percent of 12 patients.[5] MR findings in this tumor are not reported, but it is expected that MR would be inferior to CT for demonstration of bone destruction but superior to CT for demonstration of total local extent and margins of the tumor.

Therapy and Prognosis

The main form of treatment is surgery with or without local radiation therapy.[6] Overall survival is good but local recurrences may occur.

References

1. Chapman P, Carter RL, Clifford P. The diagnosis and surgical management of olfactory neuroblastoma: the role of craniofacial resection. J Laryngol Otol 1981;95:785–799.
2. Olsen KD, DeSanto LW. Olfactory neuroblastoma. Biologic and clinical behavior. Arch Otolaryngol 1983;109:797–802.
3. Becker LE, Hinton D. Primitive neuroectodermal tumors of the central nervous system. Hum Pathol 1983;14:538–550.
4. Aghadiuno PU, Thomas SM, Ogan O, et al. Olfactory neuroblastoma. A case report in an African child. J Laryngol Otol 1983;97:261–265.
5. Burke DP, Gabrielsen TO, Knake JE, et al. Radiology of olfactory neuroblastoma. Radiology 1980;137:367–372.
6. Shimada H, Chattan J, Newton WA, et al. Histopathologic prognostic factors in neuroblastic tumors: definition of subtypes of ganglioneuroblastoma and an age-linked classification of neuroblastomas. JNCI 1984;73:405–416.
7. Manelfe C, Bonafe A, Fabre P, et al. Computed tomography in olfactory neuroblastoma: one case of esthesioneuroepithelioma and four cases of esthesioneuroblastoma. J Comput Assist Tomogr 1978;2:412–420.

GANGLIOGLIOMA

Epidemiology

Gangliogliomas account for about 4 percent of all pediatric intracranial tumors. They can occur at any age but are most common over the age of 10.[1,2] About 5 percent of children will have associated congenital anomalies.

Pathology

These tumors are also called gangliocytoma. They contain both glial and ganglion (nerve) cells.[1,3] The size of the tumors vary. They can occur in any location. Cystic tumors are most common in the cerebellum and solid tumors in the temporal lobe and other lobes of the cerebrum.[1,3] Most of the tumors are low grade and relatively benign and they very rarely spread.[1–3] Hemorrhage and necrosis are very unusual.[4] In several studies, calcification has been demonstrated in about one-third of patients.[1,3] Between 30 and 50 percent may show cystic change.[3] The cystic tumors are more likely in the posterior fossa.

Clinical Presentation

Findings are usually variable and nonspecific, including signs of raised intracranial pressure, cranial nerve abnormality and convulsions.

Imaging Studies

The appearance of these tumors is quite variable, with no characteristic features (Figs. 8–9 and 8–10). On CT, the cystic lesions most commonly are of lower intensity than normal brain. The tumors demonstrate mild enhancement with intravenous contrast.[4] The solid tumors are more likely to be isodense or have increased density, with most showing mild to moderate enhancement after contrast injection.[1,3] Calcification will be identified in about one-third of patients. A tumor can, however, have almost any appearance.[2,3,5] Local invasion is uncommon.[2] On MR, the signal intensity is vari-

A B

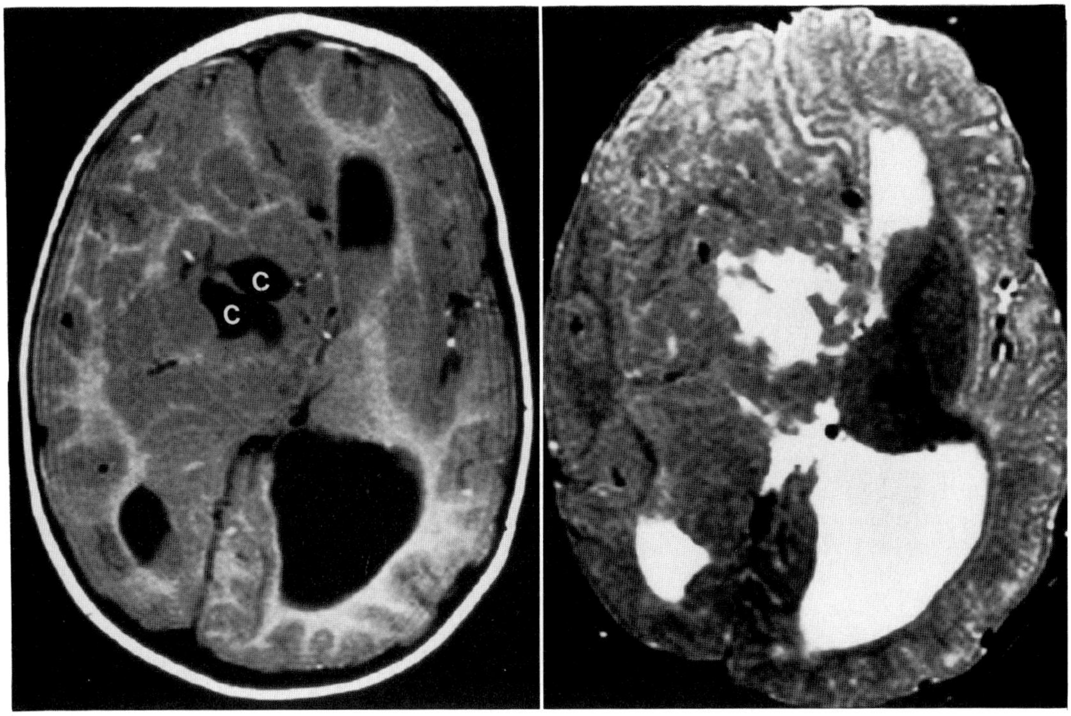

Figure 8–9. Diagnosis: Ganglioglioma.
A, MR, axial image after gadolinium-DTPA enhancement shows a large nonenhancing lesion in the region of the right basal ganglia. The mass is isointense with gray matter and contains two central cystic components (***C***). The exact boundaries of the tumor are difficult to define. ***B***, MR, T2 weighted image at the same level as ***A***. The cystic components have increased in signal intensity. The solid portion of the mass remains isointense with normal gray matter and again the boundaries of the tumor are very difficult to define.

Figure 8–10. Diagnosis: Ganglioglioma.
A, CT. Contrast enhanced. There is a cystic tumor with minimal enhancement of the posterior margin *(arrows).* It lies within the cerebellum. The lesion cannot be differentiated from a cystic astrocytoma. ***B***, MR, axial T2 weighted image. The lesion is of increased signal intensity with well-defined margins.

A B

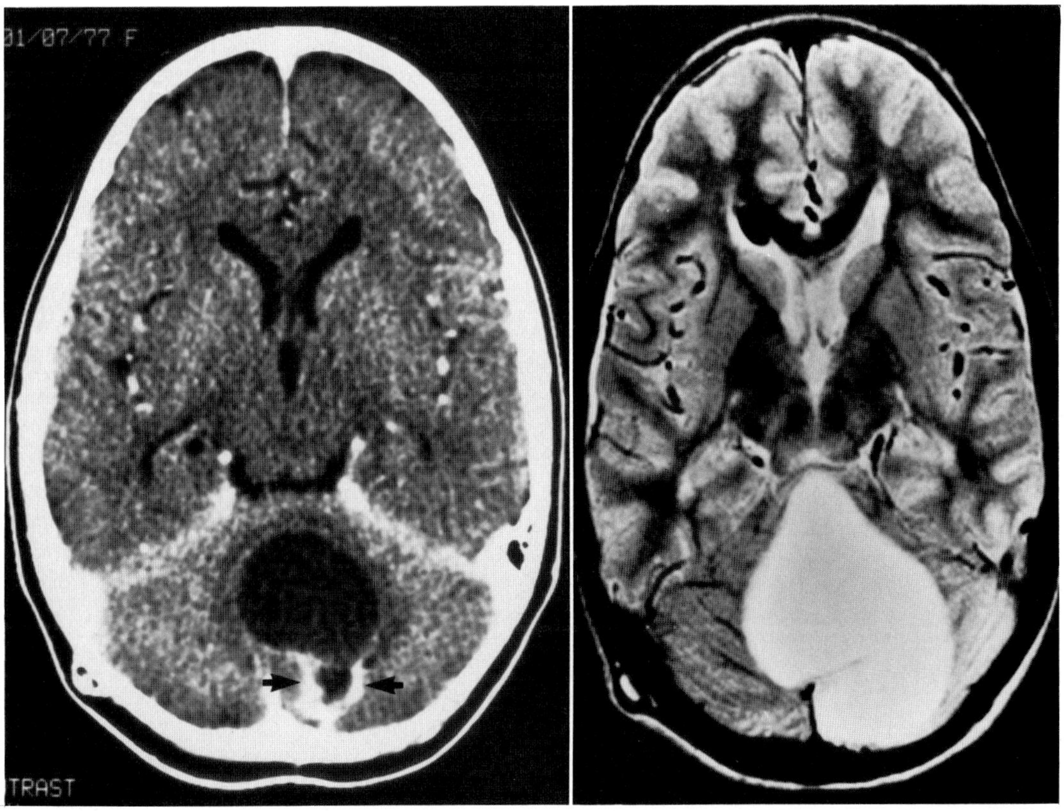

able on both T1 and T2 weighted pulse sequences[2–4] (Figs. 8–9 and 8–10). Most tumors show some areas of increased signal on T1 weighted images. Adjacent structures are displaced. Edema is minimal.[2] The margins may sometimes be difficult to see[3] (Fig. 8–9). In one patient given gadolinium-DTPA, no enhancement was identified.[3] In summary, imaging appearance on both CT and MR is variable and has no characteristic features.

Differential Diagnosis

Differential diagnosis includes most intracranial tumors. Gangliogliomas should be considered in the differential diagnosis of almost any intracranial mass.

Therapy and Prognosis

Surgery is the most effective therapy. The tumors may, however, not be completely resected, with 16 of 18 patients having some residual in one study.[2] Chemotherapy and radiation therapy are not usually used.[2] In one study, 3 of 18 patients died.[3]

References

1. Naidich TP, Zimmerman RA. Primary brain tumors in children. Semin Roentgenol 1984;19:100–114.
2. Davis P. Tumors of the brain. In: Cohen MD, Edwards MK, eds. Magnetic resonance imaging of children. Philadelphia: BC Decker, 1990;155–220.
3. Castillo M, Davis PC, Takei Y, et al. Intracranial ganglioglioma: MR, CT, and clinical findings in 18 patients. AJR 1990;154:607–612.
4. Zimmerman RA. Pediatric supratentorial tumors. Semin Roentgenol 1990;25:225–248.
5. Ambrosino MM, Hernanz-Schulman M, Genieser NB, et al. Brain tumors in infants less than a year of age. Pediatr Radiol 1988;19:6–8.

GERM CELL TUMORS

Germ cell tumors are relatively uncommon, accounting for less than 5 percent of intracranial tumors. Of all the various histologic types of germ cell tumor, the germinoma is by far the most common in the brain in children. Most of these tumors occur in the region of the pineal gland or in the suprasellar area (Fig. 8–11). Pineal tumors cause symptoms predominantly related to raised intracranial pressure. Similar symptoms may be caused by the suprasellar tumors, which in addition may cause visual or endocrine disturbance. Apart from location, there are few distinguishing features of the germ cell tumors. A variety of different appearances may be seen.

These tumors are discussed in more detail in the section on germ cell tumors in Chapter 9 and in the section on tumors of the pineal region later in this chapter.

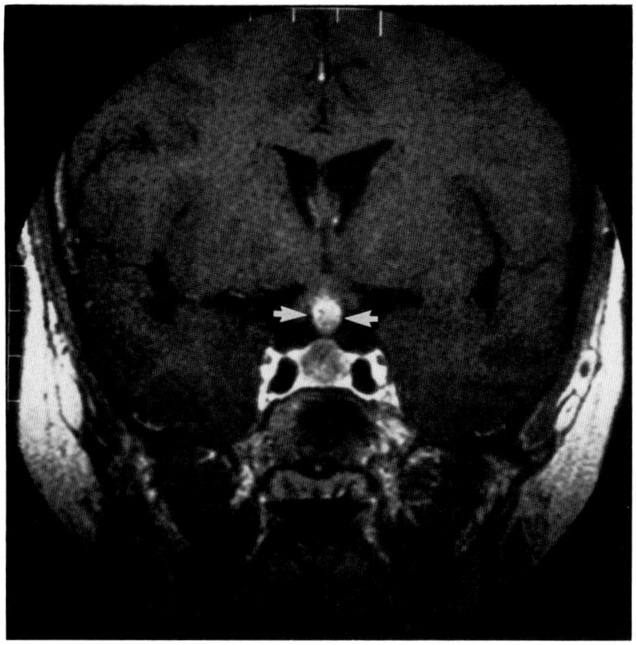

***Figure 8–11.* Diagnosis: Suprasellar germinoma. MR, T1 weighted image after gadolinium-DTPA administration. There is a small enhancing suprasellar tumor *(arrows)*.**

GLIOMA

The terminology relating to gliomas requires some discussion. Strictly speaking, glioma should refer to all tumors arising from a glial element. This would include astrocytoma and oligodendroglioma. Unfortunately, the term is sometimes loosely used interchangeably with astrocytoma. For example, astrocytomas in the cerebral hemisphere are usually termed cerebellar astrocytomas, whereas those occurring in the brain stem are usually more loosely termed brain stem gliomas. For this section the term glioma is utilized to refer predominantly to astrocytomas, and the terms astrocytoma and glioma will be used relatively loosely and can be interchanged. The much less common oligodendroglioma is discussed separately in a later section.

Astrocytomas are unusual tumors in that the epidemiology, pathology, clinical presentation, imaging findings, and prognosis vary significantly depending on the anatomic location of the tumor within the cranium (Table 8–7). Rather than describe each tumor as a completely separate entity, I have chosen to stay with the format of epidemiology, pathology, clinical findings, imaging studies, differential diagnosis, treatment, and prognosis and will discuss the variations by anatomic location under each of the main headings.

Epidemiology

Gliomas are extremely important pediatric brain tumors, accounting for about 70 percent of these tumors.[1]

TABLE 8–7
Incidence of Astrocytoma/Glioma by Anatomic Site[1–3]

Cerebrum	About 35% of all pediatric brain tumors
Visual pathways	About 5% of all pediatric brain tumors
Brain stem	About 10–20% of all pediatric brain tumors
Cerebellar	About 10–20% of all pediatric brain tumors

References
1. Walker RW, Allen JC. Pediatric brain tumors. Pediatr Ann 1983;12:383–391.
2. Heideman RL, Packer RJ, Albright LA, et al. Tumors of the central nervous system. In: Pizzo PA, Poplack DG, eds. Principles and practice of pediatric oncology. Philadelphia: JB Lippincott, 1989:505–553.
3. Smith RR. Brain stem tumors. Semin Roentgenol 1990;25:249–262.

Recent developments in imaging will cause a reevaluation of our understanding of the epidemiology of brain tumors in children. Traditionally, it has always been felt that posterior fossa tumors are far more common than supratentorial brain tumors in children. It is now felt that new imaging techniques such as MR will permit the diagnosis of many additional small low-grade astrocytomas of the cerebrum, which until the present time have never been diagnosed in childhood.[2] For example, in the screening of children with fits, MR has frequently shown these tumors in patients in whom CT scans have been completely negative.[3] As more of these children are imaged, it is believed that supratentorial cerebral astrocytomas will become the most common childhood brain tumor.[2]

The relative incidence of these tumors in different anatomic locations is given in Table 8–7.

In most children, no causative factors can be identified. There is, however, an increased incidence of gliomas in some situations. Radiation of the skull for the treatment of leukemia is associated with a significant increase of subsequent brain gliomas.[3] These tumors can occur as rapidly as 4 to 8 years after the radiation therapy and, therefore, can present while the patient is still a child.[3] There is a very strong association of astrocytomas of the optic chiasm and optic nerves with neurofibromatosis. Fifty percent of patients with these tumors have neurofibromatosis.[1] Conversely, about 5 to 10 percent of children with neurofibrosis will develop a visual glioma of the optic pathway.[1] Most of the supratentorial and cerebellar tumors present under the age of 5 years.[4] The supratentorial tumors have an additional peak in adolescence.[4] The chiasmal and optic nerve tumors have a peak at about 5 years of age,[1] and the brain stem tumors a peak between about 5 and 8 years.[5,6]

Pathology

Brain astrocytomas are separated into 4 grades, with grade I being the most well differentiated and benign (low grade) and grade IV being poorly differentiated and malignant (high grade). The term anaplastic astrocytoma is frequently used interchangeably with grade III.[7] Glioblastoma multiformae is a very malignant brain tumor and this term is used interchangeably with astrocytoma grade IV.[7] Some workers would consider glioblastoma separately from astrocytoma. For the purpose of simplicity I have chosen to include discussion of this tumor together with astrocytoma. The comments that will be made about this tumor are valid, regardless of how one might choose to classify it.

For all four stages of astrocytoma the amount of hemorrhage and necrosis present within the tumor increases significantly with increased degree of malignancy.[1,2] Low-grade tumors are not hemorrhagic at diagnosis.[2] Grade IV (glioblastoma) will frequently show hemorrhage and necrosis.[2] Calcification in these tumors is uncommon.[2] These high-grade tumors will spread in the cerebrospinal fluid.[2] Microscopically, gliomas are divided into two types: pyelocytic and fibrillary (diffuse).[1,2,8,9] The pyelocytic type are almost all low grade and relatively well defined. They are most likely to be found in the hypothalamus, cerebellum, and suprasellar area.[9] They are more likely to be partially cystic than the fibrillary tumors.[2] Fibrillary tumors occur most commonly in the cerebral hemispheres and the brain stem. As indicated by their name, they are often infiltrating, with extensive local invasion.[2,4]

CEREBRAL HEMISPHERE TUMORS

Cerebral hemisphere tumors occur predominantly in the frontal and temporal lobes, with the temporal lobe being the most common.[1,8] Occipital lobe tumors are rare.[10] They are more likely to be fibrillary in histology. Although two-thirds of cerebral astrocytomas are grade I or grade II, most of the grade III and grade IV tumors in the brain tend to occur in the cerebral hemispheres.[7,8] The glioblastomas, in addition to spread in the cerebrospinal fluid, will occasionally metastasize outside the cranium to lung, lymph nodes, liver, and bone.[8]

SUPRASELLAR TUMORS

Suprasellar tumors involve the hypothalamus, optic tracts, optic chiasm, and optic nerve. They are invariably pyelocytic and inevitably low grade in histology.[1,11] They will spread slowly between these various anatomic areas.[1] Some tumors will remain indolent for many many years, showing no change on serial imaging. They are not calcified and do not show hemorrhage or necrosis.

BRAIN STEM GLIOMAS

Brain stem gliomas can occur in the pons, medulla, or mid brain.[12] About half occur in the pons. The mid brain is the least common site. They are predominantly fibrillary.[9] About 20 percent are very benign (grade I), with up to 40 percent being very malignant (grades III or IV).[1] The likelihood of malignancy is much less with mid brain tumors than with those occurring more inferiorly.[1] A characteristic feature of brain stem gliomas is their extensive local invasion and spread.[4,8,12] Occasionally, they can extend a great distance, growing superiorly up to the thalamus or internal capsule and inferiorly into the spinal cord.[6] Also occasionally, exophytic growth may be identified; for example, a tumor may extend into the auditory canal or encase the basilar artery.[6] Because of the infiltrating growth pattern, mass effect and obstruction of the aqueduct and fourth ventricle occur relatively late and these tumors are often quite large before they cause obstruction, hydrocephalus, and clinical symptoms.[1,5] Cysts, hemorrhage, and necrosis are more likely in high-grade than in low-grade tumors.[1] Edema surrounding these tumors is minimal or absent.[13]

CEREBELLAR ASTROCYTOMAS

Cerebellar astrocytomas can arise in the vermis or hemispheres of the cerebellum. Origin in the vermis is more common.[1,14] Regardless of the location of origin, these tumors may spread to invade the other segments of the cerebellum. Eighty percent are fairly well defined, with a pyelocytic (juvenile) type of histology.[1,5] The fibrillary tumors tend to occur in older children and account for only about 20 percent of cerebellar astrocytomas.[2,8] The tumors are almost always low grade[8] and subarachnoid seeding into cerebrospinal fluid is very rare.[1] About 15 percent may show direct local meningeal invasion.[1] The fourth ventricle is rarely invaded (about 10 percent), but it is often displaced and obstructed fairly early.[1] Hydrocephalus is, therefore, common. The tumors may be solid or cystic.[1,8,14] The distinction between true cysts and solid tumors with secondary necrotic cysts is of significant clinical importance (Table 8–8). About half of the tumors will be true cysts with a single nodule of tumor in the wall. This tumor nodule may be round or flat and plaquelike. The rest of the wall of the cyst contains nonmalignant tissue so that at surgery only the tumor nodule and not the entire cyst requires resection. Cystic areas, because of necrosis, developing in previously solid tumors are, however, different in that the entire wall of the "cyst" obviously contains tumor and the surgical approach must be different.[8] The walls of the true cysts contain gliosis. They may be very vascular, which can cause enhancement on imaging. This must not be confused with tumor.[8]

GLIOMATOSIS CEREBRI

Gliomatosis cerebri is a very rare low-grade astrocytoma, which is not a focal localized tumor.[2] There is extensive tumor involving the deep white matter extending through the internal capsule and into the brain stem. All of the cerebral hemispheres are involved.[2]

TABLE 8–8
Gross Appearance of Cerebellar Astrocytoma[1]

Appearance	Percentage of Tumors
True cysts with a mural nodule	50
Solid with necrotic "cysts"	40
Completely solid	10

Reference
1. Gusnard DA. Cerebellar neoplasms in children. Semin Roentgenol 1990;25:263–278.

Clinical Presentation

These obviously depend on the anatomic location.

Cerebral hemisphere tumors may be asymptomatic for a long time. Signs are nonspecific; the most common is headache.[10] Other signs of raised intracranial pressure may also be seen. Convulsions, altered levels of consciousness, and focal signs may also occur.[4,10]

Suprasellar tumors may cause visual problems, endocrine problems because of involvement of the hypothalamus and pituitary gland, or proptosis.[1,4] Clinical stigmata of neurofibromatosis will be present in many patients. When the tumor is confined to the optic nerve, proptosis is the most common finding, occurring in 21 of 31 patients.[15] In this study, 12 patients had decreased vision and some had a squint.

Brain stem tumors cause varied symptoms. Cranial nerve abnormalities are the most common, being identified in 90 percent of patients in one study.[6,13] Signs of raised intracranial pressure may occur, but these are late findings, because obstruction occurs late with this tumor.[1] Tumors in the pons may cause personality changes.[4]

Cerebellar tumors often have prolonged nonspecific symptoms caused by raised intracranial pressure.[1] Ataxia and other specific cerebellar signs may also be found.[1]

Imaging Studies

The appearance of astrocytoma is very varied. It will depend on location, histology, and grade (Fig. 8–12). In general terms, pyelocytic tumors tend to be round or oval and well defined, show good enhancement following intravenous contrast injection, and are homogeneous (owing to absence of hemorrhage and necrosis) (Fig. 8–13). Associated edema is minimal.[2,9] Fibrillary tumors tend to show less enhancement.[2] Anaplastic tumors and glioblastoma have the most variable shape and irregular margins. Because of hemorrhage and necrosis they tend to be nonhomogeneous on CT and MR both before and after contrast administration. Edema surrounding the tumor is common.

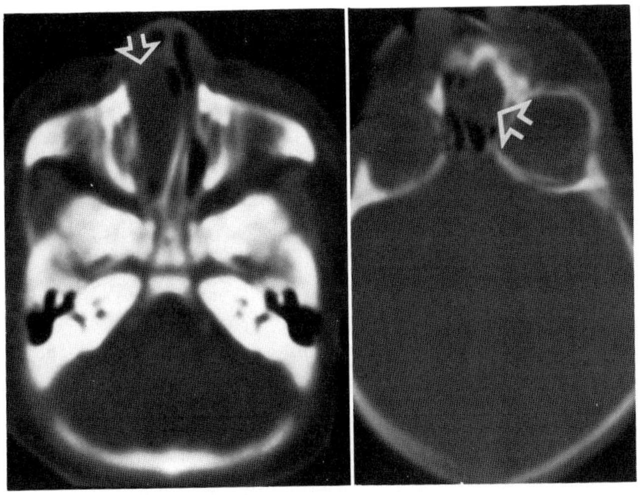

Figure 8-12. **Diagnosis: Nasal glioma.**
A **and** ***B*****, CT, axial and coronal images. There is a large soft-tissue mass** ***(open arrows)*** **in the right nasal cavity deviating the septum to the left. (From Puppala B. Nasal glioma. Clin Pediatr 1990;29:49–52.)**

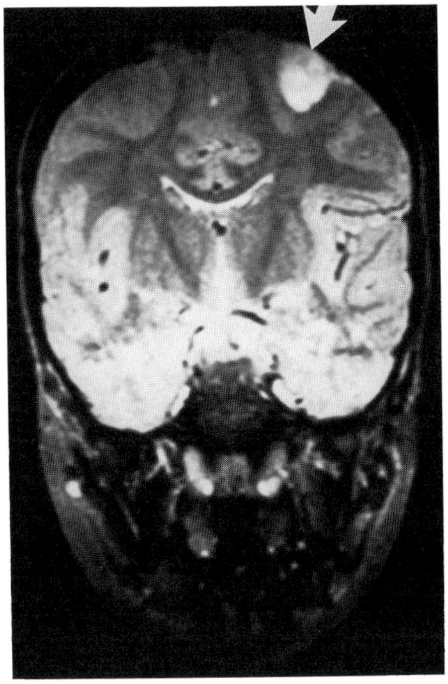

Figure 8-14. **Diagnosis: Cerebral hemisphere glioma.**
MR, T2 weighted image. Coronal plane. There is a 2 cm lesion in the left parietal lobe along the convexity ***(arrow).*** **There is no significant mass effect and no edema.**

CEREBRAL HEMISPHERE ASTROCYTOMAS

Cerebral hemisphere astrocytomas have a wide range of appearance on all imaging[2,4,12,16] (Figs. 8–14, 8–15, and 8–16). The low-grade tumors tend to be large and hypodense on CT images, showing enhancement after intravenous contrast administration.[4,16] They have little mass effect.[4] Calcification is uncommon. The high-grade tumors are more heterogeneous in appearance and show more variable enhancement.[2,12] They will show mass effect on adjacent structures and will have significant surrounding edema.[4,12] In general, the enhancing pattern is not a good predictor of malignancy.[12] On MR, the appearances are also not specific and are variable. In general, regions of soft-tissue tumor will have signal intensity consistent with prolongation of T1 and T2 relaxation times. Edema will be bright on T2 weighted images and of relatively low signal on T1 weighted images. Hemorrhage and necrosis will cause expected changes in signal intensity.[4] MR will consistently show greater extent of tumor than CT and will in many patients show lesions that have not been identified at all by CT.

Figure 8-13. **Diagnosis: Hypothalamic glioma.**
A **through** ***C*****, MR images with T1 weighting, T1 plus gadolinium-DTPA, and T2 weighting. There is a large well-defined hypothalamic tumor** ***(arrows)*** **that shows marked enhancement following gadolinium-DTPA administration and increased signal intensity with T2 weighting.**

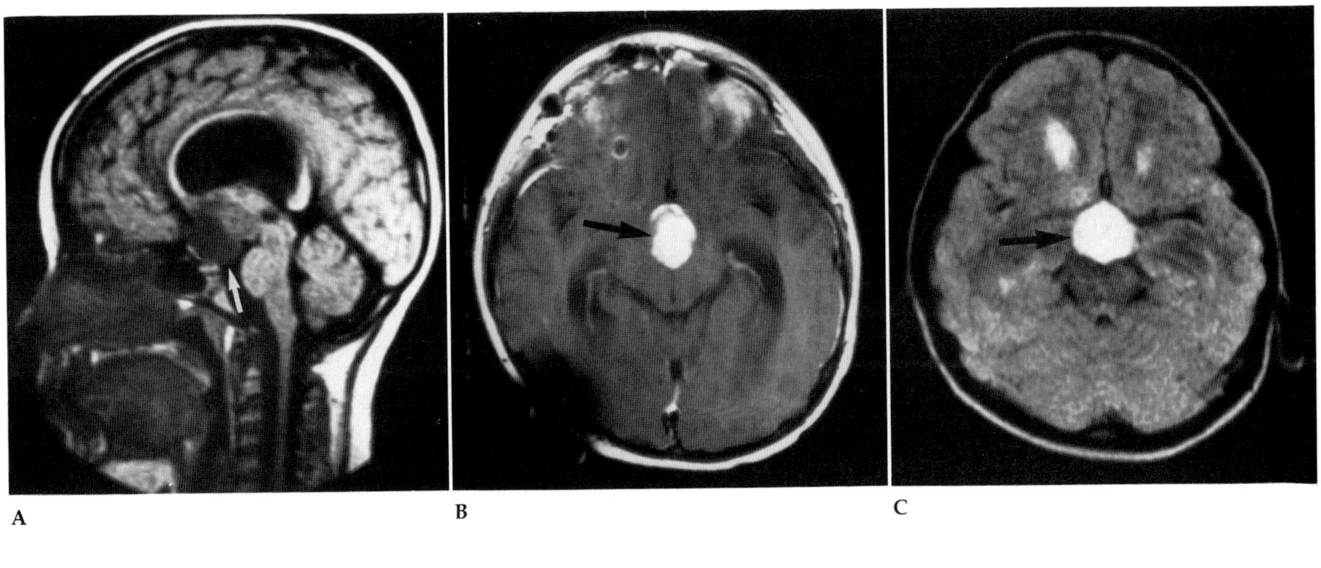

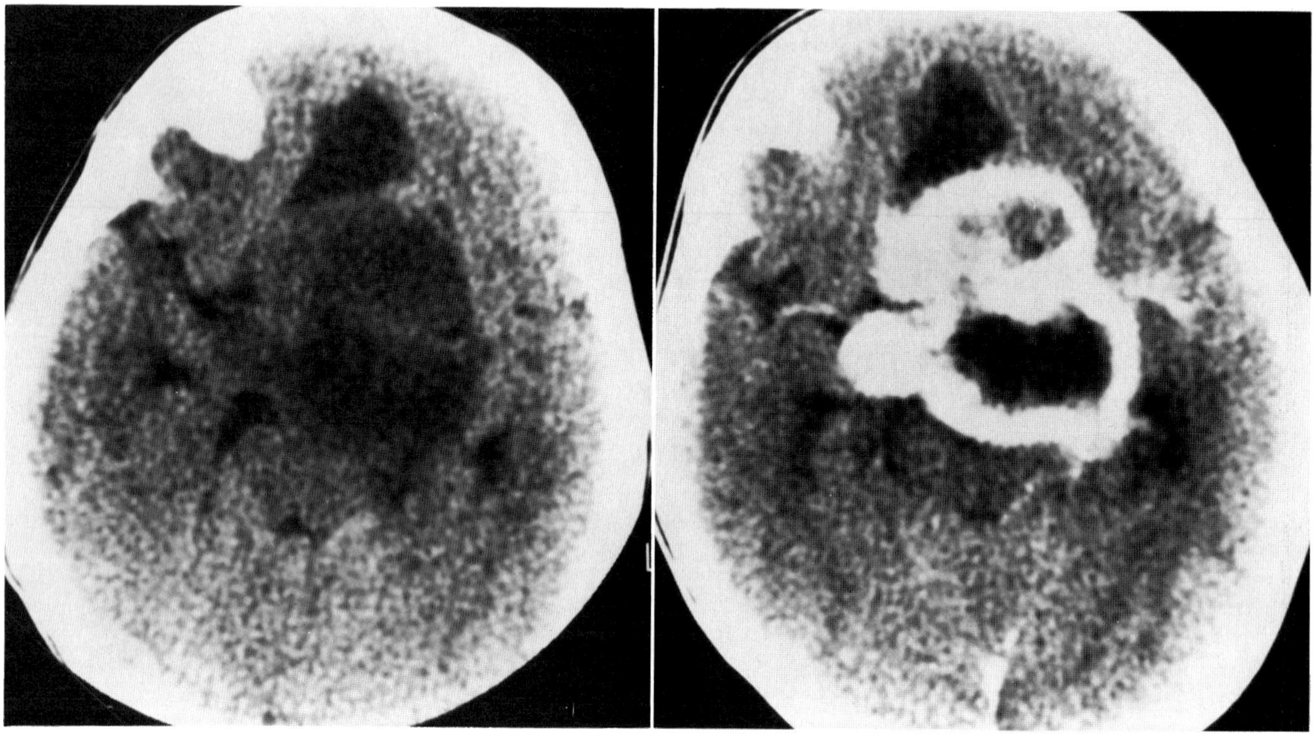

Figure 8–15. Diagnosis: Cerebral hemisphere astrocytoma.
A, CT. No contrast. There is a hypodense mass involving the frontal and parietal lobes. The boundaries are poorly defined. ***B***, CT after contrast administration. There is marked rim enhancement of the tumor with a large central nonenhancing zone of necrosis. (From Ambrosino MM. Brain tumors in infants less than one year of age. Pediatr Radiol 1988;19:6–8).

One rare associated abnormality is the presence of associated ipsilateral cerebral hemiatrophy described in one series of patients with astrocytomas of the hemispheres.[17] At this stage, note should be made of the usefulness of intraoperative ultrasound. This modality is extremely helpful in identification of tumor for biopsy or resection. In one study, the echo pattern on ultrasound was suggested to be helpful in differentiating active tumor from areas of hemorrhage or necrosis. In this particular study, areas of increased echogenicity without shadowing, seen on intraoperative ultrasound, corresponded to preoperative areas of enhancement on CT and were believed to be good areas for biopsy.[18] Note is made in this article that their findings are somewhat unusual, because literature reports of intraoperative ultrasound frequently associate echogenic areas with regions of necrosis, which are not good areas for biopsy.[18]

SUPRASELLAR AND OPTIC NERVE TUMORS

Suprasellar and optic nerve tumors can be well identified with CT or MR. In the region of the chiasm, the tumors are seen as a mass with or without extension into the optic nerves and optic tracts.[15] Tumors arising in the optic nerves may be confined to the nerves (Figs. 8–17 and 8–18) or extend into the chiasm and from there into the optic tracts. The optic nerve tumors are seen as masses or tubular or fusiform thickening of the nerve (Figs. 8–17 and 8–18). The optic foramen will often be widened.[15] The optic chiasm lesions are seen as focal mass lesions (Figs. 8–19, 8–20, and 8–21). Spread into the optic tracts is seen as a diffuse infiltrating abnormality. They can also spread locally to the orbit, pituitary fossa, and sinuses (Figs. 8–20 and 8–21). MR shows the lesions well. There is variable increase in signal intensity with T2 weighting (Figs. 8–17 and 8–18). There is also variable enhancement following gadolinium-DTPA administration (Figs. 8–18 and 8–19) and no good correlation of this enhancement with predicting behavior of the tumor.[1] MR is superior to CT for demonstrating the extent of these tumors. It is especially good for demonstrating invasion of the optic tracts in the brain. CT shows the patterns of tumor mass or infiltration described above. The lesions most commonly are isodense, showing some enhancement after intravenous contrast administration.[4] Because these tumors are frequently very low grade (astrocytes in the tumor cannot microscopically be differentiated from normal astrocytes), the true margins of these tumors may be difficult to define histologically. Similarly, on imaging, the actual margins may frequently not be accurately defined.[15]

BRAIN STEM GLIOMAS

Brain stem gliomas can be identified with CT or MR (Figs. 8–18, 8–22, 8–23, and 8–24). Some of these tumors may be completely invisible on CT yet easily seen

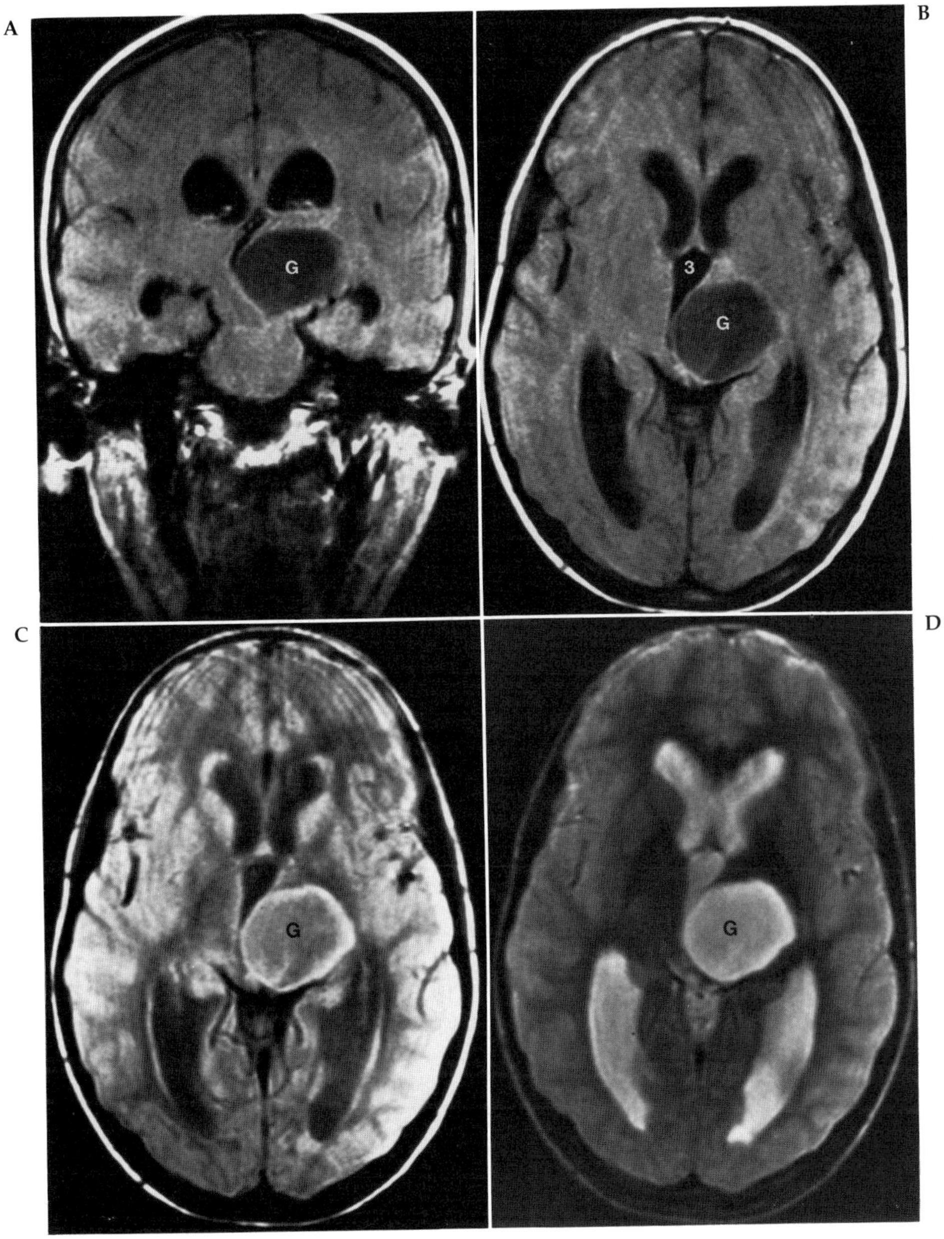

Figure 8–16. **Diagnosis: Thalamic glioma.**
***A* and *B*, MR, T1 weighted images after gadolinium-DTPA administration. These coronal and axial images show a large mass in the posterior aspect of the thalamus. It is causing compression of the posterior aspect of the third ventricle and proximal aqueduct. There is moderately severe hydrocephalus involving the third and lateral ventricles. The mass shows almost no enhancement following the gadolinium-DTPA administration. *G* = glioma. *3* = third ventricle. *C* and *D*, MR, spin density and T2 weighted images. There is progressive increase in signal intensity in the glioma. No adjacent edema is identified.**

on MR. The overall extent of the tumor is consistently shown to be greater with MR than with CT. MR is, therefore, very important for the evaluation of these tumors. Both imaging modalities show an infiltrating tumor with local spread (Fig. 8–18). The fourth ventricle is usually not invaded but is displaced[1] (Figs. 8–18 and 8–22). Exophytic growth may be identified. In one study of 34 patients,[13] imaging at the time of diagnosis revealed hydrocephalus in only 12 patients, calcification in 4, and hemorrhage in the tumor in 1.[13] In this study, the exophytic growth was shown by MR in 11 patients and by CT in 1 patient. On CT, prior to contrast administration, the tumors have very variable intensity, being described as decreased, increased, or equivalent to normal brain[1] or more commonly decreased or isointense.[5,8] Enhancement is variable, being identified in 50 percent of patients in one study.[6] Even when enhancement occurs, it may be variable in different areas of the tumor and show different patterns, including diffuse, nodular, and ring.[1,5,8] On MR, the tumors usually have

A B C

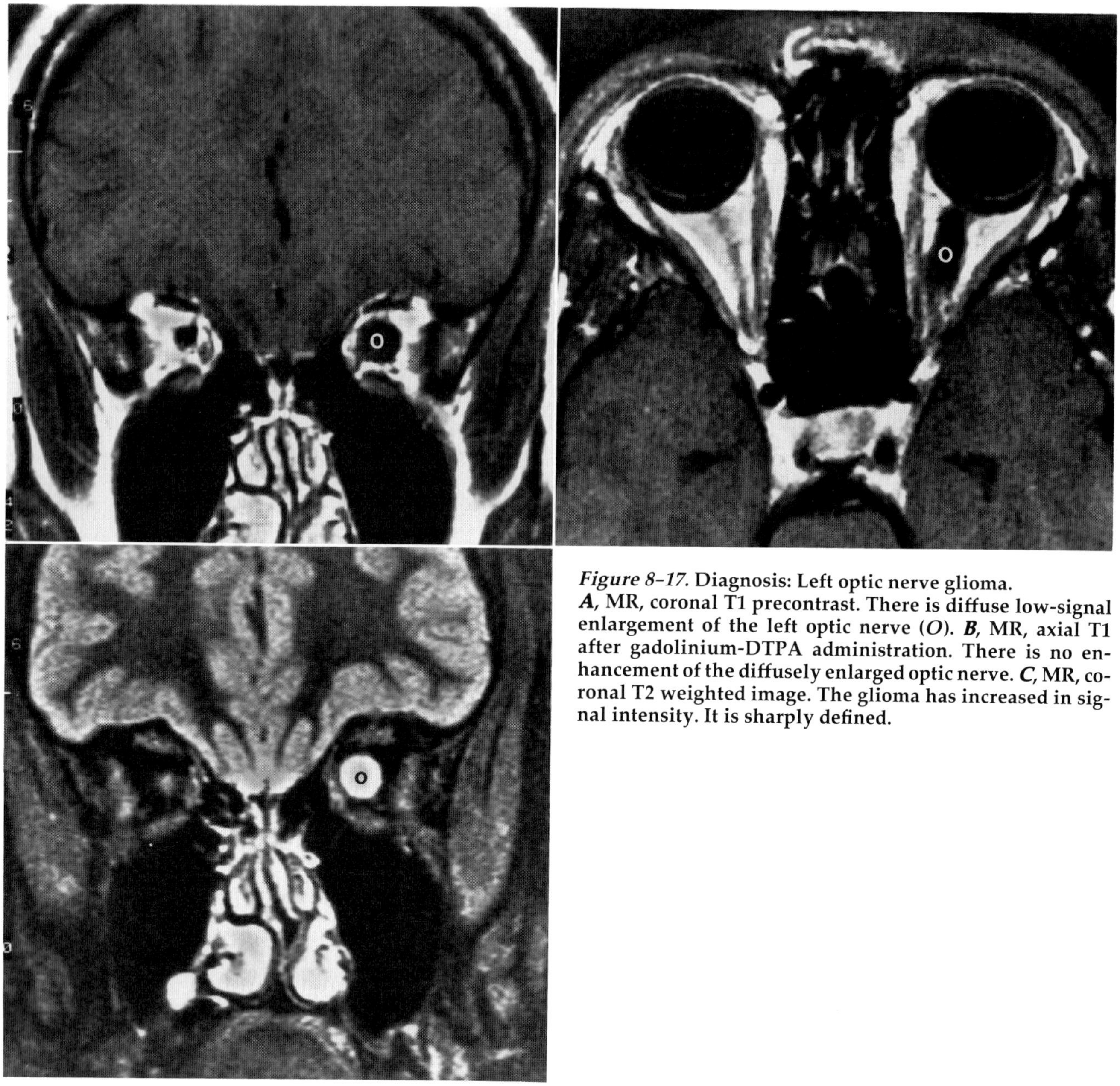

Figure 8–17. **Diagnosis: Left optic nerve glioma. *A*, MR, coronal T1 precontrast. There is diffuse low-signal enlargement of the left optic nerve (*O*). *B*, MR, axial T1 after gadolinium-DTPA administration. There is no enhancement of the diffusely enlarged optic nerve. *C*, MR, coronal T2 weighted image. The glioma has increased in signal intensity. It is sharply defined.**

low signal intensity on T1 and increased signal intensity on T2 weighted images (Figs. 8–18 and 8–23). The margins may be poorly defined because of local infiltration.[1,13] With gadolinium-DTPA only focal areas of the tumors will show enhancement[13] (Figs. 8–18, 8–19, and 8–23). Histologic correlation with gadolinium-DTPA uptake is not available. Two studies of follow-up imaging with therapy yielded helpful information,[13,19] as follows:

1. High-grade tumors regressed more quickly than low-grade tumors, with maximal response to therapy occurring within 6 months.[19]
2. All high-grade tumors recurred within 12 months.[19]
3. Some low-grade tumors recurred, often after many years.[19] With low-grade tumors, there may be slight initial increase in size of the lesion probably owing to edema.[19] Recurrence or progression may be identified on MR before new clinical signs develop.[13] New clinical signs are not always caused by tumor growth but possibly by hemorrhage or cyst formation.[13]
4. At about 4 to 6 months the clinical response correlated fairly well with MR response in 18 patients.[13] In this small series of 18 patients (utilizing hyperfractionation of radiation therapy), radiation necrosis was not seen. An increase in tumor size, and gadolinium-DTPA enhancement on MR, indicated tumor recurrence.[13]

A major problem still remaining in evaluating these tumors after therapy is differentiation of necrosis from persistent or recurrent tumor.

A B

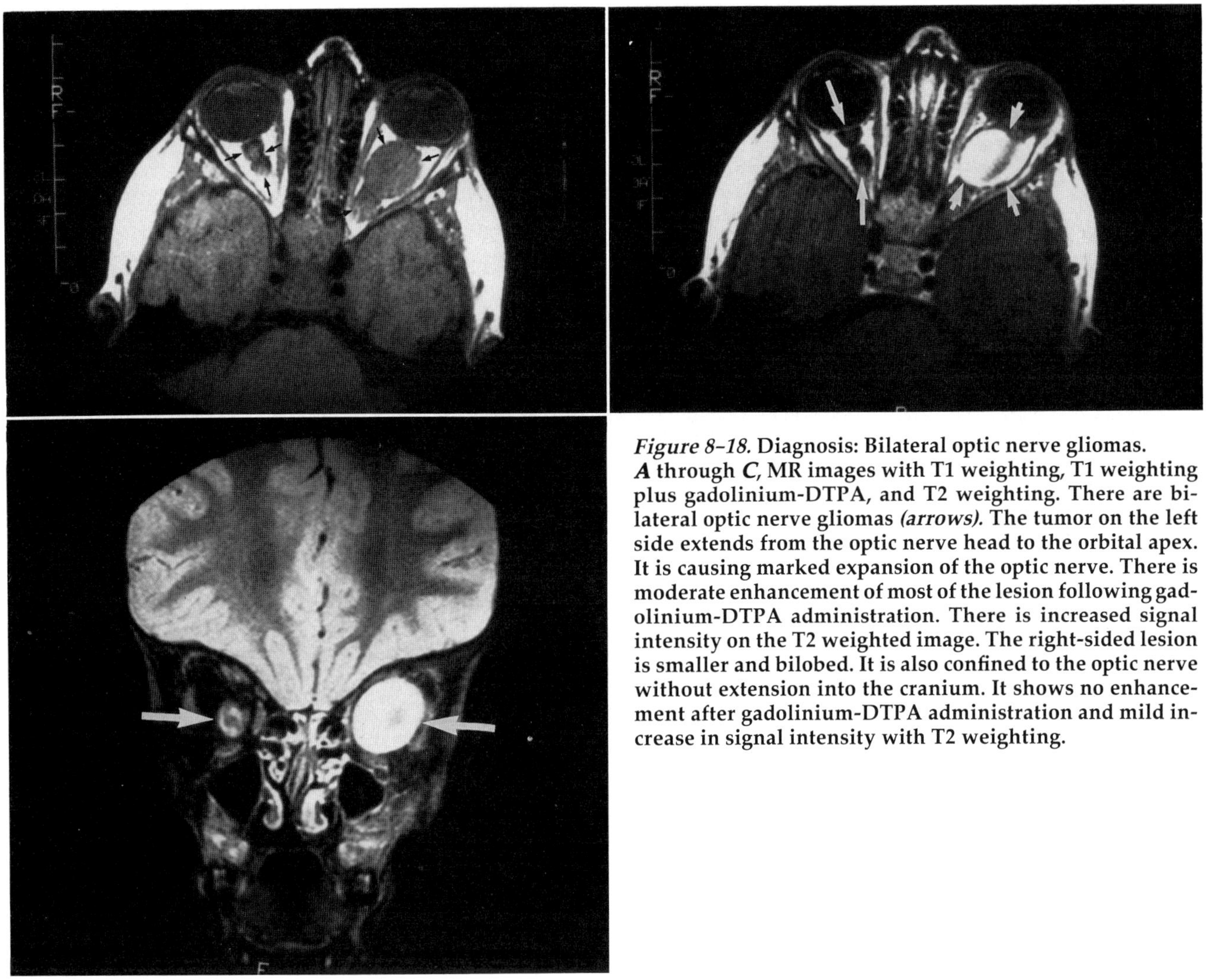

C

Figure 8–18. Diagnosis: Bilateral optic nerve gliomas.
A through ***C***, MR images with T1 weighting, T1 weighting plus gadolinium-DTPA, and T2 weighting. There are bilateral optic nerve gliomas *(arrows).* The tumor on the left side extends from the optic nerve head to the orbital apex. It is causing marked expansion of the optic nerve. There is moderate enhancement of most of the lesion following gadolinium-DTPA administration. There is increased signal intensity on the T2 weighted image. The right-sided lesion is smaller and bilobed. It is also confined to the optic nerve without extension into the cranium. It shows no enhancement after gadolinium-DTPA administration and mild increase in signal intensity with T2 weighting.

Figure 8–19. Diagnosis: Glioma of the optic chiasm.
A through ***C***, MR images with T1 weighting, T1 plus gadolinium-DTPA, and T2. There is a well-defined tumor *(arrow)* that is of very low intensity on the T1 weighted image, shows marked uniform enhancement following gadolinium-DTPA administration, and is very bright on the T2 weighted image. There is no surrounding edema.

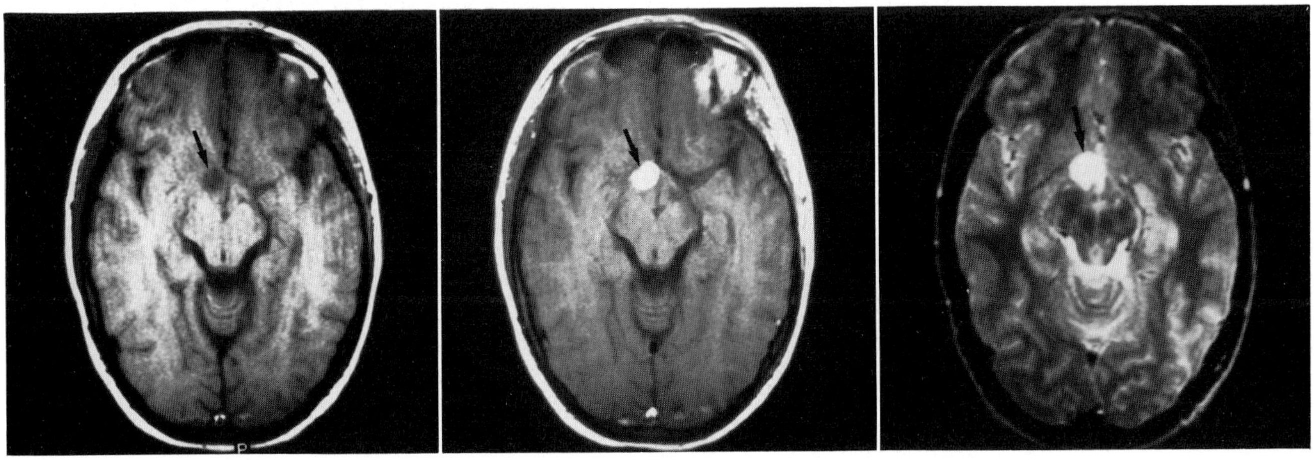

A B C

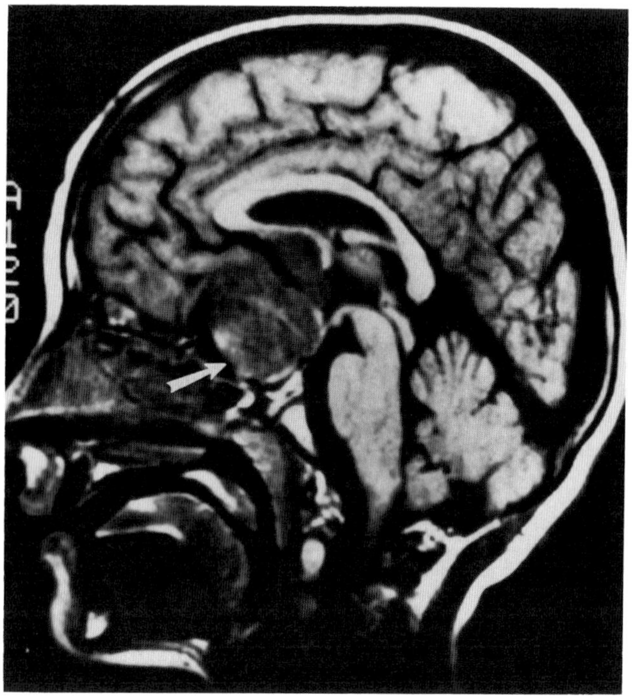

Figure 8-20. Diagnosis: Chiasmal pyelocytic astrocytoma. MR, T1 weighted image shows a large tumor *(arrow)* with downward extension into the pituitary fossa and sphenoid sinus. (From Lee YY. Juvenile pyelocytic astrocytomas. CT and MR characteristics. AJNR 1989;10:363–370.)

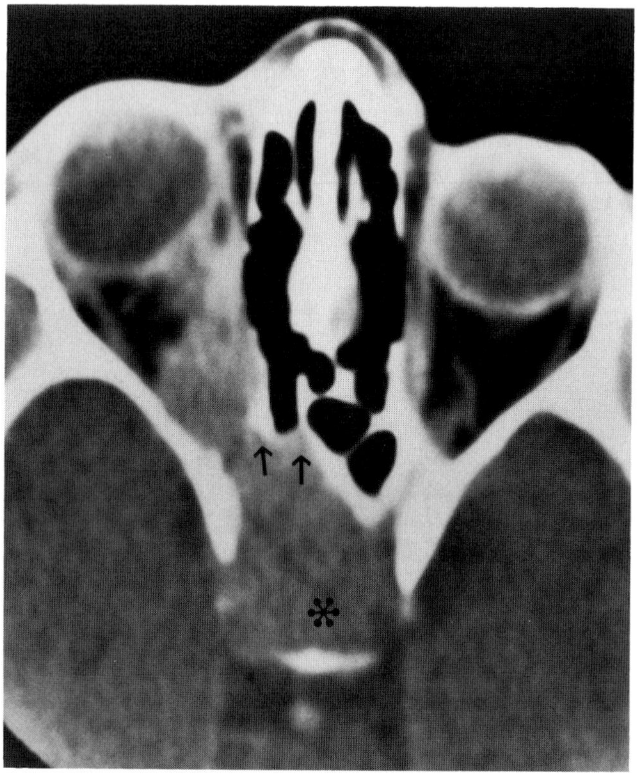

Figure 8-21. Diagnosis: Chiasmal pyelocytic astrocytoma. CT. Contrast enhanced. The astrocytoma shows anterior extension into the right orbit with erosion of the right tuberculum sellae and optic canal *(arrows).* There is downward extension into the pituitary fossa. (From Lee YY. Juvenile pyelocytic astrocytomas. CT and MR characteristics. AJNR 1989;10:363–370.)

Figure 8-22. Diagnosis: Brain stem glioma.
A and ***B,*** MR, sagittal T1 weighted images without and with gadolinium-DTPA enhancement. There is a large mass lesion centered within the pons. The tumor enhances *(arrows).* The central nonenhancing area is probably evidence of necrosis. Edema extends from the medulla up into the mesencephalon. ***C,*** MR, T2 weighted image. There is increased signal intensity from the lesion *(arrows).*

A B C

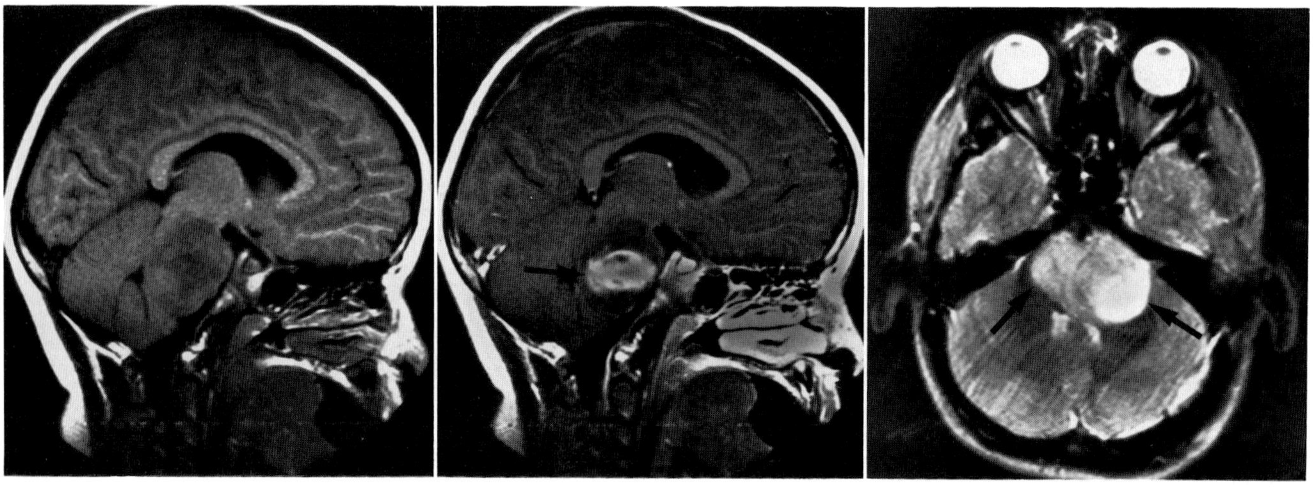

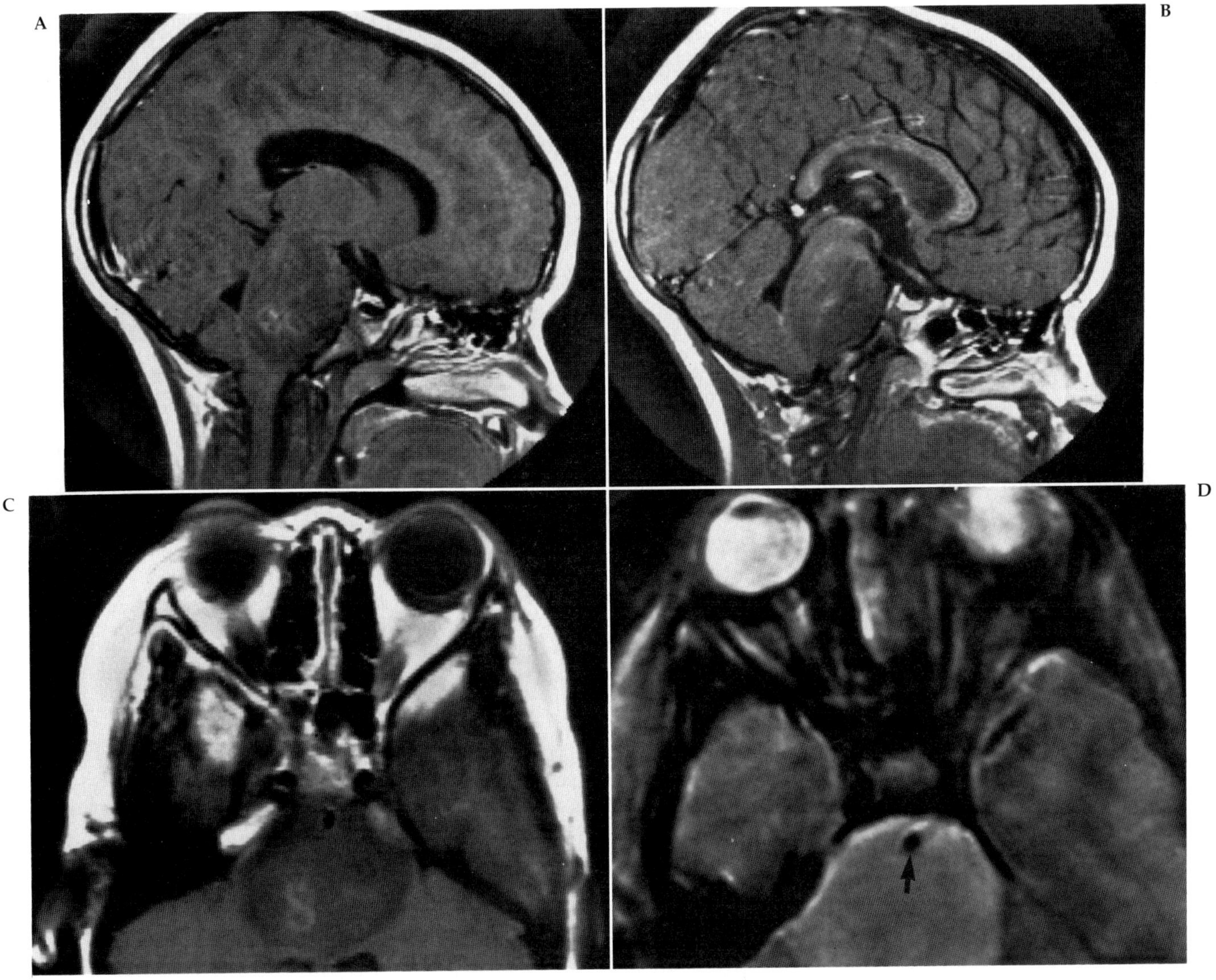

Figure 8–23. Diagnosis: Brain stem glioma.
A and ***B***, MR, sagittal images. T1 weighted after gadolinium-DTPA administration. There is a very large tumor centered in the pons. It extends superiorly into the mesencephalon. The boundaries are moderately poorly defined. Inferiorly it extends down to the foramen magnum. ***C*** and ***D***, MR, axial T1 weighted image after gadolinium-DTPA administration and axial T2 weighted image. The large tumor is better defined in this view. There is minimal enhancement with gadolinium-DTPA administration. Signal intensity is fairly uniformly bright with T2 weighting. The tumor encases the basilar artery *(arrow)*.

CEREBELLAR ASTROCYTOMAS

Cerebellar astrocytomas are well seen with CT or MR (Fig. 8–25). MR shows greater tumor extent than CT. Hydrocephalus is commonly seen with either modality (Fig. 8–25). Enhancement with contrast with either CT or MR is not a predictor of prognosis. The true cysts on CT are seen as areas of low attenuation, slightly higher than that of normal cerebrospinal fluid because of protein in the fluid[8,12] (Figs. 8–25). The soft-tissue components of the tumor will usually enhance, but this is variable[1] (Fig. 8–25). The walls of the true cysts will not enhance, whereas the walls of the necrotic cysts will show enhancement.[8,14] On MR, the cysts and tumors have signal characteristics consistent with prolonged T1 and T2 relaxation times, with the cysts being darker on T1 and brighter than tumor on T2 weighted images (Fig. 8–26). Occasionally, the cysts may contain protein, giving an increased signal intensity on T1 weighted images. Blood in the cysts is rare.[1] The soft-tissue component of the tumor may appear relatively isodense with normal cerebellum on T1 weighted images.[14]

Differential Diagnosis

Cerebral hemisphere tumor differential diagnosis includes other brain tumors such as PNET, ganglioglioma,

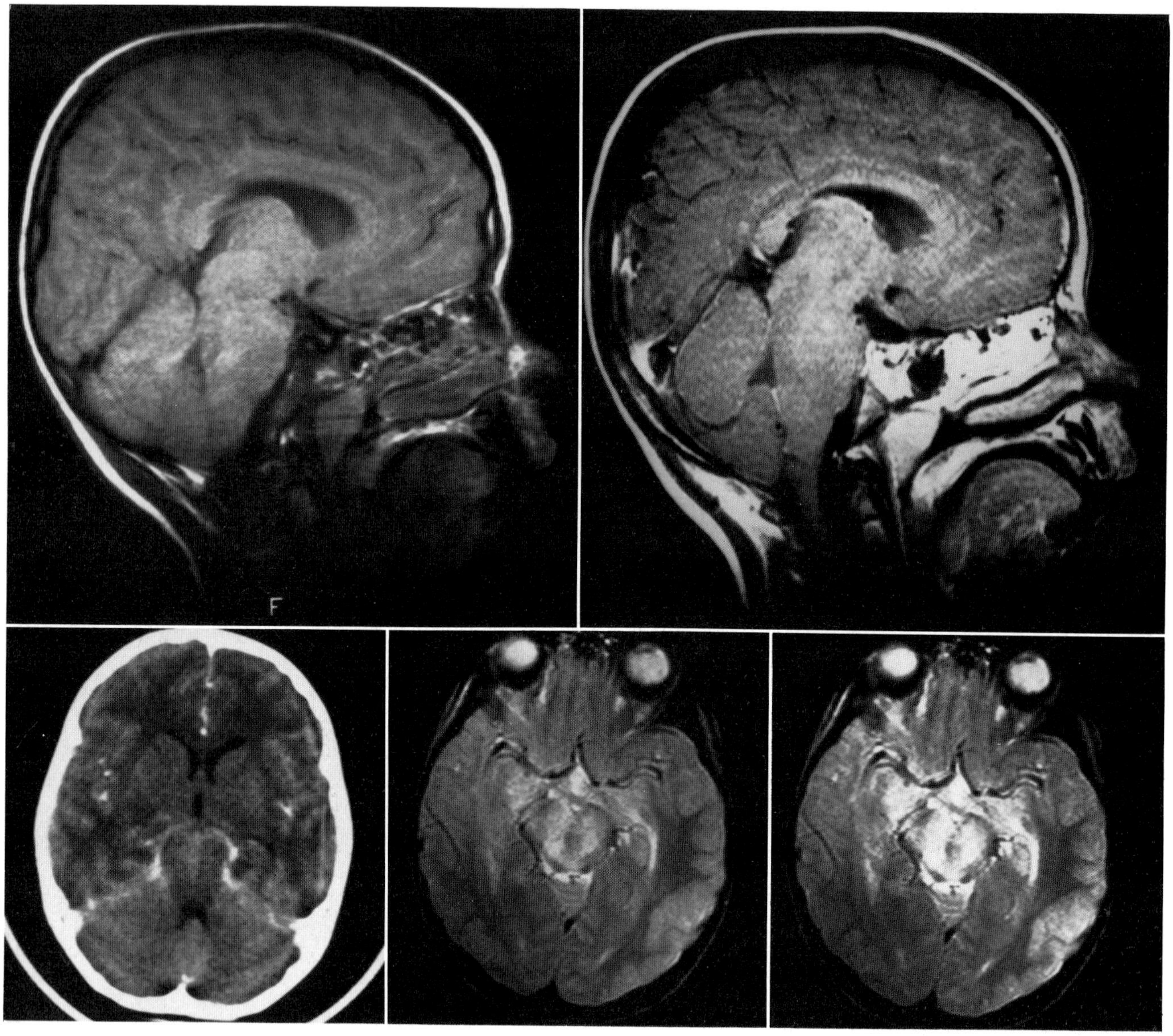

Figure 8–24. **Diagnosis: Brain stem glioma.**
***A* and *B*, MR, T1 weighted images without and with gadolinium-DTPA enhancement. There is a large mass lesion involving the midbrain, pons, and proximal medulla. It extends superiorly into the floor of the third ventricle. The margins of the tumor are very poorly defined. There is minimal enhancement with gadolinium-DTPA. *C* through *E*, Contrast-enhanced CT, spin density, and T2 weighted MR images. These all show the mass lesion. There is increasing signal intensity with T2 weighting.**

infection, infarction, and hemorrhage. Suprasellar tumor differential includes germ cell tumors. Third ventricle ependymomas may occur in the same area but these will rarely invade the chiasm.[4] Craniopharyngiomas also occur in this area but they usually displace and do not invade the chiasm.[4] In the brain stem, an "invisible" mass on CT may incorrectly be diagnosed as an aqueduct stenosis.[1] This should not be a problem with MR imaging. Hemangiomas and vascular malformations may have evidence of the presence of blood products. In this regard, MR may be particularly helpful. Abscess or viral encephalitis may look very similar.[4,8] In the cerebellum, the differential diagnosis includes medulloblastoma and ependymoma. The midline and infiltrative noncystic astrocytomas may be impossible to differentiate from these other two tumors.[1]

Therapy and Prognosis

The treatment and prognosis of these tumors depend on the histologic grade and location. Low-grade tumors will have a much more favorable outcome than high-grade tumors.

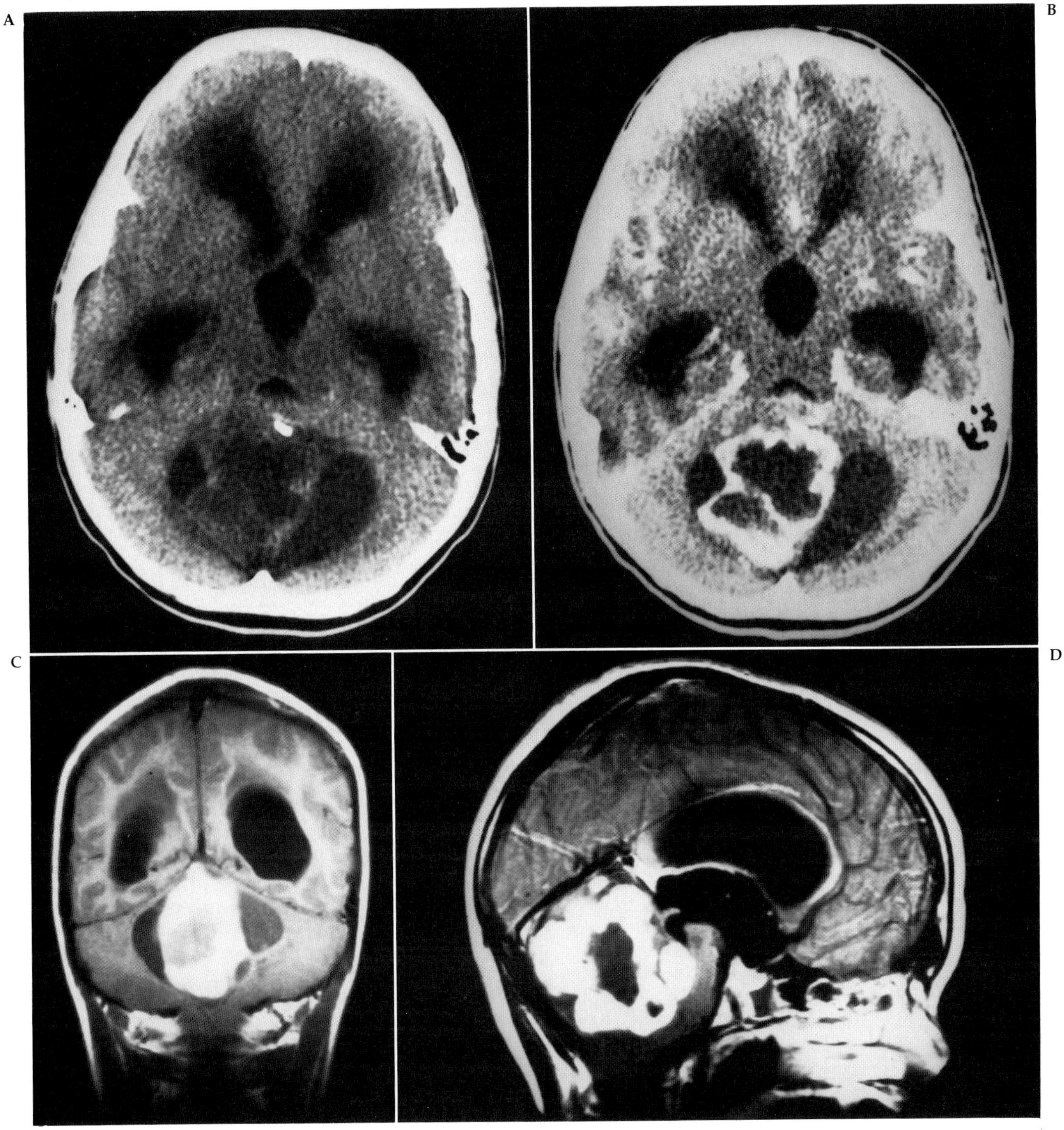

Figure 8-25. Diagnosis: Cerebellar astrocytoma.
A and ***B***, CT with and without contrast. There is a large partially cystic calcified mass in the posterior fossa. The fourth ventricle cannot be clearly identified. There is hydrocephalus involving the third and lateral ventricles. There is irregular enhancement within the tumor after contrast administration. ***C*** and ***D***, MR, T1 weighted images after gadolinium-DTPA administration. These again demonstrate a large posterior fossa mass that is mixed solid and cystic. The solid areas are showing fairly bright enhancement after contrast administration.

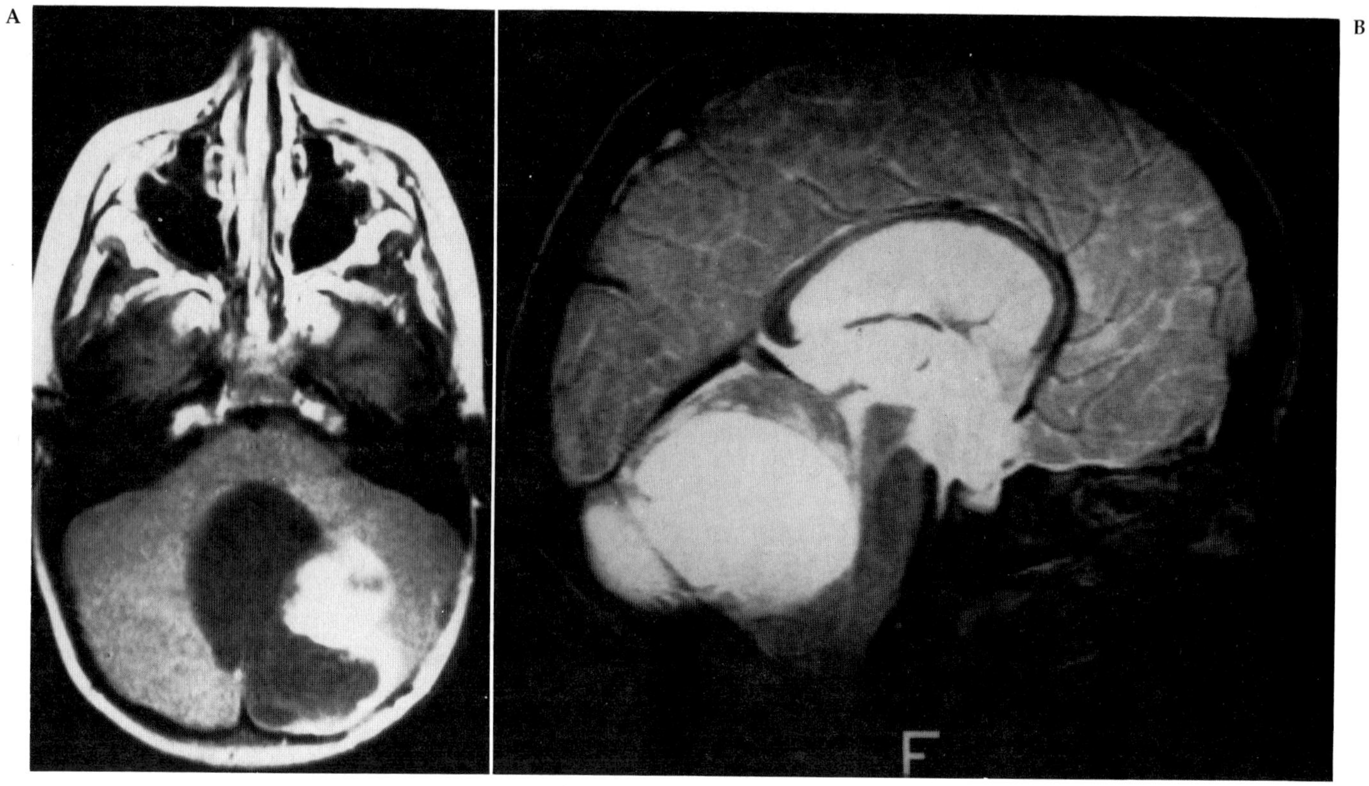

Figure 8–26. **Diagnosis: Cerebellar astrocytoma.**
***A*, MR, T1 weighted image after gadolinium-DTPA administration. There is a large solid cystic tumor with the cystic component appearing of low intensity and fairly bright enhancement in the solid component. *B*, MR, T2 weighted image. This again shows a large posterior fossa tumor. Both the solid and cystic components appear bright.**

CEREBRAL HEMISPHERE TUMORS

Surgery is most important for cerebral hemisphere and cerebellar tumors, providing complete cure in some patients when complete resection is possible.[1] Chemotherapy was shown in a CCSG study in 1976[7] to have some benefit in patients with grade III and IV tumors. Another study in 1977 showed no beneficial effect of chemotherapy for brain stem tumors. More recent studies in 1985[7,20] indicate that recently introduced aggressive chemotherapy regimes (e.g., one utilizing 8 different drugs given over a 12-hour period) does have definite effect on the tumors. Chemotherapy is of minimal use for low-grade tumors and has more effect in the high-grade tumor.[4]

Radiation therapy will have little effect on the very low-grade tumors but will cause response, but not necessarily good survival, with the more high-grade tumors. In one study, radiation therapy was found to increase relapse-free time but not survival.[2,7] Overall prognosis for grade I and II tumors is 30 to 40 percent 5-year survival, and for grade I tumors with complete resection prognosis is over 90 percent.[21] Grade III and IV tumors have less than 20 percent 5-year survival[1] and glioblastoma is almost always fatal.[22]

OPTIC NERVE AND OPTIC CHIASM TUMORS

Because of their location, surgical excision of optic nerve and optic chiasm tumors is usually impossible.[1] Because they are very low-grade tumors, they do not respond to chemotherapy or radiation therapy. There is, therefore, no good treatment.[11] In patients with purely optic nerve gliomas, resection of the nerve may be performed if the patients have severe and increasing symptoms of blindness. The surgery is performed prior to invasion of the optic chiasm, to attempt to prevent this from occurring.[15] The prognosis of these tumors without treatment is excellent so that there is a great danger of doing more harm than good with attempts at therapy. Chiasmal and brain tumors with or without brain invasion have a 50 percent, 10-year survival.[4] Those patients with optic nerve tumors alone have a 90 percent 10-year survival.[4] There is some evidence that many of these tumors will show no growth at all and become completely stable for many years. In one study of 31 patients with optic nerve gliomas, one-half showed complete stability for periods of up to 13 years.[15] There is some evidence that tumors occurring in patients with neurofibromatosis are much more likely to remain stable and not grow than tumors occurring in other patients.[15] Because these tumors may grow incredibly slowly, change in size may not be easily appreciated with serial imaging. Therefore, clinical evaluation of visual fields and the degree of proptosis must be utilized for follow-up of all these patients, in addition to imaging. The role of imaging is somewhat controversial, mainly because of the absence of any effective therapy even for those tumors shown to be growing. Because of this, many people would argue against performing routine screening in patients with neurofibromatosis for the early diagnosis of optic nerve and chiasm tumors. Again because of the absence of effective therapy, it could be argued that routine imaging in the follow-up of patients with known tumors should not be performed.

BRAIN STEM GLIOMAS

Brain stem gliomas, because of their location and infiltrating nature, are almost always not resectable.[1] In the past, many of these patients have been treated based on imaging findings alone, but more recently a trend to biopsy to confirm the diagnosis has become more widespread. The main treatment is radiation therapy,[13] with increasing hopes of improvement with aggressive chemotherapy particularly for the more high-grade tumors. Overall survival is poor, with 5-year survival being about 20 to 30 percent.[1,20,23] Prognosis is worst in the medulla, best in the brain stem, and intermediate in the pons.[4] The prognosis is also worse with extensive tumor infiltration, a high-grade histology, the presence of symptoms for less than 6 months, and the presence of cranial nerve long tract or cerebellar clinical symptoms and signs.[8,13,20,23]

CEREBELLAR ASTROCYTOMAS

Cerebellar astrocytomas have surgery as the treatment of choice. Complete resection is possible in a significant number of patients. This is more likely for the hemisphere as opposed to the midline tumors. Chemotherapy is little utilized.[1] Radiation therapy may be utilized if resection is incomplete but is usually not used if surgery is complete. No prophylactic radiation of the subarachnoid space is given.[1] Prognosis is proportional to the degree of resection. For the juvenile tumors it is over 90 percent survival.[5,8] The survival for the papillary infiltrating tumors is about 50 percent.[1,5,14] In these tumors, prognosis is even worse if there is brain stem invasion.

References

1. Davis P. Tumors of the brain. In: Cohen MD, Edwards MK, eds. Magnetic resonance imaging of children. Philadelphia: BC Decker, 1990:155–220.
2. Zimmerman RA. Pediatric supratentorial tumors. Semin Roentgenol 1990;25:225–248.
3. Shapiro S, Mealey J Jr. Sartorius C. Radiation-induced intracranial malignant gliomas. J Neurosurg 1989;71:77–82.
4. Heideman RL, Packer RJ, Albright LA, et al. Tumors of the central nervous system. In: Pizzo PA, Poplack DG, eds. Principles and practice of pediatric oncology. Philadelphia: JB Lippincott, 1989:505–553.
5. Walker RW, Allen JC. Pediatric brain tumors: Pediatr Ann 1983;12:383–391.
6. Smith RR. Brain stem tumors. Semin Roentgenol 1990;25:249–262.
7. Finlay JL, Goins SC, Uteg R, et al. Progress in the management of children with brain tumors. Hematol/Oncol Clin N Am 1987;1:753–776.
8. Naidich TP, Zimmerman RA. Primary brain tumors in children. Semin Roentgenol 1984;19:100–114.
9. Lee Y-Y, Van Tassel P, Bruner JM, et al. Juvenile pilocytic astrocytomas: CT and MR characteristics. AJNR 1989;10:363–370.
10. Qing-cheng X, Pei-yu P, Yu-shan Y, et al. A survey of 790 cases of astrocytoma. Clin Neurol Neurosurg 1990;92:27–33.
11. Listernick R, Charrow J, Greenwald MJ, et al. Optic gliomas in children with neurofibromatosis type 1. J Pediatr 1989;114:788–792.
12. Finlay JL, Goins SC. Brain tumors in children. I. Advances in diagnosis. Am J Pediatr Hematol/Oncol 1987;9:246–255.
13. Smith RR, Zimmerman RA, Packer RJ, et al. Pediatric brainstem glioma. Post-radiation clinical and MR follow-up. Neuroradiology 1990;32:265–271.
14. Gusnard DA. Cerebellar neoplasms in children. Semin Roentgenol 1990;25:263–278.
15. Wright JE, McNab AA, McDonald WI. Optic nerve glioma and the management of optic nerve tumours in the young. Br J Ophthalmol 1989;73:967–974.
16. Ambrosino MM, Hernanz-Schulman M, Genieser NB, et al. Brain tumors in infants less than a year of age. Pediatr Radiol 1988;19:6–8.
17. Mutoh K, Okuno T, Ito M, et al. Ipsilateral atrophy in children with hemispheric cerebral tumors: CT findings. J Comput Assist Tomogr 1988;12:740–743.
18. Hatfield MK, Rubin JM, Begarski SS, et al. Intraoperative sonography in low-grade gliomas. J Ultrasound Med 1989;8:131–134.
19. Wechsler-Jentzsch K, Witt JH, Fitz CR, et al. Unresectable gliomas in children: Tumor-volume response to radiation therapy. Radiology 1988;169:237–242.
20. Finlay JL, Goins SC. Brain tumors in children. III. Advances in chemotherapy. Am J Pediatr Hematol/Oncol 1987;9:264–271.
21. Dewit L, Van Der Schueren E, Ang KK, et al. Low grade astrocytoma in children treated by surgery and radiation therapy. Acta Radiol (Oncol) 1984;23:1–8.
22. Finlay JL, Uteg R, Giese WL. Brain tumors in children. II. Advances in neurosurgery and radiation oncology. AM J Pediatr Hematol/Oncol 1987;9:256–263.
23. Sanford RA, Freeman CR, Burger P, et al. Prognostic criteria for experimental protocols in pediatric brainstem gliomas. Surg Neurol 1988;30:276–280.

LYMPHOMA

Involvement of the brain in lymphoma can occur. It is much more common in adults than in children.[1] The

CNS involvement may be the primary focus of the tumor.[1] Involvement is much more common with non-Hodgkin lymphoma than with Hodgkin disease.[2] Whereas CNS involvement can be the only site of disease with non-Hodgkin lymphoma, with Hodgkin disease there is almost always tumor in multiple non-CNS sites.[2] CNS involvement may take the form of tumor within the brain itself, tumor in the meninges, or spread of tumor through the neural foramina into the epidural space.[3] Extradural spread in the spine is most likely to occur with Burkitt's lymphoma.[4] Intracranial tumor shows an increased likelihood in patients with suppressed immunity.[5]

On CT, the appearance may be nonspecific. The most common appearance is that of a focal lesion, which can be nodular. It will be isodense or of increased intensity on precontrast images and show uniform enhancement,[6] which may be quite marked.[1,5] Lesions are most likely in the cerebral hemisphere. MR will show a nonspecific mass with increased signal intensity on T2 weighted images.

Further discussion about lymphoma can be found in Chapter 5.

References

1. Egelhoff JC, Beatty EC. Primary B-cell lymphoma of the CNS in an infant. Pediatr Radiol 1989;19:204–205.
2. Sapoznik MD, Kaplan HS. Intracranial Hodgkin's disease. A report of 12 cases and review of the literature. Cancer 1983;52:1301–1307.
3. Fest T, Rozenbaum A, Cattin F, et al. Neuroblastoma-like epidural localization in non-Hodgkin's lymphoma. Neuroradiology 1988;30:569–570.
4. Dehner LP. Pediatric surgical pathology, 2nd ed. Baltimore: Williams & Wilkins, 1987:1073.
5. Pappert EJ, Parker JC, Hubbard A. Cerebral lymphoma in childhood: a diagnostic dilemma. S Med J 1989;82:1294–1298.
6. Baker L, Parker BR, Donaldson SS, et al. Staging of Hodgkin disease in children: comparison of CT and lymphography with laparotomy. AJR 1990;154:1251–1255.

MEDULLOBLASTOMA

Epidemiology

Medulloblastomas are common tumors, accounting for 10 to 25 percent of pediatric intracranial tumors.[1–3] The peak age of incidence is between 4 and 8 years, with a mean of about 6 years.[3–6] Up to 80 percent of the tumors will be found in males.[7]

Pathology

Medulloblastomas arise from an undifferentiated unknown cell of origin.[6] They are believed to be neuroectodermal tumors, but the term medulloblastoma is so well entrenched in the literature that they are still most commonly referred to by this name. Other workers have started to utilize the joint term medulloblastoma/PNET.[3]

They occur only in the posterior fossa.[4] They arise in the vermis of the cerebellum close to the roof of the fourth ventricle.[1] About 7 percent of the tumors may arise in the cerebellar hemispheres.[5] They show local spread with invasion of the fourth ventricle, adjacent cerebellar hemisphere, brain stem, and penetration into the cisterna magna.[3,5,7,8] Brain stem invasion may be seen in up to one-third of patients.[9] Fourth ventricular invasion causes early hydrocephalus, being identified in 110 of 116 patients in one series.[7] This also results in the very common spread of the tumor in the cerebrospinal fluid.[3,7,8] Between 10 and 40 percent of patients will have evidence of cerebrospinal fluid subarachnoid spread at the time of diagnosis.[1,5] This spread may be identified in the cranium or in the spinal canal. Extracranial metastases are not uncommon. Of all the intracranial tumors in children, medulloblastoma is the most likely to spread outside the CNS. The incidence of metastatic spread has been reported as low as 5 percent,[4] but up to 30 percent at some time in the illness.[1] Metastases characteristically go to bone, with over 80 percent of patients with metastatic disease having bone involvement.[1] Metastases may also be seen in decreasing order of frequency in the bone marrow, lung, liver, and lymph nodes.[1] Although there has been suggestion that spread of tumor is through cerebrospinal fluid passing out of the skull through a ventriculoperitoneal shunt, this is not the major method of spread, as 80 percent of patients with metastatic disease will have no ventriculoperitoneal shunt.[1]

Grossly, these tumors look fairly well defined but microscopically, they have poor invading margins.[8] Cysts, calcification, and necrosis are all rare prior to therapy.[4] They are very cellular tumors.[4] Various histologic variants have been described, such as melanotic tumors that contain pigment or medullomyoblastoma that contains muscle fibers.[3,4]

Clinical Presentation

Symptoms are predominantly those of raised intracranial pressure.[4] Later on ataxia and cerebellar signs develop. Focal cranial nerve signs will occur in a smaller number of patients.[4]

The cerebrospinal fluid may be examined for evidence of tumor. The demonstration of malignant cells in the cerebrospinal fluid is evidence of subarachnoid dissemination of tumor. Unfortunately, there are a large number of false negative studies, so that cerebrospinal fluid examination cannot be relied upon to exclude subarachnoid tumor. Various chemicals may be measured in the cerebrospinal fluid. Elevation of polyamines (especially putrescine) has been found to be useful, particularly for detection of tumor recurrence.[10]

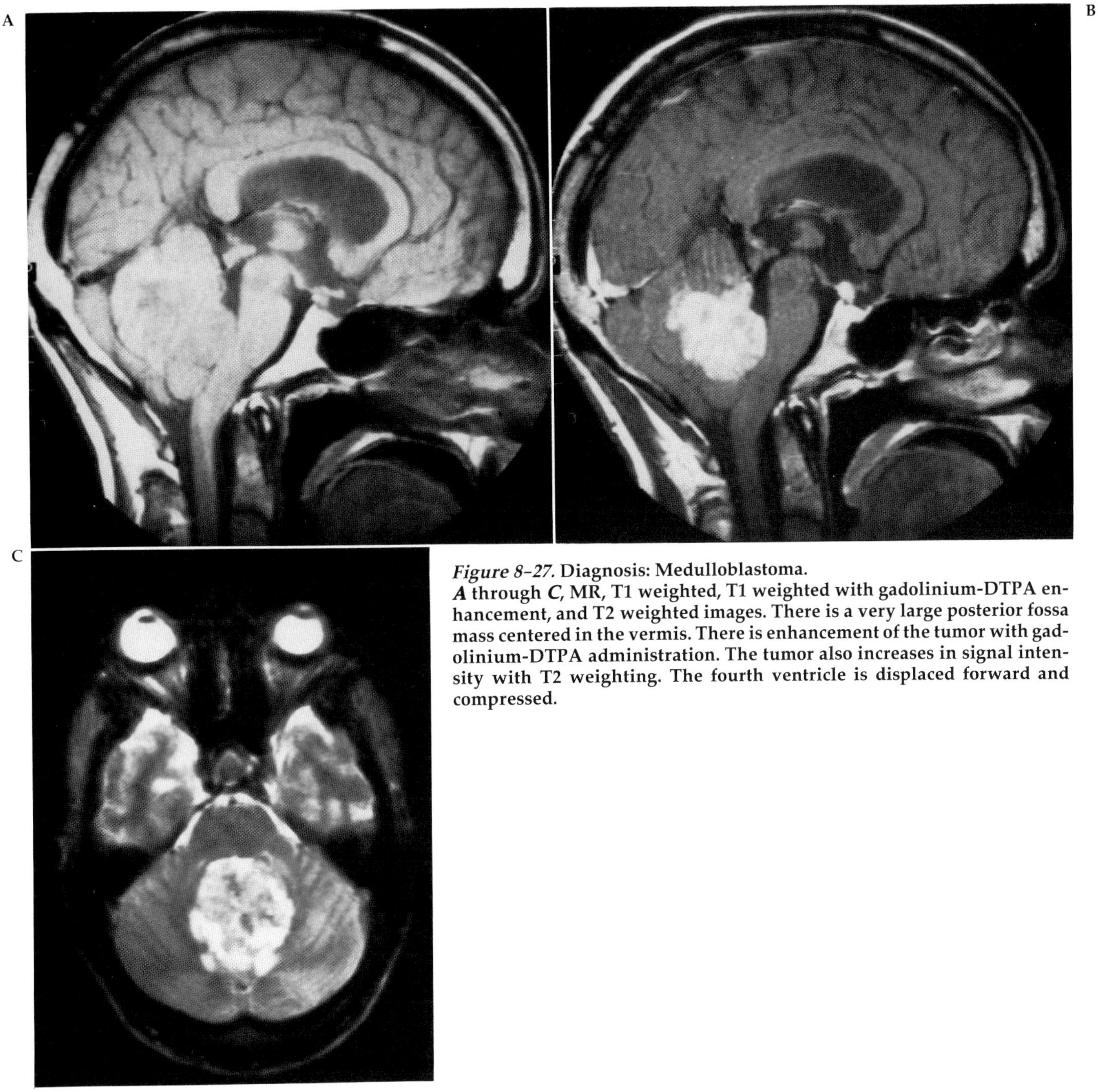

Figure 8–27. **Diagnosis: Medulloblastoma.**
A **through** ***C*****, MR, T1 weighted, T1 weighted with gadolinium-DTPA enhancement, and T2 weighted images. There is a very large posterior fossa mass centered in the vermis. There is enhancement of the tumor with gadolinium-DTPA administration. The tumor also increases in signal intensity with T2 weighting. The fourth ventricle is displaced forward and compressed.**

Imaging Studies

Medulloblastomas are easily identified on both CT and MR. They are seen as midline vermian masses with extensive local invasion (Figs. 8–27 and 8–28).

On CT, the most common appearance is that of a well-defined hyperdense mass in the vermis, with no calcification but with invasion and compression of the fourth ventricle and secondary hydrocephalus. There is moderate to marked homogeneous enhancement following intravenous contrast administration.[4,5,7,8,10] In one study of 116 patients, this fairly typical appearance was seen in about 60 percent.[7] Variations include the presence of calcification (10 to 20 percent),[7,8] cystic or necrotic areas (10 percent),[7,8] relatively poor margins, or no enhancement after intravenous contrast administration (7 percent).[7] On MR, the lesions are seen to be well defined on T1 weighted images. The intensity has been described as being decreased or equivalent to adjacent normal tissue[4] or equivalent or increased compared to

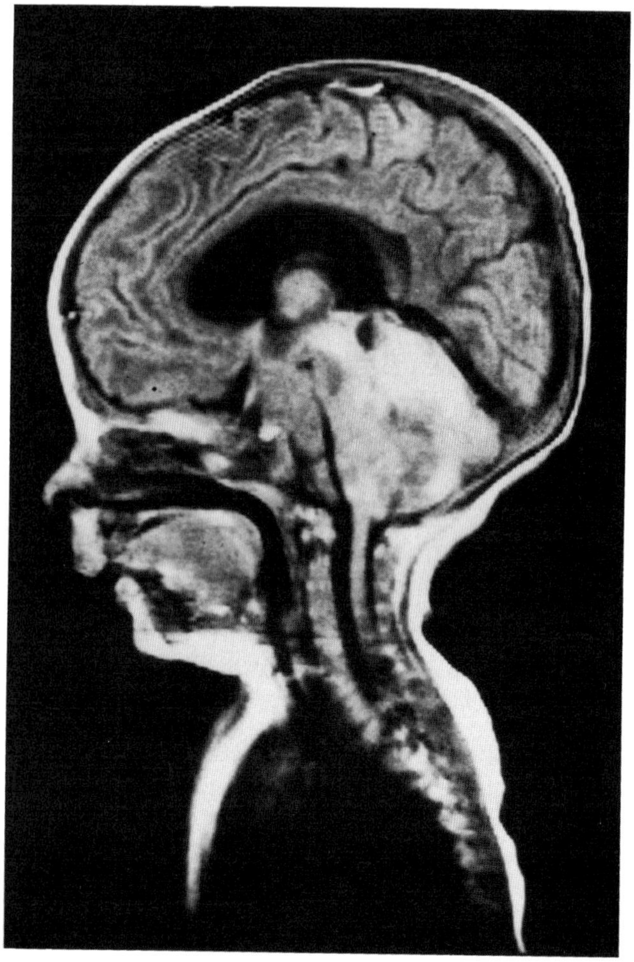

Figure 8–28. **Diagnosis: Congenital medulloblastoma. MR, sagittal T1 weighted image. There is a mixed signal intensity mass extending from the cerebellum into the brain stem. There is associated hydrocephalus. (From Buetow P. Congenital brain tumors. A review of 45 cases. AJR 1990;155:587–593.)**

normal tissue.[8] The signal intensity increases significantly on T2 weighted images,[4,8] and there is usually moderate to marked fairly uniform enhancement following gadolinium-DTPA administration.[4,8] Fourth ventricle invasion and hydrocephalus are usually seen. Atypical appearances, seen in a small number of patients, would include the presence of cysts or hemorrhage, or absence of enhancement with gadolinium-DTPA. Occasionally, the tumor may be seen to extend above the tentorium.[4] MR is probably better than CT for demonstrating the total extent of tumor. It is particularly good for demonstrating the inferior margins of the tumor, utilizing nonaxial imaging planes.

In all patients, the intracranial and spinal subarachnoid space must be evaluated for tumor spread (Fig. 8–29). Ideally, this should be performed prior to surgery. If this is not possible, one should wait for at least 2 weeks prior to screening for cerebrospinal fluid tumor spread.[8] There is a controversy regarding the optimal method of screening. As previously mentioned, cerebrospinal fluid cytology is not accurate. Traditionally, myelography has been the main method for evaluation,[1,11] but more recently MR has been utilized. Tumor in the subarachnoid space may be seen as a single nodule, multiple nodules, or extensive disease cloaking the spinal cord.[11,12] Occasionally, tumor may be seen within the spinal cord either from direct invasion or spread through the central canal.[11] The lumbosacral area is the most common area for tumor spread and the dorsum of the canal is more likely to be involved than the ventral area.[11] On myelography, the lesions may be seen as one or multiple nodules causing filling defects in the contrast column. They may also be identified by visualization of nerve root thickening, obliteration of the nerve root sheath, or cloaking around the spinal cord.[11] Occasionally, intramedullary spread will cause widening of the spinal cord.[11] On MR, the lesions may be difficult to visualize on T1 and T2 weighted pulse sequences because of similar signal intensity to cerebrospinal fluid. Utilization of gadolinium-DTPA results in enhancement of the tumor on T1 weighted images, which is well seen against the dark cerebrospinal fluid.

The theoretical advantages of MR are the strong contrast between the tumor and cerebrospinal fluid following gadolinium-DTPA administration and the ability to image in multiple planes. Unfortunately, there is some evidence that MR may miss a significant amount of tumor. In one study of 40 adults with various CNS tumors, but all with positive cerobrospinal fluid cytology indicating tumor spread into the subarachnoid space, the sensitivity of MR was less than 22 percent without gadolinium-DTPA but only increased to 36 percent following gadolinium-DTPA administration.[13] The problems with MR might be difficulty in identification of nerve root nodules, nonenhancement of metastases, or cerebrospinal fluid flow masking the presence of small metastases.[8] One difficulty in evaluation of imaging is that proof of diagnosis is frequently not available. Even cerebrospinal fluid cytology is not a solid standard, because as previously mentioned it may miss up to 50 percent of cases.[8] In one study with 5 patients having tumor demonstrated by imaging, cytology was positive in only 80 percent.[14] Difficulties in this regard are the absence of a good standard. Another problem with MR is that enhancement of a spinal lesion following gadolinium-DPTA administration is not specific for tumor. Such enhancement may occur with inflammation, following hemorrhage, or following intrathecal chemotherapy.[14]

There is no doubt that different workers will feel very strongly in favor of either myelography or MR. There is also no doubt that MR performed in specialized centers with great expertise and research interests in brain tumors will be significantly better than MR performed by the inexperienced. At the present time a good common sense approach would be to accept the philosophy that either myelography or MR might miss tumor. One should then start with either study, depending on personal preference, experience, and availability of MR,[8]

A

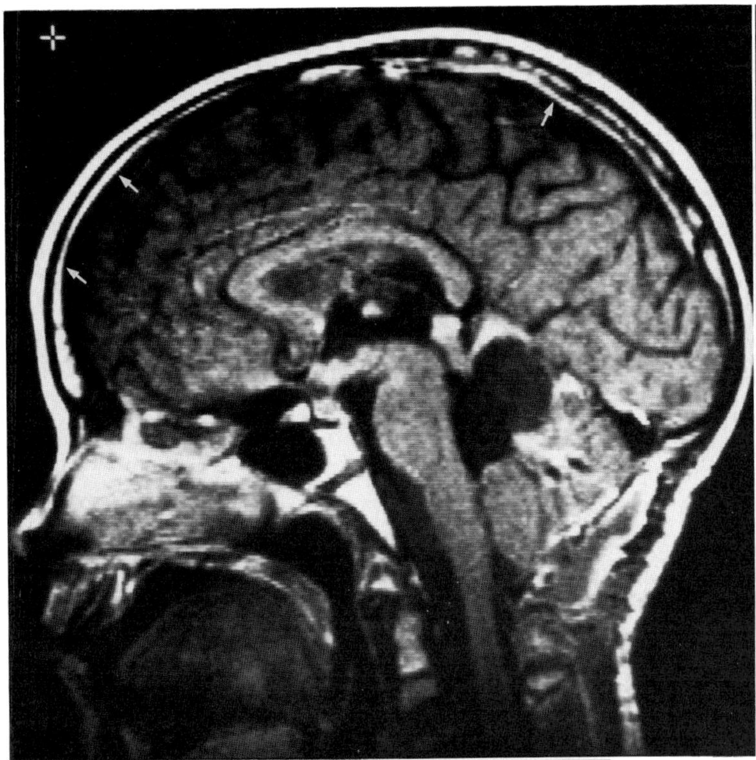

B

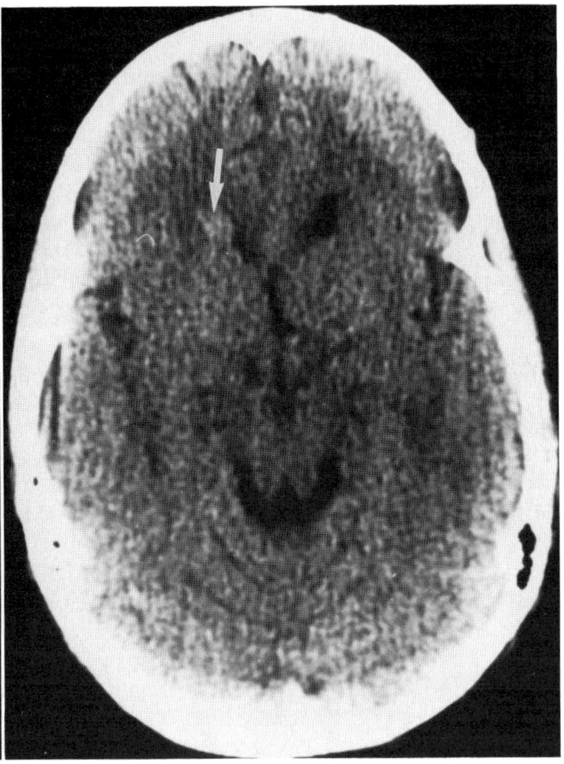

C

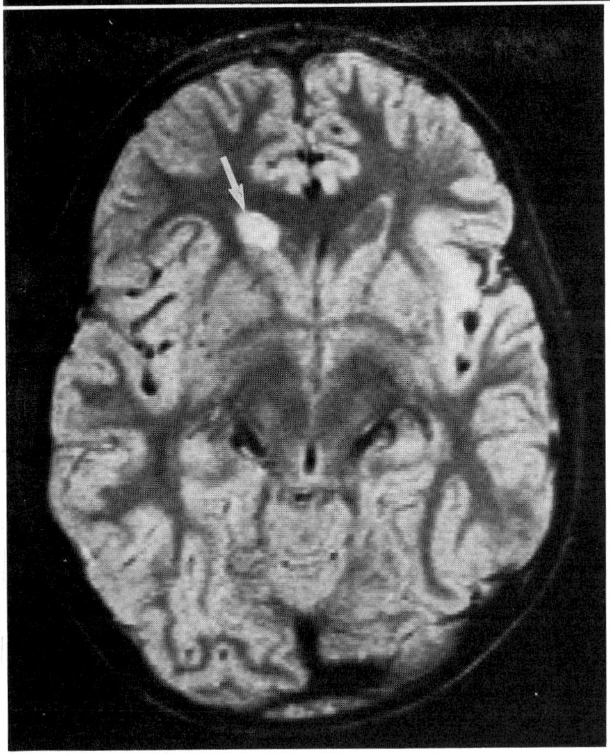

Figure 8–29. Diagnosis: Medulloblastoma. Intracranial spread. Two patients.
A, MR, sagittal T1 weighted image after gadolinium-DTPA administration. There is extensive leptomeningeal spread of tumor that is enhancing brightly *(arrows)*. ***B*** and ***C***, CT and spin-density MR images. Tumor is seen in the right frontal lobe. It is slightly hyperintense *(arrow)* on the nonenhanced CT image and bright on the spin-density MR image *(arrow)*. (From Rollins N. Recurrent medulloblastoma. AJR 1990;155:153–157.)

and then be content with a positive result obtained from either study. If the first study is negative, the opposite and second study should be performed to increase yield of positive results.[8] Ultimately I believe MR will become the clear modality of choice. Another important factor with MR is to recognize the different appearance of enhancement depending on whether one is dealing with leptomeningeal or dural abnormality. Dural abnormality is seen as a curvilinear enhancement beneath the inner table of the skull that does not follow the convolutions and gyri of the brain. Leptomeningeal enhancement is seen as lines of enhancement, or focal nodules, following the convolutions and gyri of the brain.[14]

Imaging is important to follow response of medulloblastomas to therapy. In many patients, particularly if there is some surgical doubt as to the presence or absence of residual tumor, or if it is known that residual tumor has been left behind, it is often helpful to perform imaging immediately following surgery. It is recommended that such imaging be performed within 5 days of surgery and ideally within 48 hours.[8] The reasoning for this is that after 5 days granulation tissue will develop. This will show enhancement on either CT or MR images, following contrast administration, and cannot be easily differentiated from tumor. Within 48 hours of surgery enhancing lesions are most likely to represent a residual tumor.[8]

Follow-up studies should be done regularly, the precise frequency being dependent on known presence or absence of residual tumor, potential times of change in therapy based on protocols, or the development of new clinical abnormalities. In one study utilizing CT to follow up 36 children with medulloblastoma,[15] local recurrence was identified in 20, cerebrospinal fluid recurrence in 14, and brain atrophy in 13. The cerebrospinal fluid recurrence was diffuse in half the patients and focal nodules in the other half. Nine of the 14 patients with cerebrospinal fluid recurrence had local recurrence as well, but in 5 patients the only recurrence was in the cerebrospinal fluid. Because of this, imaging must be used to screen the subarachnoid space in the cranium and spinal canal. Absence of local posterior fossa recurrence cannot be used to assume that no cerebrospinal fluid tumor is present. In this study, it was found that CSF tumor was best demonstrated on images obtained immediately after contrast injection.[15] Another study used gadolinium-DTPA to follow children with medulloblastoma.[16] In this study, all children had received surgery and radiation therapy with or without chemotherapy. Twenty-eight studies were performed as a routine and 4 because the children had new symptoms. Tumor was identified in 9 patients, indicating that the absence of clinical symptoms cannot be utilized as a justification for not performing imaging. Gadolinium-DTPA enhancement was helpful in identifying recurrence but not absolute. All of the recurrences did not enhance, and not all of the enhancing lesions were tumor. Enhancement was identified in the posterior fossa in 11 patients; tumor was identified in 9 of these 11. In the other 2 patients, the focal enhancement was believed to be the result of radiation change.[16]

Medulloblastoma is the most common CNS tumor to metastasize outside the cranium. Bones are a common site of these metastases (Fig. 8–30).

Differential Diagnosis

An astrocytoma is much more likely than a medulloblastoma to be cystic and to have its center to one side rather than in the midline. Ependymoma in the fourth ventricle may be very similar to medulloblastoma. Calcification is more common with ependymoma.[4] Encephalitis is also included in the differential.[1]

Therapy and Prognosis

Surgery is performed in all patients with attempt at resection. The surgical procedure may be complicated, because the tumor is friable and there are often poor cleavage planes between tumor and normal tissue.[17] The surgeon will always attempt to remove as much tumor as possible.[1] Prognosis is improved with successful surgery.[8]

Radiation therapy is utilized in all patients. The tumor is very sensitive to radiation therapy but relatively high doses, over 5,000 R, need to be used.[1,18] The rest of the cranium and spine are always given radiation therapy either to treat tumor or to prevent recurrence of tumor spread in the cerebrospinal fluid.[10,18] Traditionally, relatively high doses have been used. Recent protocols are attempting to utilize more aggressive chemotherapy and decrease the dose of radiation therapy. Although medulloblastoma is sensitive to radiation therapy, one problem is that the patients with the worst prognosis are often very young, at an age where maximal radiation therapy damage will occur. Use of radiation therapy definitely improves prognosis with medulloblastoma.

Chemotherapy is not believed to be of significant benefit with localized tumors.[6] In 1976, it was shown that chemotherapy was of some benefit in those children with extensive local tumor and cerebrospinal fluid spread.[18] More recent studies using more aggressive drug chemotherapy regimens may show more benefits from chemotherapy. Overall the prognosis is about a 50 percent 5-year survival,[8,17] but this has been as high as 70 percent at 5 years.[4] Unfortunately, prolonged surveillance is needed, as late recurrence can occur and survival at 10 years is definitely less common than at 5 years.[4] In one study of 44 patients, 7 had late recurrence a mean of 8 years after the initial diagnosis. In all of these 7 patients, the recurrence was in the posterior fossa with or without meningeal spread.[17] These findings mean that even with initial successful therapy, long-term imaging surveillance using CT or preferably MR is going to be needed in all of these patients. Prog-

A B C D

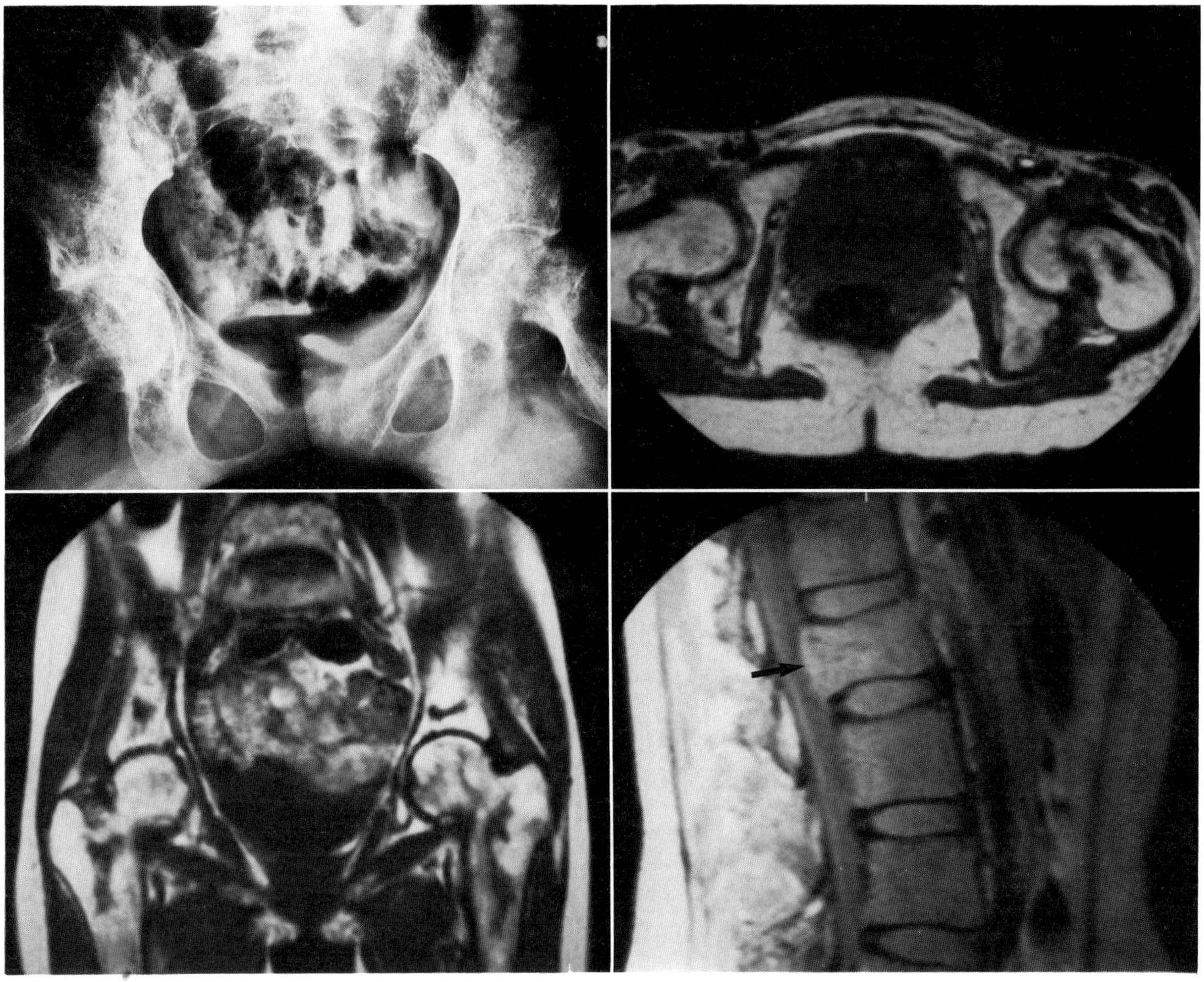

Figure 8-30. **Diagnosis: Medulloblastoma. Bone metastases.**
***A*, Plain film radiograph. Extensive ill-defined permeative lytic lesions are seen throughout the pelvis and proximal femora. *B* and *C*, MR, T1 weighted images. Multiple areas of decreased signal intensity are seen throughout the marrow. There is a pathologic fracture through the left femoral neck. *D*, MR, spin density image of the spine. A vertebral metastatic lesion is seen projecting backward into the spinal canal *(arrow)*.**

nosis is worse in patients under the age of 4 years, with cerebrospinal fluid spread, with extracranial metastases, or if the primary tumor is greater than 3 cm in diameter.[6,8]

References

1. Heideman RL, Packer RJ, Albright LA, et al. Tumors of the central nervous system. In: Pizzo PA, Poplack DG, eds. Principles and practice of pediatric oncology. Philadelphia: JB Lippincott, 1989:505–553.
2. Campbell AN, Chan HSL, Becker LE, et al. Extracranial metastases in childhood primary intracranial tumors. Cancer 1984;53:974–981.
3. Becker LE, Hinton D. Primitive neuroectodermal tumors of the central nervous system. Hum Pathol 1983;14:538–550.
4. Davis P. Tumors of the brain. In: Cohen MD, Edwards MK, eds. Magnetic resonance imaging of children. Philadelphia: BC Decker, 1990;155–220.
5. Naidich TP, Zimmerman RA. Primary brain tumors in children. Semin Roentgenol 1984;19:100–114.
6. Walker RW, Allen JC. Pediatric brain tumors. Pediatr Ann 1983;12:383–391.
7. Sandhu A, Kendall B. Computed tomography in management of medulloblastomas. Neuroradiology 1987;29:444–452.
8. Gusnard DA. Cerebellar neoplasms in children. Semin Roentgenol 1990;25:263–278.
9. Altman N, Fitz CR, Chuang S, et al. Radiologic characteristics of primitive neuroectodermal tumors in children. AJNR 1985;6:15–18.
10. Finlay JL, Goins SC. Brain tumors in children. I. Advances

A B C

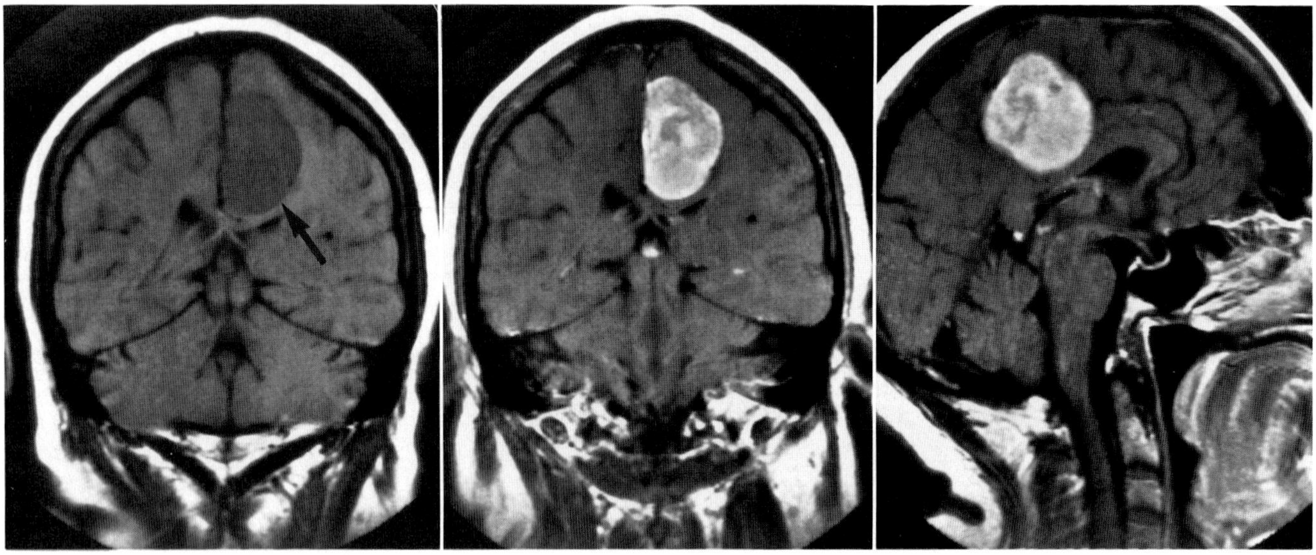

Figure 8–31. **Diagnosis: Parasigittal meningioma.**
A, **MR, coronal T1 weighted image. The tumor is well defined *(arrow)* and is of slightly lower intensity than adjacent brain. *B* and *C,* MR, coronal, and sagittal T1 weighted images after gadolinium-DTPA. There is very bright enhancement of the tumor, which is very sharply defined.**

in diagnosis. Am J Pediatr Hematol/Oncol 1987;9:246–255.

11. Stanley P, Suminski N. The incidence and distribution of spinal metastases in children with posterior fossa medulloblastomas. Am J Pediatr Hematol/Oncol 1988;10:283–287.
12. Deutsch M, Reigel DH. The value of myelography in the management of childhood medulloblastoma. Cancer 1980;45:2194–2197.
13. Yousem DM, Patrone PM, Grossman RI. Leptomeningeal metastases: MR evaluation. J Comput Assist Tomogr 1990;14:255–261.
14. Paakko E, Patronas NJ, Schellinger D. Meningeal Gd-DTPA enhancement in patients with malignancies. J Comput Assist Tomogr 1990;14:542–546.
15. Lee Y-Y, Glass JP, van Eys J, et al. Medulloblastoma in infants and children: computed tomographic follow-up after treatment. Radiology 1985;154:677–682.
16. Rollins N, Mendelsohn D, Mulne A, et al. Recurrent medulloblastoma: frequency of tumor enhancement on Gd-DTPA MR imaging. AJR 1990;155:153–157.
17. Lefkowitz IB, Packer RJ, Ryan SG, et al. Late recurrence of primitive neuroectodermal tumor/medulloblastoma. Cancer 1988;62:826–830.
18. Finlay JL, Goins SC, Uteg R, et al. Progress in the management of children with brain tumors. Hematol/Oncol Clin N Am 1987;1:753–776.

MENINGIOMA

Meningiomas are rare in children, accounting for less than 3 percent of all pediatric intracranial tumors.[1] They arise from arachnoid cells embedded in the dura. They can occur in any site, but are most common adjacent to the sagittal sinus. Because they can occur in the choroid, they can be found in the ventricles.

Pathologically, they are well-defined masses. They do not invade the brain but can cause reactive edema. They can cause adjacent reactive bone sclerosis and may occasionally invade the bone. They can cause occlusion of venous sinuses. They usually do not infiltrate.[1]

On CT, they are seen as focal mass lesions characteristically hypodense on precontrast images, with moderate enhancement after contrast administration. Calcification is common. The adjacent brain is displaced and may show reactive edema.[2] On MR, the lesions may occasionally be difficult to identify and be isointense with normal brain with all pulse sequences. They do, however, enhance well with gadolinium-DTPA so that they are easy to identify, if gadolinium-DTPA is utilized (Fig. 8–31).

Treatment of meningioma is surgical excision. Even with apparent complete resection, recurrence will occur in up to 20 percent of patients. Prognosis is very good.

Differential diagnosis is large and depends on the anatomic location of the tumor. In the ventricles, this includes choroid plexus papilloma. Although both tumors will enhance, a meningioma shows a more dense and persistent stain. In the orbit, differential diagnosis includes an optic nerve glioma. The meningiomas arise in the nerve sheath, however, and the nerve can usually be seen separately from the main tumor mass. The gliomas cause more diffuse enlargement of the nerve.

References

1. Schroeder BA, Samaraweera RN, Starshak RJ, et al. Intra-

parenchymal meningioma in a child: CT and MR findings. J Comput Assist Tomogr 1987;11:192–200.
2. David P. Tumors of the brain. In: Cohen MD, Edwards MK, eds. Magnetic resonance imaging of children. Philadelphia: BC Decker, 1990:155–220.

METASTASES

The intracranial tumors that spread in the cerebrospinal fluid are listed in Table 8–3. A variety of non-cerebrospinal fluid tumors may metastasize to the brain. An increasing number of brain metastases are being identified from solid tumors in children. The most common primary tumors are the sarcomas, including osteogenic sarcoma, Ewing sarcoma, and rhabdomyosarcoma.[1] In one study of 31 patients with metastases, most were found to be from sarcomas or germ cell tumors.[2] No CNS parenchymal metastases in this study were identified in 37 children with neuroblastoma. Primary cerebral metastases can, however, occur with neuroblastoma. Lymphoma may also cause focal CNS lesions.

Brain metastases may be single or multiple. They are seen as focal mass lesions, most commonly in areas of junctions of gray/white matter.[3,4] Hemorrhage, necrosis, calcification, and cyst formation are uncommon.[3] On CT, the most common finding is of a low-intensity lesion showing moderate to marked enhancement after contrast administration.[3] On MR, the lesion intensity is consistent with prolonged T1 and T2 relaxation times. They may, however, sometimes be missed unless gadolinium-DTPA is utilized routinely.[4]

References

1. Lewis AJ. Sarcoma metastatic to the brain. Cancer 1988;61:593–601.
2. Graus F, Walker RW, Allen JC. Brain metastases in children. J Pediatr 1983;103:558–561.
3. Pedersen H, McConnell J, Harwood-Nash D, et al. Computed tomography in intracranial, supratentorial metastases in children. Neuroradiology 1989;31:19–23.
4. Davis P. Tumors of the brain. In: Cohen MD, Edwards MK, eds. Magnetic resonance imaging of children. Philadelphia: BC Decker, 1990:155–220.

NEUROFIBROMATOSIS

Neurofibromatosis is discussed in detail in Chapter 9. The association of neurofibromatosis with glioma was discussed earlier in this chapter. In addition to a significantly increased incidence of gliomas in patients with neurofibromatosis, there is an increased incidence of cord ependymomas and other intracranial tumors.[1]

Reference

1. Davis P. Tumors of the brain. In: Cohen MD, Edwards MK, eds. Magnetic resonance imaging of children. Philadelphia: BC Decker, 1990:155–220.

OLIGODENDROGLIOMA

Oligodendroglioma is uncommon in young children and has a peak in the pediatric age group in adolescent males.[1]

It is usually a mixed glioma with oligodendrocyte cells dominating.[1] The tumor is most commonly found in the frontal or temporal lobes and never in the posterior fossa. It can look and stay benign for many years, but late recurrences occur.

On CT, oligodendrogliomas are seen as mass lesions, commonly with calcium. They have variable enhancement. Some associated edema will be seen in about one-third of patients.

Treatment is surgical resection if possible, with or without radiation therapy. There is no proven benefit for chemotherapy.

The prognosis is variable, with about a 70 percent, 5-year survival.

Reference

1. Davis P. Tumors of the brain. In: Cohen MD, Edwards MK, eds. Magnetic resonance imaging of children. Philadelphia: BC Decker, 1990:155–220.

PINEAL TUMORS

The classification of tumors occurring in the region of the pineal gland is given in Table 8–9. Germ cell tumors are the most common tumor in this region, and of these, germinoma is the most common. These tumors are discussed elsewhere.

TABLE 8–9
Classification of Tumors in the Pineal Region

Germ cell
Germinoma
Yolk sac
Teratoma
Choriocarcinoma
Pineal cell
Pineocytoma
Pineoblastoma
Other cell
Glioma
Meningioma
Cysts

Epidemiology

Pineoblastoma occurs in young males and pineocytoma in older children.[1] They are rare tumors.[2] The sex incidence is about equal.[3] A pineoblastoma may occur in association with bilateral retinoblastomas, which are usually hereditary. This association is often called a trilateral retinoblastoma.[1]

Pathology

Pineoblastomas are aggressive tumors. They are PNETs.[4,5] They may spread via the cerebrospinal fluid.[3] They are undifferentiated in appearance. They may calcify. Pineocytomas are much more benign. They also calcify. Both tumor types are rare.[2] It is important to note that calcification of the normal pineal gland is unusual in children, being present in only 12 percent under the age of 12 years and 3 percent under the age of 8 years.[3]

Clinical Presentation

Symptoms of pineal tumors, regardless of histology, are usually those of raised intracranial pressure.[3,6] Occasionally, midbrain pressure may cause a constellation of visual abnormalities.[3,6]

Imaging Studies

On CT, both pineoblastomas and pineocytomas may show calcification (Fig. 8–32). Most tumors are of increased intensity on precontrast images, showing marked enhancement following contrast injection.[3,5] Occasionally, they show a lucent center following contrast administration.[5] On MR the appearance is variable and nonspecific. MR is greater than CT for showing the total extent of the tumor. If a pineoblastoma is diagnosed, either contrast-enhanced MR or CT imaging of the rest of the cranium and spinal cord must be performed to look for cerebrospinal fluid tumor spread.

Differential Diagnosis

This includes all of the pineal region tumors (Table 8–9). Germ cell tumors account for the vast majority of these tumors. In one series of 36 children, germinomas represented 21 of 36 pineal region tumors.[6] On imaging, all of the tumors may look very similar and they cannot be differentiated one from the other. In a study of 19 children, the best predictors of histology were the age and tumor markers (cerebrospinal fluid concentrations of alpha-fetoprotein and gonadotropin). Occasionally, fat may be seen in a teratoma and if visualized it is helpful. Imaging, therefore, is very sensitive for detecting these tumors and defining their extent but poor in differentiating most of them. Pineal cysts have a low signal intensity on T1 weighted MR images. They are usually about 1 cm in size. On proton density images, they have greater signal intensity than cerebrospinal fluid and have similar signal intensity to cerebrospinal fluid on T2 weighted images. They have no adjacent mass effect. They do have pineal tissue in their walls and will, therefore, show rim enhancement after gadolinium-DTPA administration.[5]

Therapy and Prognosis

Biopsy of these tumors has been performed more frequently than previously. Whereas germ cell tumors are usually treated with radiation therapy and chemotherapy,[7] pineal cell tumors will often be treated with only

Figure 8-32. **Diagnosis: Pineocytoma.**
CT. Left image precontrast shows calcification in the pineal region. The right image shows inhomogeneous enhancement. (From Chang T. CT of pineal tumors. AJNR 1989;1039–1044.)

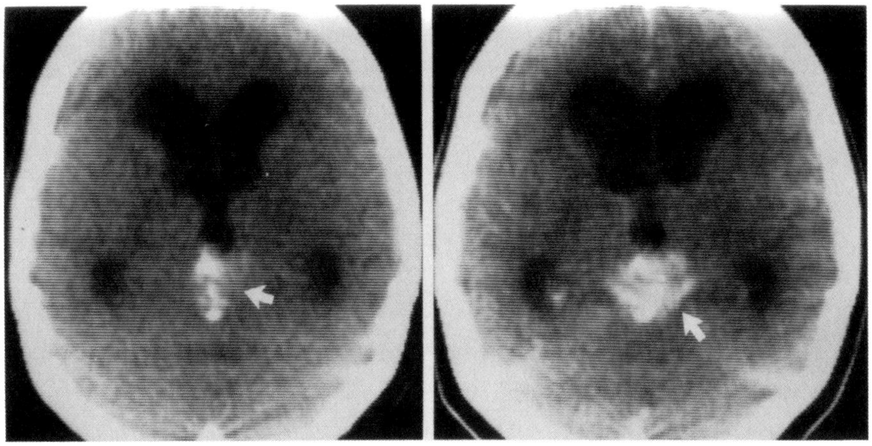

radiation therapy.[7] Prognosis with pineal cell tumors is moderate. It is not as good as with germinomas.

References
1. Davis P. Tumors of the brain. In: Cohen MD, Edwards MK, eds. Magnetic resonance imaging of children. Philadelphia: BC Decker, 1990:155–220.
2. Chang T, Teng MMH, Guo W-Y, et al. CT of pineal tumors and intracranial germ-cell tumors. AJNR 1989;10:1039–1044.
3. Zimmerman RA, Bilaniuk LT, Wood JH, et al. Computed tomography of pineal, parapineal, and histologically related tumors. Radiology 1980;137:669–677.
4. Becker LE, Hinton D. Primitive neuroectodermal tumors of the central nervous system. Hum Pathol 1983;14:538–550.
5. Zimmerman RA. Pediatric supratentorial tumors. Semin Roentgenol 1990;25:225–248.
6. Edwards MSB, Hudgins RJ, Wilson CB, et al. Pineal region tumors in children. J Neurosurg 1988;68:689–697.
7. Heideman RL, Packer RJ, Albright LA, et al. Tumors of the central nervous system. In: Pizzo PA, Poplack DG, eds. Principles and practice of pediatric oncology. Philadelphia: JB Lippincott, 1989:505–553.

PRIMITIVE NEUROECTODERMAL TUMOR

As previously discussed, many intracranial tumors such as medulloblastoma, pinealoblastoma, and retinoblastoma have been identified as being primitive neuroectodermal tumors. They have, however, been discussed under their old names, because these have widespread acceptance and because each of these tumors, in its specific site, has a different and predictable pattern of behavior. The following description refers to the remaining primitive neuroectodermal tumors (including those previously called intracranial neuroblastomas). They are predominantly lesions of the cerebral hemispheres.

Epidemiology

Seventy percent of these PNETs occur in children under the age of 6 years.[1]

Pathology

These are malignant undifferentiated tumors[1–3] arising from primitive neural tube cells.[1,2] Microscopically, they frequently contain areas of hemorrhage and necrosis.[1,3] They are often large at diagnosis, the mean diameter in one series of 30 patients being 6.5 cm.[2] Cysts will be identified in two-thirds of patients[1] and calcification in about 70 percent.[4] A thin rim of edema is sometimes seen. Hydrocephalus is common.[2] These tumors disseminate easily through the cerebrospinal fluid.[1,4–6] The most common location is superficially in the cerebral hemispheres.[1–3]

Clinical Presentation

These are nonspecific and include headache, irritability, convulsions, ataxia, hemiparesis, and papilledema.[2]

Imaging Studies

The most typical CT appearance of PNET is that of a large calcified cerebral hemisphere mass lesion with areas of cystic necrosis. It is most likely to be isointense or of increased intensity on precontrast images with moderate to marked nonhomogeneous enhancement after contrast administration[2,5,7] and showing little or no edema. Variations include low intensity on precontrast images[7] and a homogeneous enhancement following contrast.[4,7] Cerebrospinal fluid spread is common. In one study, subarachnoid tumor was identified in 9 of 13 patients.[7]

MR will show a similar large mass lesion with varying enhancement and varying signal intensities on T1 and T2 weighted images, reflecting the various internal structures of these tumors[5] (Figs. 8–33, 8–34, and 8–35).

Treatment and Prognosis

There is no effective therapy for these tumors. Surgery, radiation therapy, and chemotherapy have been tried.[2] The prognosis is poor, with less than 30 percent 5-year survival.[2,3,5,8]

References
1. Becker LE, Hinton D. Primitive neuroectodermal tumors of the central nervous system. Hum Pathol 1983;14:538–550.
2. Altman N, Fitz CR, Chuang S, et al. Radiologic characteristics of primitive neuroectodermal tumors in children. AJNR 1985;6:15–18.
3. Duffner PK, Cohen ME, Heffner RR, et al. Primitive neuroectodermal tumors of childhood. Radiology 1982;143:813.
4. Chambers EF, Turski PA, Sobel D, et al. Radiologic characteristics of primary cerebral neuroblastomas. Radiology 1981;139:101–104.
5. Davis PC, Wichman RD, Takei Y, et al. Primary cerebral neuroblastoma: CT and MR findings in 12 cases. AJNR 1990;11:115–120.
6. Figueroa RE, El Gammal T,Brooks RS, et al. MR findings on primitive neuroectodermal tumors. J Comput Assist Tomogr 1989;13:773–778.
7. Ganti SR, Silver AJ, Deifenbach P, et al. Computed tomography of primitive neuroectodermal tumors. AJNR 1983;4:819–821.
8. Heideman RL, Packer RJ, Albright LA, et al. Tumors of the central nervous system. In: Pizzo PA, Poplack DG, eds. Principles and practice of pediatric oncology. Philadelphia: JB Lippincott, 1989:505–553.

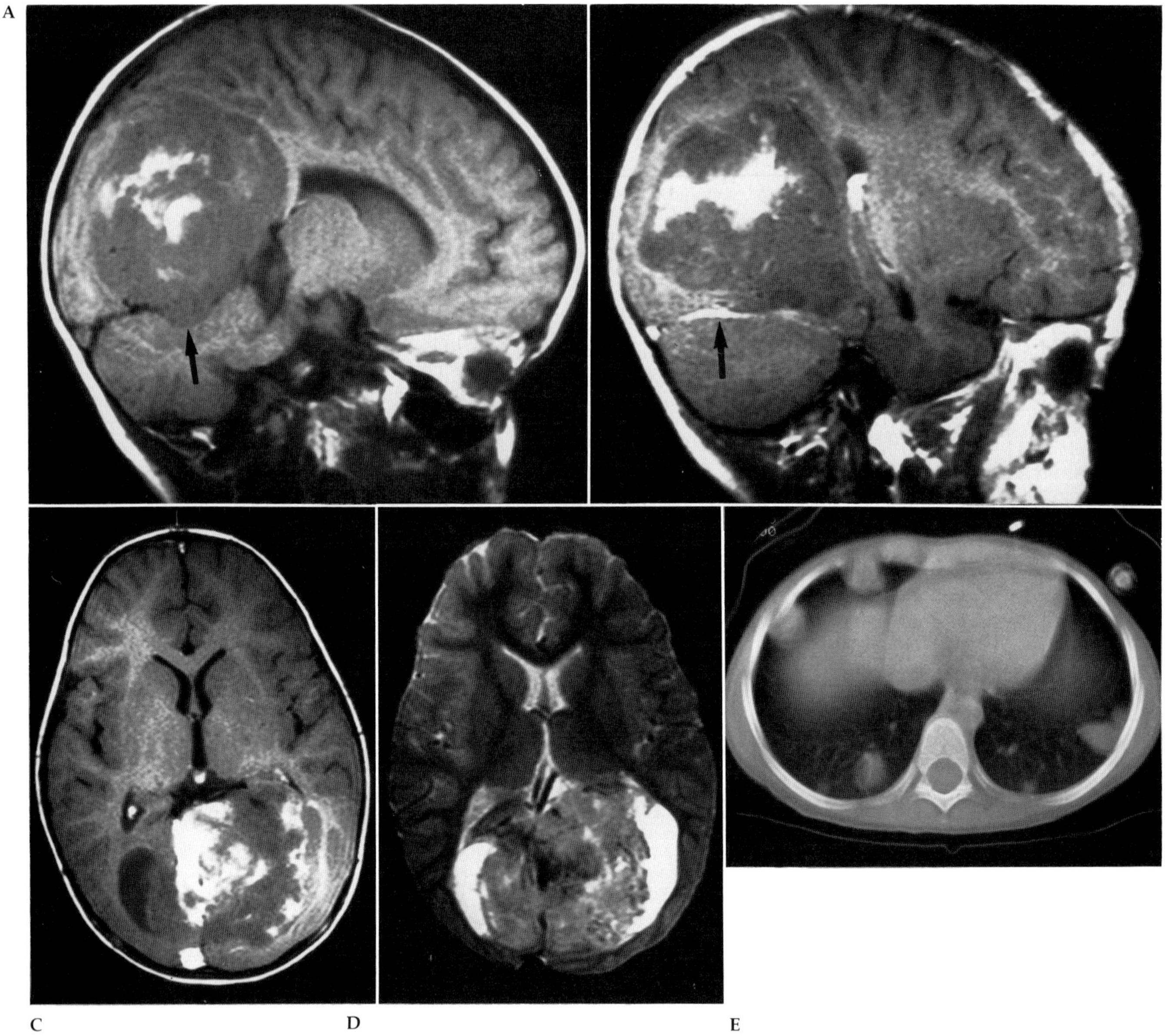

Figure 8–33. Diagnosis: Primitive neuroectodermal tumor.
A, MR, T1 weighted image. There is a large posterior tumor involving the occipital lobes but extending inferiorly through the tent into the cerebellum *(arrow).* Bright signal in the tumor represents subacute hemorrhage. ***B*** and ***C,*** MR, T1 weighted images after gadolinium-DTPA administration. There is patchy enhancement of the tumor after contrast administration. The tumor involves the torcular and the transverse sinuses *(arrow).* ***D,*** MR, T2 weighted image. There is patchy increase in signal intensity with T2 weighted imaging. The tumor is well identified. It involves both occipital lobes. Dark areas represent hemorrhage. ***E,*** Chest CT. Multiple nodular pulmonary metastases are seen.

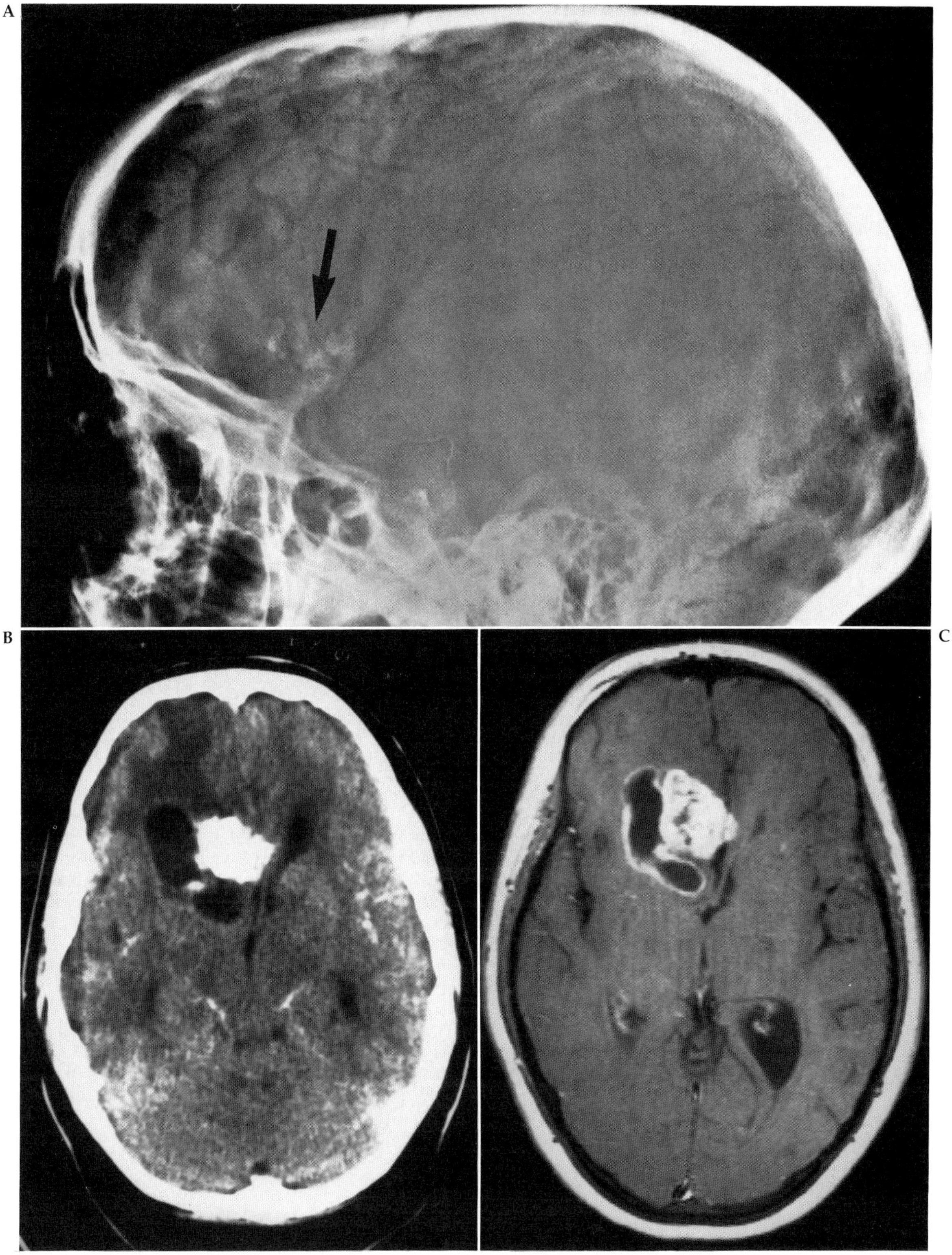

Figure 8–34. Diagnosis: Primitive neuroectodermal tumor.
A, Lateral skull radiograph. Extensive calcification *(arrow)* is identified in the frontal area. ***B***, CT. After contrast administration, there is an enhancing tumor mass with large adjacent cyst and extensive edema. ***C***, MR, T1 weighted image after gadolinium-DTPA. There is enhancement of the tumor mass and the margins of the tumor cyst. The cyst itself appears of very low signal intensity.

A B C

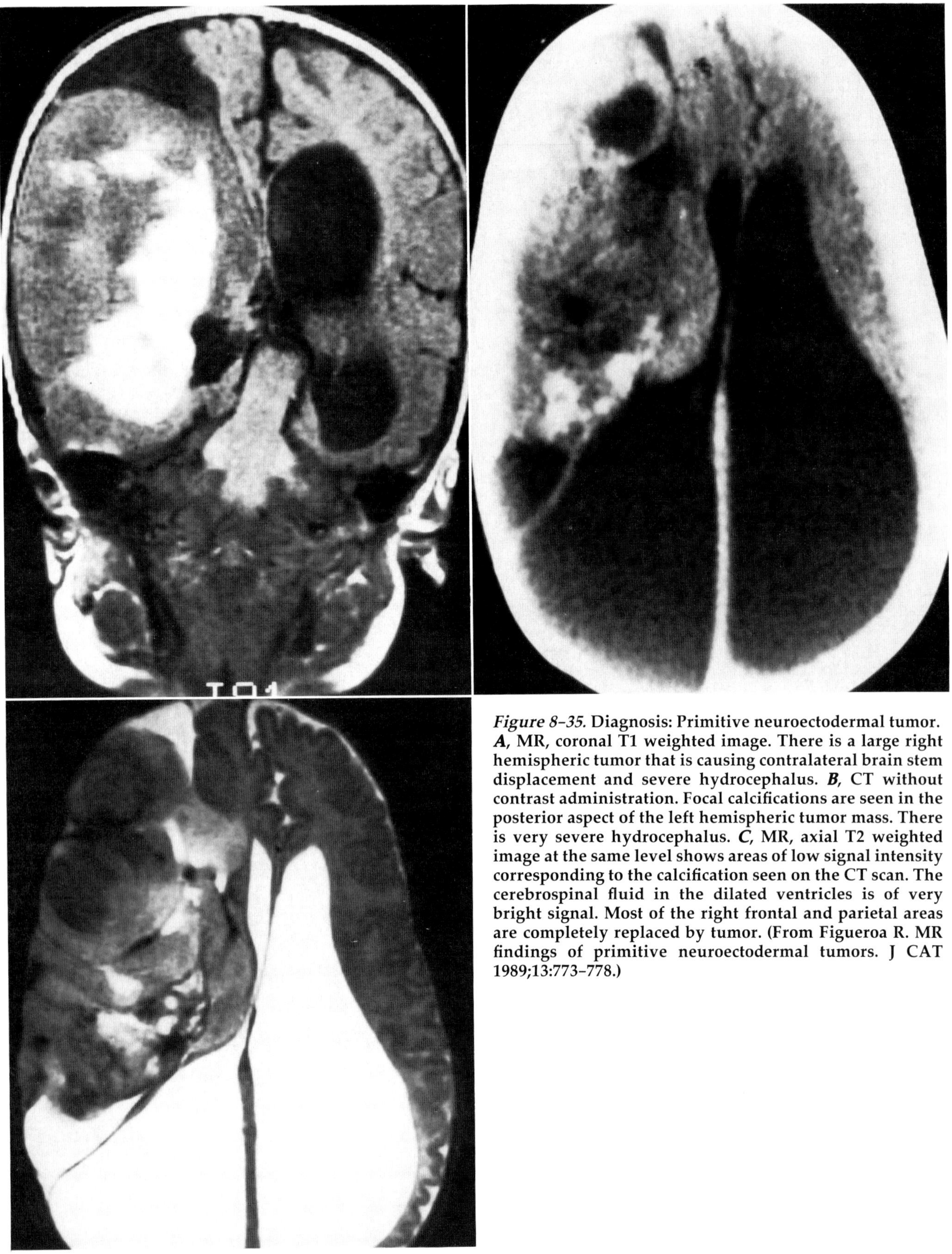

Figure 8–35. Diagnosis: Primitive neuroectodermal tumor. ***A,*** MR, coronal T1 weighted image. There is a large right hemispheric tumor that is causing contralateral brain stem displacement and severe hydrocephalus. ***B,*** CT without contrast administration. Focal calcifications are seen in the posterior aspect of the left hemispheric tumor mass. There is very severe hydrocephalus. ***C,*** MR, axial T2 weighted image at the same level shows areas of low signal intensity corresponding to the calcification seen on the CT scan. The cerebrospinal fluid in the dilated ventricles is of very bright signal. Most of the right frontal and parietal areas are completely replaced by tumor. (From Figueroa R. MR findings of primitive neuroectodermal tumors. J CAT 1989;13:773–778.)

RETINOBLASTOMA

Epidemiology

Retinoblastoma is the most common ocular tumor in children.[1] There are approximately 200 new cases per year in the United States. They occur in very young children. The average age of patients is only 13 months[1,2] and 80 percent occur in children under the age of 3 years.[1] Sixty percent of the tumors are nonhereditary. Thirty percent are hereditary, occurring as new spontaneous mutations, and 10 percent are hereditary with a positive family history.[3] The pattern of transmission is a dominant one with an 80 percent penetrance, and the abnormality is on chromosome 13.[3] The distinction between hereditary and nonhereditary tumors is extremely important. The hereditary tumors occur at an earlier age, can be bilateral, and have an increased risk of other associated malignancies. Nonhereditary tumors do not have these associations. In many patients, it is not possible to know if the tumor is hereditary or not. If there is a positive family history, it is obviously a hereditary type of tumor. If a tumor is bilateral, it is also a hereditary tumor (regardless of the family history). In all other patients, one does not know if the tumor is nonhereditary or a new mutation and, therefore, hereditary.

Pathology

Retinoblastomas are primitive neuroectodermal tumors. They grow very quickly and necrosis and calcification are common.[1,2] They seed in the aqueous and vitreous humor, spread in the orbit, spread along the optic nerve into the brain and into the cerebrospinal fluid.[1] Metastatic spread is rare, being diagnosed in only 20 percent of patients at postmortem.[4] Metastases occur to bone, brain parenchyma, and lung. When distant metastases occur, they usually appear within 2 years.[4] Twenty to 30 percent of retinoblastomas are bilateral.[1,2] About 1 percent will undergo some spontaneous necrosis and involution.

Patients with hereditary retinoblastomas have an increased incidence of second tumors. There are various different types of tumor, but osteosarcoma is the most common. Other tumors include pineoblastoma.[5] The incidence of second tumors increases with time and is increased in regions of the body that have received radiation. Seventy percent of second tumors will occur in the radiation field (radiation used to treat the retinoblastoma).[5]

In the United States, almost all the tumors are confined to the globe at the time of diagnosis. They are staged according to their local invasion and distance of spread (Table 8–10). For those tumors confined to the globe, five categories are recognized. This distinction is very helpful in predicting visual loss and in planning therapy.

TABLE 8–10
Staging of Retinoblastoma

By spread out of globe

Confined to globe	Orbit involved
Optic nerve involved	Distant metastasis

Within globe

I—1 or more tumors all <6 mm and all behind equator
II—1 or more tumors all <15 mm and all behind equator
III—any lesion anterior to equator or 1 lesion >15 mm behind equator
IV—any lesion anterior to ora serrata or >1 lesion > 15 mm behind equator
V—involvement of >1/2 of the retina or the vitreous humor

Clinical Presentation

The most common finding is leukorrhea, a white mass seen through the pupil. Other findings include squint.[3] Pain and vision loss are rare presenting symptoms, mainly because of the very young age of the affected children.[3]

Imaging Studies

Ultrasound is often used in initial investigation. The tumors are very echogenic.[2,6] Unfortunately, dense calcification may block visualization of the whole tumor and spread outside the globe is not well shown with ultrasound. CT has a very characteristic appearance. Calcification is present in over 90 percent of patients (Fig. 8–36). The pattern of calcification is very varied.[2] In 21 children, calcification was identified in at least one eye in every child, and a total of 83 percent of all tumors had calcification.[7] CT is reasonably good for demonstrating spread of the tumor, but early spread into the optic nerve may be missed.[7] MR is very good for showing the extent of the tumor. In one study of 6 patients,[8] the tumor was of equal or greater intensity than vitreous humor in 6 patients. In another series of 6 patients, on T1 weighted imaging the tumor was equal to or less than vitreous humor in signal intensity.[9] Both studies showed tumor to be of lower signal intensity than vitreous humor on T2 weighted images. Identification of calcification was much poorer on MR than CT.[8] MR was able to identify retinal effusions, hemorrhage behind the retina, and nerve spread better than CT.[8,9] Because most of the tumors are confined to the globe at diagnosis, imaging of the spinal canal is not routinely performed.

Differential Diagnosis

Any eye lesion presenting after the age of 3 years, or not containing calcium, is very unlikely to be a retinoblastoma. Differential diagnosis includes:

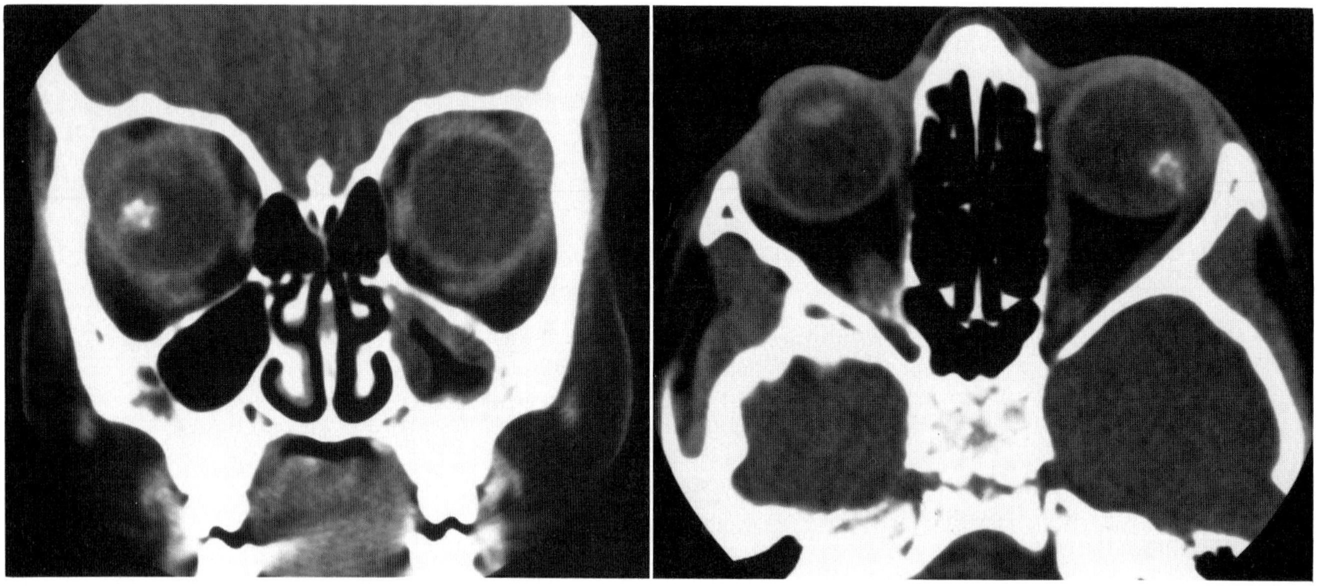

Figure 8-36. **Diagnosis: Bilateral retinoblastoma.**
***A* and *B*, CT. This shows heavily calcified tumor mass lesions in both orbits.**

1. Coates disease. This is always unilateral and usually occurs in children over the age of 4 years. In this condition, there is chronic detachment of the retina and fluid behind the retina appears very bright on T2 weighted images.
2. Retrolental fibroplasia. There is usually a positive history of oxygen administration. There is no calcification. Microphthalmia is often present.
3. Persistent hypoplastic vitreous humor.
4. Toxocara infection. In this condition, there is enhancement of the sclera on CT. There may be retinal detachment, with fluid behind the retina appearing very bright on T2 weighted images.
5. Subretinal effusion. Children with this problem do not have calcification under the age of 3 years. This condition may mimic an infiltrating retinoblastoma.[2]

Therapy and Prognosis

Surgery will cure retinoblastoma, particularly because many of the lesions are confined to the globe at the time of diagnosis. However, there are problems with surgery. The first is that with enucleation there is automatic blindness, so that surgery is rarely performed for bilateral disease. In addition, enucleation under the age of 3 years will leave a small disfiguring orbit for the rest of the patient's life. Enucleation is usually reserved for those patients with such extensive tumor that there is no chance of preserving vision, for patients with glaucoma, and for patients in whom other treatment has failed. Focal surgery using cryocoagulation or photocoagulation will be utilized for residual tumor after radiation therapy.

Radiation therapy gives a good response and is used in most cases. Unfortunately, there are complications, including a small orbit. Recent techniques attempt to confine the radiation field to the tumor limiting damage to other structures.

Chemotherapy is of little benefit and is usually only tried in patients with extraocular disease.[3]

Prognosis with regard to conservative therapy and saving of vision is proportional to the staging shown in Table 8–10. Overall survival is good. In tumors confined to the posterior aspect of the globe, it approaches 100 percent. Fortunately, most tumors are confined to the globe at diagnosis. With spread, however, prognosis drops significantly, being less than 40 percent if there is involvement of the optic nerve or the anterior part of the eye and less than 10 percent if there is distant metastatic spread. Long-term survival in patients with hereditary retinoblastoma is hampered significantly by the high incidence of later development of second tumors.

References

1. Becker LE, Hinton D. Primitive neuroectodermal tumors of the central nervous system. Hum Pathol 1983;14:538–550.
2. Mafee MF, Goldberg MF, Greenwald MJ, et al. Retinoblastoma and simulating lesions: role of CT and MR imaging. Radiol Clin N Am 1987;25:667–682.
3. Donaldson SS, Egbert PR. Retinoblastoma. In: Pizzo PA, Poplack DG, eds. Principles and practice of pediatric oncology. Philadelphia: JB Lippincott, 1989:555–568.
4. Atlas SW, Kemp SS, Rorke L, et al. Hemorrhagic intracranial retinoblastoma metastases: MR-pathology correlation. J Comput Assist Tomogr 1988;12:286–289.
5. Heideman RL, Packer RJ, Albright LA, et al. Tumors of the central nervous system. In: Pizzo PA, Poplack DG, eds. Principles and practice of pediatric oncology. Philadelphia: JB Lippincott, 1989:505–553.
6. Jooma R, Hayward RD, Grant DN. Intracranial neoplasms during the first year of life: analysis of one hundred consecutive cases. Neurosurgery 1984;14:31–41.
7. Arrigg PG, Hedges TR, Char DH. Computed tomography in the diagnosis of retinoblastoma. Br J Ophthalmol 1983;67:588–591.
8. Lee Y-Y, Glass JP, van Eys J, et al. Medulloblastoma in infants and children: computed tomographic follow-up after treatment. Radiology 1985;154:677–682.

9. Haik BG, Saint Louis L, Smith ME, et al. Magnetic resonance imaging in the evaluation of leukocoria. Ophthalmology 1985;92:1143–1152.

SPINAL TUMORS

Spinal tumors are classified as intramedullary, extramedullary intradural, and extradural.[1–4] In one study of 81 patients, 24 were intramedullary, 28 extramedullary intradural, and 29 extradural.[5]

The extradural tumors are most commonly metastatic or caused by direct invasion through the spinal foramina, e.g., with neuroblastoma or Burkitt's lymphoma.

The most common extramedullary intradural tumors are schwannomas, meningiomas, neurofibromas, and cerebrospinal fluid spread metastases.

Intramedullary spinal tumors account for about 4 to 6 percent of all CNS tumors in children.[1] They occur at a median age of about 10 years. Most are low grade. Most contain cysts. Up to 60 percent will show extensive infiltrating involvement of the cord. Two-thirds are astrocytomas and one-quarter ependymomas. All other primary intramedullary tumors are very rare. Symptoms are varied and usually insidious in onset. They include weakness, pain, sensory abnormality, sphincter problems, and gait disturbance.

Careful evaluation of plain film radiographs will demonstrate abnormality in over 50 percent of patients (widening of the spinal canal, pedicle erosions, scalloping of the posterior margins of the vertebra). Myelogram will almost always be abnormal. There will be a block at the lower end of the tumor in over 50 percent of patients, so that myelography rarely demonstrates the total extent of the tumor. MR is without question the imaging modality of choice for evaluation of medullary spinal tumors. Surgery is the mainstay of therapy of these tumors, with resection done if possible. Radiation therapy is utilized usually only for residual tumor. Prognosis is usually excellent if the tumor is resected. It is of interest that up to 15 percent of patients with primary intramedullary tumors will develop hydrocephalus, the mechanism of which is not clear.[3]

With regard to extradural metastases, the most likely diagnosis on initial presentation is Ewing tumor, neuroblastoma, or lymphoma.[6] Such metastases occurring on follow-up after initial diagnosis of the primary tumor are more likely to be caused by rhabdomyosarcoma, hepatoblastoma, or osteogenic sarcoma. With extradural metastases plain film radiographs will show bone changes in over two-thirds of the patients. A bone scan will be positive at the level of the tumor in about half the patients. As with medullary tumors, MR is probably the imaging modality of choice. CT may be particularly helpful prior to surgery in that it will show the amount of bone destruction present far better than MR. Ultrasound can show extradural spread of paraspinal tumors,[7] but I do not think it is nearly as good as CT or MR.

References

1. Heideman RL, Packer RJ, Albright LA, et al. Tumors of the central nervous system. In: Pizzo PA, Poplack DG, eds. Principles and practice of pediatric oncology. Philadelphia: JB Lippincott, 1989:505–553.
2. Iraci G. Intraspinal tumors of infancy and childhood: a review of 19 surgically verified cases. J Pediatr Surg 1966;1:534–545.
3. Oi S, Raimondi AJ. Hydrocephalus associated with intraspinal neoplasms in childhood. Am J Dis Child 1983;135:1122–1124.
4. Haft H, Ransohoff J, Carter S. Spinal cord tumors in children. Pediatrics 1959;23:1152–1159.
5. DeSousa AL, Kalsbeck JE, Mealey J, et al. Intraspinal tumors in children. A review of 81 cases. J Neurosurg 1979;51:437–445.
6. Ch'ien LT, Kalwinsky DK, Peterson G, et al. Metastatic epidural tumors in children. Med Pediatr Oncol 1982;10:455–462.
7. Zimmerman RA. Pediatric supratentorial tumors. Semin Roentgenol 1990;25:225–248.

Table 8–11 provides a summary of some characteristics of a variety of supratentorial tumors.

TABLE 8–11
Miscellaneous Notes on Supratentorial Tumors[1]

Cerebral white matter tumors
- Astrocytoma
- Ganglioglioma
- Ependymoma
- PNET
- Metastases
- Oligodendroglioma

Bleed unlikely except in low-grade astrocytoma

May not enhance on CT
- Some low-grade astrocytomas
- Some malignant gliomas

Unlikely to calcify
- Glioblastoma metastases

Only occasional calcification
- Ganglioglioma
- Low-grade astrocytoma
- PNET
- Germinoma
- Lipoma

Precontrast density compared to normal brain
- Very low—lipoma, teratoma
- < brain—glial, ganglioglioma ependymoma, metastases
- > brain—rest (mainly pineal, germ cell, choroid plexus)

Increased signal on T_1-weighted MR images
- Lipoma, dermoid, subacute bleed
- Cysts—elevated protein or cholesterol

Reference

1. Zimmerman RA. Pediatric supratentorial tumors. Semin Roentgenol 1990;25:225–248.

CHAPTER 9 TUMORS INVOLVING MULTIPLE TISSUES OR ORGANS

RHABDOMYOSARCOMA

Rhabdomyosarcoma can be found in virtually any organ or tissue in the body, and it has the most widespread distribution of any pediatric tumor. The natural history of this tumor is fascinating, because it is unique and different for each anatomic location. Awareness of the different behavior patterns of this tumor in different locations is of importance to the therapist, as the intensity of therapy needs to be tailored to the predicted behavior of the tumor. Similarly, it is of importance to the radiologist, as the imaging approach will vary depending on the anatomic location. To provide a cost-effective approach the radiologist must be aware of the regional differences of behavior of rhabdomyosarcoma.

Epidemiology

Rhabdomyosarcoma is the most common soft-tissue malignancy in children[1]; it accounts for over 50 percent of all pediatric soft-tissue sarcomas.[2] The incidence is approximately four new cases per million children under the age of 15 per year,[3] which translates to approximately 250 new cases each year in the United States.[4]

The etiology of the tumor is unknown. There have been a few reported instances of associations with disorders such as neurofibromatosis,[1,3] fetal alcohol syndrome, basal cell nevus, and congenital abnormalities of the central nervous system.[5] There is an increase in the incidence of other malignant tumors in family members of children with rhabdomyosarcoma.[6] The vast majority of rhabdomyosarcomas, however, occur without any identifiable associated disorder. There are no good biological markers for this tumor.[3]

The median age of presentation in two large series was approximately 7 years.[7,8] In 686 patients in the Intergroup Rhabdomyosarcoma Study (IRS), 4 percent occurred under the age of 1 year.[7] There are peaks in the age period 2 to 6 years and again in the age group 14 to 18 years.[1,5] Approximately 50 percent of patients will present under the age of 5 years[9] and 70 percent under the age of 10 years.[6] The peak in teenage years is in large part caused by the occurrence of paratesticular rhabdomyosarcoma.[5]

The tumor consistently shows a higher incidence in white children than black children, with the ratio being about 3:1.[7] There is also a consistent finding of 60 percent of cases occurring in males.[7,10]

> *Comment:* Rhabdomyosarcoma occurs in any location in the body and behaves differently in each location.

References

1. Agamanolis DP, Dasu S, Krill CE. Tumors of skeletal muscle. Hum Pathol 1986;17:778–795.
2. Feldman BA. Rhabdomyosarcoma of the head and neck. Laryngoscope 1982;92:424–440.
3. Malogolowkin MH, Ortega JA. Rhabdomyosarcoma of childhood. Pediatr Ann 1988;17:251–266.
4. Raney RB, Hays DM, Tefft M, et al. Rhabdomyosarcoma and the undifferentiated sarcomas. In: Pizzo PA, Poplack DG, eds. Principles and practice of pediatric oncology. Philadelphia: JB Lippincott, 1989:635–658.
5. Dehner LP. Pediatric surgical pathology, 2nd ed. Baltimore: Williams & Wilkins, 1987:208–215.
6. Maurer HM. Rhabdomyosarcoma. Curr Prob Cancer 1978;2:3–36.
7. Maurer HM, Beltangady M, Gehan EA, et al. The Intergroup Rhabdomyosarcoma Study–I. A final report. Cancer 1988;61:209–220.
8. Fernandez CH, Sutow WW, Merino OR, et al. Childhood rhabdomyosarcoma. AJR 1975;123:588–597.
9. Grosfeld JL, Weber TR, Weetman RM, et al. Rhabdomyosarcoma in childhood: analysis of survival in 98 cases. J Pediatr Surg 1983;18:141–146.
10. Caillaud JM, Gerard-Marchant R, Marsden HB, et al. Histopathological classification of childhood rhabdomyosarcoma: a report from the International Society of Pediatric Oncology Pathology Panel. Med Pediatr Oncol 1989;17:391–400.

Pathology

ANATOMIC SITE OF PRIMARY TUMOR

Most rhabdomyosarcomas do not occur in muscle; they are found in sites where muscle is not normally located.[1,2] The anatomic location of the primary tumor reported in three large series is summarized in Table 9–1. The three most common locations in descending order of frequency are the head and neck, the genitourinary system, and the extremities. The trunk and retroperitoneum are the next most common locations. In the head and neck, it is important to differentiate between a primary orbital location, a parameningeal location, and other sites. This is because the therapy of these tumors in the three different anatomic locations varies considerably. At times, with invasive tumors, it may be difficult for the radiologist to determine the exact location of origin, but with computed tomography (CT) and magnetic resonance imaging (MR) the radiologist should attempt to define the center of the tumor as accurately as possible. For the purpose of classification of head and neck rhabdomyosarcomas a parameningeal location is defined as a tumor close enough to the meninges to permit intracranial spread of the tumor. These sites are the nasopharynx, paranasal sinuses, ear, infratemporal fossa, and mastoid.[3–5] Any tumor located in one of these locations should be termed a parameningeal rhabdomyosarcoma. Of these sites the nose is the most common, followed by the sinuses, pharynx, and ear.[6] It is of interest to note that, although rare, rhabdomyosarcoma is the most common malignancy occurring in the ear in children.[6] Table 9–2 shows data collected from 202 patients with head and neck rhabdomyosarcomas in the IRS study. As can be seen, parameningeal tumors are the most common head and neck tumors.

TABLE 9–1

Rhabdomyosarcoma: Anatomic Location of Primary Tumor

Reference	Maurer	Fernandez	Grosfeld
No. of Cases	686[1]	113[2]	98[3]
Site	Percentage in Each Site		
Head & Neck			
Orbit	10	14	8
Parameningeal	14	41 (Parameningeal and Other)	14 (Parameningeal and Other)
Other	13		
Genitourinary	21	15	31
Extremity	20	14	17
Trunk	7	4	—
Retroperitoneal	8	5	—
Miscellaneous	7	7	30
	100	100	100

References

1. Maurer HM, Beltangady M, Gehan EA, et al. The Intergroup Rhabdomyosarcoma Study–I. A final report. Cancer 1988;61:209–220.
2. Fernandez CH, Sutow WW, Merino OR, et al. Childhood rhabdomyosarcoma. AJR 1975;123:588–597.
3. Grosfeld JL, Weber TR, Weetman RM, et al. Rhabdomyosarcoma in childhood: analysis of survival in 98 cases. J Pediatr Surg 1983;18:141–146.

TABLE 9–2

Distribution of 202 Head and Neck Rhabdomyosarcomas[1]

Tumor	Percentage
Parameningeal	46
Orbit	26
Other	28
	100

Reference

1. Sutow WW, Lindberg RD, Gehan EA, et al. Three-year relapse-free survival rates in childhood rhabdomyosarcoma of the head and neck. Report from the Intergroup Rhabdomyosarcoma Study. Cancer 1982;49:2217–2221.

Other than the anatomic locations listed in Table 9–1, rhabdomyosarcoma has been reported occurring in many other sites, including the heart,[7,8] the mediastinum,[7] the anus and perineal regions,[1] the biliary system,[1,9–11] and the cerebellum.[12,13]

Genitourinary rhabdomyosarcomas include those tumors arising in the bladder, prostate, spermatic cord, epididymis, testis, penis, vagina, and uterus.[14,15] In the female genitourinary tract, the two most common locations are the base of the bladder and high in the wall of the vagina. Most vaginal malignancies in female children are rhabdomyosarcomas.[15] In the male, the tumors occur commonly in the bladder, prostate, or scrotum. The term paratesticular rhabdomyosarcoma is used to designate those tumors arising in the scrotum. This term is needed because it is frequently impossible to determine whether the tumor has actually arisen from the testis, the tunica, the epididymis, or the spermatic cord. Paratesticular rhabdomyosarcomas account for about 4 percent of all these tumors.[14]

Most rhabdomyosarcomas of the gastrointestinal tract arise in the hepatobiliary system, with the common bile duct being by far the most common location (Table 9–3).

This wide variety of locations of rhabdomyosarcoma means that this tumor needs to be in the differential diagnosis of almost every nonosseous tumor mass in a child. Knowledge of the frequency of occurrence of a tumor in a particular location will help the radiologist in deciding the priority to be given to rhabdomyosarcoma in the differential diagnosis.

MACROSCOPIC APPEARANCE

Most rhabdomyosarcomas appear as nonspecific soft-tissue mass lesions.[16] They are soft, fleshy tumors[6] and lack a true capsule.[6] The margins may falsely be well defined by a pseudocapsule of compressed tissue, or no clearly defined margin may be evident. The tumors characteristically demonstrate fairly extensive local invasion and destruction of adjacent organs and tissues.[17] The term botryoid refers to a polypoid form of rhabdo-

TABLE 9–3

Distribution of 33 Hepatobiliary Rhabdomyosarcomas[1]

Location	No.
Common bile duct	23
Hepatic duct	4
Liver	4
Ampulla	1
Gallbladder	1
	33

Reference

1. Mihara S, Matsumoto H, Tikunaga F, et al. Botryoid rhabdomyosarcoma of the gallbladder in a child. Cancer 1982;49:812–818.

myosarcoma that always arises beneath a mucus membrane and then grows as a polypoid mass into an adjacent hollow structure.[1,18,19] It is seen, for example, in the bladder, vagina, and sinuses. In the head and neck, the tumors will often cause extensive local bone destruction as the soft-tissue mass expands and infiltrates. In the extremities, the tumors will displace and invade adjacent muscle. In the genitourinary system, local invasion may make the precise location of origin of the tumor difficult to determine. For example, in girls, vaginal tumors usually arise high in the anterior wall of the vagina and may invade the bladder, making differentiation from a bladder primary impossible. Similarly, in boys, it may not be possible to differentiate origin in the base of the bladder from prostatic origin.[20]

Grossly, the tumors are often necrotic and hemorrhagic.[7] The size of the tumor varies (Table 9–4). Surprisingly, paratesticular rhabdomyosarcomas are often quite large at diagnosis, with the mean diameter being 6.9 cm in one large series.[21]

At the time of diagnosis parameningeal rhabdomyosarcomas will have spread to involve the meninges from between 26 to 50 percent of cases.[7] I suspect that the wide range of incidence of meningeal involvement is in part a result of the availability of different imaging technologies over the past 20 years. CT, and particularly MR, will define penetration through the bones of the skull and soft-tissue spread of tumor into the skull vault much more readily than earlier imaging modalities allowed.

MICROSCOPY

Rhabdomyosarcoma arises from a primitive cell. The diagnosis may be difficult and there is a wide spectrum of appearance with no universally agreed criteria.[1] Errors in diagnosis are made[18] and there is some disagreement as to whether or not tumors such as undifferentiated soft-tissue sarcoma and extraosseous Ewing sarcoma should be included with rhabdomyosarcoma. These differences will account in part for the difference in reported findings with regard to the incidence, imaging appearance, treatment, and prognosis of rhabdomyosarcoma. The classic rhabdomyosarcoma is more easy to diagnose, and the appearance of Z-bands on electron microscopy and positive immune muscle antibody staining, particularly to desmoid, are features diagnostic of rhabdomyosarcoma.[2,19] Unfortunately, these findings are not present in all cases and this is when difficulties arise.

> *Comment:* Accurate pathologic diagnosis of rhabdomyosarcoma is impossible in a small number of patients.

The classic histologic classification of rhabdomyosarcoma was formulated in the 1950s[22] and has been widely utilized, particularly for the intergroup rhabdomyosarcoma studies in the United States. This classification is summarized in Table 9–5. Any particular histologic type can be found in any location but some types are more common in certain locations. There is also some correlation between histologic type and prognosis but this is by no means absolute. Another problem with

TABLE 9–4

Size of Rhabdomyosarcoma Primary Tumor on Diagnosis in 686 Cases[1]

Size (diameter)	Percentage
<3 cm	33
3–5 cm	46
>5 cm	21

Reference

1. Maurer HM, Beltangady M, Gehan EA, et al. The Intergroup Rhabdomyosarcoma Study–I. A final report. Cancer 1988;61:209–220.

TABLE 9–5

Rhabdomyosarcoma: IRS Histologic Classification and Incidence of Various Histologic Subgroups[1]

Classification	Incidence (%)
Embryonal	56
Alveolar	20
Botryoid	5
Pleomorphic	1
Undifferentiated	10
Other sarcoma	8

Reference

1. Maurer HM, Beltangady M, Gehan EA, et al. The Intergroup Rhabdomyosarcoma Study–I. A final report. Cancer 1988;61:209–220.

this classification is that it may be difficult for the pathologist to accurately place a patient into a particular group.[2]

The embryonal group represents most of the tumors in the head and neck and genitourinary tract (Table 9–5). In the paratesticular location, 90 percent of the tumors are embryonal.[21] It is the most common type in all anatomic locations except for the extremities. The botryoid type is, in fact, an embryonal rhabdomyosarcoma arising beneath mucus membranes and having a macroscopic polypoid appearance.[18] The alveolar type is the most common type in the extremities but can occur in any location. It has a worse prognosis and a higher incidence of metastases than the other type. Pleomorphic tumors probably do not occur in children, but are found in adults.[1]

Because of the difficulties with this classification, other classifications have been suggested. A European classification is summarized in Table 9–6, but I am not sure that this will gain any widespread acceptance in the United States. A new classification suggested for the intergroup rhabdomyosarcoma studies is summarized in Table 9–7; this is a complex classification, taking into account histologic, clinical, and imaging findings. The microscopic differential diagnosis of rhabdomyosarcoma includes primitive neuroectodermal tumor, extraosseous Ewing sarcoma, synovial cell sarcoma, alveolar soft-part sarcoma, hemangiopericytoma, undifferentiated sarcoma, lymphoma, and neuroblastoma.[1,2]

CLINICAL STAGING

As mentioned, a new complex integrated staging system for future studies has been suggested (see Table 9–7). At the present time, all of the intergroup rhabdomyosarcoma studies utilize the clinical staging system summarized in Table 9–8. The disadvantage of this system is its strong reliance on surgical outcome. The distribution of cases by clinical stage has remained very constant during the first three intergroup rhabdomyosarcomas studies (Table 9–9). Less than half of the patients fall into clinical stage I or II.

The clinical stage varies by anatomic site. For example, in the genitourinary system, there is a high percentage (43 percent) of stage I patients.[23] If one looks at paratesticular tumors alone, 59 percent are stage I at presentation and only 21 percent are stages III or IV. The opposite occurs in the abdomen and retroperitoneum, with none of 18 patients in one study being stage

TABLE 9–6
Suggested European Classification of Rhabdomyosarcoma[1]

Embryonal sarcoma
Embryonal rhabdomyosarcoma
- Loose
  - Botryoid
  - Nonbotryoid
- Dense
  - Poorly differentiated
  - Well differentiated
- Alveolar
- Other

Adult/pleomorphic

Reference

1. Caillaud JM, Gerard-Marchant R, Marsden HB, et al. Histopathological classification of childhood rhabdomyosarcoma: a report from the International Society of Pediatric Oncology Pathology Panel. Med Pediatr Oncol 1989;17:391–400.

TABLE 9–7
Suggested United States Staging System of Rhabdomyosarcoma[1]

Intergroup Rhabdomyosarcoma Study TGNM System

Summary of pretreatment clinical staging based on clinical, radiographic, and laboratory examination (plus histologic biopsy):

A. Localized tumor with favorable histology and clinically negative nodes
B. Locally extensive tumor with favorable histology and clinically negative lymph nodes
C. Any size tumor with clinically involved regional lymph nodes with or without unfavorable histology
D. Distant metastasis

Tumor:
- T_{site} 1—confined to anatomic site of origin; subscript indicates site
  - <5 cm in size
  - ≥5 cm in size
- T_{site} 2—extension or fixation to surrounding tissues
  - <5 cm in size
  - ≥5 cm in size

Histology:
- G1—favorable histology (mixed, undifferentiated, embryonal, botryoid, other)
- G2—unfavorable histology (alveolar)
- GX—insufficient tumor for histologic classification

Regional lymph nodes:
- N = 0—regional nodes not clinically involved
- N = 1—regional nodes clinically involved by neoplasm
- N = X—clinical status of regional nodes unknown (especially sites that preclude regional lymph node evaluation)

Metastases:
- M = 0—no distant metastasis
- M = 1_{site}—metastases present; subscript indicates site(s)

Reference

1. Raney RB, Hays DM, Tefft M, et al. Rhabdomyosarcoma and the undifferentiated sarcomas. In: Pizzo PA, Poplack DG, eds. Principles and practice of pediatric oncology. Philadelphia: JB Lippincott, 1989:635–658.

TABLE 9-8

Clinical Classification of Rhabdomyosarcoma[1,2]

Group	Clinical Features
I	Localized disease, completely resected
II	Localized disease, grossly resected with microscopic residual tumor
	Tumor with lymph node or adjacent organ involvement, completely resected with no microscopic residual tumor
	Tumor with lymph node involvement, grossly resected with microscopic residual tumor
III	Incomplete resection or biopsy with gross residual tumor
IV	Distant metastasis at the time of diagnosis

References

1. Agamanolis DP, Dasu S, Krill CE. Tumors of skeletal muscle. Hum Pathol 1986;17:778–795.
2. Maurer HM. The intergroup rhabdomyosarcoma study (NIH): objectives and clinical staging classification. J Pediatr Surg 1975;10:977–978.

TABLE 9-9

Distribution of Cases of Rhabdomyosarcoma by Clinical Stage[1]

	Study		
Clinical Stage	IRS–I	IRS–II	IRS–III
I	15	13	14
II	25	17	16
III	41	53	53
IV	19	17	17

Reference

1. Maurer HM, Beltangady M, Gehan EA, et al. The Intergroup Rhabdomyosarcoma Study–I. A final report. Cancer 1988;61:209–220.

I and 10 of the 18 patients stage IV.[21] These anatomic differences in stage represent the relative ease or difficulty of resecting the tumor based on the anatomic location.

METASTASES

The anatomic sites of metastases from rhabdomyosarcoma vary considerably. Lung and bone are the most common sites,[24] with lymph node metastases varying from extremely rare to very common depending on anatomic location of the primary tumor. Other sites of metastases include liver, marrow, and almost any other region of the body. A 1987 review of postmortem studies in 274 patients with rhabdomyosarcoma concluded that 82 percent of the deaths were caused by tumor progression.[25] Of these patients 15 percent had only local recurrence, 35 percent only metastases, and 50 percent local or metastatic tumor. Metastases were usually multiple, involved the lung most commonly, and also occurred to the bones, lymph nodes, liver, and brain. Brain metastases were much more common than previously believed. Metastases were most common for alveolar histology tumors and for primary tumors located in the extremities. Seventy-six percent of parameningeal tumors showed direct extension into the central nervous system.[25] The more specific distribution of metastases is discussed further under Imaging Studies.

References

1. Agamanolis DP, Dasu S, Krill CE. Tumors of skeletal muscle. Hum Pathol 1986;17:778–795.
2. Raney RB, Hays DM, Tefft M, et al. Rhabdomyosarcoma and the undifferentiated sarcomas. In: Pizzo PA, Poplack DG, eds. Principles and practice of pediatric oncology. Philadelphia: JB Lippincott, 1989:635–658.
3. Chan RC, Sutwo WW, Lindberg RD. Parameningeal rhabdomyosarcoma. Radiology 1979;131:211–214.
4. Latack JT, Hutchinson RJ, Heyn RM. Imaging of rhabdomyosarcomas of the head and neck. AJNR 1987;8:353–359.
5. Sutow WW, Lindberg RD, Gehan EA, et al. Three-year relapse-free survival rates in childhood rhabdomyosarcoma of the head and neck. Report from the Intergroup Rhabdomyosarcoma Study. Cancer 1982;49:2217–2221.
6. Feldman BA. Rhabdomyosarcoma of the head and neck. Laryngoscope 1982;92:424–440.
7. Malogolowkin MH, Ortega JA. Rhabdomyosarcoma of childhood. Pediatr Ann 1988;17:251–266.
8. Roy S, Bhatia R, Nanda NR. Primary rhabdomyosarcoma of the cerebellum. J Pathol 1980;132:235–241.
9. Arnaud O, Boscq M, Asquier E, et al. Embroyonal rhabdomyosarcoma of the biliary tree in children: a case report. Pediatr Radiol 1987;17:250–251.
10. Lack EE, Perez-Atayde AR, Schuster SR. Am J Surg Pathol 1981;5:643–652.
11. Mihara S, Matsumoto H, Tikunaga F, et al. Botryoid rhabdomyosarcoma of the gallbladder in a child. Cancer 1982;49:812–818.
12. Roy S, Bhatia R, Nanda NR. Primary rhabdomyosarcoma of the cerebellum. J Pathol 1980;132:235–241.
13. Shin KH, Whitehead VM. Rhabdomyosarcoma of the brain. Canad J Surg 1980;23:576–578.
14. Hamilton CR, Pinkerton R, Horwich A. The management of paratesticular rhabdomyosarcoma. Clin Radiol 1989;40:314–317.
15. La Vecchia C, Draper GJ, Franceschi S. Childhood nonovarian female genital tract cancers in Britain, 1962–1978. Descriptive epidemiology and long-term survival. Cancer 1984;54:188–192.
16. Geoffray A, Couanet D, Montagne JP, et al. Ultrasonography and computed tomography for diagnosis and follow-up of pelvic rhabdomyosarcomas in children. Pediatr Radiol 1987;17:132–136.
17. Fernandez CH, Sutow WW, Merino OR, et al. Childhood rhabdomyosarcoma. AJR 1975;123:588–597.
18. Bizer LS. Rhabdomyosarcoma. Am J Surg 1980;140:687–691.
19. Dehner LP. Pediatric surgical pathology, 2nd ed. Baltimore: Williams & Wilkins, 1987:208–215.
20. Eklof O, Brun B, Claesson I, et al. Tumours of the lower urinary tract in children. Acta Radiol Diagn 1978;19:171–185.

21. Raney RB Jr, Tefft M, Lawrence W Jr, et al. Paratesticular sarcoma in childhood and adolescence. A report from the Intergroup Rhabdomyosarcoma Studies I and II, 1973–1983. Cancer 1987;60:2337–2343.
22. Maurer HM. Rhabdomyosarcoma. Curr Prob Cancer 1978;2:3–36.
23. Maurer HM, Beltangady M, Gehan EA, et al. The Intergroup Rhabdomyosarcoma Study–I. A final report. Cancer 1988;61:209–220.
24. King DR, Clatworthy HW Jr. The pediatric patient with sarcoma. Semin Oncol 1981;8:214–221.
25. Shimada H, Newton WA Jr, Soule EH, et al. Pathology of fatal rhabdomyosarcoma. Report from Intergroup Rhabdomyosarcoma Study (IRS–I and IRS–II). Cancer 1987;59:459–465.

Clinical Presentation

The spectrum of clinical presentation of rhabdomyosarcoma is as wide as the number of sites in which this tumor may be located. In many sites, there is a nonspecific presentation of a painless mass. This is particularly true in the limbs.[1]

In the head and neck, orbital tumors may present as a superficial mass lesion or more commonly as proptosis from a tumor lying behind the globe. Other symptoms from orbital tumors include weakness of the orbital muscles, pain, headache, conjunctival edema, and decreased vision.[2] The parameningeal lesions may present late because of their deep location. In the nose, signs include respiratory difficulty, obstruction, and sinusitis.[3] Ear lesions present with signs of otitis media, with loss of hearing as an early finding. Later on there may be progressive deafness, nerve weakness (particularly of the seventh cranial nerve), and the presence of a mass in the auditory canal. Lesions in the sinuses may present very late with pain or discomfort. All the parameningeal tumors will present with signs of an intracranial mass after invasion of the cranium.

Genitourinary lesions also have a wide range of symptoms. Urinary retention is common.[4–6] Dysuria and signs of urinary tract infection may occur,[6,7] and there may be signs of fecal retention due to rectal compression.[8] Hematuria has been reported as being common[6] or only a late manifestation.[8,9] In females, vaginal tumors will present as a mass that may be prolapsing or vaginal discharge.[9,10]

Abdominal retroperitoneal rhabdomyosarcomas will present as a mass with or without pain. Biliary tumors will usually present with jaundice with or without pain.[11–13] There may, in addition, be fever and hepatomegaly.[14]

At any primary location the tumors may present with signs of disseminated malignancy such as anemia and weight loss.[15–17] Other symptoms may occur depending on the location of the tumor and its local spread.

> *Comment:* Clinical signs and symptoms of rhabdomyosarcoma are varied and nonspecific.

References

1. Raney RB, Hays DM, Tefft M, et al. Rhabdomyosarcoma and the undifferentiated sarcomas. In: Pizzo PA, Poplack DG, eds. Principles and practice of pediatric oncology. Philadelphia: JB Lippincott, 1989:635–658.
2. Vade A, Armstrong D. Orbital rhabdomyosarcoma in childhood. Radiol Clin N Am 1987;25:701–714.
3. Feldman BA. Rhabdomyosarcoma of the head and neck. Laryngoscope 1982;92:424–440.
4. Bahnson RR, Zaontz MR, Maizels M, et al. Ultrasonography and diagnosis of pediatric genitourinary rhabdomyosarcoma. Urology 1989;33:64–68.
5. Bartolozzi C, Selli C, Olmastroni M, et al. Rhabdomyosarcoma of the prostate: MR findings. AJR 1988;150:1333–1334.
6. Eklof O, Brun B, Claesson I, et al. Tumours of the lower urinary tract in children. Acta Radiol Diagn 1978;19:171–185.
7. Baker ME, Silverman PM, Korobkin M. Computed tomography of prostatic and bladder rhabdomyosarcomas. J Comput Assist Tomogr 1985;9:780–783.
8. McDougal WS, Persky L. Rhabdomyosarcoma of the bladder and prostate in children. J Urol 1980;124:882–885.
9. Hays DM. Pelvic rhabdomyosarcomas in childhood: diagnosis and concepts of management reviewed. Cancer 1980;45:1810–1814.
10. Nussbaum AR, Lebowitz RL. Interlabial masses in little girls: review and imaging recommendations. AJR 1983;141:65–71.
11. Arnaud O, Boscq M, Asquier E, et al. Embroyonal rhabdomyosarcoma of the biliary tree in children: a case report. Pediatr Radiol 1987;17:250–251.
12. Mihara S, Matsumoto H, Tikunaga F, et al. Botryoid rhabdomyosarcoma of the gallbladder in a child. Cancer 1982;49:812–818.
13. Caty MG, Oldham KT, Prochownik EV. Embryonal rhabdomyosarcoma of the ampulla of Vater with long-term survival following pancreaticoduodenectomy. J Pediatr Surg 1990;25:1256–1258.
14. Lack EE, Perez-Atayde AR, Schuster SR. Botryoid rhabdomyosarcoma of the biliary tract. Am J Surg Pathol 1981;5:643–652.
15. Etcubanas E, Peiper S, Stass S, et al. Rhabdomyosarcoma, presenting as disseminated malignancy from an unknown primary site: a retrospective study of ten pediatric cases. Med Pediatr Oncol 1989;17:39–44.
16. Almanaseer IY, Trujillo YP, Taxy JB, et al. Systemic rhabdomyosarcoma with diffuse bone marrow involvement. AJCP 1983;82:349–353.
17. Henderson DW, Raven JL, Pollard JL, et al. Bone marrow metastases in disseminated alveolar rhabdo-myosarcoma: case report with ultrastructural study and review. Pathology 1976;8:329–341.

Imaging Studies

PRIMARY TUMOR

The imaging appearance of most rhabdomyosarcomas is nonspecific. They are seen by most imaging modalities as a soft-tissue mass with varied displacement and invasion of adjacent tissues and organs. The only exception is the botryoid rhabdomyosarcoma in the base of the bladder, which has a fairly characteristic appearance. Even here, however, the findings are not pathognomonic and a similar appearance could be seen with hemorrhagic cystitis or an endodermal sinus tumor. Historically, the visualization of the soft-tissue mass has improved with the introduction of new imaging techniques. Twenty years ago the presence of the tumor was largely inferred from displacement of structures identified on such studies as intravenous urography, cystography, and barium studies. In other patients, pressure deformity or destruction of adjacent bones could be identified on plain film radiographs, suggesting the presence of an underlying tumor. With all of these modalities the actual soft-tissue tumor mass was poorly visualized.

With ultrasound the visualization of the soft-tissue tumor was greatly improved, particularly in the genitourinary system or the extremities but not in the head and neck, with the exception of some superficial soft-tissue tumors. The ultrasound appearance of rhabdomyosarcomas is very varied and nonspecific.[1] CT and MR now permit accurate delineation of total tumor extent in all sites. CT is better than MR in most cases for identification of bone destruction and this is particularly important in the skull. MR is as good as CT for demonstration of the soft-tissue mass in most patients and in some patients will better define the soft-tissue tumor, particularly when it is isointense with normal muscle on the CT scan. Calcification of the tumor is uncommon or rare.[2] In one study of 32 patients, it was not identified in any.[3] Thus the finding of calcification in a rhabdomyosarcoma, regardless of the imaging modality utilized, should raise the possibility of an alternate diagnosis. Of course, in the skull, expanded foci of destroyed bone will be identified in the tumor, but these should not be confused with primary tumor calcification.

Head and Neck Rhabdomyosarcomas. In the head and neck, CT and MR are the primary modalities to be utilized (Fig. 9–1). It is very important for treatment planning to identify the total local spread and destruction caused by the tumor. Prior to CT and MR this was extremely difficult and invasive, requiring a combination of hypocycloidal tomography, air encephalography, and angiography.[4] One of the earliest studies showing the benefits of CT in defining the extent of skull destruction and spread of rhabdomyosarcomas in 6 patients was published in 1979.[5] Most head and neck rhabdomyosarcomas appear nonhomogeneous on CT, with irregular enhancement and only moderately well-defined margins (Figs. 9–1 and 9–2). In the orbits, the lesions can be seen in the eyelid or are more deeply located. Enhancement may be the same as adjacent normal orbital muscles. The tumors usually start in an extraconal location but soon rapidly spread into the intraconal space.[6] In the ear, clouding of the mastoid sinus is often an early finding on CT; this may be accompanied by a soft-tissue mass in the middle ear.[7] Both MR and CT will show these early findings. Early bone destruction will be better defined with CT (Figs. 9–3 and 9–4). The tumors then grow, destroying bone and extending into the cranial fossa (Fig. 9–3). Occasionally, the tumor will grow through the Eustachian tube with expansion in the nasopharynx, causing a dumbbell appearance.[7] Primary tumors in the paranasal sinsues and nasopharynx will grow into the adjacent regions, destroying bone as they do so (Fig. 9–3).

As previously mentioned, CT will best define the bone destruction and MR the soft-tissue tumor (see Fig. 9–3). From a technical point of view thin slices should be obtained, particularly when subtle bone destruction or early invasion into the cranial fossa is looked for. Imaging planes should be oriented to maximize detection of abnormality so that, for example, the coronal plane is best for identification of destruction of the roof and floor of the orbit. Contrast should always be given with the CT studies to improve visualization of the soft-tissue tumor. With MR gadolinium-DTPA is particularly helpful in enhancing the soft-tissue component of the tumor on T1 weighted images while still permitting maximum anatomic definition (see Fig. 9–3). In the cranium, the tumors may invade the cavernous sinus.[8] The dura is displaced by tumor but in most cases is not penetrated.[9] With very large tumors there may be destruction of many regions of the base of the skull, orbit, and face and it may not be possible to determine the precise location of origin of the tumor.

After the tumor has been identified and defined, the most important question to be asked of imaging of most head rhabdomyosarcomas is the relationship to the bones of the base of the skull and extension of any soft-tissue tumor through these bones into the vault. This accurate definition of tumor is important, because therapeutic decisions depend upon it. For example, in patients with only invasion of the bones but no soft-tissue extension into the skull vault, it may be decided to treat the child with only systemic chemotherapy and radiation therapy but no intrathecal chemotherapy. Radiation therapy ports also require accurate definition of tumor extent.

Extremity Rhabdomyosarcomas. Extremity rhabdomyosarcomas are the most nonspecific of all rhabdomyosarcomas in their appearance. They are identified as soft-tissue masses with variable borders (Figs. 9–5, 9–6, 9–7, and 9–8). On CT, they may be of similar (Fig. 9–5) or low intensity to muscle, showing similar or greater or less enhancement with intravenous contrast than adjacent muscle. In some patients, the tumor remains isointense with muscle before and after contrast administration, and in these cases, one can identify mass effect by comparing with the opposite side, but not the actual margins of the tumor (Fig. 9–5). On MR, the tumors are somewhat variable in appearance, again depending on the amount of hemorrhage or necrosis present (Figs. 9–5 and 9–8). In general, the signal characteristics are consistent with prolongation of T1 and T2 relaxation times compared to normal muscle, with the tumor appearing of lower signal intensity than muscle on T1 and greater signal intensity on T2 weighted images (Figs. 9–5 and 9–7). Most of the tumors show enhancement following gadolinium-DTPA administra-

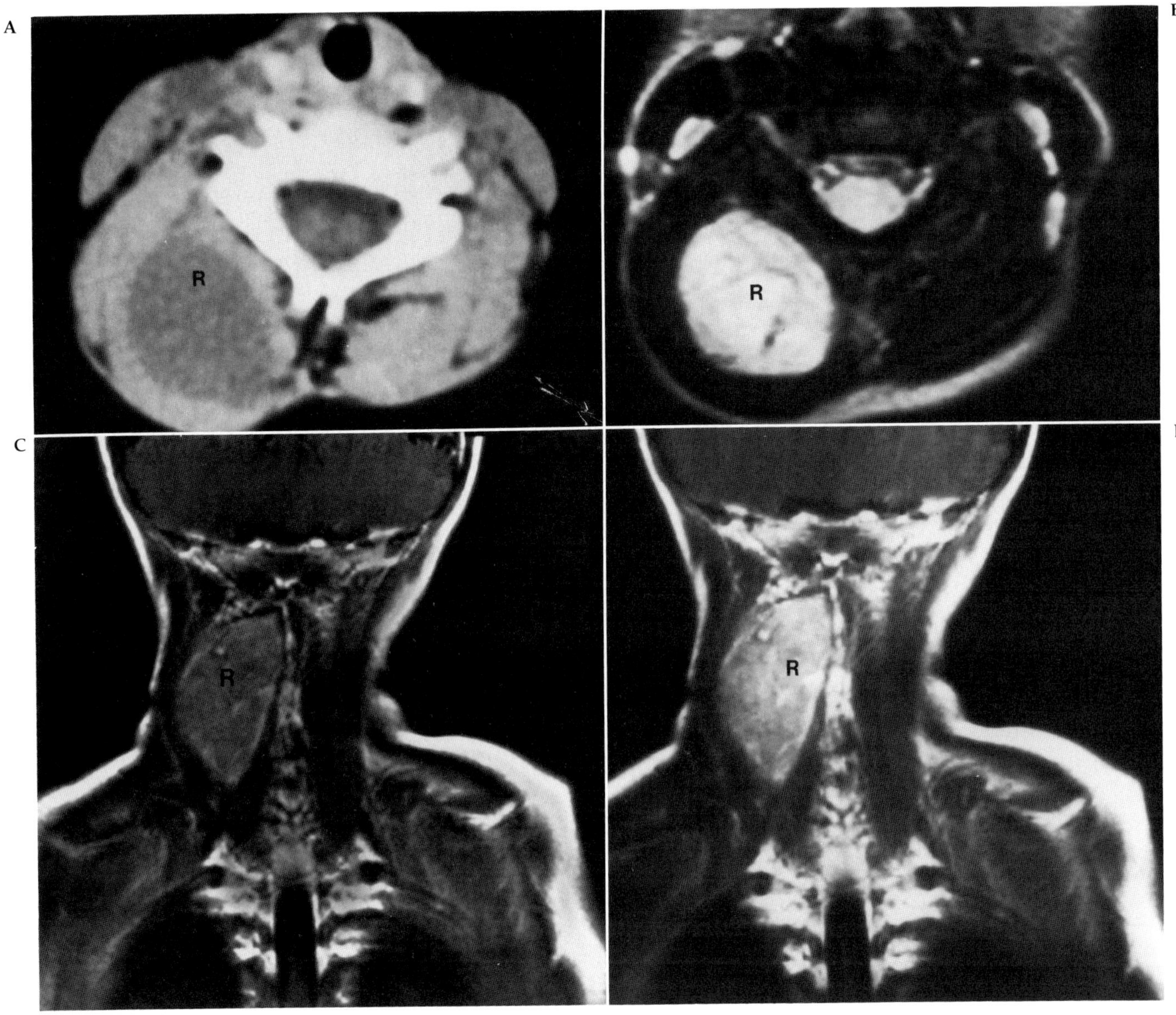

Figure 9–1. **Diagnosis: Rhabdomyosarcoma of the neck. There is a large tumor situated posterolaterally on the right side.**
***A*, CT. The rhabdomyosarcoma (*R*) is fairly well defined. *B*, MR, axial T2 weighted image. The tumor is sharply defined and of very bright signal intensity. *C* and *D*, MR, coronal T1 weighted images before and after gadolinium-DTPA administration. The tumor is well defined. It shows some enhancement following gadolinium-DTPA injection.**

tion. This enhancement may be uniform or patchy. The implications of this with regard to tissue characterization are not known.

Genitourinary Rhabdomyosarcomas. Genitourinary rhabdomyosarcomas may be identified on urography or with barium studies. In most cases, these studies provide only secondary evidence of the presence of a mass. With lesions in the base of the bladder urography will show the superior margin of the lobulated botryoid tumor very well (Fig. 9–9). The other margins of the tumor and, therefore, its total extent cannot be defined. In one study, an intravenous pyelogram was still performed in over 50 percent of cases diagnosed since the late 1970s.[10] All the information from the intravenous pyelogram is provided by MR or CT and it should now be considered an unnecessary study.

Ultrasound is particularly good for identification of lesions involving the base of the bladder.[11] These lesions are easily seen in patients presenting with urinary obstruction, as the full bladder provides a good window to the tumor.[11] Ultrasound will provide better definition of the remaining margins of genitourinary rhabdomyosarcomas than urography, but in my opinion it is not as accurate as CT or MR and I would not use it as the sole

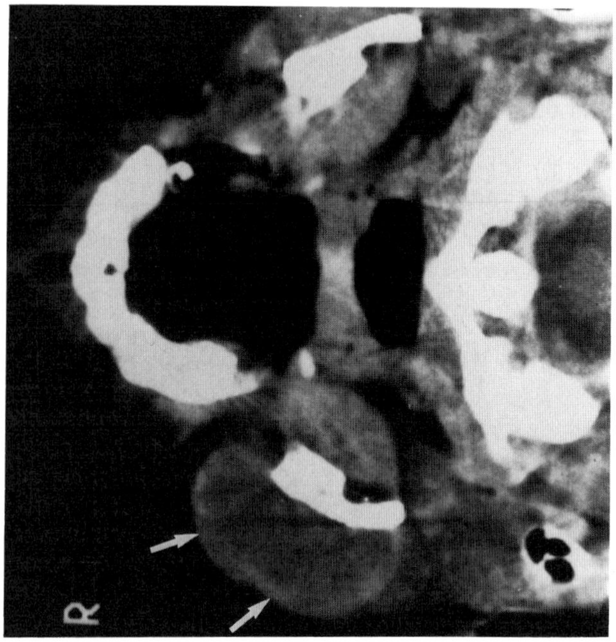

Figure 9–2. Diagnosis: Rhabdomyosarcoma of the masseter muscle.
CT. There is a large tumor *(arrows)* that has completely destroyed the masseter muscle on the right side.

A

C

E

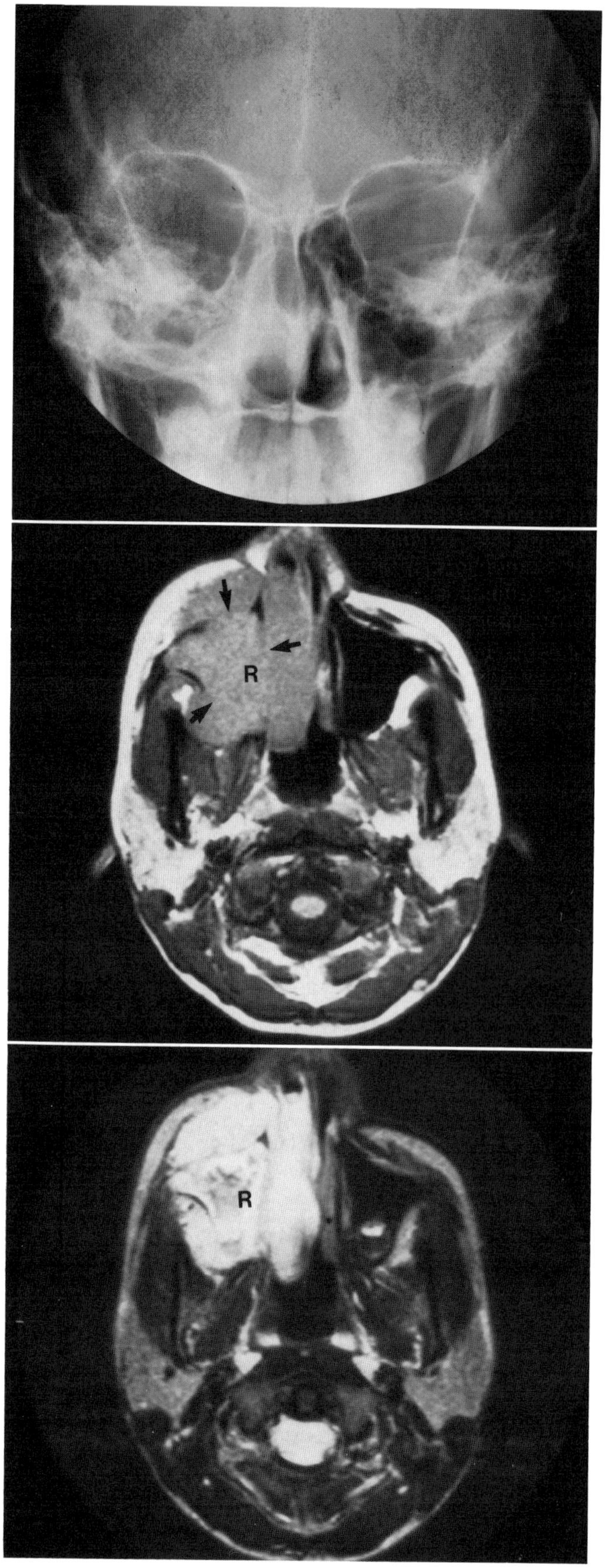

Figure 9–3. Diagnosis: Parameningeal rhabdomyosarcoma arising from the sinuses.
This study shows nice comparison between CT and MR and also between the various different pulse sequences with MR. ***A***, Plain film radiograph of face. There is opacification of the right maxillary and ethmoid sinuses with a large soft-tissue mass in the right side of the nasal cavity. ***B***, CT through the maxillary sinus. There is a large soft-tissue mass completely filling the maxillary sinus on the right side and extending to fill most of the nasal cavity on the right. There is destruction of the anterior, medial, and posterolateral walls of the maxillary sinus *(arrows)*. The tumor cannot be diffentiated from adjacent muscles, as it is of similar intensity. ***C*** through ***E***, MR, T1 weighted, T1 weighted gadolinium-DTPA enhanced, and T2 weighted images. The large tumor (*T*) is well identified. The margins are much more sharply defined than on the CT image. Penetration through the bones can be identified *(arrows)*, but the subtle bone destruction is not nearly as well seen as with CT. ***F***, CT at the level of the orbit. Tumor is seen in the orbit and in the ethmoid sinus. The medial wall of the orbit is almost completely destroyed. ***G*** through ***I***, MR images at the same level as ***G***. The images are T1 weighted, T1 weighted with gadolinium-DTPA enhancement, and T2 weighted. Once again the soft-tissue margins of the tumor are well seen with MR. The bone destruction can be diagnosed but the fine definition of the bone destruction seen on the CT image is not well seen on MR. ***R*** = rhabdomyosarcoma.

B G D H F I

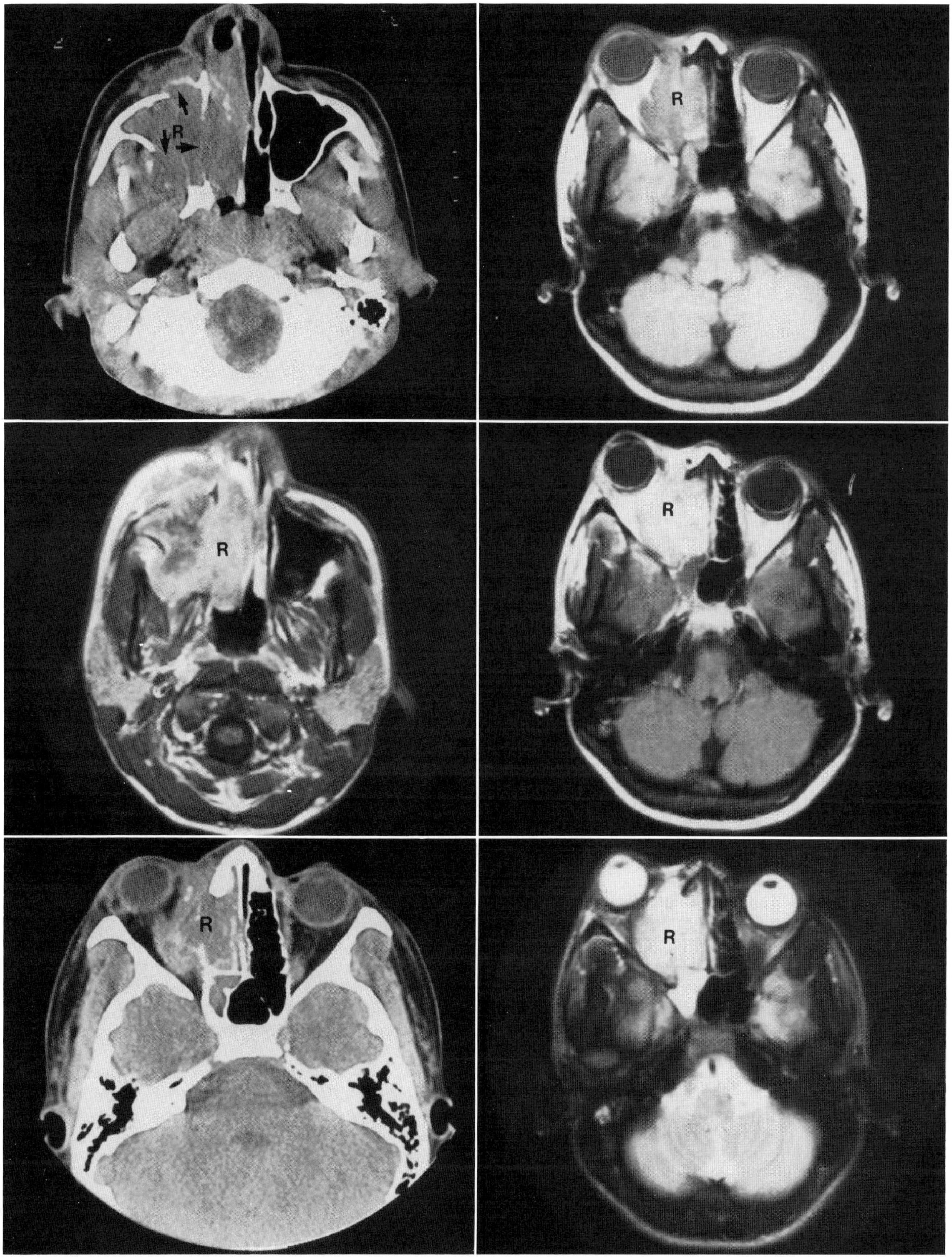

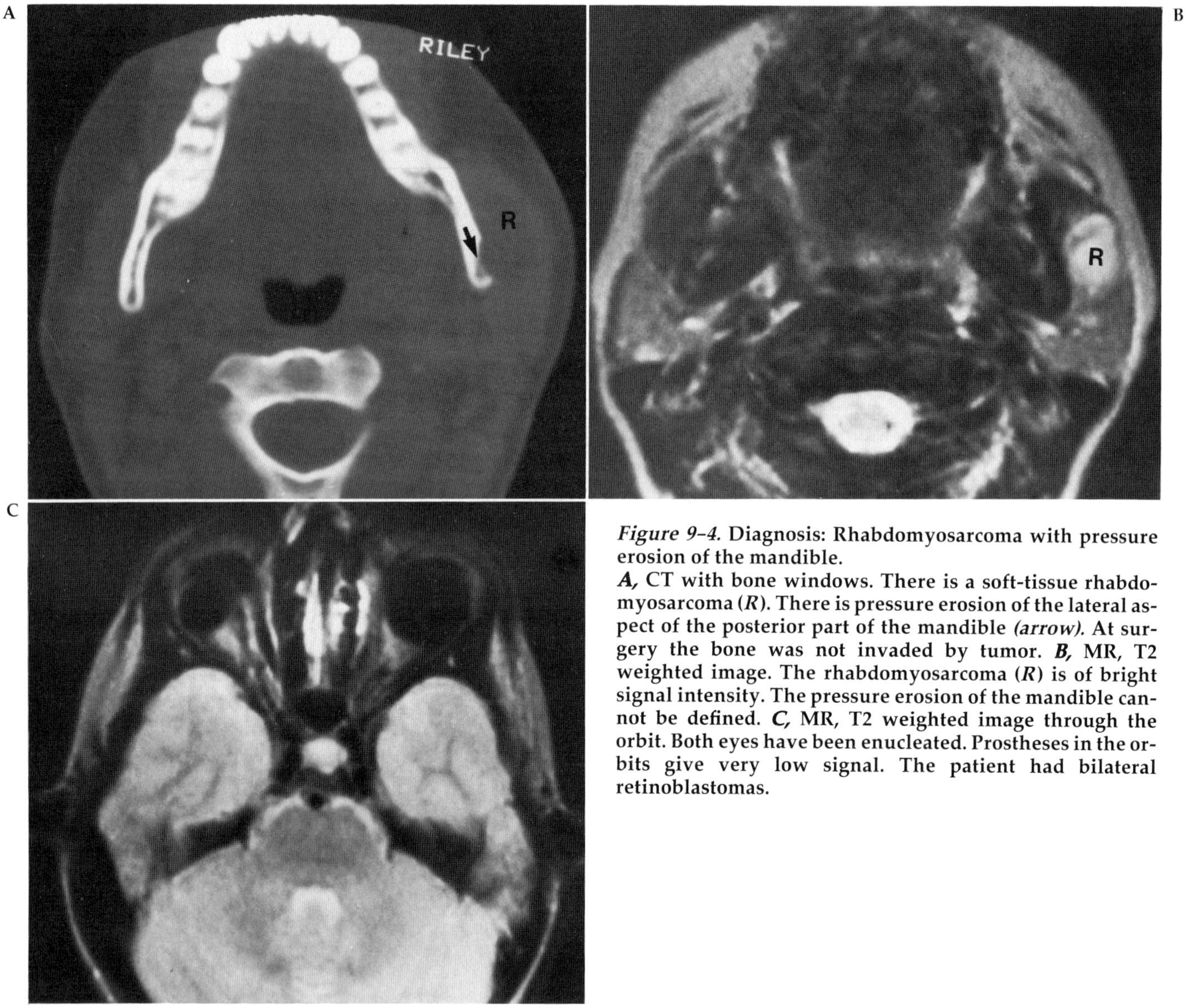

Figure 9-4. **Diagnosis: Rhabdomyosarcoma with pressure erosion of the mandible.**
A, **CT with bone windows. There is a soft-tissue rhabdomyosarcoma (*R*). There is pressure erosion of the lateral aspect of the posterior part of the mandible *(arrow).* At surgery the bone was not invaded by tumor. *B,* MR, T2 weighted image. The rhabdomyosarcoma (*R*) is of bright signal intensity. The pressure erosion of the mandible cannot be defined. *C,* MR, T2 weighted image through the orbit. Both eyes have been enucleated. Prostheses in the orbits give very low signal. The patient had bilateral retinoblastomas.**

imaging modality on initial presentation, nor would I use it for follow-up of a patient. In boys with paratesticular rhabdomyosarcomas, some patients may have no imaging studies of the primary tumor[12]; ultrasound is, however, useful and it will accurately demonstrate the presence of a solid tumor mass rather than a hydrocele in a child with scrotal swelling. Surgery would then be performed.

For bladder or prostatic primary tumors CT and MR are utilized (Figs. 9–9, 9–10, and 9–11). Prostatic tumors may invade the base of the bladder (Fig. 9–11). They will spread into adjacent tissues. They tend to displace the rectum rather than encase it with tumor. Extension into the ischiorectal fossa is not uncommon. Primary tumors in the bladder base may extend inferiorly into the prostate, and in some patients the actual site of origin may be difficult to determine. These bladder base tumors are usually botryoid in shape but may occasionally be seen as a single mass that may even be pedunculated and move. On urography, this may be confused with a ureterocele, but other imaging modalities should show that it is solid and not cystic consistency.[3] Occasionally, the main growth of a bladder base tumor may be extravesical, with only minimal indentation of the bladder base. Again CT or MR will show the large extravesical tumor component. Prior to MR, CT was utilized to demonstrate accurately spread of prostatic and bladder tumors, including invasion of the adjacent muscles and penetration through the sciatic notch or obturator foramen.[10,13] MR has been used to study genitourinary rhabdomyosarcomas.[14] MR is accurate in defining the local extent of the tumor. A particular advantage of MR when compared to CT is the ability to image in multiple planes and thereby better define interfaces that might be horizontal and thus parallel to the CT imaging plane (Figs. 9–10 and 9–11). As with the head and neck, we have found gadolinium-DTPA adminstration to be helpful in enhancing tumor contrast

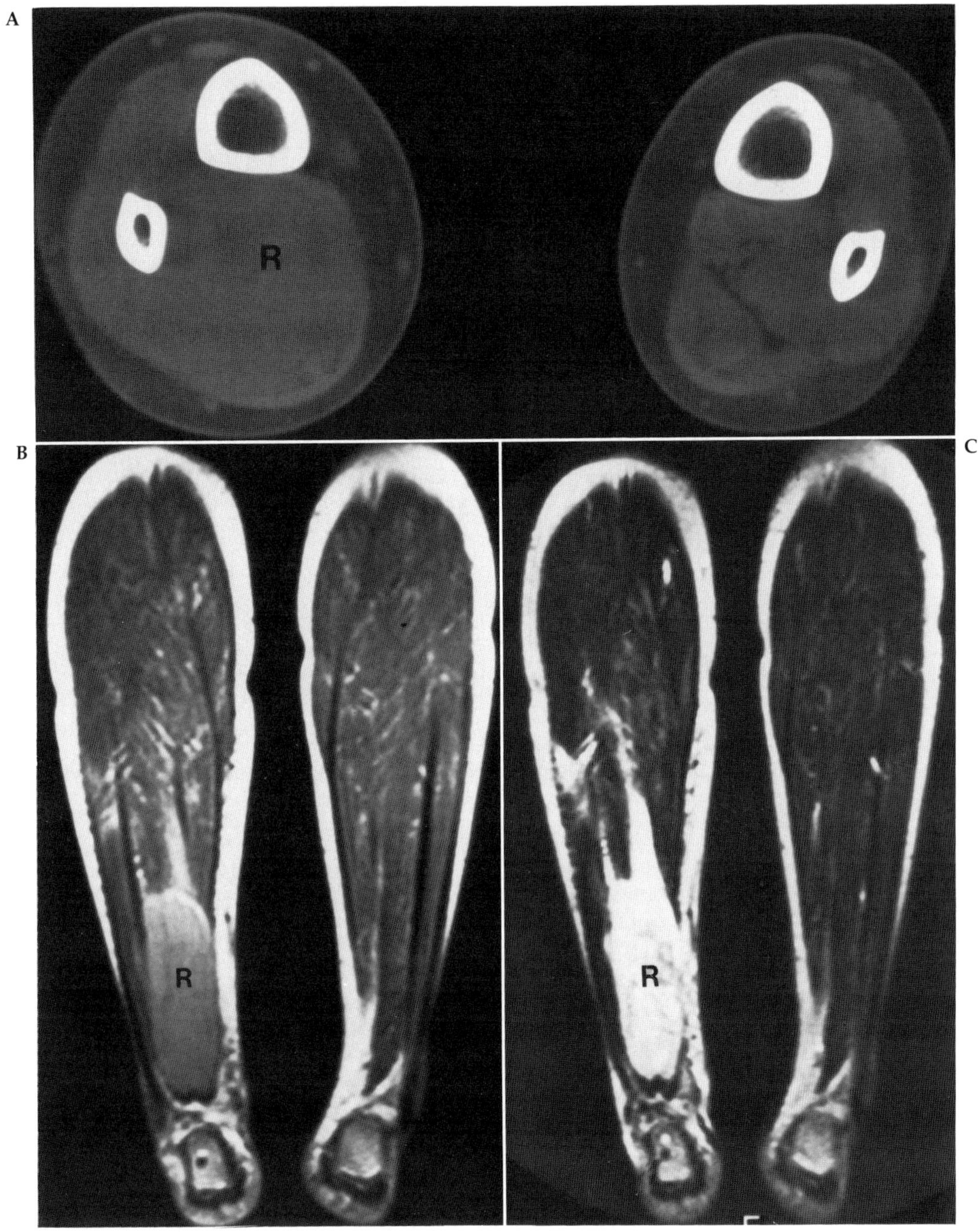

Figure 9-5. Diagnosis: Rhabdomyosarcoma of the calf.
A, CT. There is a very large soft-tissue rhabdomyosarcoma (*R*) in the posterior muscle. The tumor is of identical intensity to the adjacent muscles so that no tumor margins can be identified. ***B*** and ***C,*** MR, coronal T1 and T2 weighted images. The rhabdomyosarcoma (*R*) is clearly defined because of different signal intensity from the adjacent muscle. It is of moderate intensity on the T1 weighted image and very bright on the T2 weighted image.

on T1 weighted images while preserving the better anatomy seen with T1 as compared to T2 weighted images (Figs. 9–10 and 9–11).

In addition to the bladder base and prostate, rhabdomyosarcomas can be found in other sites in the genitourinary system, such as the testes (Fig. 9–12), penis (Fig. 9–13), and perineum (Fig. 9–14).

In females, imaging may not be able to differentiate bladder base from vaginal origin of the tumor, particularly when there has been a significant local invasion. When small, these tumors can be accurately located.

Chest and Abdomen Rhabdomyosarcomas. In the chest and abdomen, CT is probably the modality of choice for identification and definition of rhabdomyosarcomas

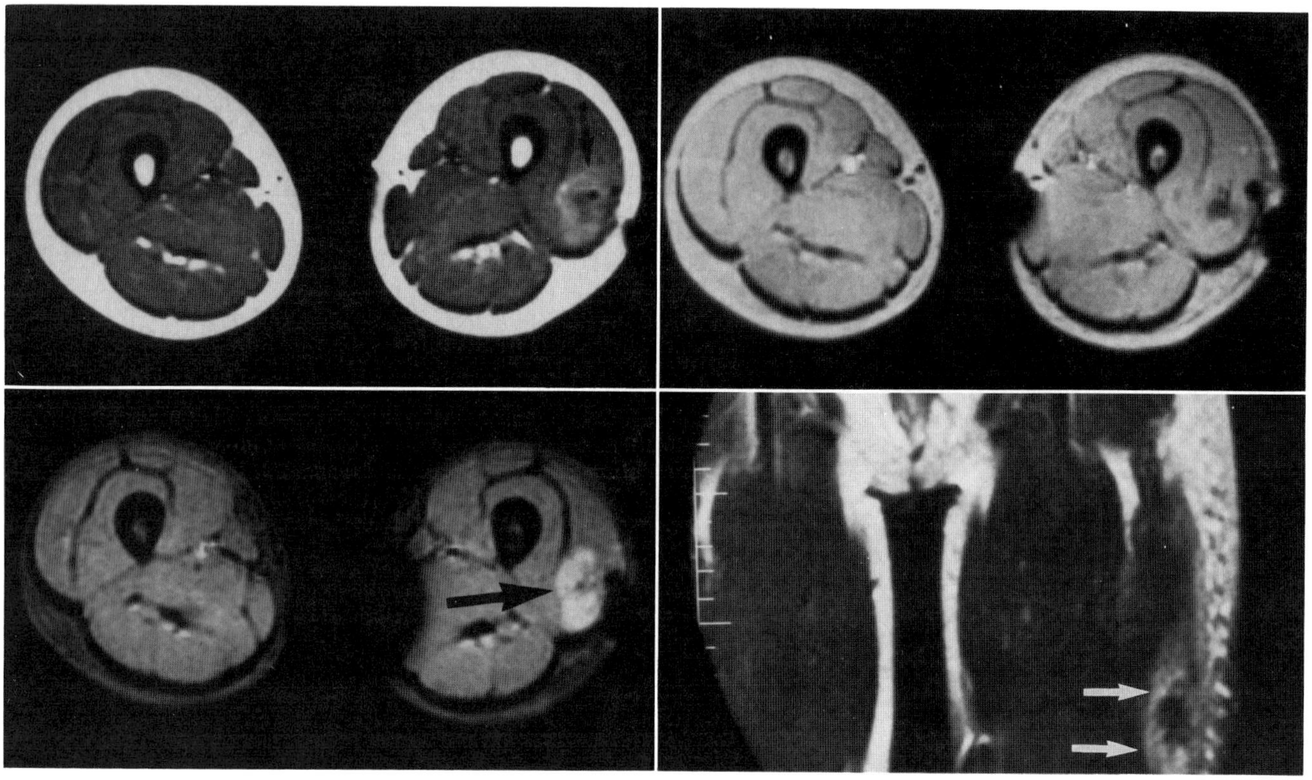

Figure 9–6. **Diagnosis: Undifferentiated sarcoma of the thigh.**
Series of MR images showing alterations in signal intensity with different pulse sequences. *A,* MR, axial T1 weighted image. The tumor involves the lateral aspect of the vastus lateralis muscle and extends into the posterior aspect of the vastus intermedus. The tumor *(arrow)* shows areas of bright signal intensity probably owing to hemorrhage and very low signal intensity probably owing to necrosis. The margins are moderately well defined. *B,* Axial field echo image with 90-degree flip angle. The tumor margins cannot be defined and most of the tumor is of similar intensity to adjacent muscle. *C,* Axial gradient echo image with 20-degree flip angle. Most of the tumor is bright on this pulse sequence. The margins of the tumor are better defined than with any of the other pulse sequences. *D,* Coronal T2 weighted image. The tumor is of mixed bright and low signal intensity probably owing to hemorrhage and necrosis within it. The margins are not as well defined as on the gradient echo image with 20-degree flip angle. All images show that the tumor is readily resectable.

(Fig. 9–15). Ultrasound or MR might be better than CT in defining small tumors arising in the diaphragm because of difficulties with CT in the horizontal imaging plane. Ultrasound is especially helpful in tumors arising in the hepatobiliary system[15] (Figs. 9–16 and 9–17). It will show a polypoid or infiltrating lesion most commonly in the common bile duct.[16,17] It will also accurately define extension of the tumor into the porta hepatis[17] or into the liver tissue,[18] and will show duct dilatation.[15,19] CT and MR would probably define these abnormalities as well, with the relative efficacy of each modality not known (Fig. 9–17). In one case, CT showed a low-density mass at the origin of the common bile duct with proximal duct distension.[15] As these tumors may become very large, the actual origin from the biliary system may be difficult to define in some patients. In these patients, the differential diagnosis would include other retroperitoneal tumors invading the liver or primary liver malignancy.[18] There are no pathogno-

Figure 9–7. **Diagnosis: Rhabdomyosarcoma of the foot.**
MR, T1 weighted image. There is a very large rhabdomyosarcoma (*R*) lying posteromedial to the first metatarsal. The tumor margins are well defined. There is no invasion of the adjacent bone. Signal intensity is slightly greater than that of normal muscle.

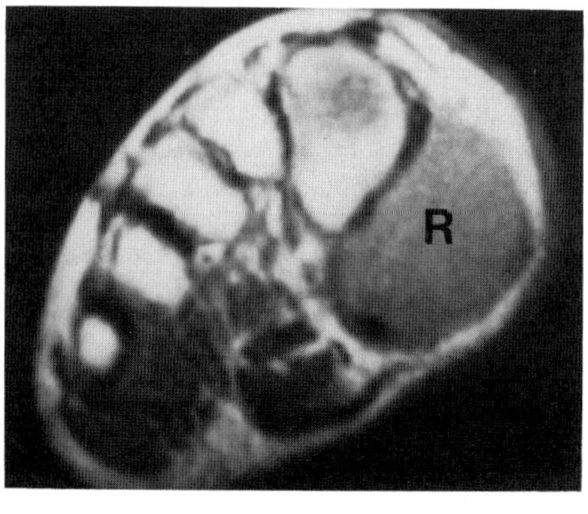

A

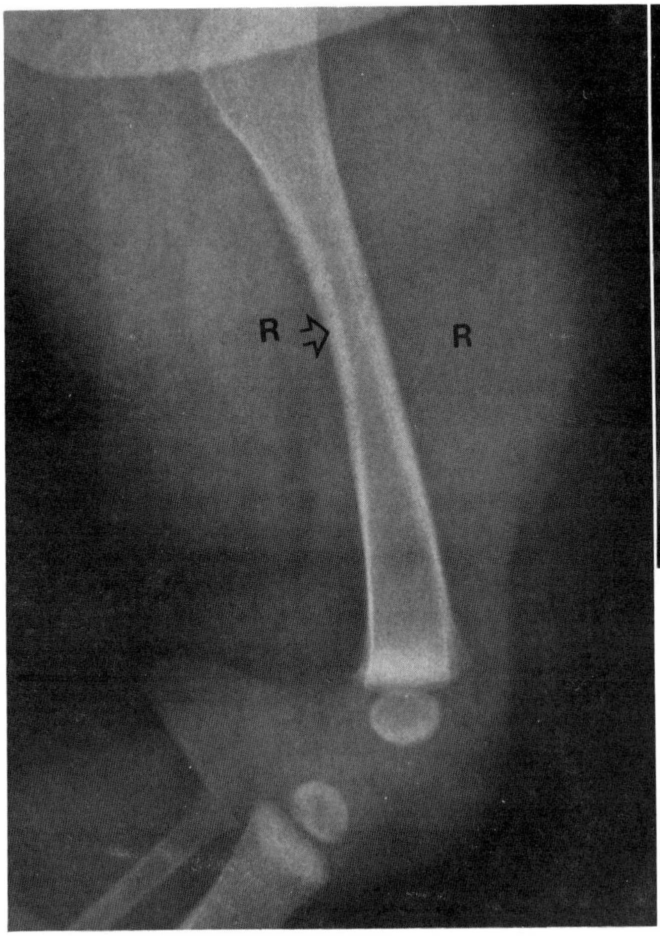

B

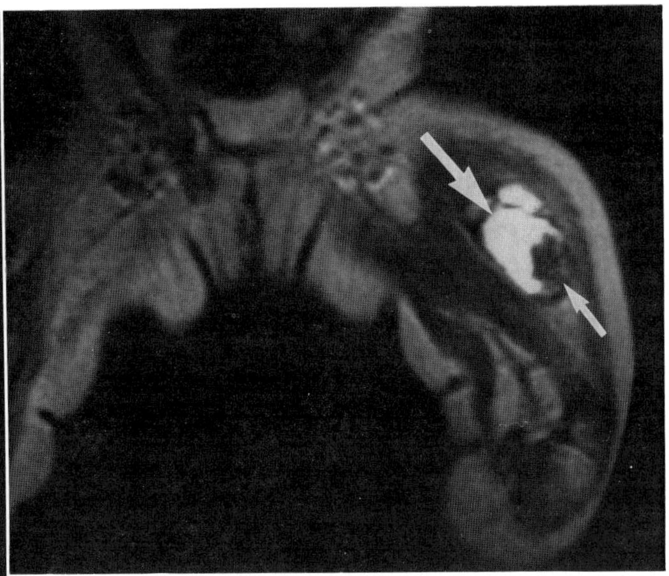

Figure 9–8. **Diagnosis: Rhabdomyosarcoma of the thigh. *A,* Plain film radiograph. A large soft-tissue rhabdomyosarcoma (*R*) is seen. It is causing mild pressure deformity of the medial aspect of the mid femur *(open arrow)*. *B,* MR, T2 weighted image. Most of the tumor is liquefied necrotic tissue and appears very bright *(large arrow)*. Hemorrhagic areas in the tumor appear of low signal intensity *(small arrow)*.**

monic features of rhabdomyosarcoma on any of the imaging modalities. On ultrasound, the lesions are solid with low or high echoes compared to normal liver. CT and MR show soft-tissue lesions with varied internal structures.

Retroperitoneal Rhabdomyosarcomas. In the rare retroperitoneal rhabdomyosarcomas, imaging will show a soft-tissue mass, but in many cases it will not be possible to differentiate this from other tumors such as neuroblastoma or lymphoma.[20]

In addition to defining the primary tumor at the time of initial diagnosis, imaging is also extremely important in monitoring the response of the primary tumor to therapy (see Fig. 9–10). Most rhabdomyosarcomas are not initially surgically resected and are treated instead with chemotherapy, radiation therapy, or both. Some surgery may be subsequently performed. Because of this, imaging is important in monitoring the response to therapy. The exception to this is the extremity, where most rhabdomyosarcomas will initially be surgically resected, and the paratesticular location, where virtually every rhabdomyosarcoma will have initial surgical resection.

The importance of imaging is illustrated by a recent European study of 96 clinical stage III patients treated with initial chemotherapy. The degree of response as measured by reduction in tumor size, after 7 weeks of chemotherapy, correlated well with survival. In those patients showing a complete response, there was 95 percent long-term survival. With those showing greater than two-thirds reduction in tumor volume, survival was 61 percent, and in those showing less than two-thirds reduction in tumor volume, survival was only 31 percent.[21] For purposes of this study volume was defined as the greatest length × width × height × pi divided by 6[21] (more accurate tumor volumes can be calculated either with CT or MR and in the future I would suggest that this be done). Accurate dimensions of irregularly shaped tumors are difficult to obtain whereas volumes calculated from the sum of cross-sectional areas × slice thickness can be very accurately and easily obtained from CT or MR. Although the results from this study are convincing, there will be patients in whom there has been a poor response as judged by tumor volume but a good response on histology because of large areas of persisting hemorrhage and necrosis in a tumor. Evaluation of tumor response should, therefore, include calculation of tumor volume and also an estimation of the percent of necrosis and hemorrhage present in the tumor.

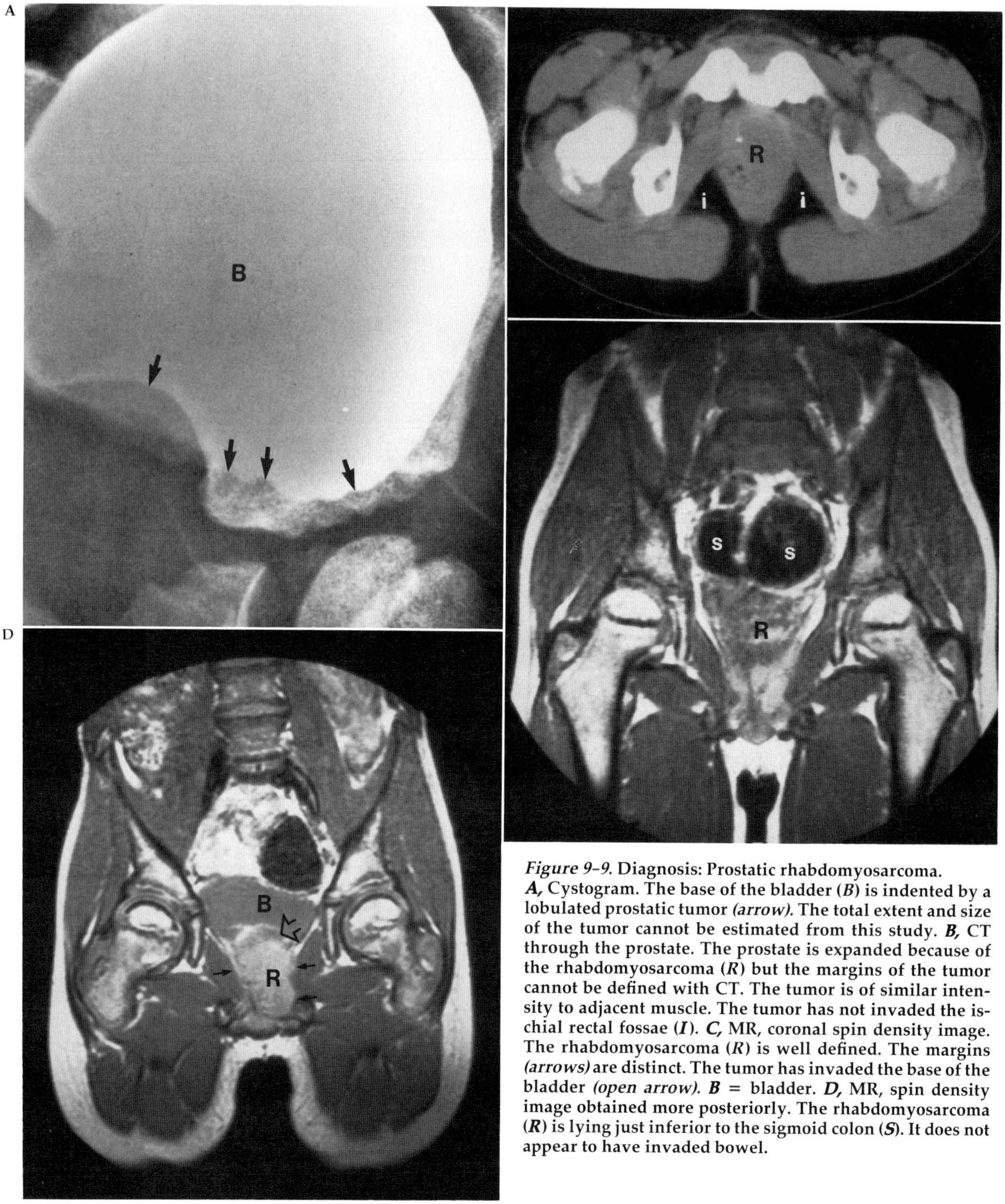

Figure 9-9. Diagnosis: Prostatic rhabdomyosarcoma. ***A,*** Cystogram. The base of the bladder (*B*) is indented by a lobulated prostatic tumor *(arrow).* The total extent and size of the tumor cannot be estimated from this study. ***B,*** CT through the prostate. The prostate is expanded because of the rhabdomyosarcoma (*R*) but the margins of the tumor cannot be defined with CT. The tumor is of similar intensity to adjacent muscle. The tumor has not invaded the ischial rectal fossae (***I***). ***C,*** MR, coronal spin density image. The rhabdomyosarcoma (*R*) is well defined. The margins *(arrows)* are distinct. The tumor has invaded the base of the bladder *(open arrow).* ***B*** = bladder. ***D,*** MR, spin density image obtained more posteriorly. The rhabdomyosarcoma (***R***) is lying just inferior to the sigmoid colon (***S***). It does not appear to have invaded bowel.

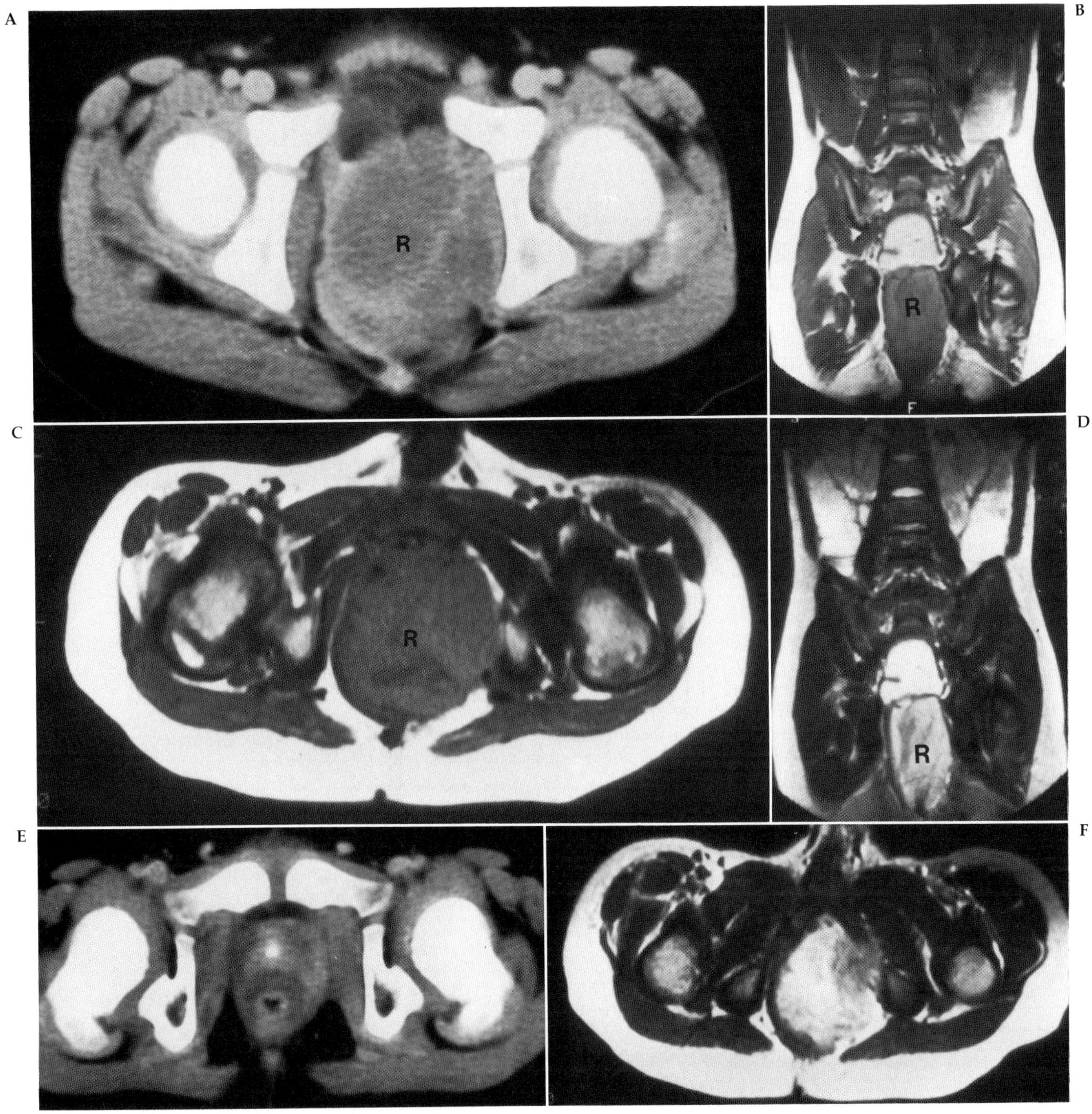

Figure 9–10. Diagnosis: Prostatic rhabdomyosarcoma.
A and ***B,*** CT and T1 weighted MR axial images. Both show the large rhabdomyosarcoma (*R*). On the CT images, it is of similar density to muscle. On the MR images, it is slightly brighter than muscle. ***C*** and ***D,*** Coronal spin density and T2 weighted images. The total extent of the rhabdomyosarcoma (*R*) is extremely well defined on both of these images. Note that signal intensity of the tumor increases with T2 weighting. ***E*** and ***F,*** CT and MR, T1 weighted image (after gadolinium-DTPA administration), obtained after chemotherapy. There has been marked reduction in size of the tumor. The gadolinium-DTPA enhancement on the MR image permits better differentiation of tumor from adjacent muscle than is identified on the CT. (Image ***F*** is slightly inferior to image ***E.***)

A B

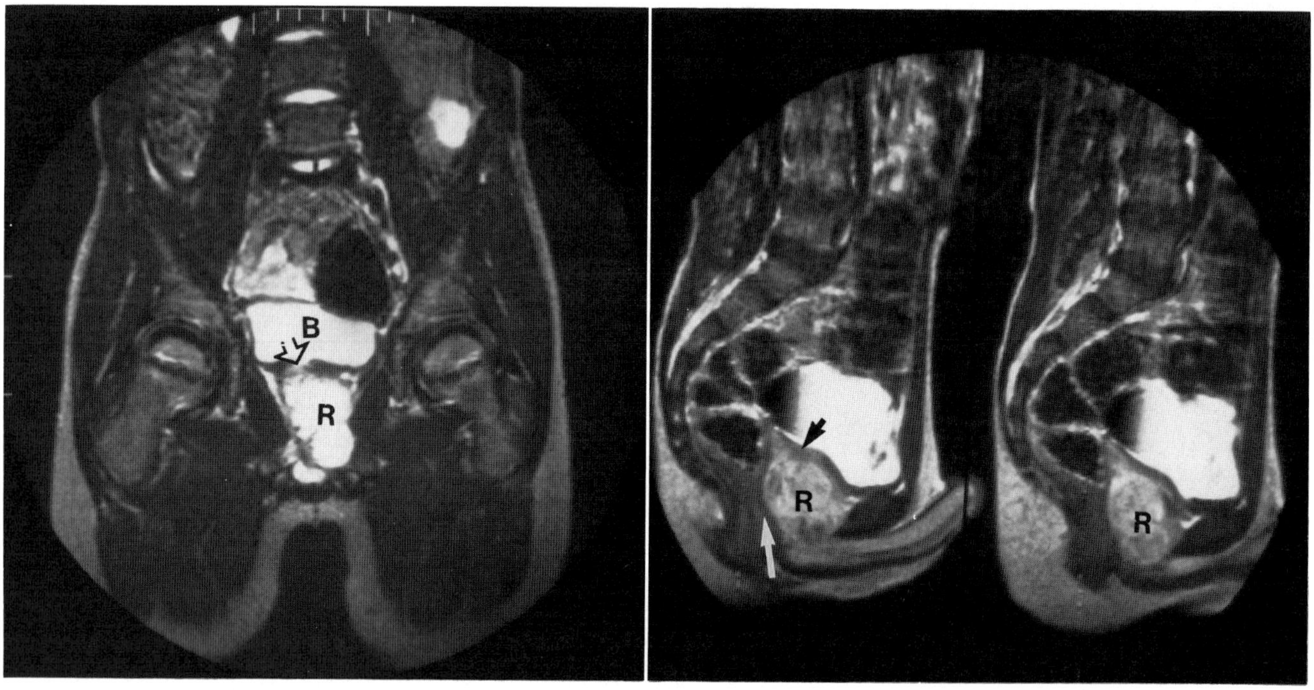

Figure 9–11. Diagnosis: Prostatic rhabdomyosarcoma.
A, MR, coronal T2 weighted image. The rhabdomyosarcoma (*R*) is lobulated and has a very irregular margin, probably indicating aggressive growth into adjacent tissue. There is invasion of the bladder base *(open arrow). B* = bladder. ***B,*** MR, T1 weighted image after gadolinium-DTPA administration. Sagittal plane. Bright signal in most of the bladder is caused by gadolinium-DTPA, which has been excreted by the kidneys. The patient is prone and a small amount of nonopacified urine is present in the posterior part of the bladder. The location and extent of rhabdomyosarcoma (***R***) is well shown. There is invasion into the bladder base *(small arrow).* The anterior rectal wall *(large arrow)* is sharply defined and has not been invaded by tumor.

Figure 9–12. Diagnosis: Rhabdomyosarcoma of the testicle with local and metastatic spread.
A, CT. The large testicular tumor *(arrow)* is seen filling the superior aspect of the right side of the scrotum. ***B*** and ***C,*** CT images. Direct local spread of the tumor has occurred through the inguinal canal *(arrows).* The tumor has spread into the pelvis and is indenting the anterolateral wall of the bladder *(open arrow).* ***D,*** CT through the lower abdomen. Large metastatic lymph node (*N*) is identified.

A B C D

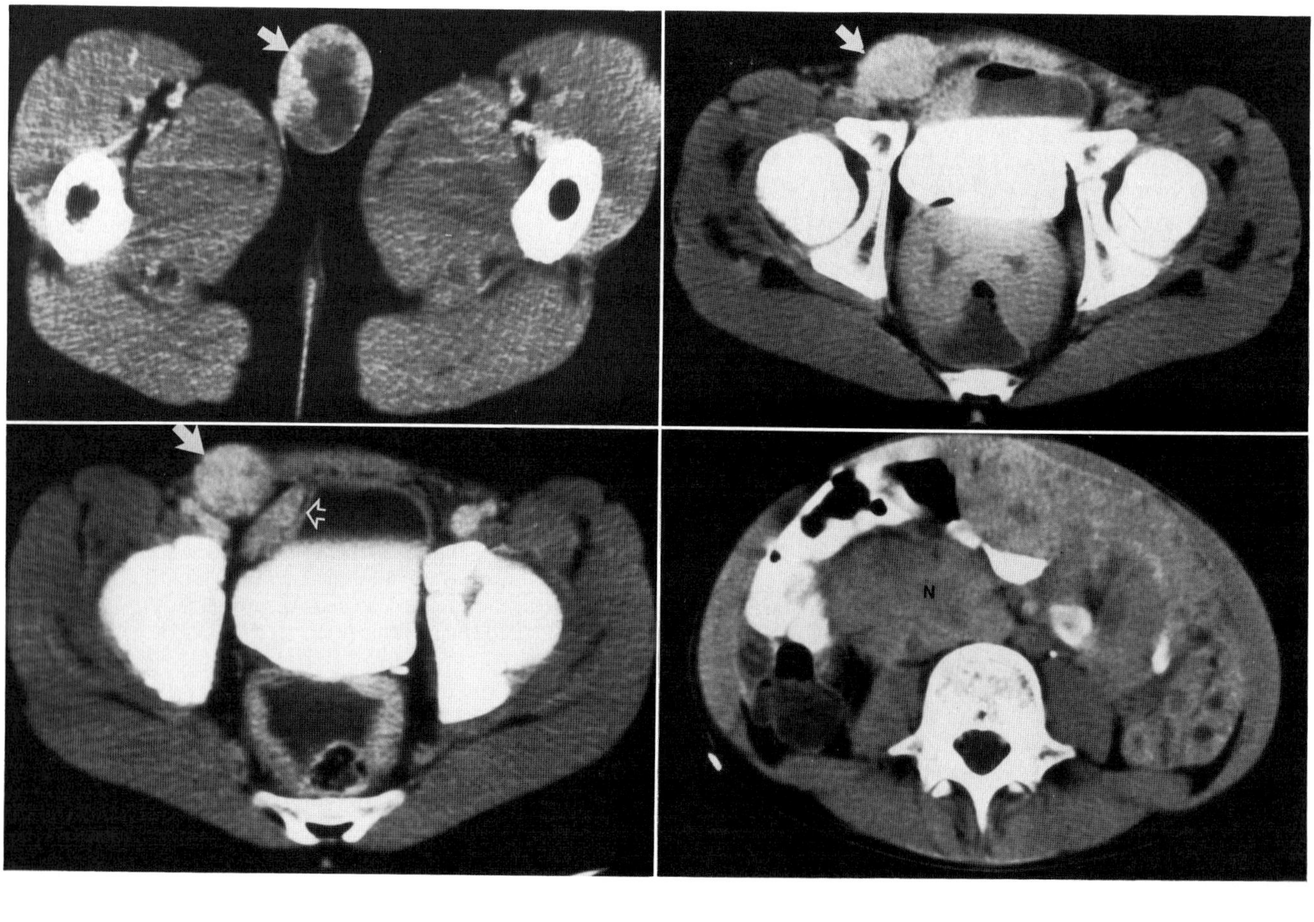

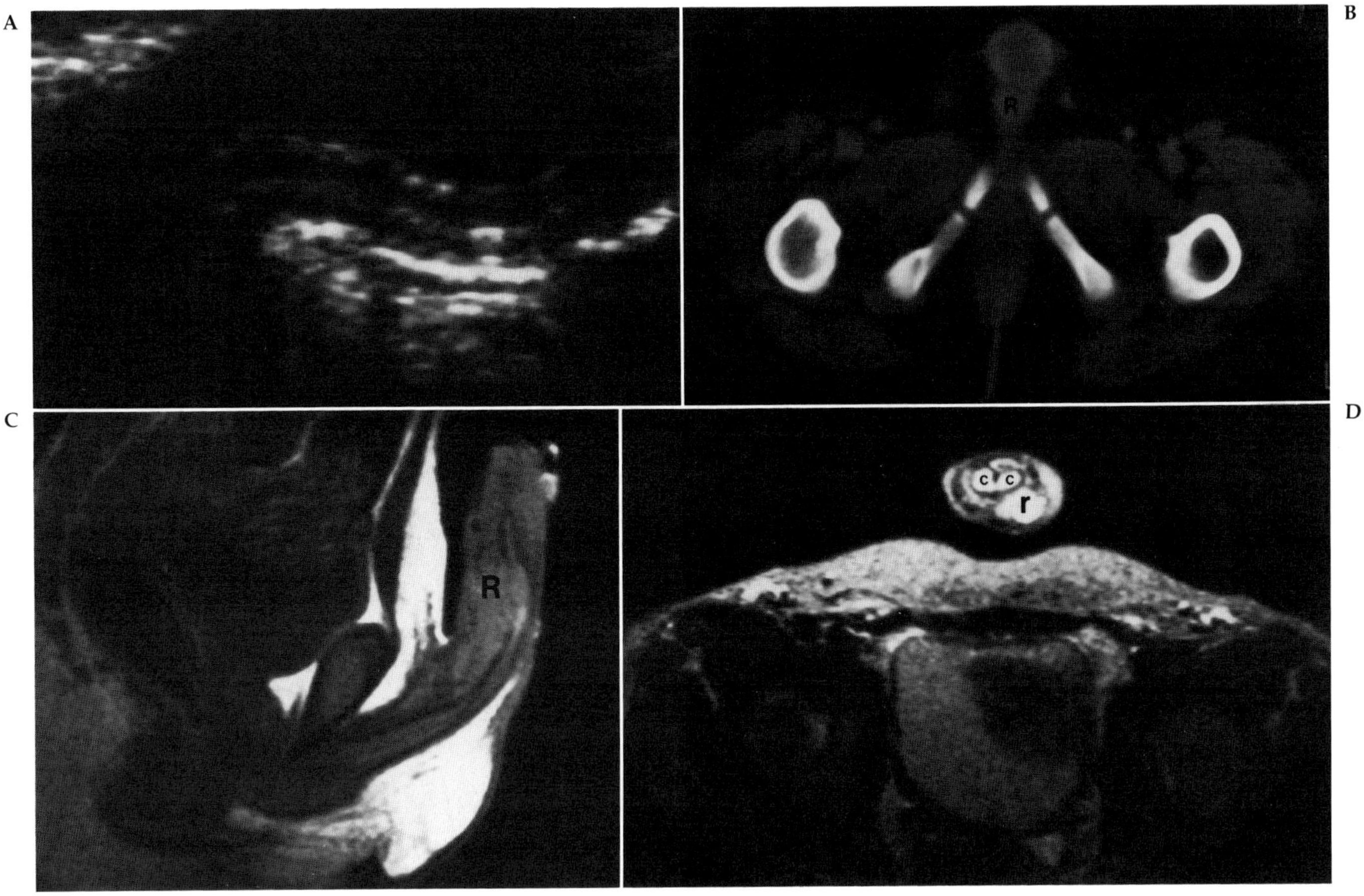

Figure 9–13. **Diagnosis: Rhabdomyosarcoma of the penis.**
A, **Longitudinal ultrasound of the penis. The tumor is very difficult to identify.** ***B,*** **CT image through the tumor. The rhabdomyosarcoma (*R*) can be identified but its precise relationship to the normal anatomic components of the penis is not well defined.** ***C,*** **MR, sagittal T1 weighted image. The rhabdomyosarcoma (*R*) can be identified. With this pulse sequence its margins are very poorly defined.** ***D,*** **MR, axial T2 weighted image. The rhabdomyosarcoma (*R*) is sharply defined. It lies in the dorsal aspect of the penis. Both corpora cavernosa (*C*) are sharply defined and clearly separate from the tumor.**

In patients in whom imaging shows apparent complete resolution of tumor, there is some debate as to whether this represents cure. It will never be possible for imaging to detect or reject the presence of microscopic tumor. The solution is either to perform surgical exploration in all these patients or to follow the patients, making final judgment dependent on the ultimate recurrence or otherwise of local tumor.

For evaluation of response to initial chemotherapy or radiation therapy, which imaging modality should be used and how frequently should imaging be performed? CT and MR are in my opinion the modalities of choice. The intensity of imaging, while tumor is still present, should be dictated by the rate of response and also by clinical decisions such as whether or not therapy will be changed depending on the result of imaging. Initially, scanning every month may be appropriate. Depending on the above factors, this interval will be increased with time. After the tumor has disappeared (following surgery, chemotherapy, or radiation therapy) or has stabilized as a residual mass, one must decide on the intensity of investigation for further follow-up. There is significant data that helps in this decision making. For example, unlike some other tumors, local recurrence with rhabdomyosarcoma is common and may occur with or without the appearance of coincident metastases (Table 9–10). Local recurrence in 686 patients occurred in between 18 and 35 percent, depending on tumor stage (see Fig. 9–16; Table 9–11). It is important to note from this table that relapse can occur with any clinical stage, although it is least common in patients with stage I disease. Thus, intensity of imaging will be greater for clinical stage IV patients, but imaging will still be performed in clinical stage I patients. Local recurrence is also extremely dependent on the anatomic site of the primary. For example, it is extremely rare in the orbit but very common with parameningeal tumors. In fact, with these latter tumors, local recurrence is even more common than metastatic recurrence.[22] Thus, parameningeal primaries should be followed closely, whereas imaging of the orbit following initial tumor control for local recurrence is a very unrewarding exercise. Similarly, local recurrence is high for extremity lesions (up to 33 percent),[23] but low for paratesticular pri-

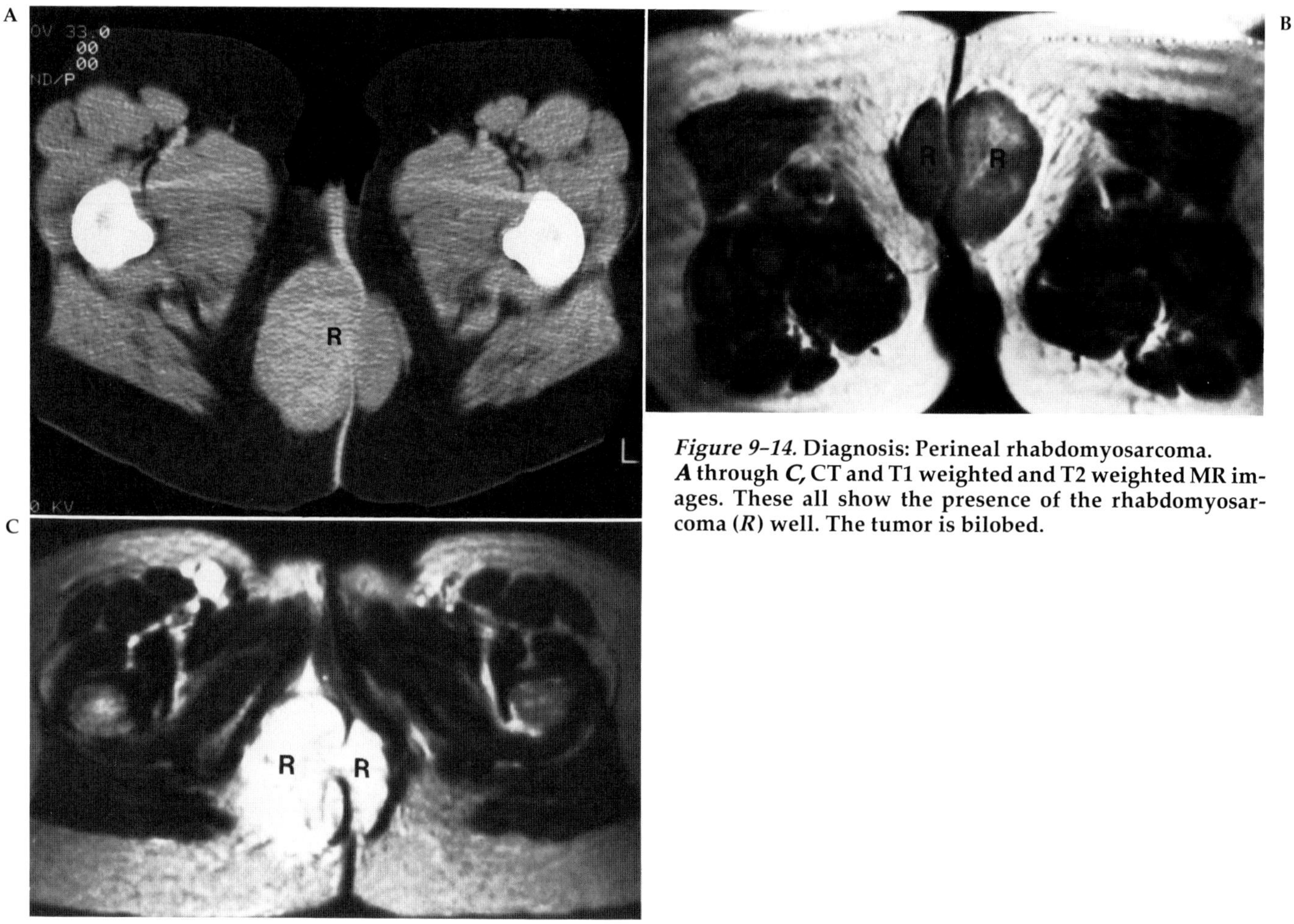

Figure 9–14. **Diagnosis: Perineal rhabdomyosarcoma. *A* through *C*, CT and T1 weighted and T2 weighted MR images. These all show the presence of the rhabdomyosarcoma (*R*) well. The tumor is bilobed.**

mary lesions. Other genitourinary primary tumors have an intermediate but significant recurrence rate.

> *Comment:* Follow-up imaging of the primary tumor is based on knowledge of the tumor stage and anatomic location.

TABLE 9–10

Tumor Recurrence in 339 Cases of Rhabdomyosarcoma: Local Relapse vs. Metastases[1]

Metastases alone	32 cases
Local recurrence	43 cases
Both local and metastatic recurrence	40 cases

Reference

1. Caillaud JM, Gerard-Marchant R, Marsden HB, et al. Histopathological classification of childhood rhabdomyosarcoma: a report from the International Society of Pediatric Oncology Pathology Panel. Med Pediatr Oncol 1989;17:391–400.

METASTASES

At the time of diagnosis between 10 and 20 percent of all patients will have metastases at some site.[2,24] The incidence of metastasis varies by anatomic location of the primary tumor. It is low for orbital primary tumors. At the other end of the spectrum, metastases were present in 58 percent of 18 patients with abdominal and retroperitoneal primary tumors at the time of diagnosis.[25] Metastatic spread is most commonly to the lung (Fig.

TABLE 9–11

Tumor Recurrence in 686 Cases of Rhabdomyosarcoma: Dependent on Stage (All Anatomic Sites)

Clinical Stage	Relapse (%)
I	18
II	28
III	25
IV	33

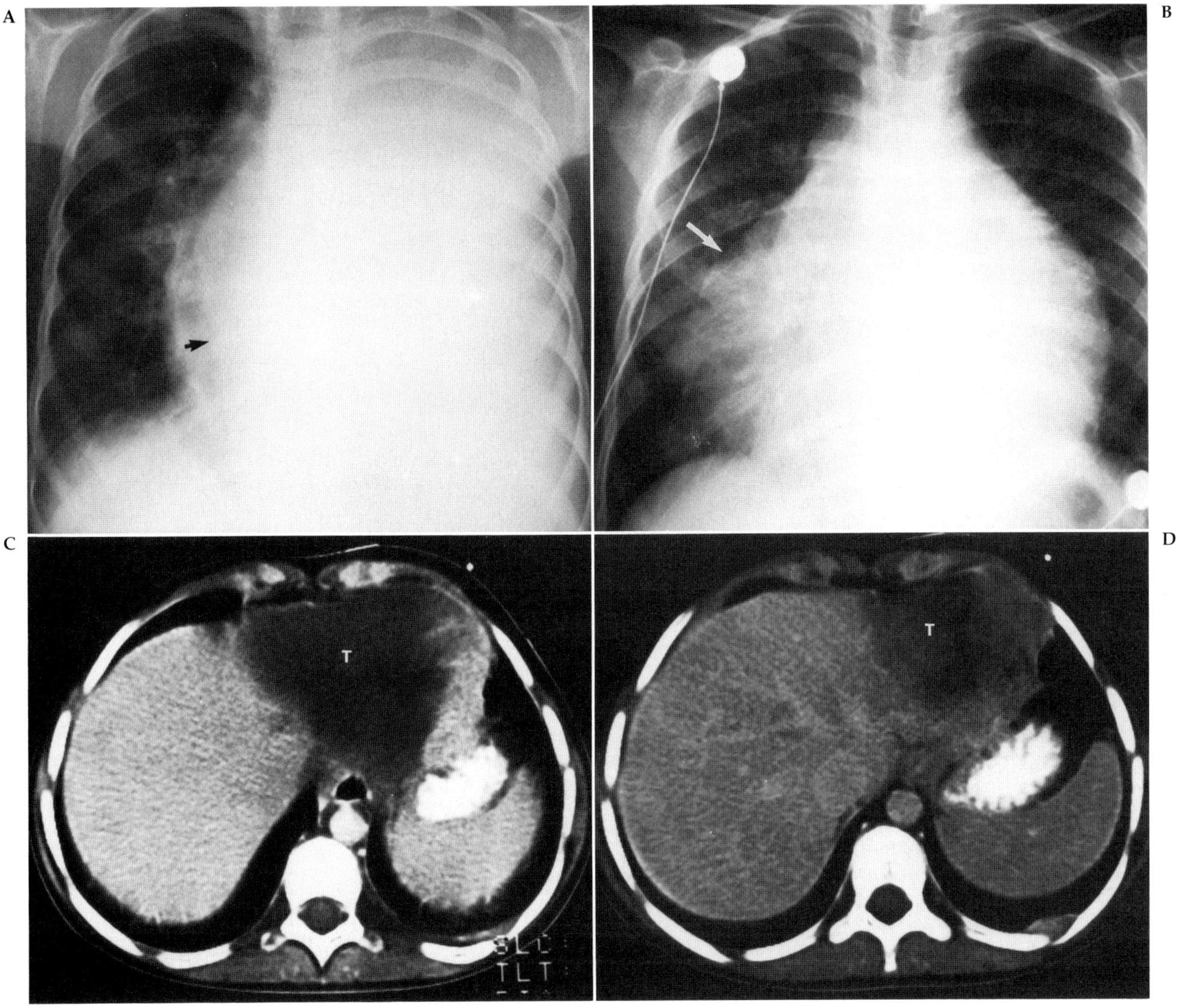

Figure 9-15. **Diagnosis: Rhabdomyosarcoma of the chest.**
A, **Chest radiograph. There is complete opacification of the left hemithorax. Tumor is seen extending across to the right side of the chest *(arrow)*. On the left side, one cannot differentiate tumor from collapsed left lung, effusion, or both. The tumor responded extremely well to initial therapy. Recurrence did, however, occur *(B, C, D)*. *B,* Chest radiograph after recurrence. There is now a large right mediastinal tumor *(arrow)*. *C* and *D,* CT images through the upper abdomen. These show that the tumor (*T*) has extended from the thorax down into the upper abdomen and across to the left side.**

9–18), bone (Figs. 9–19, 9–20, and 9–21), and lymph nodes (see Fig. 9–12). Less common sites include bone marrow and liver.[15] Metastases have been described as occasionally occurring in a wide variety of other locations, including the heart,[27] breast,[26] and soft tissues (Fig. 9–22). The brain is another not uncommon site of metastatic spread.

There is a strong relationship between the site of the primary tumor and the pattern of metastatic spread. However, in any individual patient, variations to the general pattern may occur. Tables 9–12 and 9–13 give information relating the site of metastases to the site of the primary tumor. Table 9–12 gives postmortem information. Many differences can be seen. For example, brain metastasis occurs in 7 percent of genitourinary rhabdomyosarcomas and 32 percent of extremity rhabdomyosarcomas. Lymph node metastases are rare from head and neck primary tumors but occurred in between 60 to 65 percent of extremity and genitourinary tumors. This study was performed in 1978 and the pattern of spread identified now, after different treatment regimens, could be different. In Table 9–13, information ob-

A B

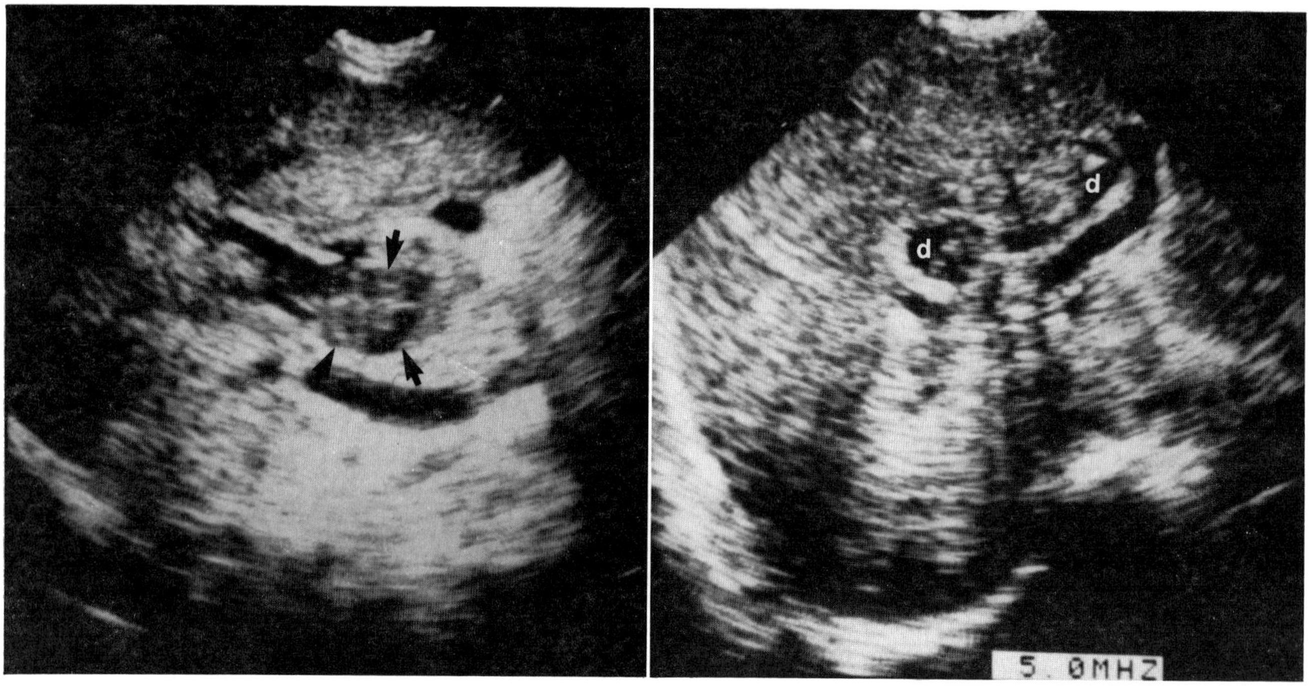

Figure 9-16. **Diagnosis: Biliary tract rhabdomyosarcoma.**
***A,* Ultrasound, oblique image. This shows the large tumor mass *(arrows)* at the hepatic hilum. *B,* Transverse sonogram. Biliary duct (*D*) dilatation is present as the result of obstruction caused by the tumor mass. (From Geoffrey A. Ultrasonography and computed tomography for diagnosis and follow-up of biliary duct rhabdomyosarcomas in children. Pediatr Radiol 1987;17:127–131.)**

tained in vivo is presented. As can be seen, lung and bone metastases can occur from any primary site of tumor. Bone marrow metastases are much more likely from genitourinary or extremity tumors. Lymph node metastases are never found with orbital primaries and rarely found with head and neck primaries but are quite common with extremity and genitourinary primary tumors.

Careful examination of Tables 9–12 and 9–13 provides no absolute criteria for different patterns of imaging evaluation for metastasis for each anatomic site. However, several clear patterns can be detected and imaging emphasis directed accordingly. There are obviously gaps in the information provided and further studies regarding the pattern of metastatic spread are needed, particularly of patients treated with modern chemotherapy. Some further information is available. For example, in a study of 30 patients with marrow metastases, it was found that 50 percent had an alveolar histology. Twenty-seven of the 30 patients had evidence of metastatic disease elsewhere. In 3 patients, however, it was the only site of metastatic disease. In all the patients, marrow metastases were diagnosed purely from marrow biopsy or aspiration and no imaging studies were performed. Perhaps with more aggressive use of imaging directed particularly at the bone marrow (either sulfur colloid bone marrow isotope scan or MR) more patients could be detected in whom bone marrow is the only site of metastatic spread. This obviously has important implications with regard to therapy and staging.

Comment: Rhabdomyosarcoma can metastasize to almost any site. Patterns of metastatic spread are dependent on location of the primary tumor.

Note should be made here of an unusual presentation of rhabdomyosarcoma. This has sometimes been

TABLE 9-12
Postmortem Location of Metastases of Rhabdomyosarcoma by Anatomic Site of Primary Tumor[1]

	Site of Primary Tumor (Percentage of Cases)			
Site of Metastasis	All Sites Combined	Head & Neck (excluding orbit)	Extremity	Genitourinary
Lung	37	25	35	35
CNS	37*	70*	32	7
Node	33	16	60	65
Bone	25	—	—	28
Liver	16	—	10	35
Marrow	7	—	—	21
Soft tissue	9	—	17	14

*Includes cases of direct invasion.
Reference
1. Maurer HM. Rhabdomyosarcoma. Curr Prob Cancer 1978;2:3–36.

A B C D

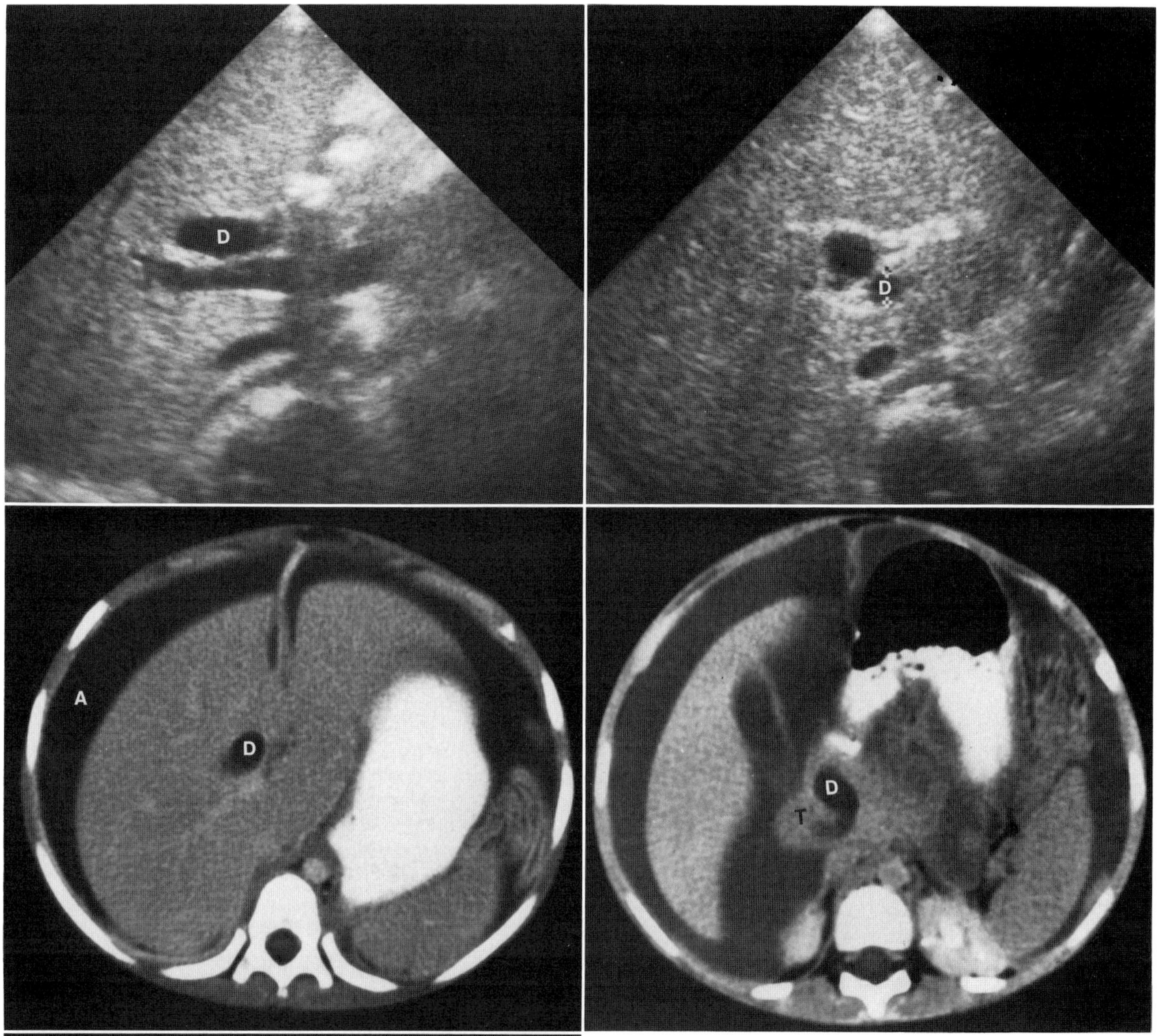

E

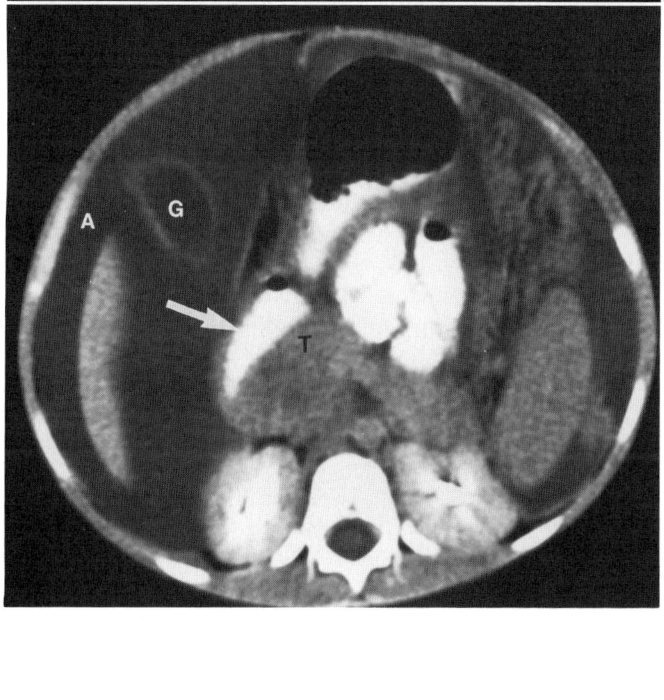

Figure 9–17. Diagnosis: Rhabdomyosarcoma of the ampulla of Vater.
A and ***B,*** Ultrasound images showing significant dilatation of the bile ducts (*D*). ***C,*** CT. This shows dilatation of the common bile duct (*D*). Ascites (*A*) is present. ***D,*** CT. At the lower end of the common bile duct, the dilated duct (*D*) is seen to narrow posteriorly as it curves toward the ampulla. A soft-tissue tumor (*T*) is seen in this region. ***E,*** CT image immediately inferior to *D.* The large soft-tissue tumor (*T*) is well seen. It was presumed to have arisen from the ampulla of Vater, but origin from the head of the pancreas cannot be differentiated. The second part of the duodenum *(arrow)* is opacified by contrast. ***A*** = ascites. ***G*** = gallbladder.

TABLE 9–13

Rhabdomyosarcoma: Site of Metastatic Spread Dependency on Location of Primary Tumor

Site of Metastasis	Location of Primary Tumor
Lung	Any site[1,2]
Bone	Any site
Bone marrow	Commonly bladder, prostate, or extremity[2]
Lymph nodes	Genitourinary
	20% have node metastases[3–6]
	(especially paratesticular)
	20–30% have node metastases[7]
	Extremity
	18% have node metastases[1]
	Trunk
	10% have node metastases[2,3]
	Head & neck
	3% have node metastases
	Orbit
	0% have node metastases[1]
Breast	Only trunk or extremity primary[8] (usually alveolar histology)
Heart	Chest, abdomen, pelvis[3]

References
1. King DR, Clatworthy HW Jr. The pediatric patient with sarcoma. Semin Oncol 1981;8:215–221.
2. Raney RB, Hays DM, Tefft M, et al. Rhabdomyosarcoma and the undifferentiated sarcomas. In: Pizzo PA, Poplack DG, eds. Principles and practice of pediatric oncology. Philadelphia: JB Lippincott, 1989:635–658.
3. Maurer HM. Rhabdomyosarcoma. Curr Prob Cancer 1978;2:3–36.
4. Fortune A, Bolton BR. Rhabdomyosarcoma of the paratesticular tissues. J Urol 1981;126:563–564.
5. Fleischmann J, Perinetti EP, Catalona WJ. Embryonal rhabdomyosarcoma of the genitourinary organs. J Urol 1981;126:389–392.
6. Tefft M, Hays D, Raney RB Jr, et al. Radiation to regional nodes for rhabdomyosarcoma of the genitourinary tract in children: is it necessary? A report from the Intergroup Rhabdomyosarcoma Study #1 (IRS–I). Cancer 1980;45:3065–3068.
7. Hamilton CR, Pinkerton R, Horwich A. The management of paratesticular rhabdomyosarcoma. Clin Radiol 1989;40:314–317.
8. Howarth CB, Caces JN, Pratt CB. Breast metastases in children with rhabdomyosarcoma. Cancer 1980;46:2520–2524.

termed systemic rhabdomyosarcoma. These patients present with widespread disseminated metastatic disease involving bone and bone marrow.[28–31] The patients are commonly teenagers. They frequently have systemic signs such as fever, weight loss, and malaise. In many of these patients, a primary tumor is not evident. Many are initially misdiagnosed. The most frequent misdiagnosis is leukemia, but these patients' diagnoses have also been initially labeled as lymphoma, neuroblastoma, and malignant histiocytosis. Imaging shows widespread evidence of bone metastases and bone marrow metastases. In some patients, there may be almost complete diffuse infiltration of the bone marrow with tumor. As mentioned, the primary tumor is not found in some patients. In others, it is found in unusual sites or sites that may be difficult to locate. I anticipate that the more widespread use of CT and MR in this small but distinct group of patients will result in detection of the primary tumor more frequently than has previously been reported.

It is difficult to know for how long patients should be followed looking for local or metastatic recurrent disease. While many patients will not relapse beyond 2 years, in the IRS–I study, 8 percent of all head and neck patients, alive and well at 2 years, relapsed beyond this time period.[22] More information, which is not available, is needed regarding late relapse, both with regard to the time and location of the relapse.

The imaging modality to be used in seeking metastasis will vary depending on the anatomic site being studied. In the lung, CT scan is without question the imaging modality of choice. For bone cortical metastases MDP technetium 99m radioisotope is the imaging modality of choice. There have been a couple of reports of radioisotope scanning missing bone lesions.[32] In one study, MDP radioisotope scan missed metastases in 4 of 13 patients and showed less abnormality than plain radiograph in 3 other patients.[33] The explanation for this is not clear. Many of the misses were close to the growth plate. With modern imaging techniques and experienced pediatric nuclear medicine radiologists, I strongly believe that radioisotope scan is superior to skeletal survey and should be the modality used. In every patient in whom the radioisotope scan is positive, plain films of the positive area should be obtained. Plain film radiographs should also be obtained in any patient having focal bone symptoms. The appearance of the metastasis on plain film radiograph varies considerably. The lesions range from lytic through mixed to more blastic. They can occur at almost any location in the skeleton. A soft-tissue mass may be present as well. Periosteal reactions are uncommon but can occasionally be present.

For the detection of bone marrow tumor in the absence of cortical invasion, sulfur colloid radioisotope scans may be helpful, although there are no reports of any large series of patients being studied with this technique. MR is extremely sensitive for detection of bone marrow metastatic disease, but, unfortunately, the entire skeleton cannot be scanned. Areas of bone marrow incorporated in MR images obtained to evaluate the primary tumor should be carefully evaluated for abnor-

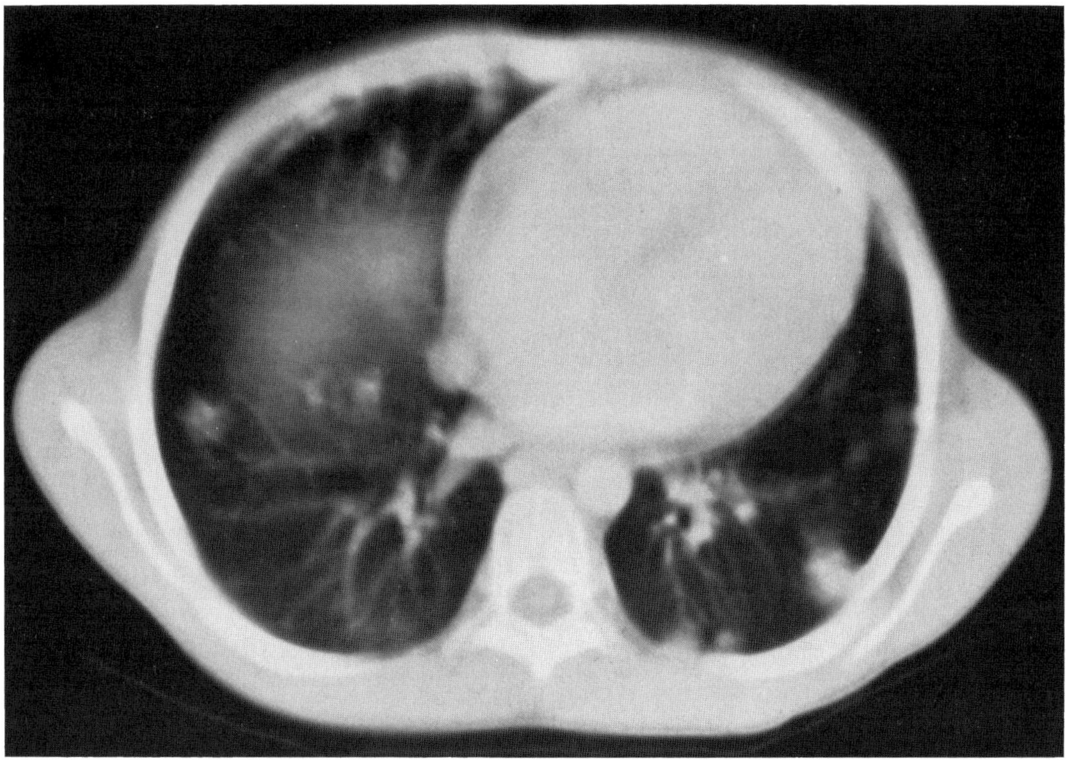

Figure 9–18. Diagnosis: Rhabdomyosarcoma lung metastases.
CT. Multiple soft-tissue metastatic nodules are seen throughout both lung fields. The appearance of these metastases is nonspecific and they cannot be differentiated from metastatic lesions from other primary tumors.

Figure 9–19. Diagnosis: Rhabdomyosarcoma. Pathologic fracture from bone metastatis.
A, Plain film radiograph. There is extensive destruction of the neck of the left femur with a pathologic fracture. ***B,*** MR, T2 weighted image. There is very bright signal intensity from the metastatis (*M*) in the femoral neck. ***C,*** MR, T1 weighted gadolinum-DTPA enhanced image. There is bright signal from the marrow in both proximal femurs. This was, in fact, caused by marrow metastases that have enhanced from the contrast. The nonenhanced image showed low intensity in these areas. The gadolinium-DTPA enhanced metastases cannot be differentiated from normal bone marrow.

A

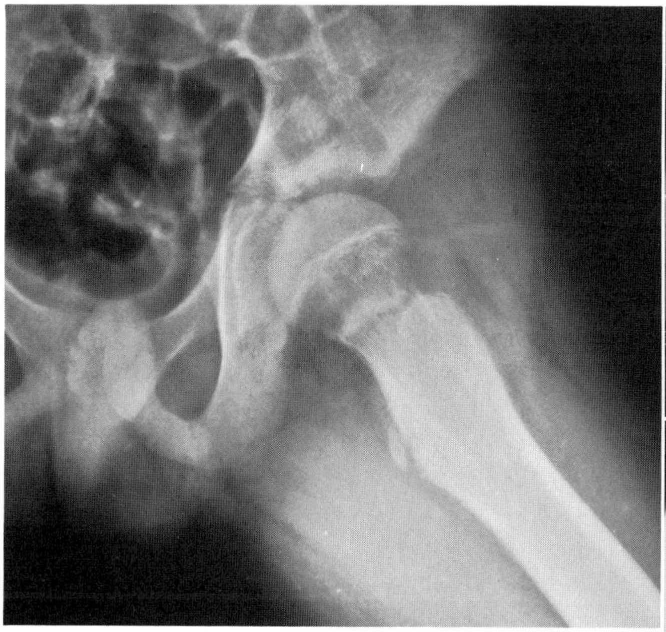

B

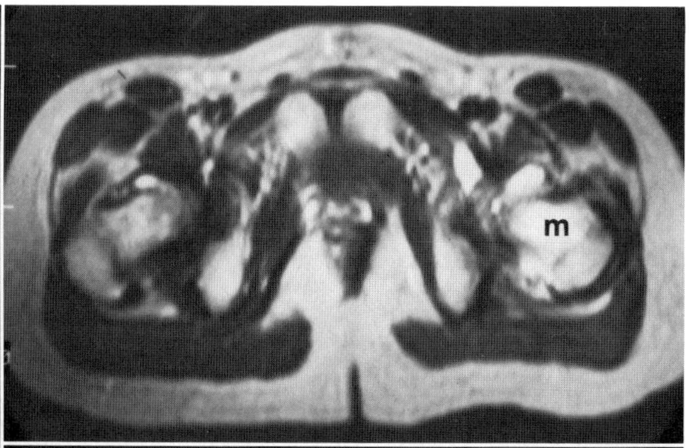

C

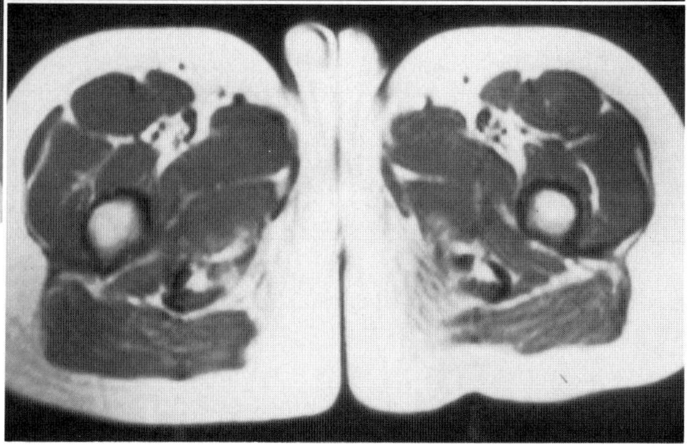

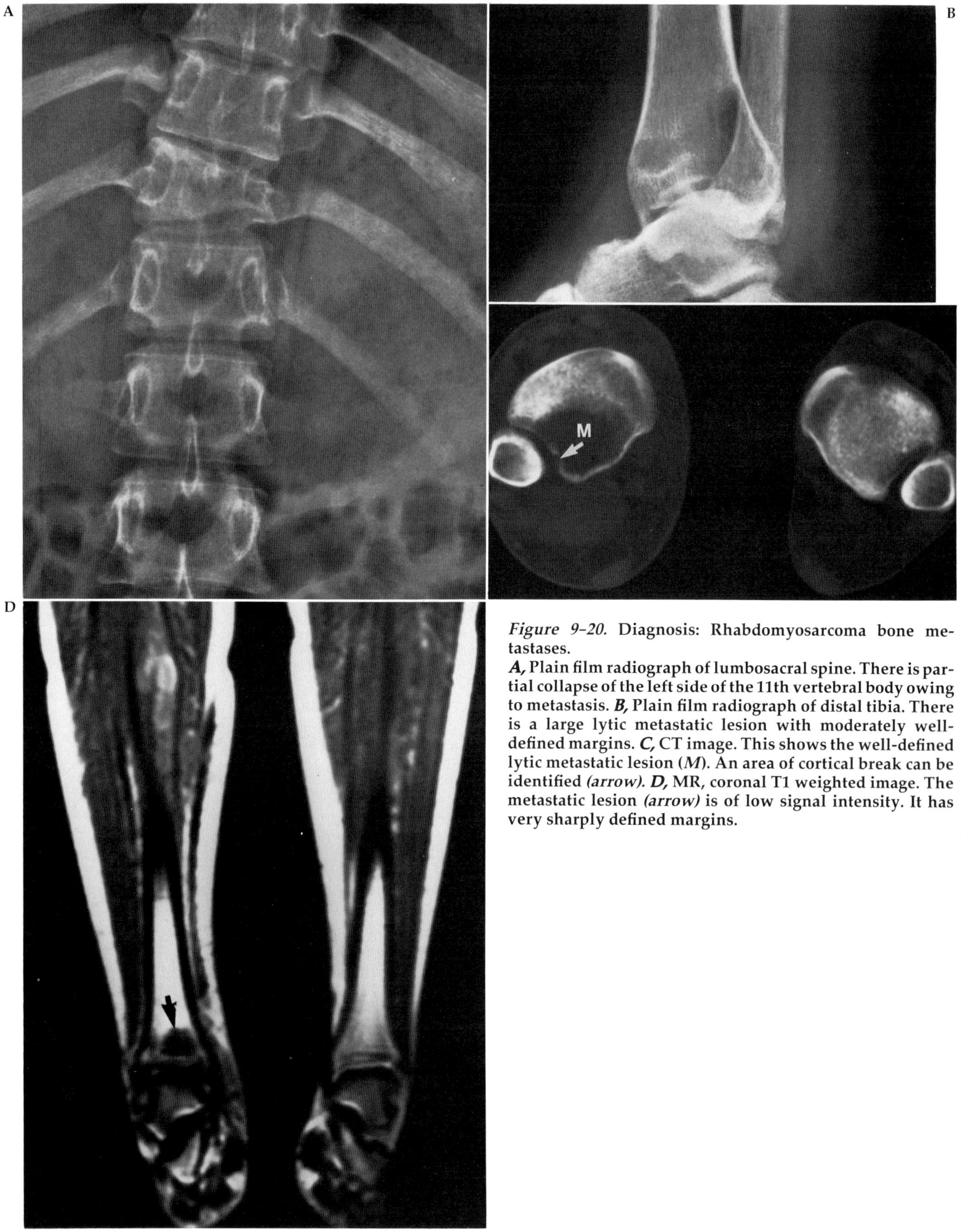

Figure 9–20. Diagnosis: Rhabdomyosarcoma bone metastases.

A, Plain film radiograph of lumbosacral spine. There is partial collapse of the left side of the 11th vertebral body owing to metastasis. ***B,*** Plain film radiograph of distal tibia. There is a large lytic metastatic lesion with moderately well-defined margins. ***C,*** CT image. This shows the well-defined lytic metastatic lesion (*M*). An area of cortical break can be identified *(arrow).* ***D,*** MR, coronal T1 weighted image. The metastatic lesion *(arrow)* is of low signal intensity. It has very sharply defined margins.

A B

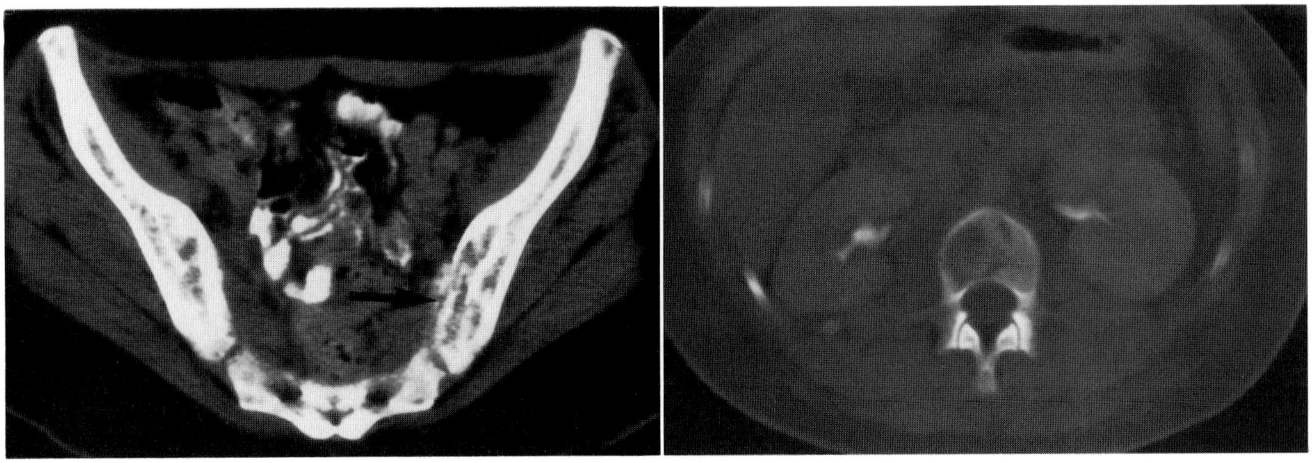

Figure 9-21. **Diagnosis: Rhabdomyosarcoma bone metastases, CT appearance.**
A, **CT through the pelvis. There is extensive poorly defined metastatic disease in the posterior half of each iliac bone. The lesions are mixed sclerotic and destructive. Some areas of cortical destruction** ***(arrow)*** **can be identified.** ***B,*** **CT through mid lumbar vertebra. A metastatic lesion involves the right two-thirds of the vertebral body. It is predominantly lytic. There is no bone expansion and no cortical destruction.**

malities in the bone marrow. These are seen as a nonspecific decrease in signal intensity compared to normal marrow on the T1 weighted images.

The incidence of liver metastatic disease is low, and most people would not recommend routine liver scanning unless the patient presents with some symptoms suggesting liver disease. The liver will, however, be partially visualized on CT scans of the chest. These visualized sections of the liver should in all cases be studied for abnormality. If imaging of the liver is to be performed, CT is probably more sensitive than liver spleen radioisotope scan. In one report of liver spleen scan in 39 patients, it detected 15 of 15 metastases but had 8 additional false positive results.[34]

Evaluation of lymph nodes for metastatic spread is more controversial. Gallium has been utilized by some workers[20] but has a low true positive and a high false negative rate[34] and I would not recommend its routine use. Lymphangiography has a few advocates but the vast majority of pediatric radiologists do not use it. If any modality is to be used for routine screening for lymph node metastases, CT is probably the modality of choice. MR may be good, but there is inadequate experience with it at this time. The problems with CT scanning are that metastatic disease may be present in lymph nodes that are not significantly enlarged, and enlarged lymph nodes may be caused by reactive hyperplasia rather than tumor metastases. Thus, CT may be

Figure 9-22. **Diagnosis: Rhabdomyosarcoma, soft-tissue and breast metastases.**
A, **CT through the lower abdomen. A well-defined metastatic nodule** ***(arrow)*** **is seen in the subcutaneous fat of the abdominal wall.** ***B,*** **CT scan through the breasts. A well-defined metastatic deposit is seen in the right breast** ***(arrow).***

A B

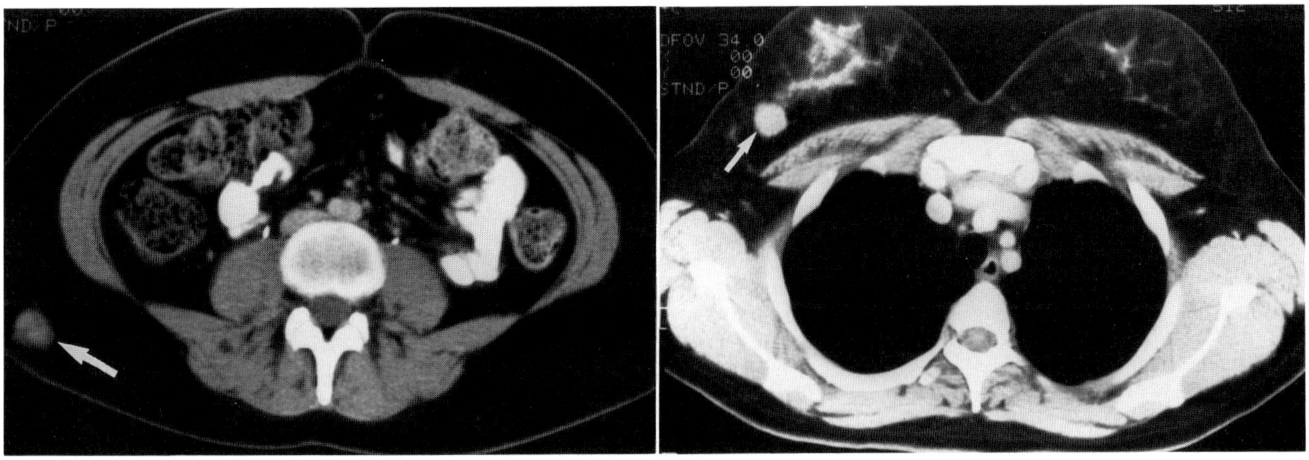

helpful in providing additional information, but it should be borne in mind that false positive and false negative results will be obtained. There are no large series reported that provide any meaningful data as to the precise accuracy of CT.

The entire question of imaging for metastatic disease is complicated, since it depends on the patient's stage, the histology and anatomic location of the primary tumor, and the accuracy of the various imaging modalities. In addition, the impact of the information on patient therapy will vary depending on the treatment protocol that the patient is on, the stage in the treatment at which the metastases are detected, and the presence or absence of known metastatic disease in other locations. It is, therefore, very difficult if not impossible to make a dogmatic statement with regard to imaging recommendations. Indeed, it would be foolish to do so, as one would either overimage some patients or underimage other patients.

Chest CT and bone radioisotope scan should be performed on presentation in all patients. Other imaging should be dictated by the location of the primary tumor. Similarly, for follow-up chest CT and bone radioisotope scan should be performed in all patients. The frequency of these studies should be determined by an institution's therapeutic protocol and the patient's response. They should be routinely repeated at times of change in therapy. They should also be repeated at times of change in clinical status. At other times the frequency could be every 3 months, every 6 months, or not at all, depending on the known potential yield, i.e., one's knowledge of the likelihood of metastases occurring at the time and location being studied.

References

1. McLeod AJ, Lewis E. Sonographic evaluation of pediatric rhabdomyosarcomas. J Ultrasound Med 1984;3:69–73.
2. Brasch RC, Kim OH, Kushner JH, et al. Ossification in a soft tissue embryonal rhabdomyosarcoma. Pediatr Radiol 1981;11:99–101.
3. Eklof O, Brun B, Claesson I, et al. Tumours of the lower urinary tract in children. Acta Radiol Diagn 1978;19:171–185.
4. Harwood-Nash DC. The radiology of rhabdomyosarcomas of the middle ear with intracranial extension in children. Clin Radiol 1971;22:321–329.
5. Danziger J, Handel SF, Jing B-S, et al. Computerized tomography in rhabdomyosarcoma of the head and neck. Cancer 1979;44:463–467.
6. Vade A, Armstrong D. Orbital rhabdomyosarcoma in childhood. Radiol Clin N Am 1987;25:701–714.
7. Latack JT, Hutchinson RJ, Heyn RM. Imaging of rhabdomyosarcomas of the head and neck. AJNR 1987;8:353–359.
8. Durham L, Mackenzie IH, Foy P. Embryonal rhabdomyosarcoma of the sphenoid sinus. J Laryngol Otol 1988;102:836–837.
9. Scotti G, Harwood-Nash DC. Computed tomography of rhabdomyosarcomas of the skull base in children. J Comput Assist Tomogr 1982;6:33–39.
10. Tannous WN, Azouz EM, Homsy YL, et al. CT and ultrasound imaging of pelvic rhabdomyosarcoma in children. A review of 56 patients. Pediatr Radiol 1989;19:530–534.
11. Bahnson RR, Zaontz MR, Maizels M, et al. Ultrasonography and diagnosis of pediatric genitourinary rhabdomyosarcoma. Urology 1989;33:64–68.
12. Raney RB Jr, Tefft M, Lawrence W Jr, et al. Paratesticular sarcoma in childhood and adolescence. A report from the Intergroup Rhabdomyosarcoma Studies I and II, 1973–1983. Cancer 1987;60:2337–2343.
13. Baker ME, Silverman PM, Korobkin M. Computed tomography of prostatic and bladder rhabdomyosarcomas. J Comput Assist Tomogr 1985;9:780–783.
14. Bartolozzi C, Selli C, Olmastroni M, et al. Rhabdomyosarcoma of the prostate: MR findings. AJR 1988;150:1333–1334.
15. Friedburg H, Kauffmann GW, Bohm N, et al. Sonographic and computed tomographic features of embryonal rhabdomyosarcoma of the biliary tract. Pediatr Radiol 1984;14:436–438.
16. Arnaud O, Boscq M, Asquier E, et al. Embroyonal rhabdomyosarcoma of the biliary tree in children: a case report. Pediatr Radiol 1987;17:250–251.
17. Mihara S, Matsumoto H, Tikunaga F, et al. Botryoid rhabdomyosarcoma of the gallbladder in a child. Cancer 1982;49:812–818.
18. Geoffray A, Couanet D, Montagne JP, et al. Ultrasonography and computed tomography for diagnosis and follow-up of biliary duct rhabdomyosarcomas in children. Pediatr Radiol 1987;17:127–131.
19. Caty MG, Oldham KT, Prochownik EV. Embryonal rhabdomyosarcoma of the ampulla of Vater with long-term survival following pancreaticoduodenectomy. J Pediatr Surg 1990;25:1256–1258.
20. Malogolowkin MH, Ortega JA. Rhabdomyosarcoma of childhood. Pediatr Ann 1988;17:251–266.
21. Treuner J, Suder J, Keim M, et al. The predictive value of initial cytostatic response in primary unresectable rhabdomyosarcoma in children. Acta Oncol 1989;28:67–71.
22. Sutow WW, Lindberg RD, Gehan EA, et al. Three-year relapse-free survival rates in childhood rhabdomyosarcoma of the head and neck. Report from the Intergroup Rhabdomyosarcoma Study. Cancer 1982;49:2217–2221.
23. Maurer HM, Beltangady M, Gehan EA, et al. The Intergroup Rhabdomyosarcoma Study–I. A final report. Cancer 1988;61:209–220.
24. Agamanolis DP, Dasu S, Krill CE. Tumors of skeletal muscle. Human Pathol 1986;17:778–795.
25. Ransom JL, Pratt CB, Hustu HO, et al. Retroperitoneal rhabdomyosarcoma in children. Cancer 1980;45:845–850.
26. Howarth CB, Caces JN, Pratt CB. Breast metastases in children with rhabdomyosarcoma. Cancer 1980;46:2520–2524.
27. Krous HF, Sexauer CL. Embryonal rhabdomyosarcoma arising within a congenital bronchogenic cyst in a child. J Pediatr Surg 1981;16:506–508.
28. Etcubanas E, Peiper S, Stass S, et al. Rhabdomyosarcoma, presenting as disseminated malignancy from an unknown primary site: a retrospective study of ten pediatric cases. Med Pediatr Oncol 1989;17:39–44.
29. Almanaseer IY, Trujillo YP, Taxy JB, et al. Systemic rhabdomyosarcoma with diffuse bone marrow involvement. AJCP 1983;82:349–353.
30. Henderson DW, Raven JL, Pollard JL, et al. Bone marrow metastases in disseminated alveolar rhabdo-myosarcoma: case report with ultrastructural study and review. Pathology 1976;8:329–341.

31. Dehner LP. Pediatric surgical pathology, 2nd ed. Baltimore: Williams & Wilkins, 1987:208–215.
32. Dillon E, Parkin GJS. The role of diagnostic radiology in the diagnosis and management of rhabdomyosarcoma in young persons. Clin Radiol 1978;29:53–59.
33. Quddus FF, Espinola D, Kramer SS, et al. Comparison between x-ray and bone scan detection of bone metastases in patients with rhabdomyosarcoma. Med Pediatr Oncol 1983;11:125–129.
34. Weinblatt ME, Miller JH. Radionuclide scanning in children with rhabdomyosarcoma. Med Pediatr Oncol 1981;9:293–301.

Differential Diagnosis

Some of the more common or important disorders to be considered in the differential diagnosis for varying anatomic sites are listed in Table 9–14. Many of these tumors are described in detail in other sections. For any particular site one should consider the patient's age, clinical and laboratory findings, appearance of the abnormality, patterns of spread. In many patients, biopsy will be required to differentiate rhabdomyosarcoma from benign lesions. Obviously, in all patients in whom a malignancy is suspected, biopsy will be performed.

TABLE 9–14
Differential Diagnosis for Rhabdomyosarcoma

Location of Rhabdomyosarcoma	Differential Diagnosis
Bladder/prostate	Ureterocele
	Hemorrhagic cystitis
	Germ cell tumor
	Polyp
	Hemangioma
Vagina	Urethral prolapse
	Polyp
	Hydrometrocolpos
	Yolk sac tumor
	Cyst
Paratesticular	Hydrocele
	Infection
	Germ cell tumor
Head	Lymphoma
	Ewing sarcoma
	Osteogenic
	Juvenile angiofibroma
	Yolk sac tumor
	Histiocytosis
	Neuroblastoma
Retroperitoneum	Neuroblastoma
	Lymphoma
	Germ cell tumor
Orbit	Intraconal
	Glioma
	Lymphangioma
	Extraconal
	Lymphoma neuroblastoma
	Leukemia
	Histiocytosis
	Other
	Lacrimal carcinoma
	Pseudotumor
	Teratoma
Any site	Abscess
	Hematoma

Therapy and Prognosis

Obviously, with a tumor occurring in many sites in the body the treatment will vary by anatomic location. The factors influencing therapy will include the accessibility of the lesion to the desired therapy and a knowledge of the natural history of the tumor in each location. For example, while complete surgical excision is always desirable, in many locations (other than the paratesticular or extremity tumors), complete surgical excision is impossible without mutilation. Chemotherapy should reach tumors in the entire body, but those parameningeal tumors that have spread into the extradural space seem particularly resistent to chemotherapy. Rhabdomyosarcoma is moderately but not excessively sensitive to radiation therapy. This means that high doses of radiation therapy need to be utilized to treat this tumor. Radiation therapy is, therefore, limited in specific sensitive anatomic locations or in young children in whom the complications from radiation therapy are greater. An example of the effect of anatomic location is the orbit; in this location, prognosis is excellent and current therapeutic attempts are trying to cut back on therapy to retain excellent survival and reduce complications of therapy. In the retroperitoneum, on the other hand, the prognosis is terrible and current therapeutic efforts are directed toward intensification of therapy.

The prognosis for survival with rhabdomyosarcoma has improved dramatically. Prior to 20 years ago, prognosis was uniformly terrible, with reported survival in the range of 10 to 20 percent.[1,2] Overall survival for all stages and all anatomic locations improved to about 55 percent for the IRS–I study conducted between 1972 and 1978. Subsequent IRS–II and IRS–III studies have shown overall survival of 65 percent and subsequently 73 percent.[3] There has thus been a significant improvement in survival with the introduction of chemotherapy and the more widespread use of radiation therapy. Survival is also improved because delayed surgery (after tumor shrinkage by chemotherapy or radiation therapy) has permitted resection of more tumors than previously.

The information with regard to overall survival does not tell the entire story, as the survival is heavily dependent on stage and anatomic location. Survival by clinical stage and by anatomic site is given in Tables 9–15 and 9–16. As can be seen, survival ranges from 88 percent for stage I to 32 percent for stage IV. Similarly, with anatomic site survival ranges from 46 percent in the retroperitoneum to 93 percent in the orbit. The data presented from the large number of patients in the IRS

TABLE 9-15
Rhabdomyosarcoma: Survival by Clinical Stage for Intergroup Studies[1]

Stage	IRS–I (%)	IRS–II (%)
I	80	88
II	72	77
III	52	68
IV	20	32

Reference
1. Maurer HM, Beltangady M, Gehan EA, et al. The Intergroup Rhabdomyosarcoma Study–I. A final report. Cancer 1988;61:209–220.

TABLE 9-16
Rhabdomyosarcoma: 3 Year Survival (IRS–II) by Anatomic Site

Site	Percentage
Orbit	93
Paratesticular	80
Parameningeal	71
Other head and neck	69
Other genitourinary	64
Trunk	57
Extremities	56
Retroperitoneum	46

studies has also been borne out in smaller studies. For example, the good survival rate in paratesticular tumors has been confirmed as ranging from 73 to 89 percent.[4,5] The prognosis for retroperitoneal tumors has been as low as 22 percent survival.[6] Several other points of importance with regard to prognosis are not brought out in the tables. Much of the failure of improvement in therapy over the last 20 years has been in patients with stage IV disease, and it is in this group that the least progress has been made. Another important point is that relapse is a very poor prognostic sign, and overall survival at 2 years following relapse in any location is only 17 percent.[3] Prognosis for biliary rhabdomyosarcoma is poor, not from metastatic disease, but from the devastating results of extensive local tumor invasion.[7]

> *Comment:* For rhabdomyosarcoma recovery after relapse is very unlikely.

The relative roles of chemotherapy, radiation therapy, and surgery are changing. Initially, surgery was the mainstay of therapy and prognosis prior to chemotherapy was awful. Surgery then went through a phase of radical resections, but the emphasis with current protocols is to maximize the benefits and effects of chemotherapy, hoping to minimize the severe handicap and mutilation that high doses of radiation therapy and surgery in difficult locations can cause.

This is best explained using the example of *non*paratesticular genitourinary tumors. These tumors can be cured with extensive pelvic organ resection and chemotherapy. They can also be cured with high doses of radiation therapy. Both the surgery and radiation therapy result in severe loss of normal bodily functions. Current objectives are to shrink the tumor maximally with chemotherapy, consolidate this with radiation therapy, and then utilize more delayed surgery to attempt complete resection of residual tumor without sacrificing major organs or body functions. A wide range of drugs are utilized for rhabdomyosarcoma therapy, including vincristine, actinomycin, cyclophosphamide,[8] and more recently cysplatinum, etoposide, and ifosphamide.[8,9] Radiation therapy dose needs to be above 4,500 R,[8] with a higher dose for treatment of gross rather than microscopic disease.

A large number of important therapeutic principles and recent therapeutic changes impact on imaging and these need to be discussed.

1. Chemotherapy is poor for treatment of parameningeal tumors after spread into the extradural space.[10] Imaging demonstration of such spread is, therefore, of critical importance. Prophylactic central nervous system radiation therapy and intrathecal chemotherapy for all parameningeal tumors decreased the meningeal relapse rate from 23 to 6 percent[8] and increased the 3-year survival from 33 to 63 percent. Current protocols are evaluating reduction in the use of prophylactic central nervous system radiation and intrathecal chemotherapy by utilizing more localized radiation therapy and intrathecal therapy only after demonstration of extradural spread. Imaging is crucial to evaluate this.
2. As previously mentioned, bladder, prostatic, and vaginal rhabdomyosarcomas are now being treated with initial aggressive chemotherapy.[11] Imaging is of critical importance in evaluating the residual tumor following chemotherapy so that the surgeon has the best possible opportunity of resecting the tumor completely without causing unacceptable damage to vital organs.
3. Delayed surgery is becoming more widely used in other locations as well, and imaging must demonstrate the extent of tumor and also if possible differentiate between residual active tumor and fibrosis and necrosis.
4. Radiation therapy is used for almost all rhabdomyosarcomas. It is used to treat the local tumor, regardless of whether prior surgery or chemotherapy has been used. The only exception is a stage I nonalveolar tumor. Knowledge of this means that secondary effects of radiation therapy should be looked for on imaging in all patients except stage I nonalveolar patients. This could be important; for example, abnormality detected in the bone marrow might be caused by radiation therapy and not tumor. Similarly, soft-tissue edema from radiation therapy should not be confused with tumor spread.
5. Surgical technique for treatment of paratesticular tumors is important.[5,12] If an inguinal approach is used and the spermatic cord is resected with the adjacent tes-

ticle, local recurrence is rare. If the tumor is resected through a transscrotal approach, local recurrence is common. Traditionally, clinical examination was used to detect local recurrence, but more sensitive imaging with MR and new high-resolution ultrasound might permit earlier detection of such local recurrence in patients in whom transscrotal surgery was performed.

6. Since chemotherapy is given to all patients with paratesticular tumors, lymph node abdominal dissection is now seldom performed. Because of this, imaging of the abdominal nodes may be much less important, as the surgeon's attention does not need to be drawn to large lymph nodes. There is some debate as to whether or not debulking of large abdominal lymph nodes affected with metastatic tumor affects prognosis. If the final decision is that it does, imaging to detect such nodes and to direct surgery becomes more important.
7. A study in 1989[13] of trunk and extremity rhabdomyosarcomas indicated that survival was improved if primary re-excision was performed. This means that if the initial resection of a tumor indicated the presence of microscopic residual, a second surgical procedure with wider excision was performed. While imaging cannot detect the microscopic residual following the initial surgical procedure, it is hoped that new imaging techniques, particularly MR, will more accurately define the total spread of infiltrating tumors. If the surgeon were to resect all of the abnormality identified on MR, perhaps the number of patients with microscopic residual could be significantly reduced and, therefore, the number of patients requiring the trauma and expense of a second surgical procedure could be decreased.
8. Surgical excision of a tumor is still the initial treatment of choice when this is possible. New imaging techniques should more accurately determine the resectability of tumor.
9. The prognosis in patients with local relapse is poor and extensive surgery is indicated in these patients. Again imaging is important in defining the total extent of the tumor.[15]

A report in 1989[16] cautioned that even the approach of initial chemotherapy with delayed surgery may still have problems. First, microscopic residual tumor may still be left behind and second, function of organs may still be impaired. Thus the delayed surgery is still not free of problems. Again imaging is important to maximize the likelihood of a satisfactory surgical outcome.

References

1. King DR, Clatworthy HW Jr. The pediatric patient with sarcoma. Semin Oncol 1981;8:215–221.
2. Agamanolis DP, Dasu S, Krill CE. Tumors of skeletal muscle. Hum Pathol 1986;17:778–795.
3. Maurer HM, Beltangady M, Gehan EA, et al. The Intergroup Rhabdomyosarcoma Study-I. A final report. Cancer 1988;61:209–220.
4. Olney LE, Narayana A, Loening S, et al. Intrascrotal rhabdomyosarcoma. Urology 1979;14:113–125.
5. Raney RB Jr, Tefft M, Lawrence W Jr, et al. Paratesticular sarcoma in childhood and adolescence. A report from the Intergroup Rhabdomyosarcoma Studies I and II, 1973–1983. Cancer 1987;60:2337–2343.
6. Ransom JL, Pratt CB, Hustu HO, et al. Retroperitoneal rhabdomyosarcoma in children. Cancer 1980;45:845–850.
7. Lack EE, Perez-Atayde AR, Schuster SR. Am J Surg Pathol 1981;5:643–652.
8. Malogolowkin MH, Ortega JA. Rhabdomyosarcoma of childhood. Pediatr Ann 1988;17:251–266.
9. Maurer HM. Rhabdomyosarcoma. Curr Prob Cancer 1978;2:3–36.
10. Grosfeld JL, Weber TR, Weetman RM, et al. Rhabdomyosarcoma in childhood: analysis of survival in 98 cases. J Pediatr Surg 1983;18:141–146.
11. Hays DM. Pelvic rhabdomyosarcomas in childhood: diagnosis and concepts of management reviewed. Cancer 1980;45:1810–1814.
12. Hamilton CR, Pinkerton R, Horwich A. The management of paratesticular rhabdomyosarcoma. Clin Radiol 1989;40:314–317.
13. Hays DM, Lawrence W Jr, Wharam M, et al. Primary reexcision for patients with "microscopic residual" tumor following initial excision of sarcomas of trunk and extremity sites. J Pediatr Surg 1989;24:5–10.
14. Johnson DE, McHugh TA, Jaffe N. Paratesticular rhabdomyosarcoma in childhood. J Urol 1982;128:1275–1276.
15. Raney RB, Hays DM, Tefft M, et al. Rhabdomyosarcoma and the undifferentiated sarcomas. In: Pizzo PA, Poplack DG, eds. Principles and practice of pediatric oncology. Philadelphia: JB Lippincott, 1989:635–658.
16. McLorie GA, Abara OE, Churchill BM, et al. Rhabdomyosarcoma of the prostate in childhood: current challenges. J Pediatr Surg 1989;24:977–981.

FIBROMATOSIS

Because of the extremely confusing classification of this group of disorders in the literature, the radiologist may experience fear and frustration when confronted with a patient with fibromatosis. Fibromatosis refers to a group of very rare soft-tissue tumors, and the experience of any individual institution in dealing with these abnormalities is limited.

The fibromatoses may be defined as nonmetastasizing proliferative fibroblastic tumors that usually invade locally[1–3] (Fig. 9–23).

Because of their tendency to invade adjacent tissues, they should not be called fibromas. They do not metastasize, so the term fibrosarcoma is inappropriate. Significant causes of confusion with these tumors are that the aggressiveness of the histologic appearance varies considerably from patient to patient and that there is poor correlation between the histology and the clinical behavior of the tumor. At one end of the spectrum some of these tumors may appear identical to a fibrosarcoma histologically, and in some patients the final diagnosis is only made retrospectively after the clinical behavior (metastatis or no metastasis) of the tumor has been observed.

Grossly, these tumors are poorly defined infiltrating

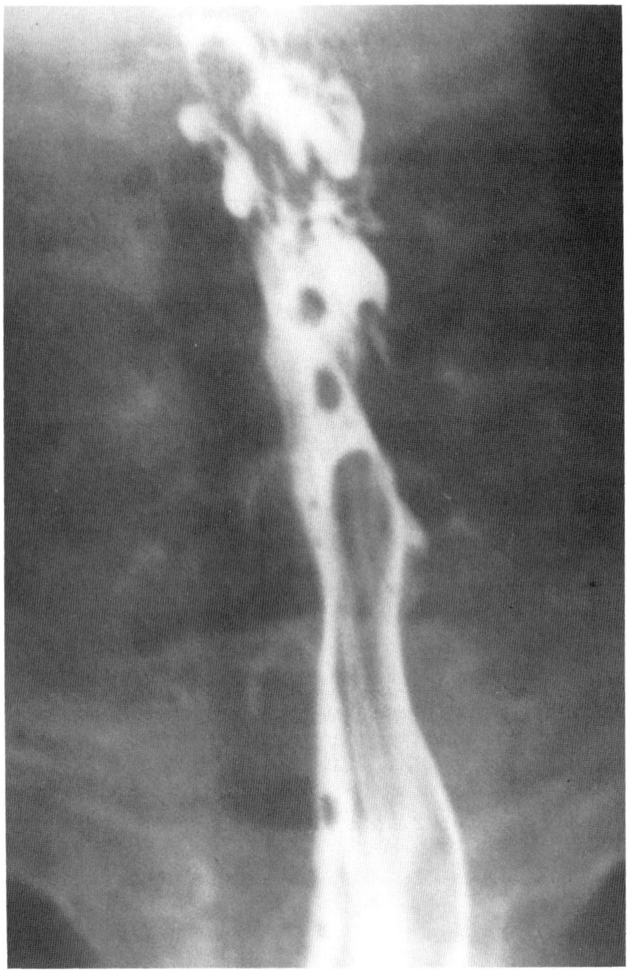

Figure 9-23. **Diagnosis: Aggressive fibromatosis involving the esophagus. 4-year-old girl with dysphagia. Barium swallow. The patient has a cervical soft-tissue mass that is invading the esophageal wall, causing nodular filling defects. The lesion has not penetrated through the mucosa. (From Wolf Y. Dysphagia in a child with aggressive fibromatosis of the esophagus. J Pediatr Surg 1989;24:1137–1139.)**

lesions. They tend to be firm and homogeneous without significant areas of hemorrhage or necrosis.

Classification of fibromatosis is exceedingly complex and is complicated by the fact that the same term will be used by different authors to mean different things. Fortunately, from a radiologic viewpoint the classification of these diseases can be simplified, and a simple workable classification is presented in Table 9–17. As can be seen from Table 9–18, the age of presentation of children with fibromatosis falls into two distinct groups. The first group presents under the age of 1 year and forms the congenital group in the classification in Table 9–17. The second group presents after the age of 3 years, with over 50 percent presenting after the age of 6 years. These form the second group in the classification in Table 9–17. In order to help the radiologist, consulting the literature with these patients I have listed the synonyms for each of the various types of tumor that have been used in the literature.

TABLE 9–17
Classification of Fibromatosis

Group	Synonyms in Literature
I. Congenital fibromatosis	
Focal	Fibromatosis colli Congenital fibrosarcoma Fibrous hematoma of infancy
Multiple	
Without visceral involvement	Aggressive infantile Multiple fibromatosis[1] Diffuse infantile fibromatosis Infantile myofibromatosis[2]
With visceral involvement	Generalized fibromatosis[1] Infantile myofibromatosis[3]
II. Aggressive fibromatosis	Infantile fibrosarcoma[4] Fibromatosis[5] Musculoaponeurotic fibromatosis[5] Extra-abdominal desmoid[6]

References

1. Dehner LP. Pediatric surgical pathology, 2nd ed. Baltimore: Williams & Wilkins, 1987:885–886, 1002–1003.
2. Wiswell TE, Davis J, Cunningham BE, et al. Infantile myofibromatosis: the most common fibrous tumor of infancy. J Pediatr Surg 1988;23:314–318.
3. Lawrence MAJ, Burgess PA, Quilligan JJ, et al. Congenital multiple fibromatosis (infantile myofibromatosis). Arch Otolaryngol Head Neck Surg 1988;114:207–209.
4. Sartoris DJ, Arkoff RS, Parker BR. Aggressive fibromatosis of the mandible in childhood. Skeletal Radiol 1983;10:154–156.
5. Rao BN, Horowitz ME, Parham DM, et al. Challenges in the treatment of childhood fibromatosis. Arch Surg 1987;122:1296–1299.
6. Griffiths HJ, Robinson K, Bonfiglio TA. Aggressive fibromatosis. Skeletal Radiol 1983;9:179–184.

TABLE 9–18
Age of Presentation of 66 Children with Fibromatosis[1]

Age	Percentage
Less 1 yr	23
1–2 yrs	5
3–5 yrs	18
6–10 yrs	24
11–15 yrs	30

Reference

1. Dehner LP, Askin FB. Tumors of fibrous tissue origin in childhood. A clinicopathologic study of cutaneous and soft tissue neoplasms in 66 children. Cancer 1976;38:888–900.

Comment: Fibromatosis can be classified as congenital or aggressive.

CONGENITAL FIBROMATOSIS

Congenital fibromatosis may be focal or multiple. Multiple lesions may occur with or without visceral organ involvement (see Table 9–17). They occur in children under the age of 1 year. They may frequently be diagnosed at the time of birth.

The focal lesions occur predominantly in the soft tissues. They are most commonly found in the head and neck (one-third of cases) or in the leg (one-third of cases),[4] but they can occur at any site in the body.[5] They lie deep in the soft tissues and are usually not attached to skin. Imaging studies will reveal a nonspecific soft-tissue mass. Occasionally, these lesions will cause secondary pressure effects and erosion of adjacent bone. In one 8-month-old infant, there was destruction with periosteal reaction of the adjacent mandible.[6] In another study of two patients,[7] soft-tissue masses adjacent to the ends of long bones caused adjacent erosion and sclerosis, with a fairly characteristic angulation of the adjacent ends of the bone probably representing the effects of longstanding pressure. These focal lesions are treated by surgical resection. In one study of 3 patients, no recurrence was identified.[8] My impression from the literature is that focal congenital fibromatosis is the least common form that is found. While single lesions most commonly occur in the soft tissues, they can occasionally (less than 10 percent) be found as single bone lesions.[1]

The multiple form of congenital fibromatosis is divided into two groups, depending on the presence or absence of visceral involvement. This distinction is important, because the prognosis is much worse if visceral involvement is present. In one study, reviewing 170 patients in the literature, 158 were under the age of 1 year. Seventy-three percent died if there was visceral involvement, whereas the mortality without visceral involvement was 15 percent.[8] All the patients have subcutaneous nodules and multiple bone lesions. Visceral involvement when present can affect any organ. Typically, patients with congenital multiple fibromatosis will present at birth. Lesions may appear in the first few months of life (Fig. 9–24), and preexisting lesions will often show increase in size during this period. Following this, there is frequently spontaneous involution of the lesions,[1,9,10] and this is particularly evident in the bone (Fig. 9–24). Some reports in the literature state that this spontaneous involution is only seen in patients without visceral involvement. I suspect, however, that the two types of tumor are biologically similar, with death occurring in patients with visceral involvement before involution can occur. Death in these patients does not appear to be caused by a more aggressive metastatic behavior of the tumor but rather simply by the local effects of the tumor being much more serious to the patient when vital organs are involved than when bones or soft tissues are. Some reports of metastases in patients with congenital multiple fibromatosis[11] are much more likely to represent multifocal primary tumors than true metastatic spread.

The radiographic appearance of the multiple congenital fibromatosis lesions have been well described in the bone (see Fig. 9–24), with very few descriptions of lesions appearing in the organs. Most of the imaging has involved plain film radiography, with few if any reports of CT or MR. Bone lesions in congenital multiple fibromatosis are almost always multiple. They are typically lytic metaphyseal lesions, which can be symmetrical and may have an adjacent periosteal reaction[9] (Fig. 9–24). In one newborn patient, the multiple lytic lesions had slightly permeative margins with extensive periosteal reactions and one pathologic fracture.[1] This patient also had multiple lytic skull lesions that were well defined. In another child with a soft-tissue facial lesion, multiple metaphyseal lucent lesions were identified at birth[10]; at the age of 2½ years these had almost all completely resolved. In another patient, who presented with a foot soft-tissue lesion at 3 weeks of age, the patient had a much more aggressive appearance in the metaphyses, with extensive destruction, some expansion, and very widespread periosteal reaction. In another patient, aged 1 month,[12] the lesions were much less aggressive, occurring in the diametaphyseal areas of the long bones, the flat bones, and the spine. They had more well-defined sclerotic margins and some bony expansion.[12] A review of the literature of the appearance of these lesions in 12 patients[13] indicates that there is a significant variation in the number and site of the lesions. This review confirms the varied degree of aggressiveness in appearance of the lesions.

The differential diagnosis of the bone lesions includes metastases from neuroblastoma, histiocytosis X, multiple hemangiomas, congenital syphillis, and multifocal osteomyelitis. The lungs of one patient, with postmortem confirmation of the presence of fibromatosis, were initially normal at birth but soon demonstrated a fine reticular nodular pattern that progressed to more coalescent larger lesions. The appearance was nonspecific.[14] It is important to note that the lesions did not appear as well-defined focal nodules.

AGGRESSIVE FIBROMATOSIS

There are a number of reports of this disorder.[2,6,15–24] The lesions can occur in any site. In 20 children, they were found in the head and neck in 7, in the trunk of 6, and in the extremities in 7.[22] In another study of 13 patients, 7 lesions occurred in the leg and 3 in the arm. They are almost always single lesions, with less than 10 percent being multifocal.[22] Most of the lesions arise in the deep soft tissues or in the facial area. Occasionally, they can invade visceral organs, with one patient having a lesion invading the cervical esophagus and causing dysphagia[20] and another patient having a lesion causing obstruction of the duodenum.[17] The median age of presentation in one study of 20 children was 9 years. The most common presentation is that of a mass, with pain being present in only 6 of 20 children.[22]

A B

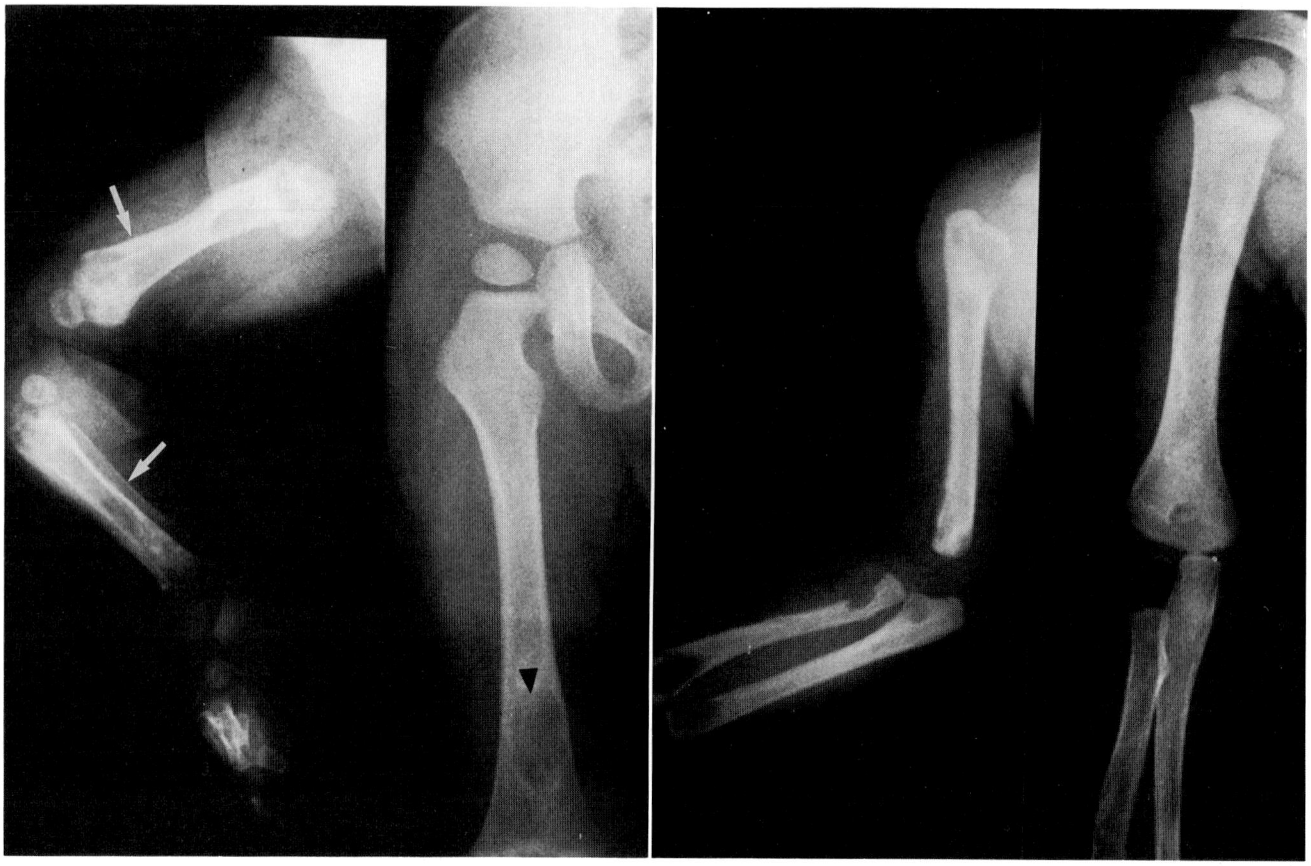

Figure 9–24. **Diagnosis: Congenital generalized fibromatosis.**
A, **The left image of the femur and tibia were obtained at birth. There are extensive lesions predominantly involving the metaphyses. They are lytic in appearance. There is marked periosteal reaction on both the tibia and femur *(arrows).* The right-hand image of the femur was obtained at age 22 months. There has been marked spontaneous improvement. There is a residual lytic lesion in the lower metaphysis *(arrowhead)* but no other abnormality. *B,* Plain film radiograph of the arm. The left image was obtained at birth. There are multiple lytic lesions in the metaphyses of all the forearm bones. The right image was obtained 18 months later. Most of the bone lesions have shown spontaneous disappearance. (From Chan YF. Congenital generalized fibromatosis with predominant osseous involvement in a Chinese newborn. J Pediatr Orthoped 1989;9:64–68.)**

Imaging is extremely important in the evaluation of aggressive fibromatosis, being needed to define the tumor extent for the surgeon. Plain film radiographs will show the soft-tissue abnormality in most but not all patients. Adjacent bone destruction will be seen. The total extent of the destruction, particularly in the skull and facial bones, will not be demonstrated by the plain film radiograph. In the skull, these lesions can be particularly invasive and destructive.[11,18,22] On CT, they appear as relatively homogeneous soft-tissue abnormalities with poorly defined margins. The intensity has been described as less than normal muscle[15] or similar to normal muscle[19] prior to contrast administration. Following contrast injection, enhancement varies from little[15] to moderate.[19] A wide spectrum of different patterns of enhancement is identified, probably representing the varied percentage of cellularity and fibrosis in the tumor. CT is the modality of choice for definition of the total extent of bone invasion and destruction. In another study of CT of 9 patients, considerable variation was found. Before contrast administration, the tumor appeared brigher than muscle in 3 and less bright than muscle in one. Following contrast administration, enhancement was minimal to moderate and homogeneous or heterogeneous. In this study of 9 patients, no correlation was found between the CT appearance and the histology (necrosis, vascularity, fibrosis, cellularity).[23]

Angiography is not routinely utilized for evaluation of fibromatosis, but in one study, some mild increase in vascularity was identified in 7 of 8 patients.[19]

There are a number of reports of the MR appearance of aggressive fibromatosis. On T1 weighted images, the lesions appear of lower signal intensity than muscle, because of the presence of the fibrous tissue.[25] I would expect the degree of enhancement following gadolinium-DTPA to be little. On T2 weighted imaging, the appearance of the lesion varies.[18,25,26] Compared to T1 weighted images there may be little, mild, or moderate increase in signal intensity with T2 weighting (Fig. 9–25). They are not all of low signal intensity, like fibrous scar tissue. In one patient with a primary lesion in the anterior two-thirds of the tongue, the lesion was moderately well defined and homogeneous, with no surrounding edema, which was thought to be helpful in differentiating it from infection. The accuracy of the MR definition of the margins was evidenced by the absence of recurrence following surgical resection.[18] Although no large series of patients have been reported, I would predict that MR will be the most effective imaging modality for defining the extent of these tumors and that it will result in a decrease in the incidence of local recurrence.

Surgery is the most important modality for treatment of aggressive fibromatosis. Radiation has been utilized with some success. In one study of 16 patients, mainly adult, there was good local control in some with radiation therapy.[24] In another study of 12 patients, some local control was obtained utilizing very high doses, greater than 5,800 R.[16] Chemotherapy has occasionally been utilized[6] but it is not particularly effective. Recurrence after surgery may be identified in up to 50 percent of cases.[2] In one 17-year-old patient with a forearm lesion, multiple recurrences and multiple more proximal amputations were not successful in achieving a cure.[2] The reasons for surgical failure and recurrence are twofold. First, the lesions, particularly in the skull, may not be amenable to complete surgical excision without extreme patient mutilation. In other sites, however, the fine infiltrative pattern of the tumor may not be appreciated, so that adequately wide margins of excision may not be utilized. With wide resection cure can be achieved.[6,18] In one study of patients in whom the surgeon believed good margins had been achieved, recurrence occurred in 1 of 11 patients.[22]

The most important factor in treatment is surgery and the surgeon is heavily reliant on the radiologist for defining the extent of the tumor. The prognosis in aggressive fibromatosis is completely dependent on the potential complete resectability of the tumor. It is not dependent on histology.

Comment: Aggressive fibromatosis is very difficult to excise completely because of infiltrating local spread.

References

1. Chan Y-F, Lau JHK, Tong CY. Congenital generalized fi-

Figure 9-25. **Diagnosis: Aggressive fibromatosis.**
***A* and *B,* Sagittal MR, T1, and T2 weighted images. The fibromatosis (*F*) appears as a fairly well-defined lesion. Some of the margins are irregular. The lesion is of low intensity on the T1 weighted image and very bright on the T2 weighted image. This is active growing cellular fibrous tissue and it therefore appears bright on the T2 weighted image. It is unlike fibrous scar tissue, which appears dark on T2 weighted images.**

A

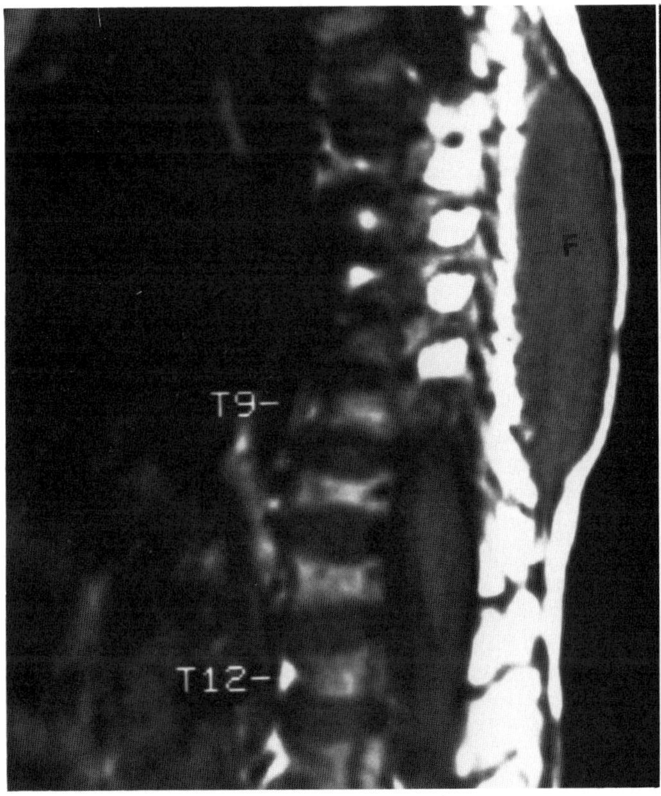

B

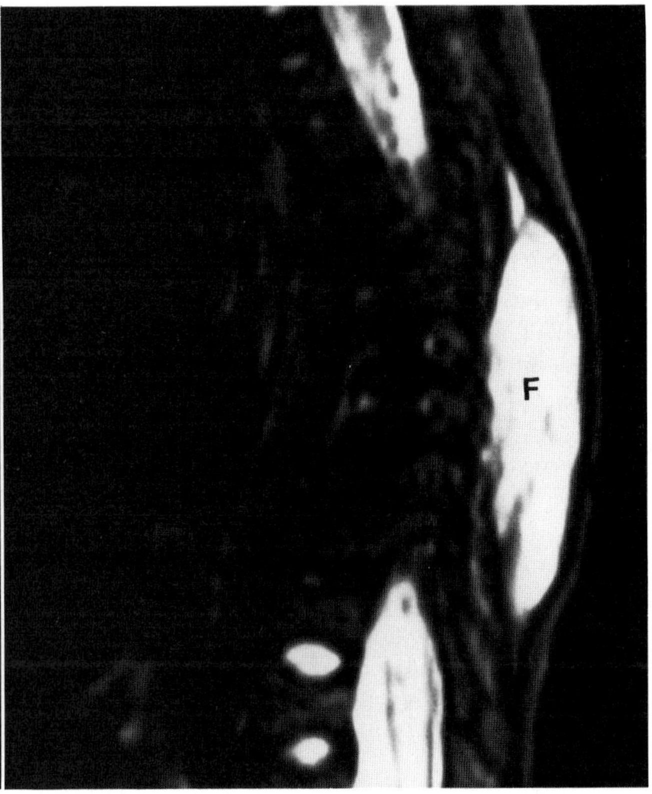

bromatosis with predominant osseous involvement in a Chinese newborn. J Pediatr Orthoped 1989;9:64–68.
2. Griffiths HJ, Robinson K, Bonfiglio TA. Aggressive fibromatosis. Skeletal Radiol 1983;9:179–184.
3. Dehner LP, Askin FB. Tumors of fibrous tissue origin in childhood. A clinicopathologic study of cutaneous and soft tissue neoplasms in 66 children. Cancer 1976;38:888–900.
4. Dehner LP. Pediatric surgical pathology, 2nd ed. Baltimore: Williams & Wilkins, 1987;885–886, 1002–1003.
5. Goslee L, Clermont V, Bernstein J, et al. Superficial connective tissue tumors in early infancy. A study of fibromatosis and lipoblastomatosis. J Pediatr 1964;65:377–387.
6. Sartoris DJ, Arkoff RS, Parker BR. Aggressive fibromatosis of the mandible in childhood. Skeletal Radiol 1983;10:154–156.
7. Capusten BM, Azouz EM, Rosman MA. Fibromatosis of bone in children. Radiology 1984;152:693–694.
8. Wiswell TE, Davis J, Cunningham BE, et al. Infantile myofibromatosis: the most common fibrous tumor of infancy. J Pediatr Surg 1988;23:314–318.
9. Kumar R, Madewell JE, Lindell MM, et al. Fibrous lesions of bones. RadioGraphics 1990;10:237–256.
10. Lawrence MAJ, Burgess PA, Quilligan JJ, et al. Congenital multiple fibromatosis (infantile myofibromatosis). Arch Otolaryngol Head Neck Surg 1988;114:207–209.
11. Shankwiler RA, Athey PA, Lamki N. Aggressive infantile fibromatosis pulmonary metastases documented by plain film and computed tomography. Clin Imag 1989;13:127–129.
12. Condon VR, Allen RP. Congenital generalized fibromatosis. Radiology 1961;76:444–448.
13. Baer JW, Radkowski MA. Congenital multiple fibromatosis. A case report with review of the world literature. AJR 1973;118:200–205.
14. Morettin LB, Mueller E, Schreiber M. Generalized hamartomatosis (congenital generalized fibromatosis). AJR 1972;114:722–734.
15. Campbell AN, Chan HSL, Daneman A, et al. Agressive fibromatosis in childhood: computed tomographic findings in three patients. CT 1983;7:109–113.
16. Greenberg HM, Goebel R, Weichselbaums, et al. Radiation therapy in the treatment of aggressive fibromatoses. Int J Radiat Oncol Biol Phys 1981;7:305–310.
17. Canioni D, Fekete C, Nezelof C. Solitary intestinal fibromatosis: a rare cause of neonatal obstruction. Pediatr Pathol 1989;9:719–724.
18. Chen PC, Ball WS, Towbin RB. Aggressive fibromatosis of the tongue: MR demonstration. J Comput Assist Tomogr 1989;13:343–345.
19. Hudson TM, Vandergriend RA, Springfield DS, et al. Aggressive fibromatosis: evaluation by computed tomography and angiography. Radiology 1984;150:495–501.
20. Wolf Y, Katz S, Lax E, et al. Dysphagia in a child with aggressive fibromatosis of the esophagus. J Pediatr Surg 1989;24:1137–1139.
21. Fu Y-S, Perzin KH. Nonepithelial tumors of the nasal cavity, paranasal sinuses and nasopharynx. A clinicopathologic study. VI. Fibrous tissue tumors (fibroma, fibromatosis, fibrosarcoma). Cancer 1976;37:2912–2928.
22. Rao BN, Horowitz ME, Parham DM, et al. Challenges in the treatment of childhood fibromatosis. Arch Surg 1987;122:1296–1299.
23. Francis IR, Dorovini-Zis K, Glazer GM, et al. The fibromatoses: CT-pathologic correlation. AJR 1986;147:1063–1066.
24. Wara WM, Phillips TL, Hill DR, et al. Desmoid tumors—treatment and prognosis. Radiology 1977;124:225–226.
25. Aisen AM, Martel W, Braunstein EM, et al. MRI and CT evaluation of primary bone and soft-tissue tumors. AJR 1986;146:749–756.
26. Sundaram M, McGuire MH, Schajowicz F. Soft-tissue masses: histologic basis for decreased signal (short T2) on T2-weighted MR images. AJR 1987;148:1247–1250.

GERM CELL TUMORS

Germ cell tumors are uncommon and their histologic classification is complicated, with considerable disagreement existing. In addition to there being a wide range of different histologic tumors, they may occur at many different sites in the body, and the behavior and appearance of the tumors will vary considerably depending on the anatomic location. There is also confusion with regard to the definition of malignancy. For example, should immature teratomas be considered benign or malignant lesions? Fortunately, by making a few generalizations and simplifications, the whole subject of germ cell tumors can be brought under control.

Epidemiology

Germ cell tumors account for approximately 3 percent of all pediatric cancers.[1] The most common age of presentation and the sex difference with these tumors are summarized in Table 9–19. It is immediately apparent that the age of presentation is greatly dependent on the anatomic location. Sacrococcygeal and head and neck teratomas usually present in the newborn period. Most of the other germ cell tumors are disorders of the very young, occurring under the age of 2 years. The major exception to this is the ovary, where most lesions present around the age of puberty. A significant number of testicular lesions may also be found in this age group. With regard to sex distribution the germ cell tumors are extremely unusual in that there is a marked predilection for either boys or girls and this is very heavily dependent on anatomic location. For example, over 80 percent of sacrococcygeal teratomas and most of the retroperitoneal teratomas occur in females. By contrast, almost all of the mediastinal yolk sac tumors and gastric teratomas occur in males.

The etiology of germ cell tumors is not known. A positive family history has been obtained in 6 families with presacral teratomas,[2] and there have been several reports of increased association of germ cell tumors with a wide variety of congenital anomalies,[3–5] with such abnormalities being identified in as many as 17 percent of 126 patients in one large series.[6]

TABLE 9–19
Germ Cell Tumors: Age and Sex Epidemiology

Tumor Type	Sex Differences	Age
Sacrococcygeal teratoma	80% female[1–3]	Most newborn[4]
Yolk sac: testis	—	Mean 17 mos[5] 80% under 2 yrs[6]
Yolk sac: nongonadal	—	Mean 21 mos[5,7]
Yolk sac: mediastinal	>90% male[8,9]	Any age, commonly <1 yr[4]
Gastric teratoma	90% male[10]	90% under 1 yr[10]
Retroperitoneal teratoma	75% female[11]	50% under 6 mos[11] Mean 5 mos[4]
Ovarian teratoma	—	Puberty[4]
Head & neck teratoma	—	Newborn[4]
All teratomas	Female more common	50% newborn

References
1. Dehner LP. Gonadal and extragonadal germ cell neoplasia of childhood. Hum Pathol 1983;14:493–511.
2. Grosfeld JL, Ballantine TVN, Lowe D, et al. Benign and malignant teratomas in children: analysis of 85 patients. Surgery 1976;80:297–305.
3. Noseworthy J, Lack EE, Kozakewich HPW, et al. Sacrococcygeal germ cell tumors in childhood: an updated experience with 118 patients. J Pediatr Surg 1981;16:358–364.
4. Tapper D, Lack EE. Teratomas in infancy and childhood. A 54-year experience at the Children's Hospital Medical Center. Ann Surg 1983;198:398–409.
5. Kaplan GW, Cromie WC, Kelalis PP, et al. Prepubertal yolk sac testicular tumors—report of the testicular tumor registry. J Urol 1988;140:1109–1112.
6. Huddart SN, Mann JR, Gornall P, et al. The UK Children's Cancer Study Group: testicular malignant germ cell tumours 1979–1988. J Pediatr Surg 1990;25:406–410.
7. O'Sullivan P, Daneman A, Chan HSL, et al. Extragonadal endodermal sinus tumors in children: a review of 24 cases. Pediatr Radiol 1983;13:249–257.
8. Truong LD, Harris L, Mattioli C, et al. Endodermal sinus tumor of the mediastinum. A report of seven cases and review of the literature. Cancer 1986;58:730–739.
9. Fox MA, Vix VA. Endodermal sinus (yolk sac) tumors of the anterior mediastinum. AJR 1980;135:291–294.
10. Cairo MS, Grosfeld JL, Weetman RM. Gastric teratoma: unusual cause for bleeding of the upper gastrointestinal tract in the newborn. Pediatrics 1981;67:721–724.
11. Davidson AJ, Hartman DS, Goldman SM. Mature teratoma of the retroperitoneum: radiologic, pathologic, and clinical correlation. Radiology 1989;172:421–425.

References
1. Ablin A, Isaacs H. In: Pizzo PA, Poplack DG, eds. Principles and practice of pediatric oncology. Philadelphia: JB Lippincott, 1989:713–731.
2. Hunt PT, Davidson KC, Ashcraft DW, et al. Radiography of hereditary presacral teratoma. Radiology 1977;122:187–191.
3. Huddart SN, Mann JR, Gornall P, et al. The UK Children's Cancer Study Group: testicular malignant germ cell tumours 1979–1988. J Pediatr Surg 1990;25:406–410.
4. Sakashita S, Koyanagi T, Tsuji I, et al. Congenital anomalies in children with testicular germ cell tumor. J Urol 1980;124:889–891.
5. Tagawa T, Mimaki T, Ono J, et al. Aicardi syndrome associated with an embryonal carcinoma. Pediatr Neurol 1989;5:45–47.
6. Mann JR, Pearson D, Barrett A, et al. Results of the United Kingdom Children's Cancer Study Group's Malignant Germ Cell Tumor Studies. Cancer 1989;63:1657–1667.

Pathology

Germ cell tumor is an all-embracing term and includes a variety of different tumors linked together because of overlapping histology and common origin. All germ cell tumors arise from primordial germ cells of the yolk sac that normally migrate to the gonads but can have their migration arrested along the route of passage or may occasionally occur in ectopic sites.[1–4] Most of these tumors are always malignant but some, for example a teratoma, may be mature (benign) or malignant. Most malignant teratomas contain tissues of other types of germ cell tumor. Some publications will term these lesions malignant teratomas while most authorities would classify them by the more malignant tissue. For example, a teratoma showing areas of endodermal sinus tumor would be called an endodermal sinus tumor. One of the more widely accepted classifications of germ cell tumors is presented in Table 9–20. The following points should be noted.

1. Only teratomas and yolk sac tumors occur in children with any significant frequency. For practical purposes most of the rest of the descriptions of germ cell tumors refer only to these two tumor types.
2. The term yolk sac tumor is synonymous with endodermal sinus tumor. Most authorities would include infantile embryonal carcinoma with yolk sac tumor[4] and for this reason the term infantile embryonal sarcoma does not appear separately in the table.
3. Germinoma has previously been called seminoma in the testicle and dysgerminoma in the ovary. The term germinoma should be used for these tumors regardless of site. In pubertal children, they are most common in the ovary in girls and in the pineal gland in boys.[2] They are found less frequently in the anterior mediastinum and testis in adolescence.[2]
4. Choriocarcinoma is very rare in children. It is usually seen in the age group 15 to 19 years and occurs in the pineal gland, anterior mediastinum, and ovary.[2] Very occasionally, metastases from a placental primary may be identified in the newborn.
5. Gonadoblastoma is a very rare benign tumor that almost only occurs in dysgenetic gonads (abnormal gonads in children with true or pseudohermaphroditism). Forty percent are bilateral. Their importance is that up to 30 percent of patients will have an associated additional germinoma present as well.[5]
6. Adult embryonal carcinoma almost never occurs in children and will not be mentioned further.

Not all germ cell tumors are malignant. Most teratomas are benign. All yolk sac tumors should be considered malignant. The likelihood of a germ cell tumor being malignant is very much dependent on its anatomic site (Table 9–21). It is important for the radiologist to be aware of this variation in malignancy. It is obviously wasteful to indulge in an expensive exercise of imaging for metastases from a germ-cell tumor that, by its location, is certain to be benign (head and neck and gastric teratomas). Conversely, in other locations, for example, the testis, the lesions are invariably malignant and this information should result in a different imaging approach. Not only is the likelihood of malignancy dependent on anatomic site, but for sacrococcygeal tumors, it is heavily dependent on the patient's age. In the first few weeks of life, less than 2 percent of these tumors will be malignant.[2] The likelihood of malignancy being present increases rapidly with age, with the exact incidence of malignancy varying from series to series. For example, in one report, 50 percent of sacrococcygeal teratomas over the age of 2 months were malignant.[5]

The anatomic location of germ cell tumors is varied. The sites of occurrence of germ cell tumors are summarized in Tables 9–22, 9–23, and 9–24. As can be seen, the ovary, testis, and sacrococcygeal area are the most common locations. When one breaks down the tumors into yolk sac tumor, teratoma, or a combination of all germ cell tumors, the results of distribution vary some-

TABLE 9–20
Histologic Classification of Germ Cell Tumors[1,2]

Teratoma
  Mature
  Immature
Germinoma
Adult embryonal carcinoma
Yolk sac tumor (endodermal sinus tumor)
Choriocarcinoma
Gonadoblastoma
Mixed germ cell

References
1. Dehner LP. Gonadal and extragonadal germ cell neoplasia of childhood. Hum Pathol 1983;14:493–511.
2. Mann JR, Pearson D, Barrett A, et al. Results of the United Kingdom Children's Cancer Study Group's Malignant Germ Cell Tumor Studies. Cancer 1989;63:1657–1667.

TABLE 9–21
Likelihood of Malignancy in Pediatric Germ Cell Tumors

Anatomic Site	Likelihood of Malignancy
Sacrococcygeal	Age dependent[1] Newborn—1 month 2% malignant[2] Over 1 month 71% malignant Overall—13% malignant[3]
Testis	Over 80% malignant[3]
Ovary	Over 2/3 benign[3,4]
Head and Neck	Usually benign[1]
Vagina	Usually malignant[1]
Retroperitoneum	$<$10% malignant[4]
Gastric	All benign[4]
Anterior mediastinum	20% malignant[5]

References
1. Ablin A, Isaacs H. In: Pizzo PA, Poplack DG, eds. Principles and practice of pediatric oncology. Philadelphia: JB Lippincott, 1989;713–731.
2. Dehner LP. Gonadal and extragonadal germ cell neoplasia of childhood. Hum Pathol 1983;14:493–511.
3. Billmire DF, Grosfeld JL. Teratomas in childhood: analysis of 142 cases. J Pediatr Surg 1986;21:548–551.
4. Tapper D, Lack EE. Teratomas in infancy and childhood. A 54-year experience at the Children's Hospital Medical Center. Ann Surg 1983;198:398–409.
5. Filler RM, Simpson JS, Ein SH. Mediastinal masses in infants and children. Pediatr Clin N Am 1979;26:677–690.

TABLE 9–22
Pediatric Germ Cell Tumors: Anatomic Distribution

References	Brodeur	Dehner	Mann	Hawkins
No. of Cases	57[1]	526[2]	156[3]	89[4]
Site	All Germ Cell Tumors (%)		Only Malignant Germ Cell Tumors (%)	
Sacrococcygeal	23	42	16	29
Ovary	37	24	24	37
Testis	19	9	48	13
Retroperitoneum	14	4	2	—
Mediastinum	7	7	4	—
Other	—	14	24	21

References
1. Brodeur GM, Howarth CB, Pratt CB, et al. Malignant germ cell tumors in 57 children and adolescents. Cancer 1981;48:1890–1898.
2. Dehner LP. Gonadal and extragonadal germ cell neoplasia of childhood. Hum Pathol 1983;14:493–511.
3. Mann JR, Pearson D, Barrett A, et al. Results of the United Kingdom Children's Cancer Study Group's Malignant Germ Cell Tumor Studies. Cancer 1989;63:1657–1667.
4. Hawkins EP, Finegold MJ, Hawkins HK, et al. Nongerminomatous malignant germ cell tumors in children. A review of 89 cases from the Pediatric Oncology Group, 1971–1984. Cancer 1986;58:2579–2584.

what. In addition, the anatomic distribution will vary depending on whether the researcher includes all germ cell tumors in the data or only malignant germ cell tumors (Table 9–22). Other variations of anatomic site distribution reported in the literature can be accounted for by differences in regional referral patterns, the population age served by a center, the histologic classification utilized, and the criteria used for differentiating benign from malignant tumors. Rare sites of some of these tumors are listed, together with appropriate references, in Tables 9–23 and 9–24.

Staging of germ cell tumors is a problem and it is important for the radiologist to be aware that there is no universally accepted staging system. Some institutions adopt different staging systems for different anatomic locations of the tumor. One classification that has been used for some collaborative studies is presented in Table 9–25. For sacrococcygeal teratoma a very useful classification based purely on the anatomic spread of the tumor is widely utilized[2,6–8] (Table 9–26). This classification depends on the anatomic extent of the tumor. It is important, first, because the extent of tumor determines the most appropriate surgical approach, and second, because the incidence of malignancy varies depending on the stage. For example, only 8 percent of predominantly external sacrococcygeal teratomas are malignant. This incidence of malignancy increases to 34 percent for those tumors spreading through the pelvis into the abdomen. In addition to this increased malignancy seen with more widespread extent of the tumor, patients with purely presacral teratomas and no external component also have a high incidence of malignancy. Recurrence of a sacrococcygeal teratoma is more likely to be malignant than the originally resected tumor. For example, in one study, the original tumor was a benign teratoma, with recurrence in 5 patients being malignant teratoma.[7] This knowledge is important to the surgeon, as every effort must be made at the time of original surgery to minimize the likelihood of recurrence.

Tumor markers are important in the management of germ cell tumors. Two markers are routinely evaluated. These are human chorionic gonadotrophin (HCG) and alpha-fetoprotein (αFP). HCG has a half-life of 45 minutes. It is elevated only in patients with choriocarcinoma and as this is a very rare tumor in children estimation of HCG is of limited value.[5] Alpha-fetoprotein is an alpha 1 globulin and is the main normally occurring serum protein in the fetus.[5] It has a half-life of about 5 days. Its concentration in the serum is increased in patients with hepatomas, hepatitis, some gastrointestinal tumors, and yolk sac tumors. It is not increased with dysgerminomas, choriocarcinomas, or mature teratomas.[5] It is reliably and consistently elevated in patients with yolk sac tumors.[9–13] In one large series, it was elevated in 100 percent of 94 such patients.[14] The degree of elevation of alpha-fetoprotein has no relationship to tumor prognosis. The finding of elevated alpha-fetoprotein is very helpful, however, in the differential diagnosis of a tumor. It is also extremely helpful to serially measure concentrations of alpha-fetoprotein after therapy. Levels return to normal with satisfactory response to therapy and become elevated very quickly with tumor relapse. The importance of this finding is that it

TABLE 9-23
Pediatric Teratoma: Anatomic Distribution

Reference	Tapper 245 Cases[1]		Billmire 142 Cases[2]	
Anatomic Location	No.	Percentage	No.	Percentage
Sacrococcygeal	102	40	84	58
Ovary	95	37	15	12
Head and neck	14	5	3	3
Retroperitoneum	12	5	7	4
Anterior mediastinum	11	4	14	10
Testis	8	4	15	12
CNS	9	3	—	—
Liver	2	1	—	—
Other*	2	1	4	2

*Other sites include pericardium,[3,4] stomach,[1,5] diaphragm,[6] pancreas,[5] mesentery,[10] intradural,[8] posterior mediastinum,[8,9–11] and orbit.[12]

References
1. Tapper D, Lack EE. Teratomas in infancy and childhood. A 54-year experience at the Children's Hospital Medical Center. Ann Surg 1983;198:398–409.
2. Billmire DF, Grosfeld JL. Teratomas in childhood: analysis of 142 cases. J Pediatr Surg 1986;21:548–551.
3. Banfield J. Intrapericardial teratoma: a new and treatable cause of hydrops fetalis. Am J Dis Child 1980;134:1174–1175.
4. Sumner TE, Crowe JE, Klein A, et al. Intrapericardial teratoma in infancy. Pediatr Radiol 1980;10:51–53.
5. Bowen B, Ros PR, McCarthy MJ, et al. Gastrointestinal teratomas: CT and US appearance with pathologic correlation. Radiology 1987;162:431–433.
6. Muller NL. CT features of cystic teratoma of the diaphragm. J Comput Assist Tomogr 1986;10:325–326.
7. Prieto ML, Casanova A, Delgado J, et al. Cystic teratoma of the mesentery. Pediatr Radiol 1989;19:439.
8. Smoker WRK, Biller J, Moore SA, et al. Intradural spinal teratoma: case report and review of the literature. AJNR 1986;7:905–910.
9. Ruzal-Shapiro C, Abramson SJ, Berdon WE. Posterior mediastinal cystic teratoma surrounded by fat in a 13 month old boy. Pediatr Radiol 1989;20:107–109.
10. Vade A, Nolan J. Posterior mediastinal teratoma involving the esophagus. Gastrointest Radiol 1989;14:106–108.
11. Weinberg B, Rose JS, Efremidis SC, et al. Posterior mediastinal teratoma (cystic dermoid): diagnosis by computerized tomography. Chest 1980;77:694–695.
12. Weiss AH, Greenwald MJ, Margo CE, et al. Primary and secondary orbital teratomas. J Pediatr Ophthalmol 1989;26:44–49.

raises the question as to how intensively imaging should be used in following up patients with yolk sac tumors. If the alpha-fetoprotein is normal, one could make an argument for not performing any imaging follow-up studies. This would obviously have significant cost advantages to the patient.

Comment: In pediatric germ cell tumors, only teratomas and yolk sac tumors are of major importance.

Tumor malignancy depends on the anatomic site and the patient's age.

Alpha-fetoprotein is an extremely accurate marker for evaluation of the status of a yolk sac tumor.

References
1. Olsen MM, Raffensperger JG, Gonzalez-Crussi F, et al. Endodermal sinus tumor: a clinical and pathological correlation. J Pediatr Surg 1982;17:832–840.
2. Dehner LP. Gonadal and extragonadal germ cell neoplasia of childhood. Hum Pathol 1983;14:493–511.
3. Brodeur GM, Howarth CB, Pratt CB, et al. Malignant germ cell tumors in 57 children and adolescents. Cancer 1981;48:1890–1898.
4. Tumor Board of the Children's Hospital of Philadelphia. Med Pediatr Oncol 1987;15:96–101.
5. Ablin A, Isaacs H. In: Pizzo PA, Poplack DG, eds. Principles and practice of pediatric oncology. Philadelphia: JB Lippincott, 1989:713–731.
6. Altman RP, Randolph JA, Lilly JR. Sacrococcygeal tera-

TABLE 9-24
Yolk Sac Tumor: Anatomic Location[1,2]

Most Common	Less Common	Rare
Ovary	Mediastinum	Penis[3]
Testis	Vagina	Pericardium[4]
Sacrococcygeal	Liver	Prostate
	Head & neck	Sinus[1]
		Mandible[5]

References
1. O'Sullivan P, Daneman A, Chan HSL, et al. Extragonadal endodermal sinus tumors in children: a review of 24 cases. Pediatr Radiol 1983;13:249–257.
2. Dehner LP. Gonadal and extragonadal germ cell neoplasia of childhood. Hum Pathol 1983;14:493–511.
3. Kennedy K, Larson A. Congenital endodermal sinus tumor of the penis. J Ped Surg 1987;22:791–792.
4. Banfield J. Intrapericardial teratoma: a new and treatable cause of hydrops fetalis. Am J Dis Child, 1980;134:1174–1175.
5. Shebib S, Sabbah R, Sackey K, et al. Endodermal sinus tumor (yolk sac) in infants and children. Am J Ped Hematol Oncol 1989;11:36–39.

TABLE 9-25
Classification of Germ Cell Tumors[1,2]

Stage	Description
I	Localized with or without local node involvement—complete resection
II	Localized with or without local node involvement—microscopic residual
III	Gross residual and/or nodes >2 cm diameter and/or malignant cells in ascites or pleural fluid
IV	Disseminated metastases

References
1. Brodeur GM, Howarth CB, Pratt CB, et al. Malignant germ cell tumors in 57 children and adolescents. Cancer 1981;48:1890–1898.
2. Diez B, Richard L. Malignant germ cell sacrococcygeal tumors in children. Acta Oncol 1989;28:249–251.

toma: American Academy of Pediatric Surgical Section Survey. J Pediatr Surg 1974;9:389–398.
7. Billmire DF, Grosfeld JL. Teratomas in childhood: analysis of 142 cases. J Pediatr Surg 1986;21:548–551.
8. Schey WL, Shkolnik A, White H. Clinical and radiographic considerations of sacrococcygeal teratomas: an analysis of 26 new cases and review of the literature. Radiology 1977;125:189–195.
9. Kaplan GW, Cromie WC, Kelalis PP, et al. Prepubertal yolk sac testicular tumors—report of the testicular tumor registry. J Urol 1988;140:1109–1112.
10. Sham JST, Chan FL, Choi PHK, et al. Primary mediastinal endodermal sinus tumors: CT evaluation. Clin Imag 1989;13:299–304.
11. Sham JST, Chiu CSW, Lau WH, et al. Experience with the management of primary endodermal sinus tumor of the mediastinum. Cancer 1989;64:756–761.
12. Shebib S, Sabbah RS, Sackey K, et al. Endodermal sinus (yolk sac) tumor in infants and children. Am J Pediatr Hematol/Oncol 1989;11:36–39.
13. Truong LD, Harris L, Mattioli C, et al. Endodermal sinus tumor of the mediastinum. A report of seven cases and review of the literature. Cancer 1986;58:730–739.
14. Mann JR, Pearson D, Barrett A, et al. Results of the United Kingdom Children's Cancer Study Group's Malignant Germ Cell Tumor Studies. Cancer 1989;63:1657–1667.

Clinical Presentation

Most germ cell tumors present with signs and symptoms of the local tumor mass. Presentation with diffuse metastatic disease is decidedly uncommon. The presenting symptoms are varied, reflecting the multitude of anatomic locations of the primary tumor. Sacrococcygeal teratomas most often present as an easily detectable exophytic mass that is almost always very large. Very rarely anterovenous shunting within the tumor may cause high-output cardiac failure.[1] The diagnosis is usually obvious. In the small number of sacrococcygeal teratomas in which the tumor is entirely presacral, the diagnosis may be delayed[2] and symptoms will include difficulty with urination or defecation or urinary infection. Testicular tumors most often present as a painless mass.[3] Attention is occasionally drawn to the mass by

TABLE 9-26
Classification of Sacrococcygeal Teratoma and Likelihood of Malignancy[1–4]

Stage	Incidence (%)	Malignancy (%)
I, Predominantly external	49	8
II, External with pelvic component	34	21
III, External with pelvic and abdominal component	8.0	34
IV, Presacral (no external component)	9.0	38

References
1. Altman RP, Randolph JA, Lilly JR. Sacrococcygeal teratoma: American Academy of Pediatric Surgical Section Survey. J Pediatr Surg 1974;9:389–398.
2. Dehner LP. Gonadal and extragonadal germ cell neoplasia of childhood. Hum Pathol 1983;14:493–511.
3. Billmire DF, Grosfeld JL. Teratomas in childhood: analysis of 142 cases. J Pediatr Surg 1986;21:548–551.
4. Schey WL, Shkolnik A, White H. Clinical and radiographic considerations of sacrococcygeal teratomas: an analysis of 26 new cases and review of the literature. Radiology 1977;125:189–195.

accidental trauma. A hydrocele may be present, leading to earlier detection of a clinical mass than would otherwise occur. Ovarian teratomas are usually found as an incidental mass and are, therefore, frequently large at the time of diagnosis.[4,5] Pain can occur. The causes of pain include torsion, hemorrhage within the tumor, or compression of adjacent structures. Retroperitoneal teratomas may be found as an incidental mass.[6] They can cause pain. They may present with signs of bowel compression and obstruction and have occasionally caused hypertension from kidney compression.[7] Gastric teratomas will cause feeding difficulty; a mass may be detected. Occasionally, these patients may present with bleeding.[8] Vaginal tumors present with a prolapsing vulvar mass, bleeding, or discharge.[9] In the mediastinum, the tumors are often very large at the time of diagnosis and grow very quickly. They may occasionally be an incidental finding on a chest radiograph but frequently will cause respiratory distress, dyspnea, wheezing, or evidence of vessel obstruction.[10–13] Rarely they may cause hemoptysis because of bronchial erosion.[14]

References

1. Bond SJ, Harrison MR, Schmidt KG, et al. Death due to high-output cardiac failure in fetal sacrococcygeal teratoma. J Pediatr Surg 1990;25:1287–1291.
2. Malone PS, Duffy PG, Ransley PG. Urinary tract obstruction secondary to presacral teratoma: a missed diagnosis. J Urol 1989;142:1047–1049.
3. Kaplan GW, Cromie WC, Kelalis PP, et al. Prepubertal yolk sac testicular tumors—report of the testicular tumor registry. J Urol 1988;140:1109–1112.
4. Siegel MJ, McAlister WH, Shackelford GD. Radiographic findings in ovarian teratomas in children. AJR 1978;131:613–616.
5. Calame JJ, Schaberg A. Solid teratomas and mixed mullerian tumors of the ovary: a clinical, histological, and immunocytochemical comparative study. Gynecol Oncol 1989;33:212–221.
6. Davidson AJ, Hartman DS, Goldman SM. Mature teratoma of the retroperitoneum: radiologic, pathologic, and clinical correlation. Radiology 1989;172:421–425.
7. Schey WL, Vesely JJ, Radkowski MA. Shard-like calcifications in retroperitoneal teratomas. Pediatr Radiol 1986;16:82–84.
8. Bowen B, Ros PR, McCarthy MJ, et al. Gastrointestinal teratomas: CT and US appearance with pathologic correlation. Radiology 1987;162:431–433.
9. Collins HS, Burke TW, Heller PB, et al. Endodermal sinus tumor of the infant vagina treated exclusively by chemotherapy. Obstet Gynecol 1989;73:507–509.
10. Kenny JB, Carty HML. Infants presenting with respiratory distress due to anterior mediastinal teratomas: a report of three cases and a review of the literature. Br J Radiol 1988;61:241–244.
11. Filler RM, Simpson JS, Ein SH. Mediastinal masses in infants and children. Pediatr Clin N Am 1979;26:677–690.
12. Grosfeld JL, Ballantine TVN, Lowe D, et al. Benign and malignant teratomas in children: analysis of 85 patients. Surgery 1976;80:297–305.
13. Sham JST, Chiu CSW, Lau WH, et al. Experience with the management of primary endodermal sinus tumor of the mediastinum. Cancer 1989;64:756–761.
14. Robertson JM, Fee HJ, Mulder DG. Mediastinal teratoma causing life-threatening hemoptysis. Am J Dis Child 1981;135:148–150.

Imaging Studies

SPECIFIC IMAGING MODALITIES

A wide variety of different imaging modalities may be used to evaluate patients with germ cell tumors. The intensity of investigation and the choice of modality will vary from site to site. However, a few general comments can be made about the various modalities. In some areas, no imaging of the primary tumor will be performed. This is particularly true of the testicle and many of these lesions have traditionally been resected without any imaging. This is probably an incorrect approach and ultrasound should be utilized for initial evaluation of all testicular masses to distinguish solid or partially solid tumors from simple fluid collection such as hydrocele. It must, however, be conceded that this differentiation can frequently be made clinically.

Plain Film Radiograph. A plain film radiograph will be performed in most patients with germ cell tumor. It is not particularly helpful. In many patients, it may be normal. Signs of displacement and compression of adjacent structures may be seen and evidence of bone abnormality will very occasionally be identified. The primary mass lesion is most likely to be identified in the chest but not when it is very small (Figs. 9–26, 9–27, 9–28, and 9–29). In the chest, pleural effusions may also be seen. In the very young infant, errors in diagnosis may occur in the chest. For example, in 3 babies with anterior mediastinal teratomas, the diagnosis on the chest radiograph was initially missed in 2 of the 3 patients. The teratoma was misdiagnosed as a normal but prominent thymus.[1] In older children, this is not a problem.[2] The most common abnormality seen on plain film

Figure 9–26. **Diagnosis: Mediastinal teratoma.**
2-year-old presenting with wheeze. *A* and *B,* AP and lateral chest radiographs. There is a very large right-sided mass filling most of the hemithorax. The underlying lung is completely collapsed and this accounts for the limited mediastinal shift. *C,* Ultrasound. This shows the main component of the tumor to be predominantly cystic. The cystic fluid does contain a few echoes. *D* and *E,* MR, T1 weighted axial and coronal images. These show the massive tumor filling most of the right hemithorax. The tumor is predominantly homogeneous mottled low signal from the cyst containing debris. *F,* MR, T2 weighted axial image. Most of the lesion is very bright because of the fluid within it. Some anterior parts of the lesion are not quite as bright, and these represent the more solid components of the tumor. At surgery the lesion was found to be well encapsulated and was completely excised. It was a benign teratoma.

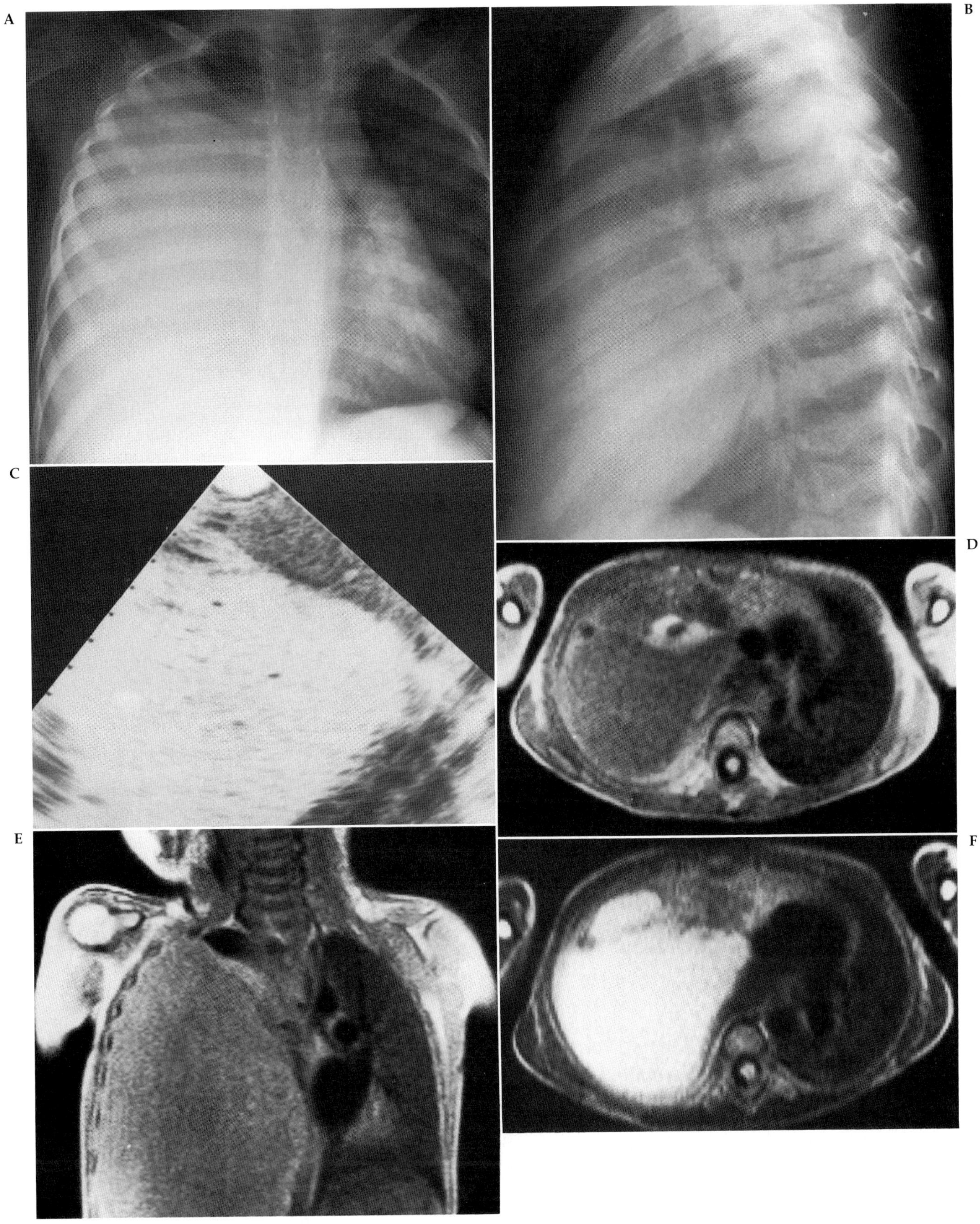
A
B
C
D
E
F

A B C D E F

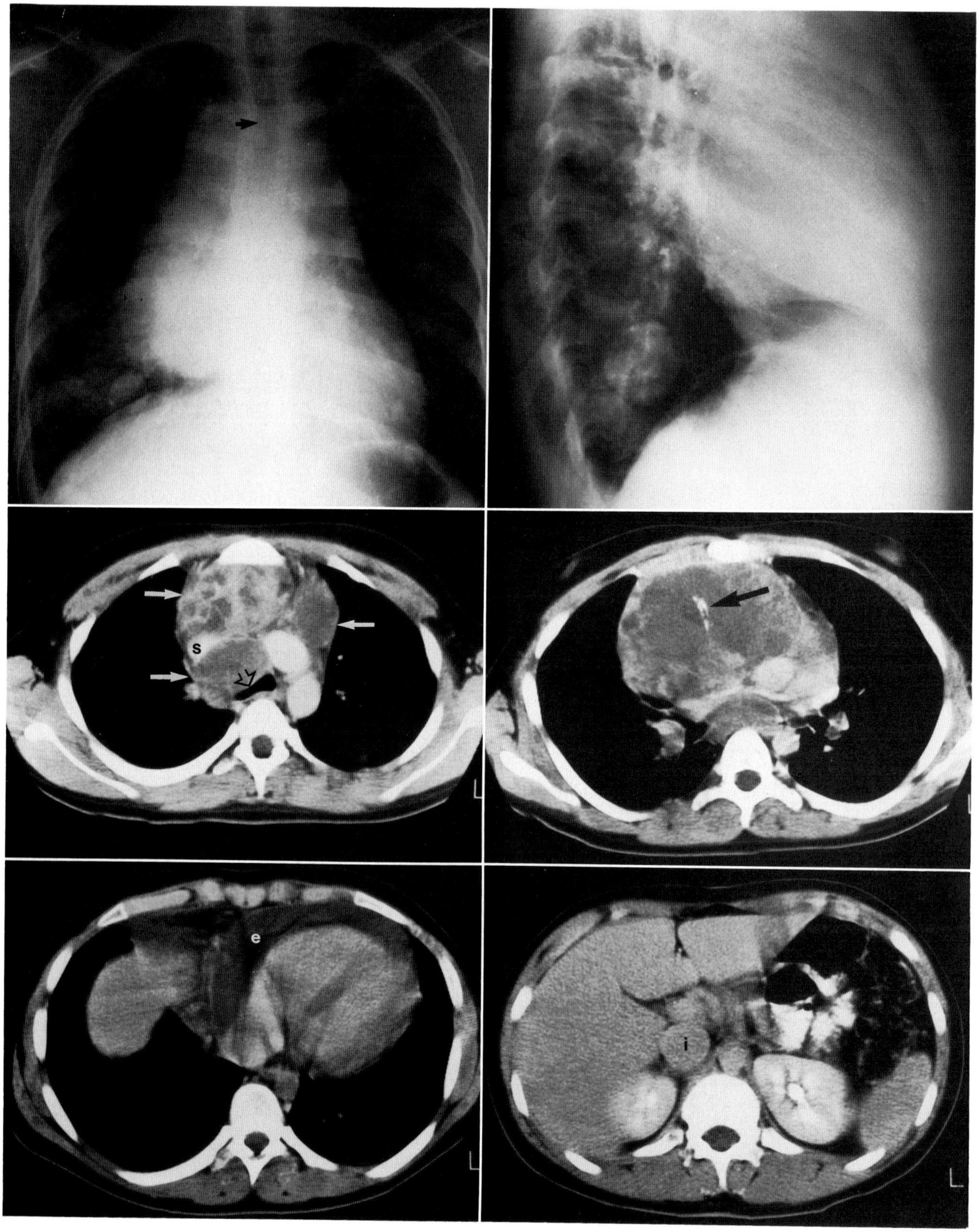

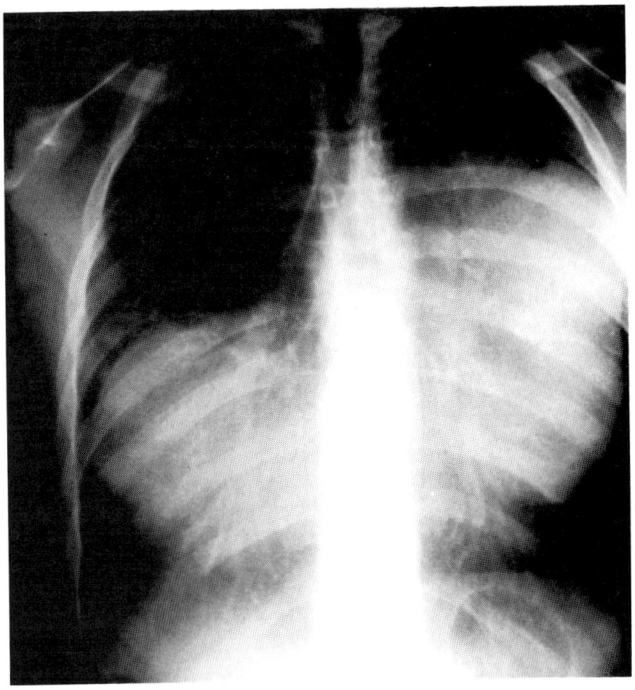

Figure 9-28. **Diagnosis: Mediastinal yolk sac tumor. Chest radiograph. There is a massive mediastinal tumor that involves the left mid and right lower thorax. There are no specific features on the plain film radiograph to suggest the correct diagnosis.**

radiograph is calcification. In some small series, calcification was not identified in any patients.[1,2] In other series, the incidence of calcification detected on plain films has ranged from 30 percent of mediastinal teratomas,[3] 35 percent of teratomas,[4] 34 percent of 118 sacrococcygeal teratomas,[5] 40 percent of mediastinal teratomas,[6] 68 percent of 23 ovarian teratomas in children,[7] 70 percent of ovarian teratomas,[6] and 85 percent of retroperitoneal teratomas.[6] The appearance of the calcification is usually nonspecific and the differential diagnosis will include a wide range of pathologies in which calcium can be identified. Occasionally, the calcification in retroperitoneal teratomas will have pathognomonic dense sheetlike appearance with sharp margins.[8] In other patients, the calcification will take the form of clearly defined teeth or bone segments and again the appearance is usually pathognomonic for teratoma.[7]

Ultrasound. Ultrasound is widely recommended as the initial investigation of choice for children with abdominal tumors (Figs. 9–30 and 9–31). It has many significant drawbacks in the evaluation of germ cell tumors and, particularly in the pelvis, where germ cell tumors are most common and where benign cystic masses are less common than in the upper abdomen, it might be argued that ultrasound need not be performed. My reason for this statement is that regardless of the findings on ultrasound, CT will be performed in all cases and the CT will be expected to provide more information than the ultrasound. While ultrasound will almost always detect the tumor mass, it cannot identify specific features that are so helpful in making the diagnosis of germ cell tumor on the imaging study.

First, ultrasound cannot detect fat.[9,10] This is because fat has a very variable appearance on ultrasound. The echogenicity of fat ranges from very low to very high, and in no patient can fat be accurately characterized. Second, ultrasound will miss areas of calcification. Large or moderately large regions of calcium will be identified on ultrasound by their high echogenic appearance and distal shadowing. In all studies, however, when ultrasound is compared with CT, it is inferior for calcium detection. For example, in one study, it missed calcium in 3 of 17 patients in whom it was seen on CT.[11] In another study, it missed calcification in 4 patients.[12] Third, nodules of tumor projecting into the lumen of cystic filled spaces are not as clearly seen with ultrasound as with CT.[11,12] In a recent study using state-of-the-art ultrasound equipment, mural nodules, compared to pathology, were missed in 10 of 17 patients by ultrasound[11] (Fig. 9–31). This problem is worse in children than in adults. In an ultrasound study diagnosing ovarian teratomas, the diagnostic features in prepubertal girls were compared with those in postpubertal people. In the 17 patients studied, mural nodules and areas of shadowing were much less commonly identified in the prepubertal girls. In addition, more of the prepubertal girls had an absence of cystic areas in the teratoma.[11]

CT. CT, by contrast with ultrasound, is excellent in identification of those features that characterize many of the germ cell tumors. These are areas of cysts, calcification, and the presence of fat (Figs. 9–24, 9–27, 9–30, 9–32, and 9–33). All can be well identified and accurately characterized with CT. With regard to CT technique, it is most helpful for accurate identification of calcium to scan the tumor initially without administration of intravenous contrast. Slice thickness should vary between 5 and 10 mm depending on the anatomic lo-

Figure 9-27. **Diagnosis: Mediastinal yolk sac tumor.**
***A* and *B,* AP and lateral chest radiograph. There is a large right-sided mediastinal tumor. It is compressing and indenting the trachea *(arrow)*. *C,* CT. There is a very large mediastinal mass involving the anterior and mid mediastinum *(arrows)*. It is compressing the origin of the right main stem bronchus *(open arrow)*. It completely encases the superior vena cava (*S*), which is narrowed but patent. *D,* More inferior CT image. Large areas of low intensity within the tumor are evidence of fat. A small focus of calcification is well defined *(arrow)*. *E,* The tumor has invaded the pericardium and is causing an extensive pericardial effusion (*E*). This is obstructing venous return from the superior vena cava. *F,* CT through the upper abdomen. The inferior vena cava (*I*) is markedly distended because of obstruction from the pericardial effusion.**

A

B

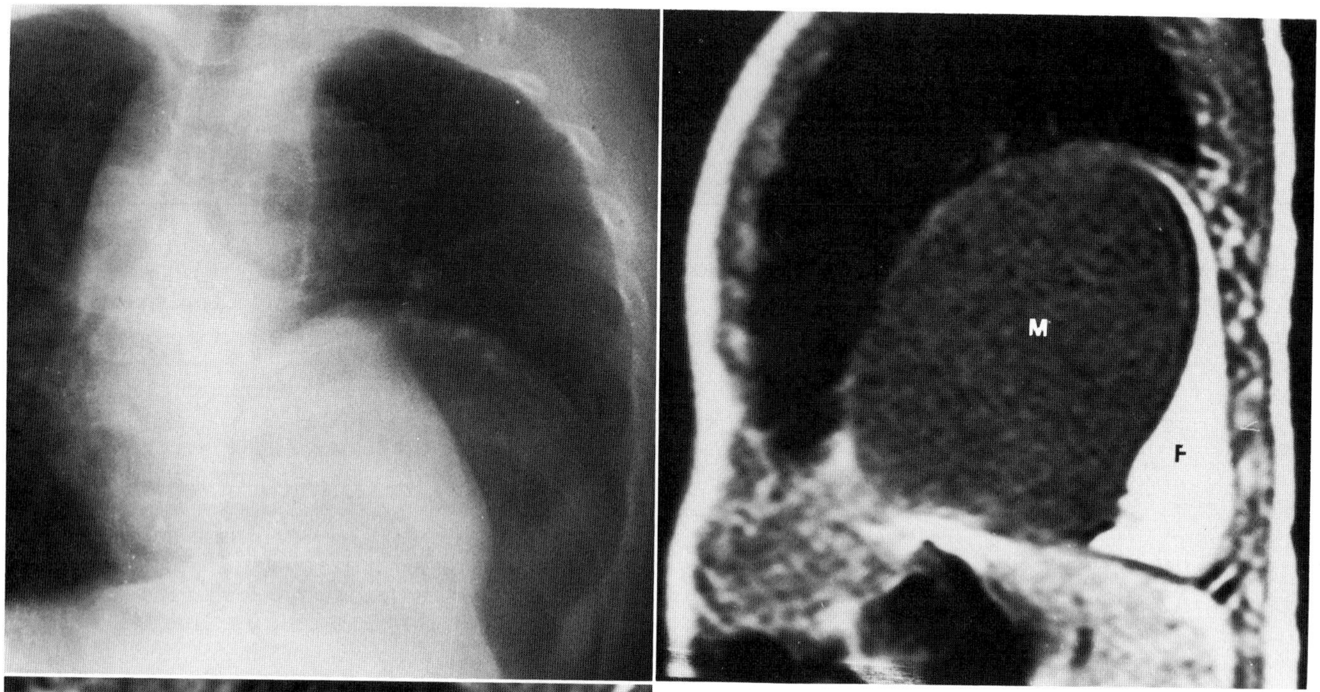

C

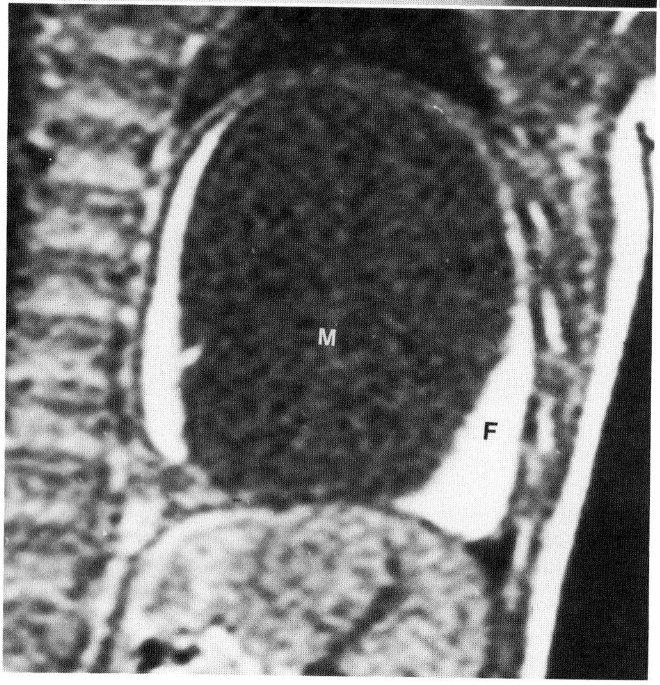

Figure 9-29. **Diagnosis: Posterior mediastinal teratoma. *A,* Chest radiograph. There is a large mass behind the heart. The ribs appear normal. No calcification is seen within the mass. *B* and *C,* Axial and coronal T1 weighted MR images. Most of the mass (*M*) is of low intensity compatible with fluid. There is surrounding bright signal from fat (*F*), which suggests the correct diagnosis of teratoma. (From Shapiro CR, Abramson SJ, Berdon WE. Posterior mediastinal cystic teratoma surrounded by fat. Pediatr Radiol 1989;20:107–109.)**

cation and the overall size of the tumor. Direct coronal or sagittal imaging is easily performed in very young infants. This technique is frequently forgotton but is particularly helpful in some patients, particularly in regard to defining the spread of sacrococcygeal tumor into the pelvis and abdomen.[13]

As has been mentioned, CT has consistently been found to be superior to ultrasound for the characterization of most germ cell tumors.[9,12] In addition to the above-described features of germ cell tumors, occasionally a fluid fluid level can be identified by CT. It is also, but less often, seen on ultrasound. This is because of layering of semisolid fat on other fluids. CT provides all that is needed of an imaging modality. It defines the extent of the tumor, monitors response to therapy, and can be used for detection of recurrence. In regard to recurrence, the appearance on CT may occasionally be confusing. In one study of 14 patients, enlarging masses were identified while the patients were on chemotherapy. In none of these patients did the serum concentration of alpha-fetoprotein rise. The sites of the lesions were in the chest and retroperitoneum. At surgery the

A B C

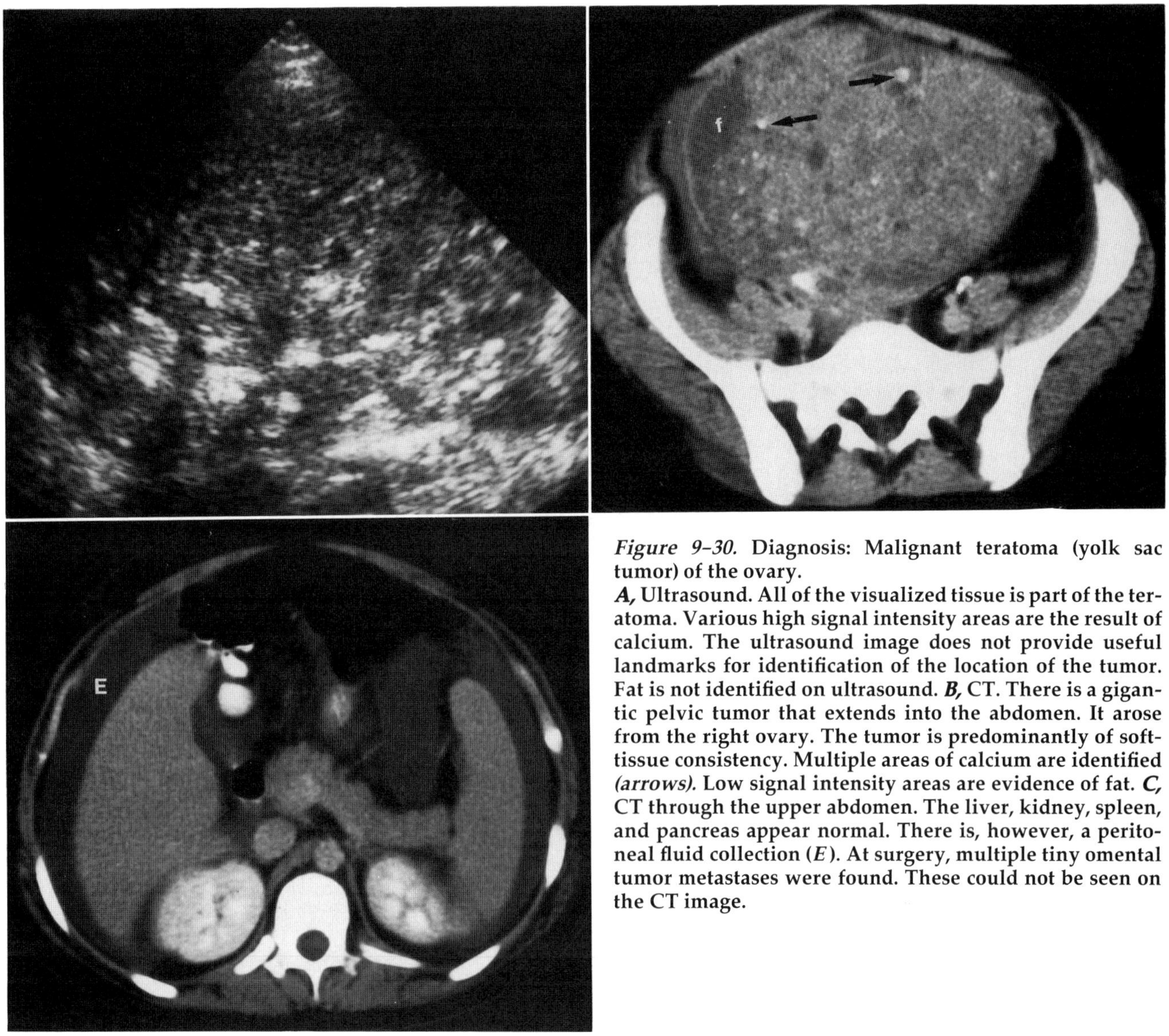

Figure 9–30. **Diagnosis: Malignant teratoma (yolk sac tumor) of the ovary.**
A, **Ultrasound. All of the visualized tissue is part of the teratoma. Various high signal intensity areas are the result of calcium. The ultrasound image does not provide useful landmarks for identification of the location of the tumor. Fat is not identified on ultrasound.** ***B,*** **CT. There is a gigantic pelvic tumor that extends into the abdomen. It arose from the right ovary. The tumor is predominantly of soft-tissue consistency. Multiple areas of calcium are identified** ***(arrows).*** **Low signal intensity areas are evidence of fat.** ***C,*** **CT through the upper abdomen. The liver, kidney, spleen, and pancreas appear normal. There is, however, a peritoneal fluid collection (*E*). At surgery, multiple tiny omental tumor metastases were found. These could not be seen on the CT image.**

enlarging lesions were all found to be benign and mature teratomas in the site of previous malignant germ cell tumors.[14] The study again stresses the importance and value of using estimations of alpha-fetoprotein concentrations in the blood in following up patients with malignant germ cell tumors. It should be stressed that the features of calcification, cysts, and fat will only be found in teratomas and not other germ cell tumors. Pure yolk sac tumors appear as nonspecific soft-tissue mass lesions. It is important to remember, however, that a significant percentage of yolk sac tumors are found as a portion or segment of a larger teratoma.

> *Comment:* CT is at present the major modality for imaging germ cell tumors.

MR. MR has also been utilized to evaluate patients with germ cell tumors[15–17] (Figs. 9–32, 9–33, 9–34, and 9–35). There is good correlation between the findings seen on CT and those identified on MR.[17] There are no large series comparing MR and CT. MR will be less accurate than CT for the identification of small to moderate-sized areas of calcification. In most patients, MR will accurately characterize fluid and fat. Although never reported, I would anticipate that occasionally difficulties may be encountered in misdiagnosing regions of hemorrhage as fat. This is because both fat and blood of intermediate age can have high signal intensity on T1 weighted images. In these patients, it will be critical for both T1 and T2 weighted MR images to be obtained in the same imaging plane so that specific focal areas of the tumor can be compared from one image to the other. In

A

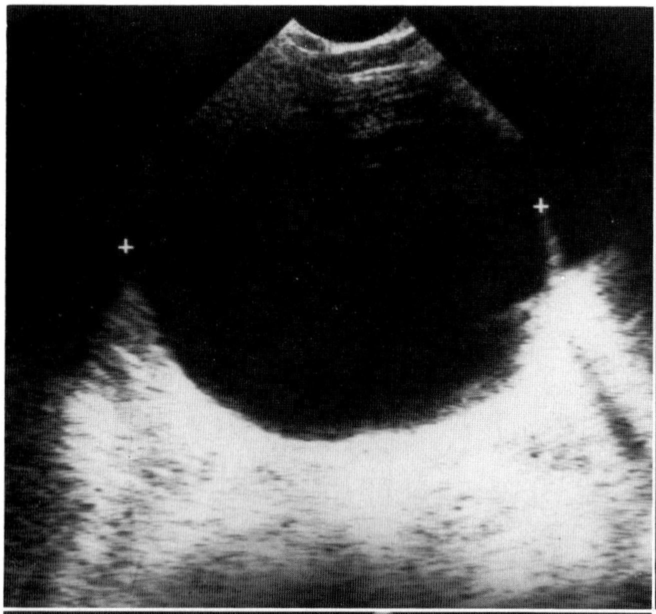

B

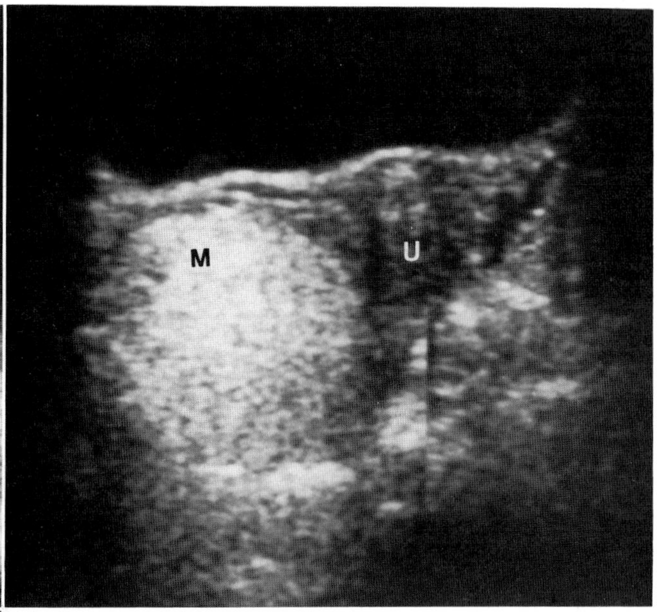

C

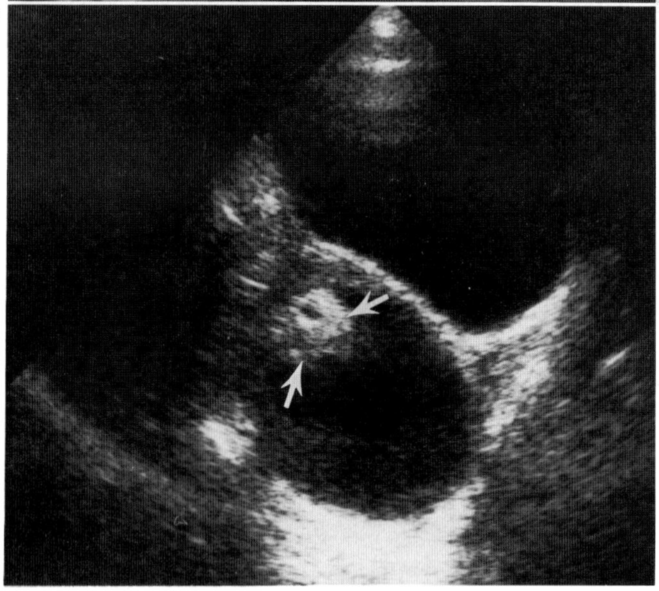

Figure 9–31. **Diagnosis: Ovarian teratoma. Three different cases.**
Ultrasound findings. *A,* 10-year-old girl. Transverse sonogram shows a large anechoic mass with a very thin wall. The tumor was almost completely cystic. *B,* Solid teratoma in a 15-year-old girl. Transverse sonogram of the pelvis shows an echogenic mass (*M*). It is inseparable from the right ovary. *U* = uterus. *C,* Complex teratoma with a mural nodule in an 11-year-old girl. Longitudinal sonogram through the left adnexa shows a complex mass with an echogenic mural component *(arrows)* in the wall. A portion of the left adnexa was seen at pathologic examination. (From Sisler CL, Siegel MJ. Ovarian teratomas. A comparison of the sonographic appearance in prepubertal and postpubertal girls. AJR 1990;154:139–141.)

this way, errors regarding characterization of tissue based on their signal intensity will be minimized. On the MR images, fluid will have a low signal intensity on T1 and a very high signal intensity, greater than fat, on T2 weighted images. Soft-tissue components of the tumor will be similar to, greater, or less than muscle on T1 weighted images, and show increase in signal intensity, but below that of fat, on T2 weighted images. Fat will in general appear of bright signal on T1 and T2 weighted images. The signal intensity from the fat will vary, however, depending on whether the fat is solid or fluid and also depending on whether the fat is mixed with other tissues (e.g., hair and soft tissue) or whether it is uniform fat. Areas of calcification will be of low signal on T1 and T2 weighted images. Blood, as mentioned above, will have a variable appearance depending on its age. In most patients, I would anticipate CT and MR as being somewhat complementary, with CT having a distinct advantage in those patients in whom the plain film radiograph has not previously identified calcification in the tumor. In a few patients, MR will be expected to offer distinct advantages. For example, in the detection of invasion of the spinal canal with sacrococcygeal teratoma (this is rare) or in defining the operability of large tumors, particularly their relationship to major adjacent vessels.

Angiography. Angiography has no place in the routine evaluation of germ cell tumors. It has, however, previously been utilized. Reported studies indicate that most of these tumors are very vascular. At one time angiography was utilized to define the vascular supply to sacrococcygeal teratomas.[18] These tumors have a varied

A

B

C

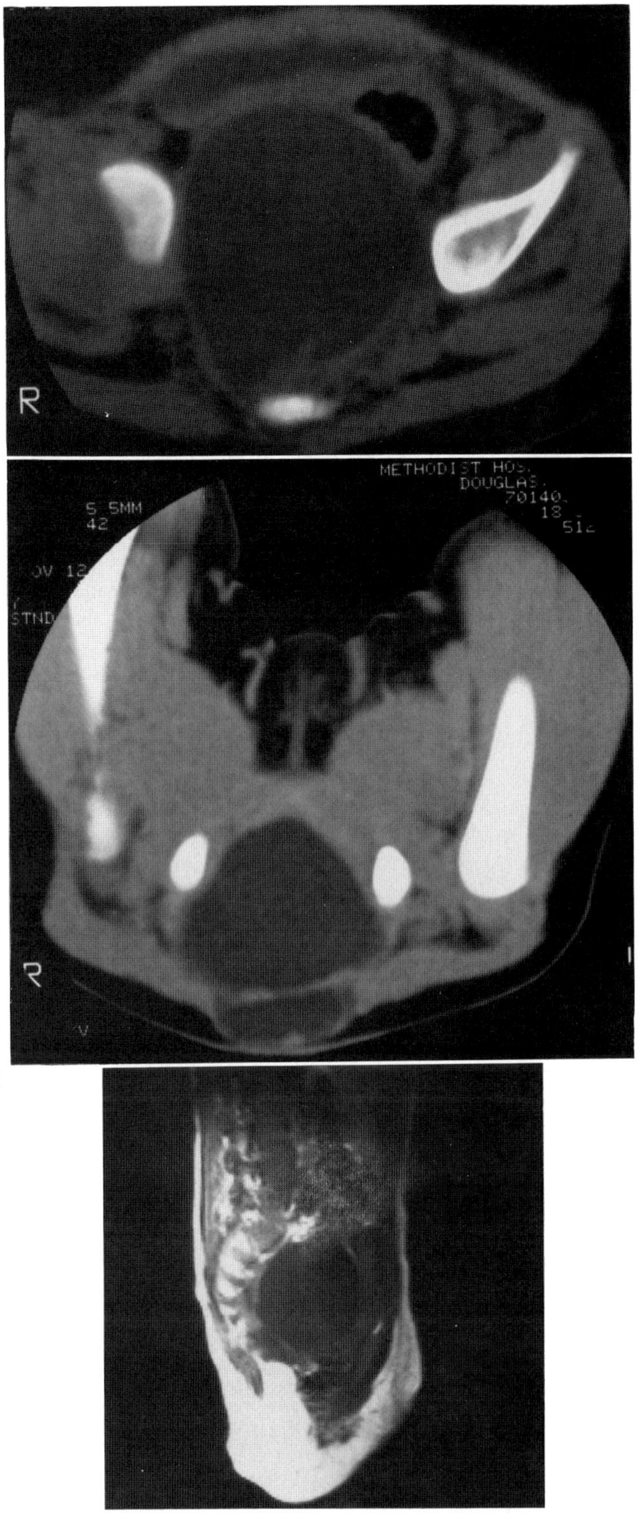

Figure 9-32. **Diagnosis: Sacrococcygeal teratoma with yolk sac tumor.**
A **and** ***B,*** **CT scan at birth. There is a large almost cystic mass that extends around the coccyx. This was not completely excised.** ***C,*** **MR sagittal T1 weighted image 6 months later. There is a recurrent mass anterior to the sacrum. It has a large cyst with a smaller soft-tissue component between the cyst and the sacrum. This contained elements of mature teratoma and yolk sac tumor.**

blood supply from the internal iliac, femoral, and middle sacral arteries. They are all very vascular and all have arteriovenous shunts within them.[18] Angiography does not play a role in the evaluation of these patients at the present time.

> *Comment:* No imaging modality can predict the likelihood of malignancy in a germ cell tumor. The most accurate nonhistologic way of predicting malignancy is by demonstrating elevated blood concentrations of alpha-fetoprotein.

IMAGING BY ANATOMIC SITE

Sacrococcygeal Teratoma. Sacrococcygeal teratomas, with the exception of pure presacral tumors, are readily apparent at birth. They may occasionally be confused with very low-lying meningomyeloceles and rarely in one patient with a meconium pseudocyst penetrating beyond the buttock.[19] Imaging can easily differentiate these disorders (Fig. 9–36). On ultrasound or CT, the lesions are large. Cystic areas can be identified in them (see Fig 9–32). In one study of 5 patients, CT identified cysts in all, fat in 3 of 5, and calcium in 3 of 5. CT, ultrasound, or MR can all be utilized to evaluate the spread into the pelvis or the abdomen (see Figs. 9–32, 9–34, and 9–35).

Pictorially, sagittal images obtained with CT or MR are probably of most help to the surgeon. CT will be the best modality for identification of the rare patient in whom bone is invaded. MR would be the modality of choice for identification of the rare patient with spinal canal invasion. The patient with a purely presacral teratoma will be more difficult to evaluate. This may occur as a localized lesion or may be associated as part of a triad with congenital anomalies of the sacrum (especially a scimitar shape), and an anorectal malformation. In patients with this triad, the presacral mass may be a teratoma but it is not always so. It may be a duplication cyst of the rectum or an anterior meningocele. Very occasionally, a teratoma may be found together with an anterior meningocele in association with anorectal malformation and sacral anomalies. Ultrasound can identify a purely cystic lesion such as an anterior meningocele or a rectal duplication cyst. CT can also characterize this finding. It may show characteristic features diagnostic of a teratoma. It can also be utilized to better define the perineal musculature. Accurate characterization of an anterior meningocele may require the injection of subarachnoid water-soluble nonionic contrast. MR, while not as good as CT for characterization of the teratoma, will with sagittal imaging show continuity of an anterior meningomyelocele with the spinal canal without requirement for contrast injection. It will also be excellent for evaluation of the pelvic musculature seen in association with anorectal malformation.

All patients with a sacrococcygeal teratoma and those in whom such a lesion is suspected because of associated sacral and anorectal malformations, should

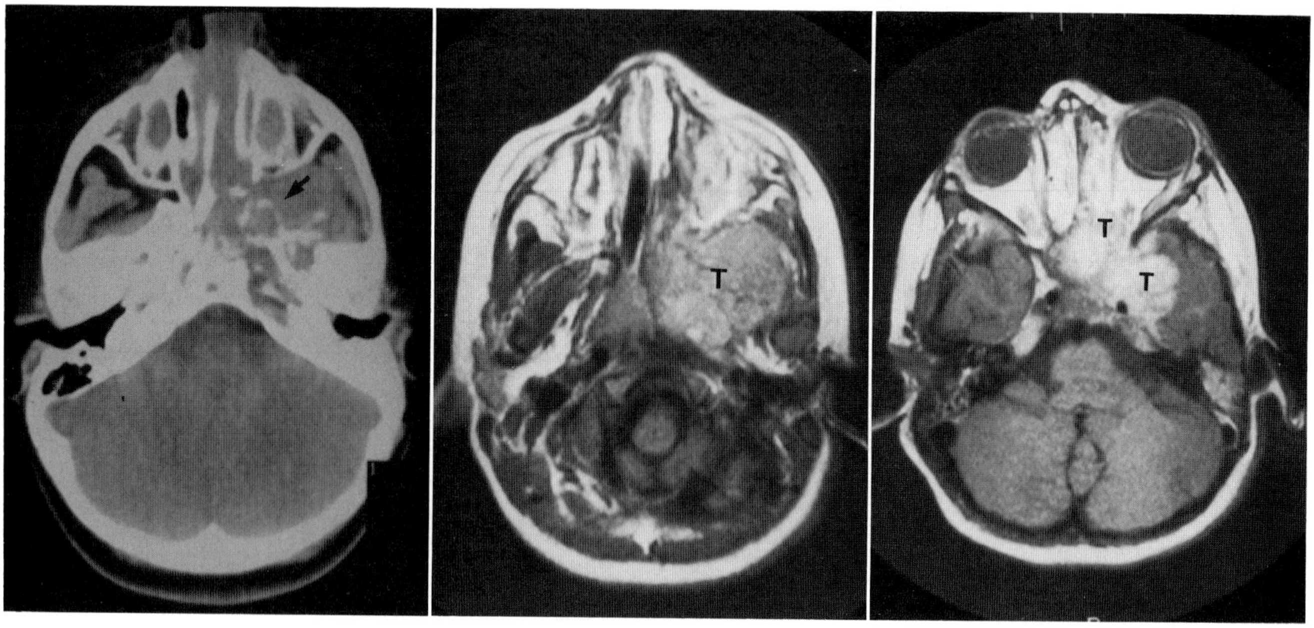

Figure 9–33. **Diagnosis: Yolk sac tumor of the face.**
***A,* CT. There is a large tumor mass involving the nose and roof of the orbit. There is extensive bony destruction *(arrow)* of the base of the skull with invasion of the tumor into the middle fossa. *B* and *C,* MR, T1 weighted images before and after gadolinium-DTPA administration. The images are at different levels. There is a large tumor (*T*) that extends from the nose through the base of the skull into the middle cranial fossa. It enhances with gadolinum-DTPA.**

probably have a CT scan performed. Some might prefer to perform an MR. It should not truly be necessary to perform both studies, except perhaps in very selected patients. The role of ultrasound is limited because of the advantages of the other two modalities. Imaging cannot differentiate benign sacrococcygeal teratomas from those in which some malignant degeneration has occurred (Figs. 9–32 and 9–37).

Testicular Lesions. As mentioned, testicular lesions may not be imaged. Most testicular lesions are pure yolk sac tumors without evidence of teratoma. Imaging will show a mass lesion in relationship to the testis. This should be readily identifiable with ultrasound, CT, or MR. There are no series reported comparing these modalities.

Ovarian Tumors. Most ovarian germ cell tumors are teratomas or are partly teratoma (see Figs. 9–30 and 9–31). CT is excellent in identifying the features that

Figure 9–34. **Diagnosis: Sacrococcygeal teratoma in a newborn.**
MR, sagittal spin density image. The large sacrococcygeal teratoma (*T*) extends from the lower abdomen through the pelvis and below the buttocks.

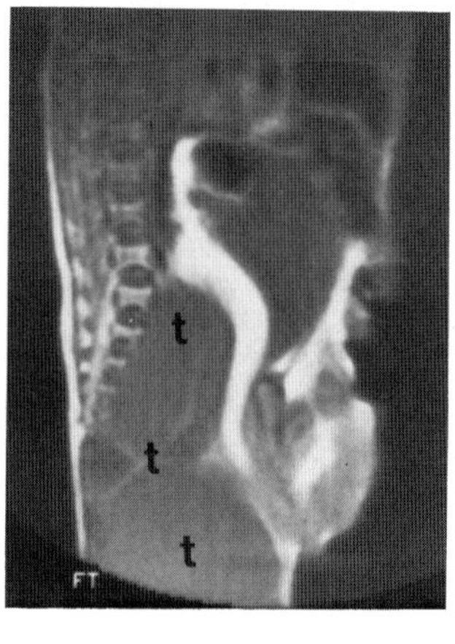

Figure 9–35. **Diagnosis: Perineal yolk sac tumor in a 2-year-old.**
MR, sagittal spin density image. There is a very large bilobed tumor (*T*) that is of moderate signal intensity. Note the close association of the tumor to the coccyx. There are no specific features to suggest the correct diagnosis.

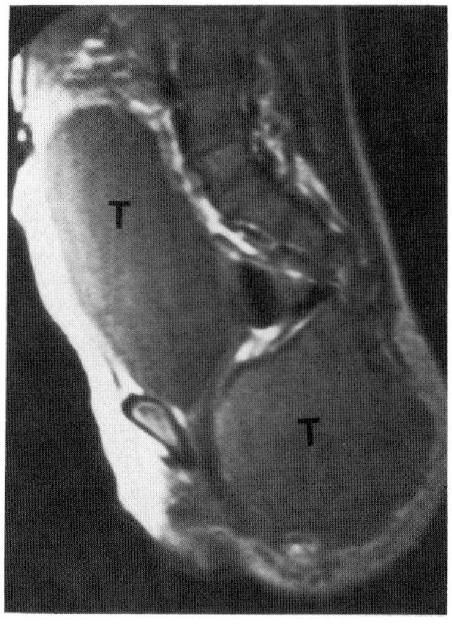

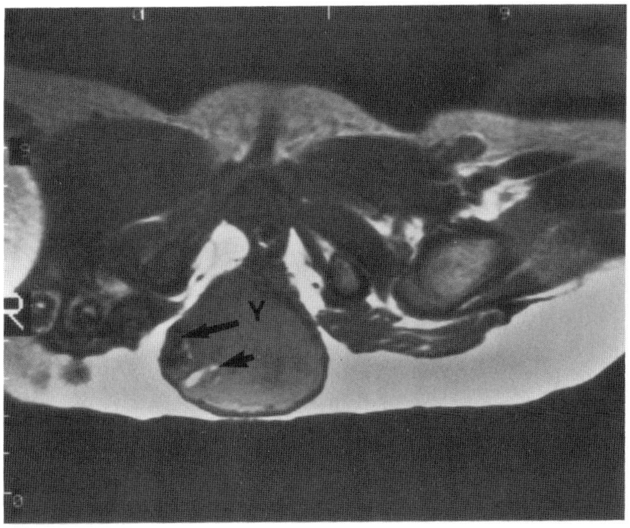

Figure 9-36. **Diagnosis: Yolk sac tumor of the perineum. MR, axial T1 weighted image. The yolk sac tumor (*Y*) is very well defined. It is, in fact, a mixed teratoma with components of yolk sac tumor. Fat *(small arrow)* appears of very bright signal intensity and calcium *(large arrow)* of very low signal intensity. Note that the fat and calcium cannot be characterized with complete confidence, as fluid could cause low signal intensity and hemorrhage high signal intensity with this pulse sequence.**

allow characterization of the tumor. In one study of 40 patients with ovarian teratoma, CT permitted a definitive preoperative diagnosis to be made in 98 percent of these patients. The mean size was 8 cm. All patients had cysts that were unilocular or multilocular. CT identified the tumor in 100 percent of cases, fat in 93 percent, calcification or a tooth in 56 percent, a fat fluid level in 12 percent, and soft-tissue nodules protruding into the cystic spaces in 81 percent. Ultrasound will identify the features seen on CT, but with a diminished accuracy. Imaging cannot identify malignancy, but in some patients, signs suggestive of malignancy may be seen. These signs include marked irregularity of the soft-tissue component of the tumor, penetration of the tumor into the adjacent soft tissues, free peritoneal fluid, and enlarged regional lymph nodes.[9] Some ovaries with tumors will undergo torsion. There is some debate with regard to the accuracy of imaging in defining torsion. Torsion may be suggested by thickening of the wall of the tumor, increased thickness of the Fallopian tube, and the presence of free peritoneal fluid.[9] In a series of young girls presenting with ovarian torsion, ultrasound was not able to differentiate those ovaries that were normal but had torsion from those ovaries that contained a teratoma and underwent torsion.[20] One important but often overlooked fact is that the ovary is frequently an intra-abdominal organ. In 9 of 23 children, ovarian teratomas were located in the abdomen and not in the pelvis,[7] so that an ovarian teratoma, particularly in very young children, should be part of the differential diagnosis of all abdominal mass lesions.

Teratomas of the Abdomen and Retroperitoneum. In the abdomen and retroperitoneum, teratomas are well seen with CT[21,22] (Fig. 9–38). In one study of 23 children with benign retroperitoneal teratomas, CT accurately identified a complex mass lesion in 100 percent, fluid in all of the tumors, fat in 61 percent, calcification in 70 percent, and soft-tissue protrusions into the cysts in 50 percent.

Figure 9-37. **Diagnosis: Gluteal adenocarcinoma in a recurrent teratoma. 2-year-old child with previous sacrococcygeal teratoma. CT. There is a large gluteal soft-tissue mass *(arrows)* that is completely nonspecific in appearance.**

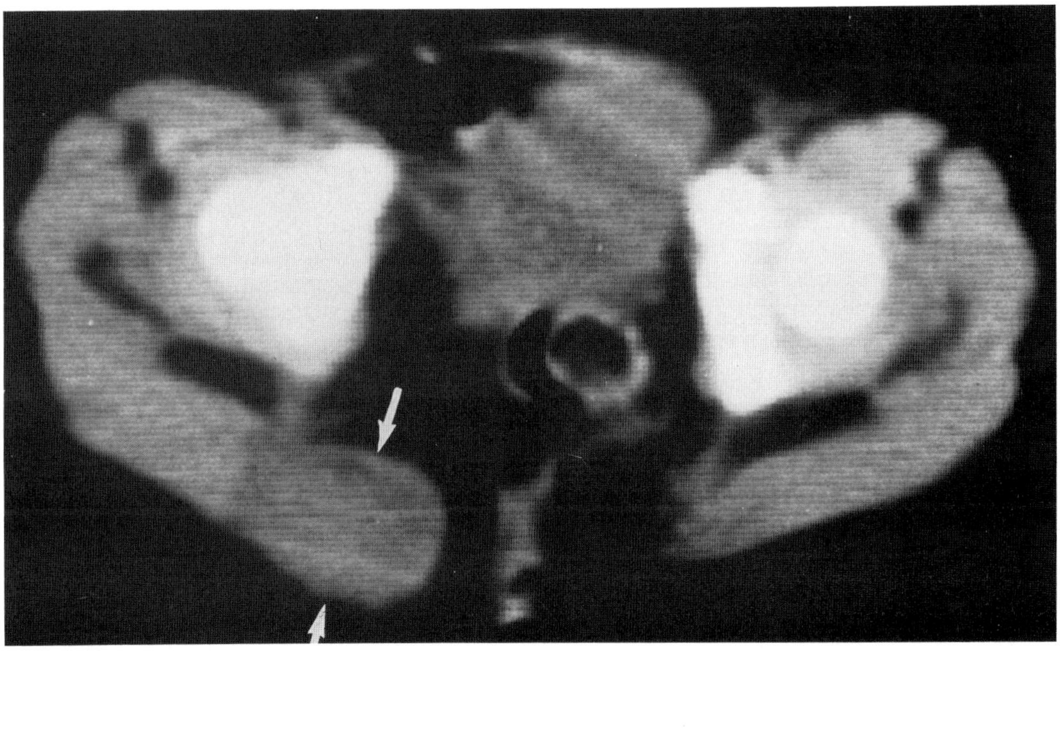

A B C

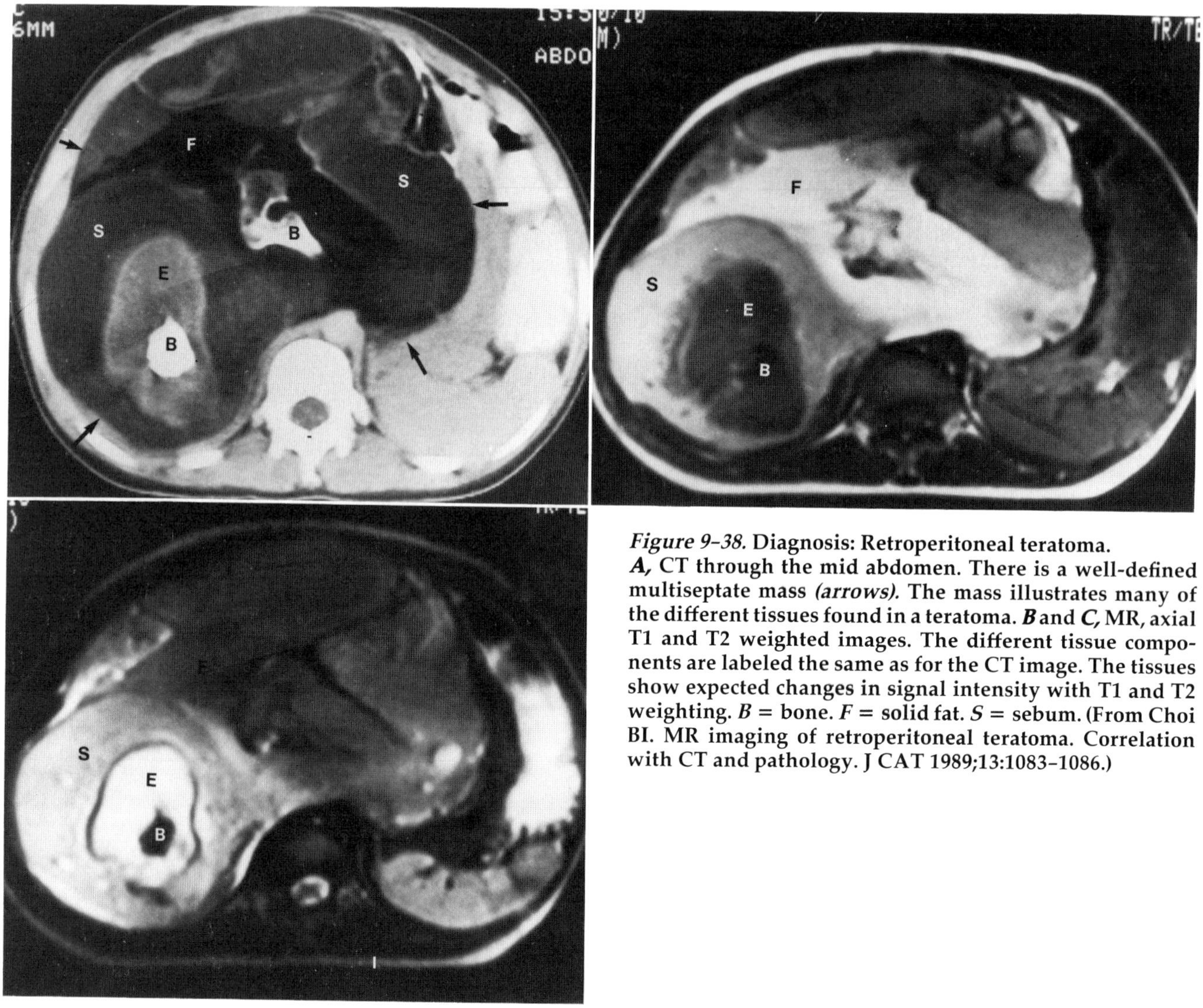

Figure 9–38. **Diagnosis: Retroperitoneal teratoma. *A,* CT through the mid abdomen. There is a well-defined multiseptate mass *(arrows).* The mass illustrates many of the different tissues found in a teratoma. *B* and *C,* MR, axial T1 and T2 weighted images. The different tissue components are labeled the same as for the CT image. The tissues show expected changes in signal intensity with T1 and T2 weighting. *B* = bone. *F* = solid fat. *S* = sebum. (From Choi BI. MR imaging of retroperitoneal teratoma. Correlation with CT and pathology. J CAT 1989;13:1083–1086.)**

All the lesions had sharp margins with patchy enhancement following intravenous contrast. Similar findings were obtained in another study of 5 patients.[21] Ultrasound has also been utilized to diagnose abdominal and retroperitoneal teratomas.[8,21,23] These tumors can occur in any site in the abdomen. If calcium, fat, and fluid are identified, the specific diagnosis is easy, but the precise organ of origin may not be clearly evident. Gastric teratoma might be suggested by clinical symptoms of feeding difficulty. Barium study or CT contrast study will show a filling defect in the stomach. These lesions usually have a large exophytic soft-tissue component.[21,24] Other abdominal teratomas, such as those arising in the mesentery, have no specific features to identify the precise location of origin.

Mediastinal Teratomas. Mediastinal teratomas usually occur in the anterior mediastinum[25–27] (see Figs. 9–26, 9–27, and 9–28). They are usually very large at the time of diagnosis, contain calcium, and may have large areas of necrosis.[25,26] In one series of 5 patients,[28] calcium was present in only 2 patients and fat in none. All the tumors were nonhomogeneous on CT with irregular enhancement. The malignant tumors may be extensively locally invasive with penetration into the intercostal muscles and infiltration of the mediastinal structures, and may cause pleural or even pericardial effusions[28] (see Fig. 9–27). In the young infants in whom there is difficulty in differentiating a teratoma from an enlarged thymus on the chest radiograph, ultrasound provides a very quick and simple method of differentiating these structures (see Fig. 9–26). Thymus will have a uniformly normal echogenicity. The teratomas will show areas of fluid and in many cases can be identified separate from the thymus. Although it is generally accepted that mediastinal teratomas occur in the anterior mediastinum, they can occasionally be located in the posterior mediastinum (Figs. 9–26 and 9–29). In two reported patients,[24,29] they were located on the left side behind the heart. In one patient, there was only a single large cyst with no calcification. The diagnosis was suggested by the identification of a thin rim of fatty tissue seen on MR (Fig. 9–29). This was present only in retrospect on the CT scan.[15] In the anterior mediastinum, the pattern of calcification may occasionally be helpful in differentiating teratoma from thymoma. In the latter, the calcification characteristically has an eggshell appearance, which is not seen with germ cell tumor.

Germ cell tumors may occur in other locations. In the face, teratomas are sometimes seen in the region of the nose (see Fig. 9–33). These lesions can be large and deforming and the differential diagnosis would include an encephalocele. With an encephalocele fluid in the lesion will be of similar intensity to that in cerebrospinal fluid and a defect in the base of the skull will usually be identifiable. Orbital teratomas have been described in two newborns[30] (Fig. 9–39). These tumors were large and caused extreme proptosis. They contain calcium, fat, and cysts and can be easily diagnosed with CT. Despite their very large size, they do not cause bone destruction nor do they have any intracranial spread.[30] Intracranial teratomas are most commonly suprasellar or pineal in location (Fig. 9–40).

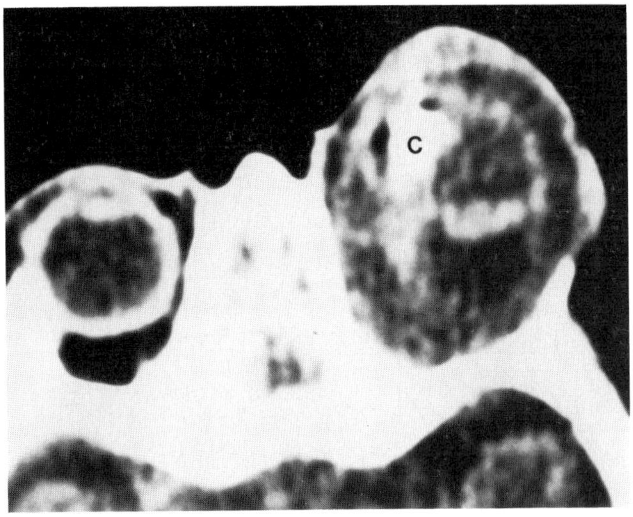

Figure 9–39. **Diagnosis: Orbital teratoma in a newborn. CT. There is a large mass occupying most of the left orbit and displacing the eye forward. Calcium (*C*) is identified in the mass. The boundaries of the lesion are poorly defined. (From Weiss A. Primary and secondary orbital teratomas. J Pediatr Ophthalmol 1989;26:44–49.)**

IMAGING OF METASTASES

Metastases do not play a critical role in germ cell tumors. This is unlike other tumors, such as Wilms tumor, neuroblastoma, rhabdomyosarcoma, or primary bone tumors, for which a great deal of time and effort is ex-

Figure 9–40. **Diagnosis: Suprasellar germinoma.**
A, **CT noncontrast scan. There is a high-density mass lesion *(arrows)* in the suprasellar area. *B,* CT after contrast. The mass lesion shows homogeneous intense enhancement *(arrows).* (From Chang T. CT of pineal and intracranial germ cell tumors. AJNR 1989;10:1039–1044.)**

A

B

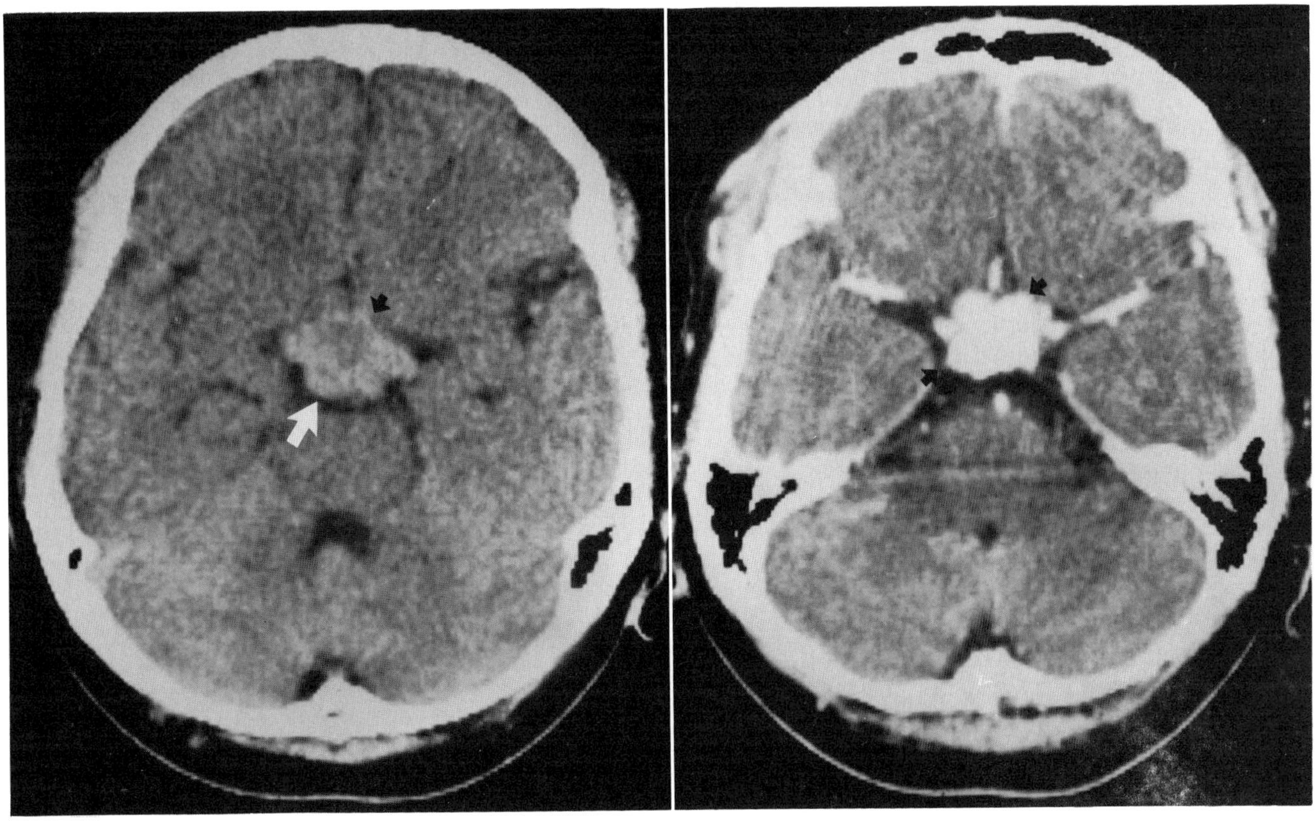

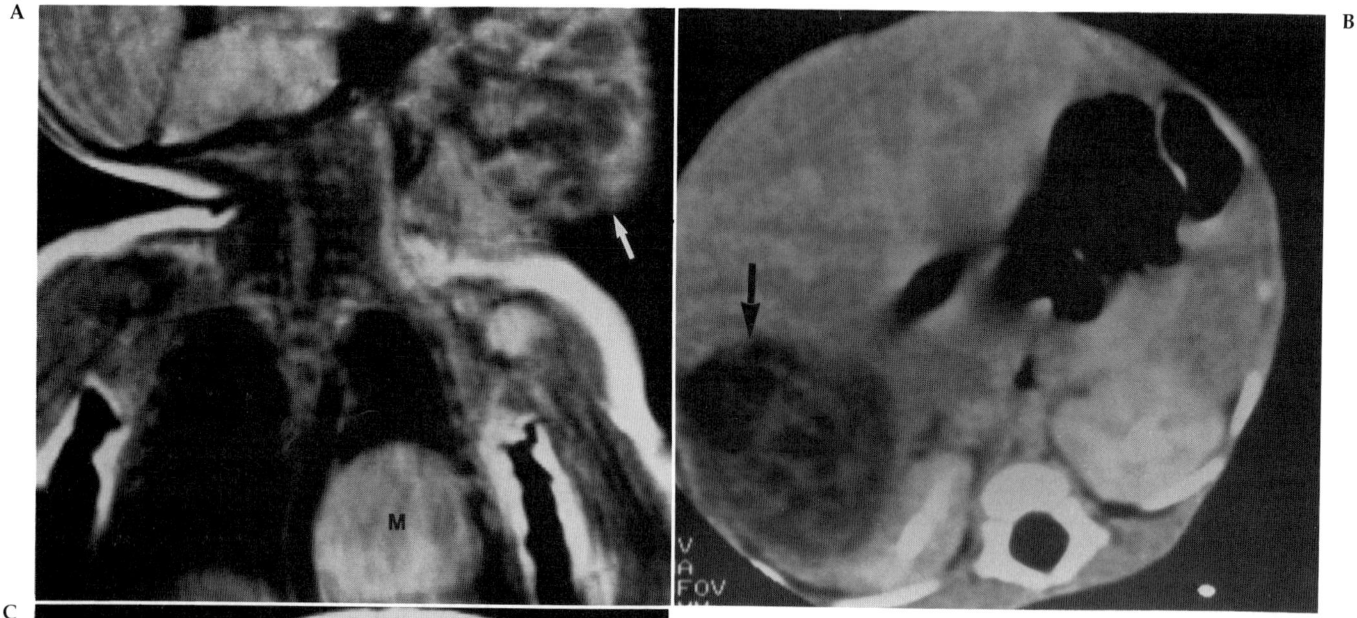

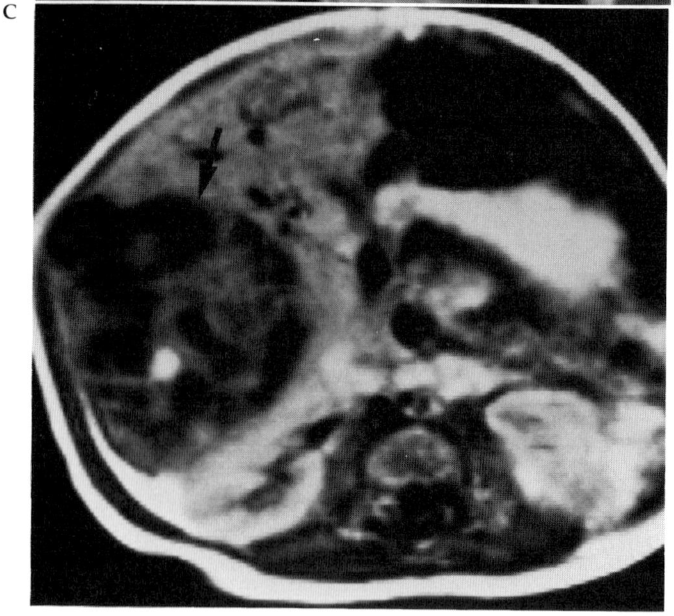

Figure 9–41. Diagnosis: Teratoma with metastases to lung and liver. Newborn infant.
A, Coronal MR image. There is a large neck primary malignant teratoma *(arrow).* There is a large metastasis (*M*) to the left lung. ***B,*** CT of liver. There is a large metastatic lesion in the right lobe of the liver *(arrow).* ***C,*** Axial MR 3 weeks later. There is marked increase in size of the metastatic lesion in the right lobe of the liver *(arrow).* (From Touran T, Applebaum H, et al. Congenital metastatic cervical teratoma. J Pediatr Surg 1989;24:21–23.)

pended in seeking metastases and the results of whose investigations are of critical importance. There are a number of reasons for this. First, metastatic spread in germ cell tumors is not as common as with some of the other tumors. One reason for this is that benign lesions are included in any series of germ cell tumors. This has to be the situation, because in most patients there are no reliable methods for differentiating accurately every benign from malignant lesion. In addition, it is known that initially benign lesions may recur locally as malignant lesions. Therefore, with germ cell tumors the distinction between benign and malignant is not as clear-cut as with other tumors. Another reason might be that metastatic spread is most frequently to local lymph nodes rather than to widely disseminated locations. Other sites of metastases do, however, occur (Figs. 9–41, 9–42, and 9–43). Finally, there are no good large studies cor-

Figure 9–42. Diagnosis: Malignant teratoma lung metastases. This is the same patient illustrated in Figure 9–27. Multiple lung nodules are identified. The appearance of these nodules is nonspecific and the nature of the primary tumor cannot be predicted from their appearance.

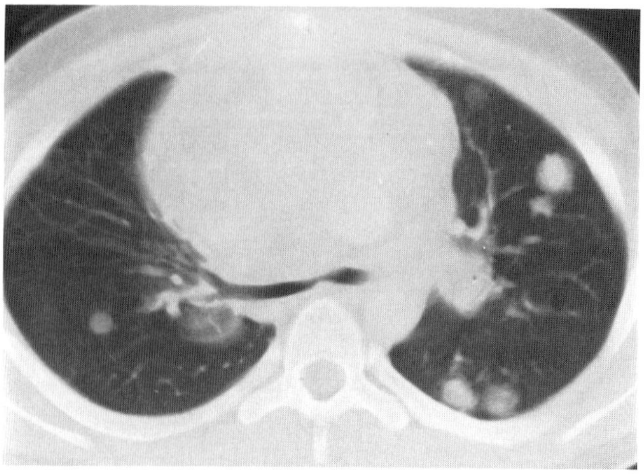

relating the detection of metastasis with prognosis, and with the exception of stage I testicular yolk sac tumors, all patients receive chemotherapy. Therapy, therefore, may not be greatly altered merely because of the identification of metastatic disease.

Unfortunately, there is not a great deal of helpful information in the literature to guide the radiologist with regard to imaging. Local node involvement will obviously vary depending on the site of the primary. With regard to more distant metastases we do not know if there is any significant difference in the pattern of metastatic spread, depending on the site of origin of the primary tumor. We also do not know the incidence of metastatic disease in various sites at the time of diagnosis, nor do we have much useful information regarding the pattern of metastatic relapse on follow-up. We do know that recurrence, either local or metastatic, almost invariably occurs within 2 years of original diagnosis,[31] so that it is probably inappropriate to continue routine screening for metastatic disease beyond this time period.

The pattern of metastatic spread in 33 germ cell tumors in one small series of 33 patients is summarized in Table 9–27. It is not known if this pattern would be true in a larger series and how it would vary for different anatomic primary sites. Two interesting studies with large series of patients with primary yolk sac tumors of the testicle have recently been published.[32,33] Unlike as in adults, the vast majority of testicular yolk sac tumors in children are confined to the testis and are stage I (80 percent).[34] The results of imaging studies seeking metastatic disease on initial presentation in 246 patients with testicular yolk sac tumor are summarized in Table 9–28. As can be seen, the positive yield in return for a considerable financial expenditure is extremely low. In addition, the number of false positives is high. These reflect the inability of imaging to differentiate enlargement of lymph nodes from tumor from enlargement of lymph nodes owing to inflammation. The results of these studies might suggest that no imaging or limited imaging should be performed in patients presenting with testicular yolk sac tumor.

This argument can be further extended when one introduces the factor of measurements of alpha-fetoprotein. In the United Kingdom study of 70 patients,[32] no child was ever found to have identifiable tumor and a normal serum alpha-fetoprotein concentration. Knowing that most testicular yolk sac tumors are stage I, that they can be accurately followed with alpha-fetoprotein, and that the results of large imaging

TABLE 9–27

Location of Distant Metastases from Germ Cell Tumors in 33 Patients with Metastasis*[1]

Location	No. of Patients
Lung	25
Pleura	17
Liver	22
CNS	13
Bone	3

*Rarely metastases will occur in bowel, spleen, diaphragm, adrenal gland, and pericardium.

Reference

1. Brodeur GM, Howarth CB, Pratt CB, et al. Malignant germ cell tumors in 57 children and adolescents. Cancer 1981;48:1890–1898.

TABLE 9–28

Low Yield of Imaging for Metastases from Testicular Yolk Sac Malignancy in Children

	Total No. of Patients	
Study and Positive Yield	Huddart 70*[1]	Kaplan 176[2]
Chest radiograph	0 of 68	7 of 165 (3 were false positive)
IVP	0 of 19	—
Abdominal ultrasound	2 of 19	1 of 20 (it was false positive)
CT lung	2 of 25	—
CT abdomen	4 of 37 (2 were false positive)	5 of 85 (2 were false positive)

*12% had metastases at diagnosis.

References

1. Huddart SN, Mann JR, Gornall P, et al. The UK Children's Cancer Study Group: testicular malignant germ cell tumours 1979–1989. J Pediatr Surg 1990;25:406–410.
2. Kaplan GW, Cromie WC, Kelalis PP, et al. Prepubertal yolk sac testicular tumors—report of the testicular tumor registry. J Urol 1988;140:1109–1112.

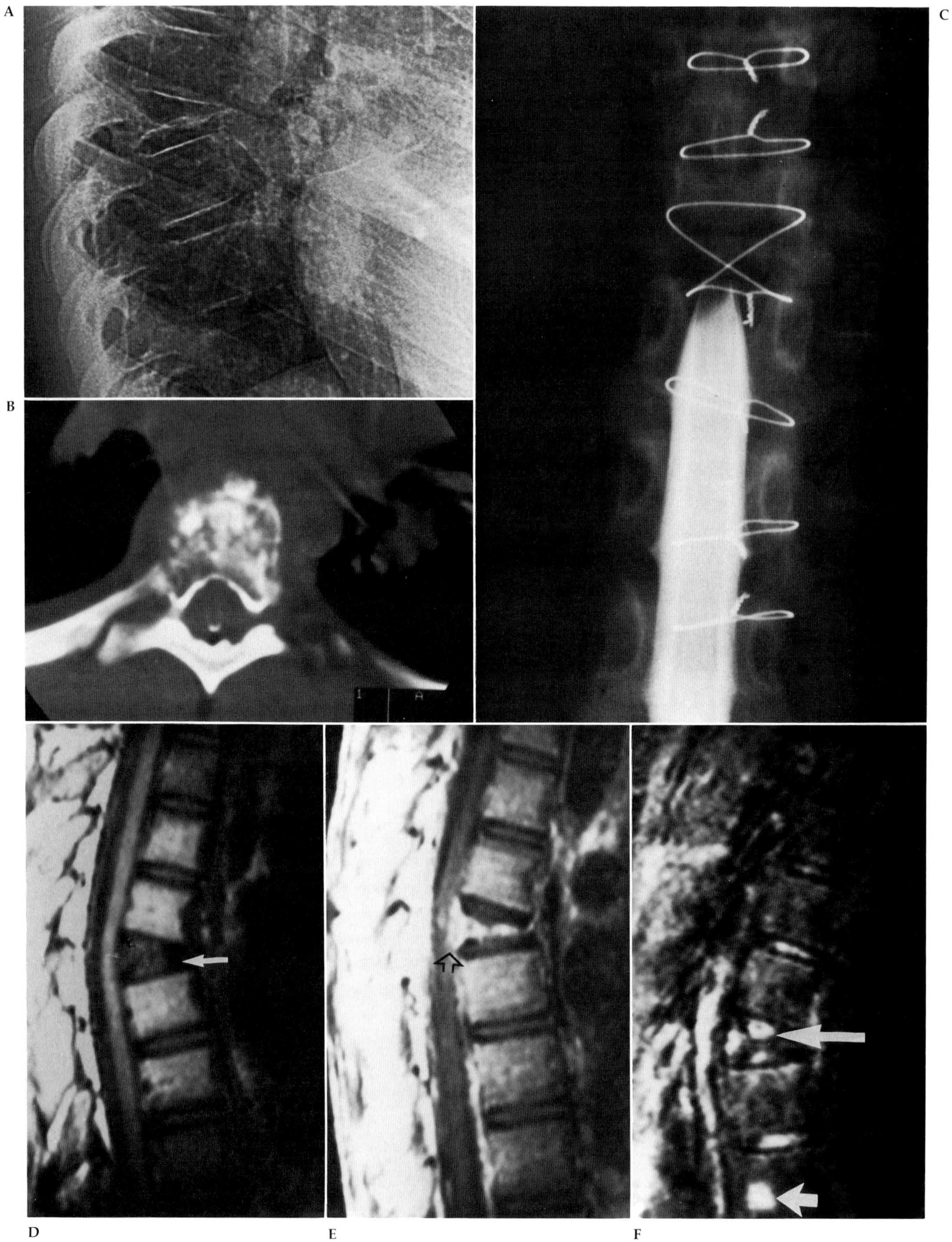
A
B
C
D
E
F

Figure 9–43. **Diagnosis: Bone metastases from yolk sac tumor. This is the same patient illustrated in Figure 9–28.**
A, **Plain film radiograph. There is almost complete collapse of one of the mid thoracic vertebrae. The other vertebrae are demineralized but without focal abnormality.** ***B,*** **CT through the collapsed vertebra. There is extensive destruction of the body of this vertebra.** ***C,*** **Myelogram. There is complete block at the level of the vertebral metastasis.** ***D*** **and** ***E,*** **MR, T1 weighted images before and after gadolinium-DTPA administration. The collapsed vertebra is well identified** ***(arrow).*** **There is enhancement of the tumor in this collapsed vertebra with gadolinium-DTPA administration. Soft-tissue component of the tumor is seen extending posteriorly, compressing the adjacent spinal cord** ***(open arrow).*** ***F,*** **MR, STIR pulse sequence. Bright signal is seen in the metastasis in the collapsed vertebra** ***(large arrow).*** **Another metastasis is seen in a vertebra two levels inferiorly** ***(small arrow).***

studies are extremely low, one could argue in favor of performing no imaging in these patients. One could resect the primary tumor and monitor alpha-fetoprotein levels for 4 to 6 weeks. In the majority of patients, these levels will return to normal and no further imaging would be done.[32,35] In those few patients in whom the alpha-fetoprotein level remained high, one could then perform a search for metastatic disease, starting with CT of the pelvis, abdomen, and chest. I think that this is an entirely appropriate approach in the routine clinical setting. In a research environment, to maximize further knowledge with regard to these tumors, it still might be appropriate to perform CT of the chest, abdomen, and pelvis on initial presentation. Certainly for further follow-up I would strongly suggest that no imaging be done unless alpha-fetoprotein levels start to rise beyond the normal range.

Less information is available with regard to metastases from malignant germ cell tumors in other locations. As almost all of the malignancies in children contain yolk sac tumor, it should be possible to apply a reasoning to the nontesticular tumors similar to that we have utilized for testicular tumors. In another study of nongonadal yolk sac tumors, metastases were present on diagnosis in 13 of 24 patients. These metastases were in the lung (8), lymph nodes (5), bone (1), and liver (1).[33] More work in this area is needed, however, before dogmatic statements can be made.

With regard to the screening protocol to be utilized at the time of diagnosis and with regard to recommendations for routine follow-up both with regard to anatomic site and frequency of imaging, no firm recommendations can be given. The only conclusion I can draw from the literature is that intensity of metastatic search for germ cell tumors should be much less than one would utilize for other tumors.

References

1. Filler RM, Simpson JS, Ein SH. Mediastinal masses in infants and children. Pediatr Clin N Am 1979;26:677–690.
2. Fox MA, Vix VA. Endodermal sinus (yolk sac) tumors of the anterior mediastinum. AJR 1980;135:291–294.
3. Dehner LP. Gonadal and extragonadal germ cell neoplasia of childhood. Hum Pathol 1983;14:493–511.
4. Grosfeld JL, Ballantine TVN, Lowe D, et al. Benign and malignant teratomas in children: analysis of 85 patients. Surgery 1976;80:297–305.
5. Noseworthy J, Lack EE, Kozakewich HPW, et al. Sacrococcygeal germ cell tumors in childhood: an updated experience with 118 patients. J Pediatr Surg 1981;16:358–364.
6. Billmire DF, Grosfeld JL. Teratomas in childhood: analysis of 142 cases. J Pediatr Surg 1986;21:548–551.
7. Siegel MJ, McAlister WH, Shackelford GD. Radiographic findings in ovarian teratomas in children. AJR 1978;131:613–616.
8. Schey WL, Vesely JJ, Radkowski MA. Shard-like calcifications in retroperitoneal teratomas. Pediatr Radiol 1986;16:82–84.
9. Buy J-N, Ghossain MA, Moss AA, et al. Cystic teratoma of the ovary: CT detection. Radiology 1989;171:697–701.
10. Davidson AJ, Hartman DS, Goldman SM. Mature teratoma of the retroperitoneum: radiologic, pathologic, and clinical correlation. Radiology 1989;172:421–425.
11. Sisler CL, Siegel MJ. Ovarian teratomas: a comparison of the sonographic appearance in prepubertal and postpubertal girls. AJR 1990;154:139–141.
12. Sheth S, Fishman EK, Buck JL, et al. The variable sonographic appearances of ovarian teratomas: correlation with CT. AJR 1988;151:331–334.
13. Feldberg MAM, van Waes PFGM, Hendriks MJ. Direct multiplanar CT findings in cystic teratoma of the ovary. J Comput Assist Tomogr 1984;8:1131–1135.
14. Panicek DM, Toner GC, Heelan TR, et al. Nonseminomatous germ cell tumors: enlarging masses despite chemotherapy. Radiology 1990;175:499–502.
15. Ruzal-Shapiro C, Abramson SJ, Berdon WE. Posterior mediastinal cystic teratoma surrounded by fat in a 13 month old boy. Pediatr Radiol 1989;20:107–109.
16. Touran T, Applebaum H, Frost DB, et al. Congenital metastatic cervical teratoma: diagnostic and management considerations. J Pediatr Surg 1989;24:21–23.
17. Choi BI, Chi JG, Kim SH, et al. MR imaging of retroperitoneal teratoma: correlation with CT and pathology. J Comput Assist Tomogr 1989;13:1083–1086.
18. Smith WL, Stokka C, Franken EA Jr. Anteriography of sacrococcygeal teratomas. Radiology 1980;137:653–655.
19. West DK, Touloukian RJ. Meconium pseudocyst presenting as a buttock mass. J Pediatr Surg 1988;23:864–865.
20. Graif M, Itzchak Y. Sonographic evaluation of ovarian torsion in childhood and adolescence. AJR 1988;150:647–649.
21. Bowen B, Ros PR, McCarthy MJ, et al. Gastrointestinal teratomas: CT and US appearance with pathologic correlation. Radiology 1987;162:431–433.
22. Davidson AJ, Hartman DS, Goldman SM. Mature teratoma of the retroperitoneum: radiologic, pathologic, and clinical correlation. Radiology 1989;172:421–425.
23. Prieto ML, Casanova A, Delgado J, et al. Cystic teratoma of the mesentery. Pediatr Radiol 1989;19:439.
24. Cairo MS, Grosfeld JL, Weetman RM. Gastric teratoma:

unusual cause for bleeding of the upper gastrointestinal tract in the newborn. Pediatrics 1981;67:721–724.
25. Hijiya N, Horikawa R, Matsushita T, et al. Malignant mediastinal germ-cell tumors in childhood: a report of two cases achieving long-term disease-free survival. Am J Pediatr Hematol/Oncol 1989;11:437–440.
26. Ihmeidan IH, Tehranzadeh J, Mnaymneh W, et al. Case report 434. Skeletal Radiol 1987;16:568–572.
27. Truong LD, Harris L, Mattioli C, et al. Endodermal sinus tumor of the mediastinum. A report of seven cases and review of the literature. Cancer 1986;58:730–739.
28. Sham JST, Chan FL, Choi PHK, et al. Primary mediastinal endodermal sinus tumors: CT evaluation. Clin Imag 1989;13:299–304.
29. Weinberg B, Rose JS, Efremidis SC, et al. Posterior mediastinal teratoma (cystic dermoid): diagnosis by computerized tomography. Chest 1980;77:694–695.
30. Weiss AH, Greenwald MJ, Margo CE, et al. Primary and secondary orbital teratomas. J Pediatr Ophthalmol 1989;26:44–49.
31. Brodeur GM, Howarth CB, Pratt CB, et al. Malignant germ cell tumors in 57 children and adolescents. Cancer 1981;48:1890–1898.
32. Huddart SN, Mann JR, Gornall P, et al. The UK Children's Cancer Study Group: testicular malignant germ cell tumours 1979–1988. J Pediatr Surg 1990;25:406–410.
33. Kaplan GW, Cromie WC, Kelalis PP, et al. Prepubertal yolk sac testicular teratomas—report of the testicular tumor registry. J Urol 1988;140:1109–1112.
34. Flamant F, Nihoul-Fekete C, Patte C, et al. Optimal treatment of clinical stage I yolk sac tumor of the testis in children. J Pediatr Surg 1986;21:108–111.
35. Fernandes ET, Etcubanas E, Bar BN, et al. Two decades of experience with testicular tumors in children at St Jude Children's Research Hospital. J Pediatr Surg 1989;24:677–682.

TABLE 9–29
Survival of 126 Children with Malignant Germ Cell Tumors[1]

By Site			By Stage		
	No.	Survival (%)		No.	Survival (%)
Testis	59	100	I	62	97
Vagina, uterus, prostate	4	100	II	14	86
			III	18	83
Ovary	25	88	IV	16	72
Thorax	5	40			

Reference
1. Mann JR, Pearson D, Barrett A, et al. Results of the United Kingdom Children's Cancer Study Group's Malignant Germ Cell Tumor Studies. Cancer 1989;63:1657–1667.

Therapy and Prognosis

Prior to the 1960s malignant germ cell tumors, with the exception of those that could initially be completely resected, were uniformly fatal.[1] With the introduction of chemotherapy, prognosis has improved considerably. In the pre-1980 era, it had improved to approximately 42 percent overall.[2] The most recent data published in 1989 shows that for many of these tumors the prognosis is extremely good (Table 9–29). The prognosis is best for the genitourinary primary tumors[3,4] and not as good in other locations.[3,5–7] The prognosis is not dependent on the tumor histology and is the same for pure yolk sac tumors as it is for yolk sac tumor mixed with teratoma.[8]

With regard to therapy, radiation therapy is little utilized in the frontline management of germ cell tumors.[2,9] Most patients are treated with both surgery and chemotherapy. The only exception to this is stage I testicular yolk sac tumor for which surgery alone can be curative.[2,10] Chemotherapy is effective in germ cell tumors.[3,5,11,12] A very wide range of chemotherapeutic agents can be utilized. These include vincristine, actinomycin, cyclophosphamide, and cisplatinum. The combination of vinblastine, bleomycin, and cisplatinum used in adults has been found to be toxic in children.[11,13] Current trials with chemotherapy are exploring the use of new agents and more intense use of existing agents for poor-prognosis tumors.

Surgical excision of all tumors is performed when possible. Most of the testicular, genitourinary, ovarian, and sacrococcygeal tumors can be completely excised. The same is true of most abdominal lesions. In the anterior mediastinum, the tumors are frequently large and infiltrating and cannot be resected on initial surgery prior to chemotherapy. There is some debate regarding the need to perform lymph node dissection for children with testicular yolk sac tumor. Arguments against performing this surgery routinely are the fact that lymph node metastases are much less common in children than in adults and that there are significant complications of extensive lymph node resection in the retroperitoneum. As discussed in the section on metastases, one common approach is to resect the primary tumor and then only to seek additional tumor with imaging, surgery, or both if the alpha-fetoprotein concentration in the blood fails to return to normal following tumor resection.[10,13–15] As all germ cell tumors have a potential for recurrence, which may be malignant, initial surgery should attempt to achieve wide resection. Imaging is thus important in defining the total extent of the tumor prior to surgical resection. One important technical note is that for sacrococcygeal teratoma, if the coccyx is not excised with the tumor, the incidence of local recurrence is extremely high.[8]

References
1. Tumor Board of the Children's Hospital of Philadelphia. Med Pediatr Oncol 1987;15:96–101.
2. Brodeur GM, Howarth CB, Pratt CB, et al. Malignant

germ cell tumors in 57 children and adolescents. Cancer 1981;48:1890–1898.
3. Mann JR, Pearson D, Barrett A, et al. Results of the United Kingdom Children's Cancer Study Group's Malignant Germ Cell Tumor Studies. Cancer 1989;63:1657–1667.
4. Dehner LP. Gonadal and extragonadal germ cell neoplasia of childhood. Hum Pathol 1983;14:493–511.
5. Sham JST, Chiu CSW, Lau WH, et al. Experience with the management of primary endodermal sinus tumor of the mediastinum. Cancer 1989;64:756–761.
6. Truong LD, Harris L, Mattioli C, et al. Endodermal sinus tumor of the mediastinum. A report of seven cases and review of the literature. Cancer 1986;58:730–739.
7. O'Sullivan P, Daneman A, Chan HSL, et al. Extragonadal endodermal sinus tumors in children: a review of 24 cases. Pediatr Radiol 1983;13:249–257.
8. Hawkins EP, Finegold MJ, Hawkins HK, et al. Nongerminomatous malignant germ cell tumors in children. A review of 89 cases from the Pediatric Oncology Group, 1971–1984. Cancer 1986;58:2579–2584.
9. Ablin A, Isaacs H. In: Pizzo PA, Poplack DG, eds. Principles and practice of pediatric oncology. Philadelphia: JB Lippincott, 1989:713–731.
10. Flamant F, Nihoul-Fekete C, Patte C, et al. Optimal treatment of clinical stage I yolk sac tumor of the testis in children. J Pediatr Surg 1986;21:108–111.
11. Collins HS, Burke TW, Heller PB, et al. Endodermal sinus tumor of the infant vagina treated exclusively by chemotherapy. Obstet Gynecol 1989;73:507–509.
12. Diez B, Richard L. Malignant germ cell sacrococcygeal tumors in children. Acta Oncol 1989;28:249–251.
13. Huddart SN, Mann JR, Gornall P, et al. The UK Children's Cancer Study Group: testicular malignant germ cell tumours 1979–1988. J Pediatr Surg 1990;25:406–410.
14. Kaplan GW, Cromie WC, Kelalis PP, et al. Prepubertal yolk sac testicular tumors—report of the testicular tumor registry. J Urol 1988;140:1109–1112.
15. Exelby PR. Testis cancer in children. Semin Oncol 1979;6:116–126.

NEUROFIBROMATOSIS

Epidemiology

Neurofibromatosis occurs in approximately 1 out of 3,000 children.[1] It is an autosomal dominant disorder with a high mutation rate.[2,3] The abnormal gene is located on chromosome 17.[2] It is included in this book because of its association with many malignant tumors.

Neurofibromatosis is classified into type I, which is von Recklinghausen's disease, and type II, which is bilateral acoustic neuromas occurring in adults. The rest of this section deals only with type I neurofibromatosis.

The criteria for the diagnosis of neurofibromatosis is summarized in Table 9–30.[2] Some clinical stigma of the disease are present in 100 percent of children by the age of 5. Skin lesions develop first, usually by the first year, with neurofibromas developing about the age of puberty.[2]

TABLE 9–30
Diagnostic Criteria for Neurofibromatosis, Type I

The diagnostic criteria are met in an individual if two or more of the following are found:
- >6 café au lait macules >5 mm in greatest diameter in prepubertal individuals and >15 mm in greatest diameter in postpubertal individuals
- >2 neurofibromas of any type or one plexiform neurofibroma
- Freckling in the axillary or inguinal regions
- Optic glioma
- >2 Lisch nodules (iris hamartomas)
- A distinctive osseous lesion such as sphenoid dysplasia or thinning of long bone cortex with or without pseudoarthrosis
- A first-degree relative (parent, sibling, or offspring) with type I by the above criteria

DISEASE DISTRIBUTION AND MANIFESTATIONS

Neurofibromatosis is a diffuse mesenchymal abnormality affecting virtually every structure of the body. The imaging findings reflect the wide diversity of specific disorders that occur in association with neurofibromatosis. This section describes the distribution and relative incidence of these disorders. The actual appearance of the disorders, on imaging, is not described here. The appearance of the various tumors associated with neurofibromatosis is discussed in the relevant sections pertaining to each of these tumors.

Central Nervous System. Fifty percent of children have a head circumference greater than the 97th percentile.[2] Lesions found within the cranium include gliomas (especially of the optic nerve, cerebellar astrocytomas, glioblastoma). In addition, areas of heterotopia may frequently be identified.[4] In a study of 53 patients with a mean age of 18 years, single intracranial lesions were found in 32, mulitple lesions in 14, and no abnormality in 7.[4] Routine screening, especially with MR, will frequently identify central nervous system lesions in the absence of any clinical abnormality.[5]

Orbit. In many patients, there is hypoplasia of the greater wing of the sphenoid bone with elevation of the lesser wing,[1] causing lateral displacement of the oblique line on the frontal skull radiograph. The middle cranial fossa appears enlarged, as does the size of the orbit. The ethmoid and maxillary sinuses are decreased in size. In addition, herniation of the subarachnoid space causes pulsations that increase the overall size of the orbit.[3] The presence of neurofibromas in the orbit may cause proptosis.[2]

Spine.[2,3,5] Kyphoscoliosis is common. Dural ectasia can cause posterior scalloping of the vertebral bodies. The intervertebral foramina may be enlarged owing either to bulging of the dura, forming lateral meningoceles, or to neurofibromas of the nerves passing through the foramina.

Bone. Pseudoarthroses, particularly of the tibia, are characteristic.[1] In the ribs, notching or a twisted ribbon appearance may be identified.[3] Cystic or fibrotic lesions in the medulla may also be identified.[3]

Other Findings. These include renal artery stenosis, pheochromocytomas, carcinoids of the duodenum, serosal or submucosal neurofibromas in the bowel.

Most of the above complications of neurofibromatosis can occur at any age. Occasionally, the age of the patient is helpful. For example, pseudoarthroses do not occur under the age of 5 years, large skull plexiform neurofibromatoses usually occur under the age of 1 year, and endocrine associated tumors never occur under the age of 10 years.

The differential diagnosis includes McCune Albright syndrome (fibrous dysplasia, skin pigmentation, and precocious puberty) and Watson syndrome (café au lait spots, decreased IQ, and pulmonary stenosis).

> *Comment:* Neurofibromas are benign but the recognition of the presence of neurofibromatosis is important because of the increased incidence of many different malignant tumors with this syndrome.

References

1. Editorial. Neurofibromatosis. Lancet 1987;(Mar 21):663–664.
2. Huson SM. Recent developments in the diagnosis and management of neurofibromatosis. Arch Dis Childh 1989;64:745–749.
3. Klatte EC, Franken EA, Smith JA. The radiographic spectrum in neurofibromatosis. Semin Roentgenol 1976;11:17–33.
4. Bognanno JR, Edwards MK, Lee TA, et al. Cranial MR imaging in neurofibromatosis. AJR 1988;151:381–388.
5. Gray J, Swaiman KF. Brain tumors in children with neurofibromatosis: computed tomography and magnetic resonance imaging. Pediatr Neurol 1987;3:335–341.

NEUROFIBROSARCOMA[1–4]

Neurofibrosarcoma goes by many other names, including malignant schwannoma, malignant nerve sheath tumor, and neurogenic sarcoma.

Epidemiology

Neurofibrosarcoma occurs in up to 15 percent of children with von Recklinghausen's disease.[1] In children, most neurofibrosarcomas are often associated with von Recklinghausen's disease, although this is not true in adults. In one series of 139 children with peripheral neurogenic tumors, 43 percent of the tumors were neurofibrosarcomas.[2] The median age at presentation in two series was about 12 years.[2,4]

Pathology

The tumors arise in nerve sheaths. They can be multiple and can occur in any location. In one series of 24 patients, 42 percent were in the extremities, 21 percent on the trunk, and 25 percent in the retroperitoneal area.[4] These tumors grow quickly and most are over 6 cm in size at the time of diagnosis.[2] They may occur independently or arise in a preexisting neurofibroma.[2] Metastases are present in about 10 percent of patients at the time of diagnosis.[1] Metastases most commonly go to lung, liver, and bone. Local recurrence is common following resection. Note that as these tumors may arise in preexisting neurofibromas, local biopsy may miss areas of malignancy.

Clinical Presentation

Findings are usually those of a rapidly growing mass lesion.

Imaging Studies

The tumors are nonhomogeneous and are identified as a nonspecific mass lesion on ultrasound, CT, or MR (Figs. 9–44, 9–45, and 9–46). There are no specific distinguishing features. The margins of the tumor vary. Erosion of adjacent bone may be present. Metastases may be seen (Fig. 9–47). In general terms, imaging cannot differentiate benign from malignant lesions. In one study, however, it was suggested that the presence of gallium uptake in the tumor is strongly suggestive of the presence of malignancy.[3] No series have yet been published using MR to study neurofibrosarcoma, but it is anticipated that MR will prove extremely helpful for defining the extent of these lesions prior to surgical resection. The tumors cannot be differentiated from other malignant soft-tissue malignancies (Fig. 9–48).

Therapy and Prognosis

The treatment of neurofibrosarcoma is surgical excision. Complete resection is extremely important for survival. In one series of 24 patients, 3-year survival was 37 percent. In this series, all 12 of 24 patients with gross residual disease following initial surgery died.[4] Although surgery is the main form of therapy, recent work indicates some favorable response to chemotherapeutic agents such as ifosphomide and etoposide.[1]

References

1. Miser JS, Triche TJ, Pritchard DJ, et al. Ewing's sarcoma and the nonrhabdomyosarcoma soft tissue sarcomas of

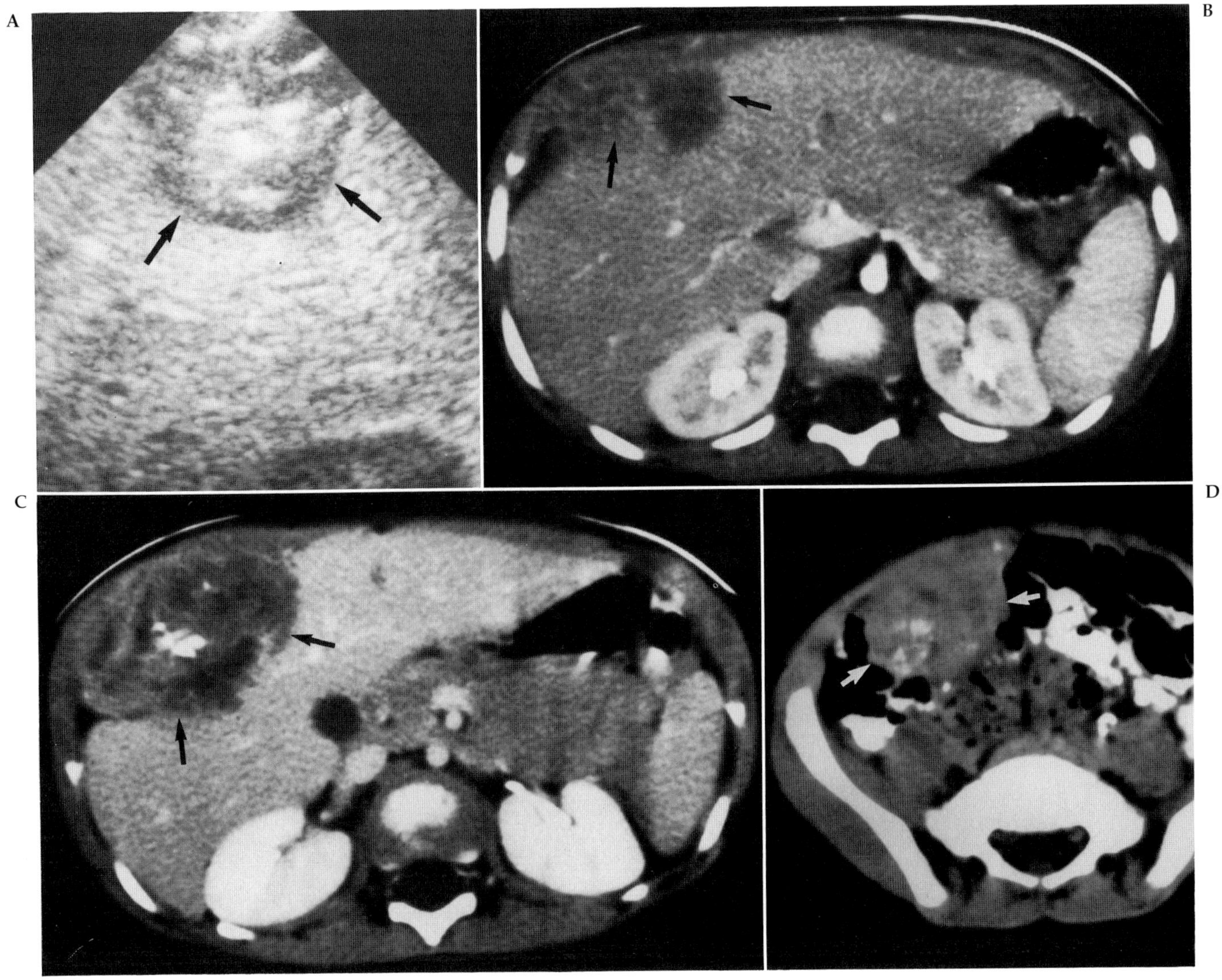

Figure 9–44. Diagnosis: Malignant schwannoma of the anterior abdominal wall.
A, Ultrasound. There is a large tumor mass *(arrows)* extending from the anterior abdominal wall and indenting the anterior surface of the liver. ***B*** and ***C,*** CT images. These show the anterior abdominal wall mass *(arrows)* indenting the anterior surface of the liver. Calcium is seen in the center of the lesion. On imaging, it was not possible to differentiate an anterior abdominal wall tumor from a primary liver tumor. At surgery, the liver was not invaded by the tumor. ***D,*** CT of tumor recurrence. One year after initial surgery recurrent tumor is identified in the anterior abdominal wall of the lower abdomen *(arrows).*

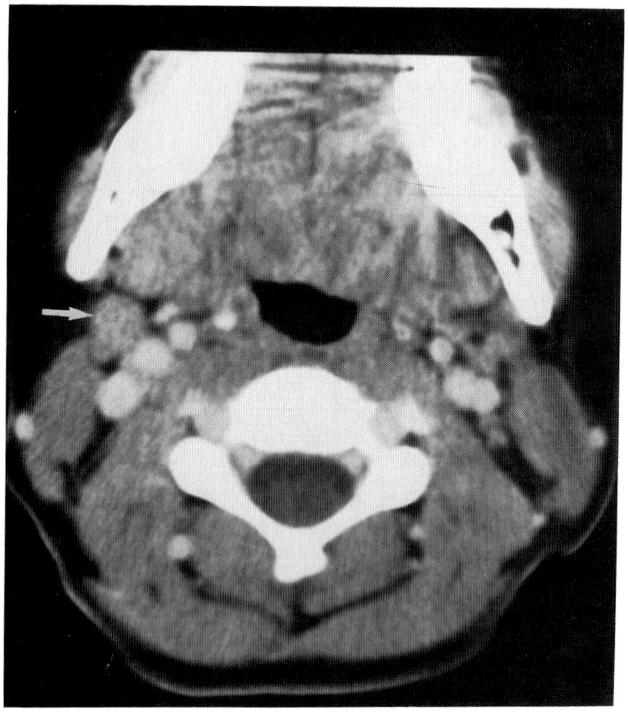

Figure 9-45. Diagnosis: Malignant schwannoma node metastasis.
There is an enlarged lymph node *(arrow)* at the bifurcation of the carotid artery on the right. The appearance of this lymph node with metastatic tumor is completely nonspecific.

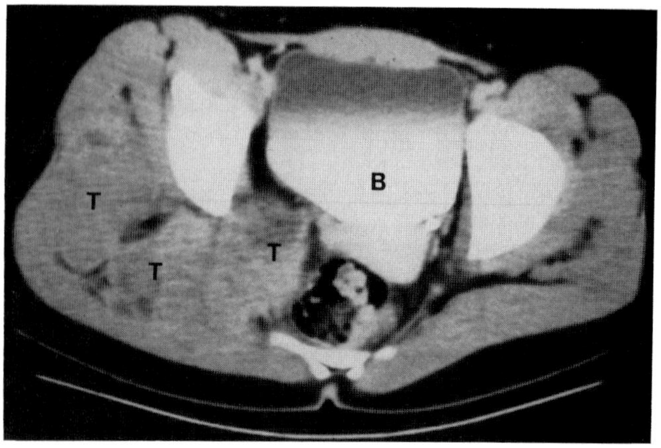

Figure 9-46. Diagnosis: Neurofibrosarcoma of the buttocks. There is a very large tumor (*T*) extending from the buttock through the sciatic notch into the pelvis. It is indenting the posterolateral aspect of the right side of the bladder (*B*). The appearance of this tumor is nonspecific and it cannot be differentiated from other soft-tissue tumors such as rhabdomyosarcoma or nonosseous Ewing sarcoma.

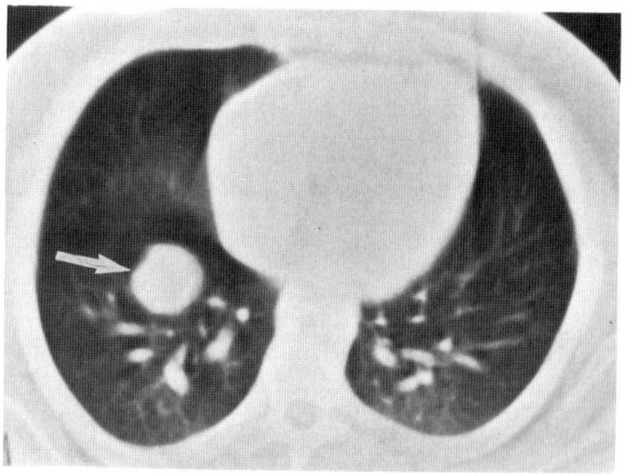

Figure 9-47. Diagnosis: Malignant schwannoma pulmonary metastasis.
There is a large single metastasis in the right lower lobe *(arrow)*.

Figure 9-48. Diagnosis: Leiomyosarcoma of the thigh.
There is a very well-defined soft-tissue tumor lying in the subcutaneous tissues of the thigh. The appearance of this lesion is nonspecific and cannot be differentiated from other soft-tissue tumors such as malignant schwannoma or rhabdomyosarcoma.

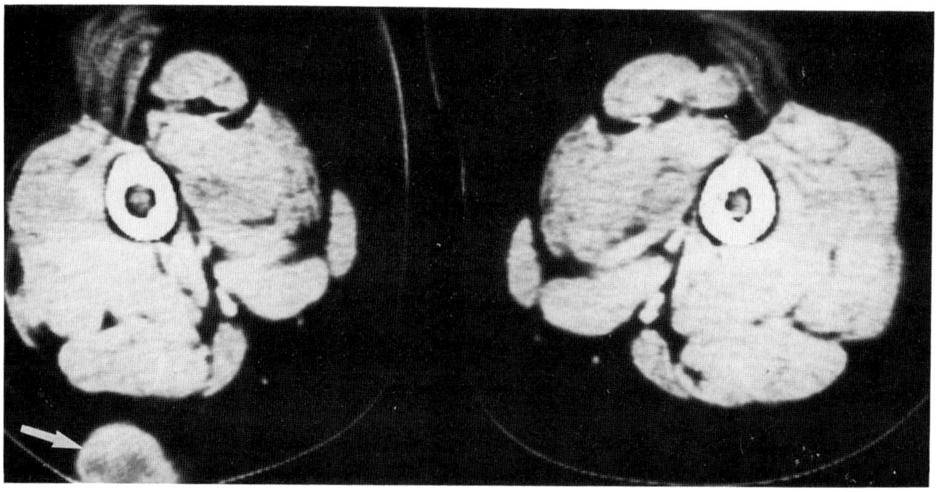

childhood. In: Pizzo PA, Poplack DG, eds. Principles and practice of pediatric oncology. Philadelphia: JB Lippincott, 1989:659–688.
2. Coffin CM, Dehner LP. Peripheral neurogenic tumors of the soft tissues in children and adolescents: a clinicopathologic study of 139 cases. Pediatr Pathol 1989;9:387–407.
3. Levine E, Huntrakoon M, Wetzel LH. Malignant nerve-sheath neoplasms in neurofibromatosis: distinction from benign tumors by using imaging techniques. AJR 1987;149:1059–1064.
4. Raney B, Schnaufer L, Ziegler M, et al. Treatment of children with neurogenic sarcoma. Experience at the Children's Hospital of Philadelphia, 1958–1984. Cancer 1987;59:1–5

MULTIPLE ENDOCRINE NEOPLASIA SYNDROME[1]

Multiple endocrine neoplasia is a series of disorders that are autosomal dominant in nature. They are classified as follows.

Type I (Wermer). This has adenomas of the pituitary, parathyroid, pancreas, and adrenal glands, and also carcinoid tumors.

Type II (Sipple disease). This is a combination of medullary thyroid carcinoma, pheochromocytoma, and parathyroid tumors.

Type II-B. This has the tumors as type II with multiple ganglioneuromas. These ganglioneuromas occur in the gastrointestinal tract, causing multiple areas of segmental bowel dilatation, disordered motility, and constipation. The appearances may be very similar to Hirschsprung's disease.

Reference

1. Demos TC, Blonder J, Schey WL, et al. Multiple endocrine neoplasia (MEN) syndrome. Type IIB: gastrointestinal manifestations. AJR 1983;140:73–78.

MALIGNANT MELANOMA[1]

Malignant melanoma is a very rare disorder in children. A review of 33 cases identified a mean age of 12 years with a male predominance. In this series, 13 lesions were in the extremities, 10 in the trunk, and 7 in the head and neck. At the diagnosis, 17 were localized, 10 had lymph node spread, and 6 disseminated disease.

The imaging appearance of metastatic disease is not specific (Fig. 9–49). Mortality in this series was about 40 percent.

Reference

1. Rao BN, Hayes, FA, Pratt CB, et al. Malignant melanoma in children: its management and prognosis. J Pediatr Surg 1990;25:198–203.

Figure 9–49. **Diagnosis: Malignant melanoma lymph node metastasis.**
CT. The affected lymph node *(circle)* is markedly enlarged and homogeneous in appearance. It is of slightly lower density than adjacent muscle.

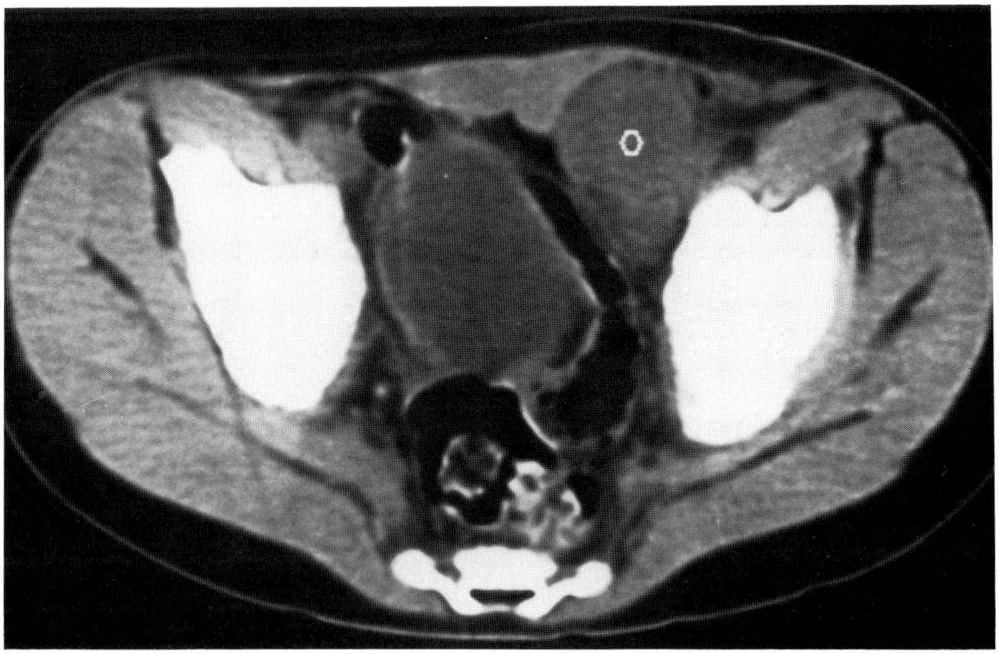

APPENDIX 1
DIFFERENTIAL DIAGNOSIS

Large Facial Destructive Tumors
- Ewing sarcoma
- Teratoma
- Rhabdomyosarcoma
- Lymphoma
- Aggressive fibromatosis

Orbital Masses
- Preseptal (anterior to globe)
  - Rhabdomyosarcoma
  - Lymphangioma
  - Hemangioma
  - Histiocytosis
  - Infection
  - Leukemia
  - Lymphoma
  - Dermoid
  - Lacrimal gland carcinoma
- Intraconal
  - Optic nerve glioma
  - Lymphangioma
  - Hemangioma
  - Nerve cyst
  - Pseudotumor
- Muscle
  - Leukemia
- Extraconal
  - Neuroblastoma
  - Rhabdomyosarcoma
  - Lymphangioma
  - Hemangioma
  - Histiocytosis
  - Infection
  - Leukemia
  - Dermoid
  - Osteoma
  - Pseudotumor
  - Teratoma

Cystic Neck Tumor
- Lymphoma
- Abscess
- Cystic hygroma
- Dermoid
- Thyroglossal cyst

Massive Chest Tumor
- Rhabdomyosarcoma
- Malignant teratoma
- Mesenchymal hamartoma
- Ewing tumor

Anterior Mediastinal Mass
- Teratoma
- Lymphoma
- Enlarged thymus
- Hemangioma
- Cystic hygroma
- Abscess
- Seminoma
- Yolk sac tumor
- Thymolipoma
- Thymic cyst

Middle Mediastinal Mass
- Bronchogenic cyst
- Lymphoma
- Inflammatory adenopathy
- Pericardial cyst
- Teratoma
- Rhabdomyosarcoma

Posterior Mediastinal Mass
- Neuroblastoma
- Enlarged thymus
- Teratoma
- Duplication cyst
- Pheochromocytoma
- Malignant schwannoma

Cystic Abdominal Tumor
- Duplication cyst
- Teratoma
- Lymphangioma
- Abscess
- Localized ascites
- Volvulus
- Wilms tumor

Presacral Mass
- Meningocele
- Hamartoma
- Teratoma
- Yolk sac tumor
- Rhabdomyosarcoma
- Neuroblastoma
- Abscess
- Duplication cyst

Retroperitoneal Tumor
- Wilms tumor
- Neuroblastoma
- Germ cell tumor
- Adrenal cell carcinoma
- Giant lipoma
- Lymphoma
- Pancreatic tumor
- Rhabdomyosarcoma
- Teratoma

Nontumor Soft-tissue Masses
- Nodular fascitis
- Fibromatosis colli
- Myositis ossificans
- Focal myositis
- Abscess
- Hematoma
- Parasite infection

Tumors with Bone Destruction (Non-Bone Primary)
- Rhabdomyosarcoma
- Neuroblastoma
- Leukemia
- Lymphoma
- Histiocytosis

Small Round Cell Tumors of Childhood
- Ewing sarcoma
- Neuroblastoma
- Enchondral lymphoma
- Rhabdomyosarcoma
- Small cell osteosarcoma
- Mesenchymal chondrosarcoma
- Primitive neuroectodermal tumor (PNET)

APPENDIX 2
TUMOR EMERGENCIES[1]

Superior Vena Cava Obstruction
 Most non-Hodgkin lymphoma
 Other, neuroblastoma, Hodgkin, teratoma

Tracheal Compression
 Hodgkin
 NHL
 Neuroblastoma
 Teratoma

Pericardial Effusion & Tamponade
 Wilms
 non-Hodgkin lymphoma
 Rhabdomyosarcoma
 Teratoma

Oesophagitis
 Leukemia

Obstruction
 Intussusception
 Typhlitis

Perirectal Abscess
 Chronic neutropenia

Massive Enlarged Liver
 IV-S neuroblastoma

Hemorrhagic Pancreatitis
 Leukemia asparaginas treatment

Hemorrhage Cystitis
 Cyclophosphamide and ifosphamide

Acute Loss of Consciousness
 Bleed, metastases, infection, metabolic, hydrocephalus

Cord Compression
 Epidural by far most common

Tumor Lysis Syndrome
 (Increased urate, potassium, and phosphate concentration in serum)
 Lymphoma (especially Burkitt's)

Hypercalcemia
 Leukemia, non-Hodgkin lymphoma, neuroblastoma, Ewing, rhabdoid renal tumor

Urine Retention
 Pelvic mass
 Spinal tumor

Reference

1. Lange B, D'Angio G, Ross AJ, et al. Oncologic emergencies. In: Pizzo PA, Poplack DG, eds. Principles and practice of pediatric oncology. Philadelphia: JB Lippincott, 1989:799–822.

APPENDIX 3
PATHOLOGIC GRADING OF SOLID CHILDHOOD MALIGNANCIES[1]

Tumors with a Reliable Correlation Between Grade and Prognosis

Rhabdomyosarcoma (embryonal versus alveolar)
Wilms tumor (favorable versus unfavorable histology)
Malignant lymphoma (Hodgkin disease versus non-Hodgkin lymphoma, small noncleaved cell versus small convoluted cell versus large noncleaved cell)
Other soft-tissue sarcomas
- Fibrosarcoma
- Synovial sarcoma
- Malignant fibrous histiocytoma

Neuroblastoma (poorly differentiated versus ganglioneuroblastoma, nodular versus diffuse, stroma-rich versus stroma-poor, high or low MKI)
Hepatoblastoma (embryonal versus fetal)
Immature teratoma of ovary (degree of immaturity)
Astrocytoma

Tumors with Questionable Correlation or No Correlation Between Grade and Prognosis

Peripheral and central primitive neuroectodermal tumors (Askin tumor, medulloblastoma)
Endodermal sinus tumor
Alveolar soft part sarcoma
Ewing sarcoma
Osteosarcoma (exclusive of special subtypes and responses to chemotherapy)
Adrenal cortical carcinoma
Hepatocellular carcinoma (exclusive of fibrolamellar carcinoma)

Reference

1. Dehner LP. Classic neuroblastoma: Histopathologic grading as a prognostic indicator. The Shimada System and its progenitors. Am J Pediatr Hematol/Oncol 1988;10:143–154.

APPENDIX 4

LABORATORY DIAGNOSTIC METHODS FOR PEDIATRIC TUMORS[1]

Light microscopy
Electron microscopy
Immunocytochemistry
  "Staining" of paraffin tissue sections with specific "labeled" antibodies, e.g., to neuron specific enolase
Immunophenotyping
  "Staining" of frozen sections with "labeled" monoclonal antibodies
Cytogenetics
  Alteration in chromosomes
Molecular genetics
  Analysis of DNA, e.g., N myc amplification
Biochemical analysis
  Of tumor cells in culture, e.g., enzymes
  Of body fluids for products secreted by tumor in vivo, e.g., vinylmandelic acid

Reference

1. Triche TJ, Cavazzana AO. In: Pizzo PA, Poplack DG, eds. Principles and Practice of Pediatric Oncology. Philadelphia: JB Lippincott, 1989;93–125.

INDEX

Page numbers in italic type indicate illustrations.

C

H

I

K

L

M

N

R

U

V

W

Y

Z